# Core Topics in Paediatric Anaesthesia

Second Edition

# Core Topics in Paediatric Anaesthesia

## Second Edition

Edited by

**James Ip**
Great Ormond Street Hospital for Children, London

**Grant Stuart**
Great Ormond Street Hospital for Children, London

**Isabeau Walker**
Great Ormond Street Hospital for Children, London

**Ian James**
Great Ormond Street Hospital for Children, London

CAMBRIDGE
UNIVERSITY PRESS

CAMBRIDGE
UNIVERSITY PRESS

Shaftesbury Road, Cambridge CB2 8EA, United Kingdom

One Liberty Plaza, 20th Floor, New York, NY 10006, USA

477 Williamstown Road, Port Melbourne, VIC 3207, Australia

314–321, 3rd Floor, Plot 3, Splendor Forum, Jasola District Centre,
New Delhi – 110025, India

103 Penang Road, #05–06/07, Visioncrest Commercial, Singapore 238467

Cambridge University Press is part of Cambridge University Press & Assessment, a department of the University of Cambridge.

We share the University's mission to contribute to society through the pursuit of education, learning and research at the highest international levels of excellence.

www.cambridge.org
Information on this title: www.cambridge.org/9781108845304

DOI: 10.1017/9781108955409



When citing this work, please include a reference to the DOI 10.1017/9781108955409

First published 2013
Second edition 2025

*A catalogue record for this publication is available from the British Library*

*A Cataloging-in-Publication data record for this book is available from the Library of Congress*

ISBN 978-1-108-84530-4 Hardback

# Contents

# Contributors

**Nargis Ahmad**
Consultant Anaesthetist, Great Ormond Street Hospital for Children NHS Foundation Trust, London, UK

**Usman Ali**
Consultant Anaesthetist, Great Ormond Street Hospital for Children NHS Foundation Trust, London, UK

**Alistair Baxter**
Consultant Anaesthetist, Royal Hospital for Sick Children, NHS Lothian, Edinburgh, UK

**James Bennett**
Consultant Anaesthetist, Birmingham Children's Hospital NHS Foundation Trust, Birmingham, UK

**Samantha Black**
Consultant Paediatric and Perioperative Anaesthetist, Medway NHS Foundation Trust, UK

**Peter Bromley**
Consultant Anaesthetist, Birmingham Children's Hospital NHS Foundation Trust, Birmingham, UK

**David Chisolm**
Consultant Anaesthetist, The Royal Marsden Hospital NHS Foundation Trust, London, UK

**Ben Clevenger**
Consultant Anaesthetist, Royal National Orthopaedic Hospital NHS Trust, London, UK

**Marc Cohen**
Consultant Anaesthetist, Great Ormond Street Hospital for Children NHS Foundation Trust, London, UK

**Philip Cunnington**
Consultant Anaesthetist, Great Ormond Street Hospital for Children NHS Foundation Trust, London, UK

**Pamela Cupples**
Consultant Anaesthetist, Great Ormond Street Hospital for Children NHS Foundation Trust, London, UK

**Joy Dawes**
Consultant Anaesthetist, Great Ormond Street Hospital for Children NHS Foundation Trust, London, UK

**David de Beer**
Consultant Anaesthetist, Great Ormond Street Hospital for Children NHS Foundation Trust, London, UK

**Graham Derrick**
Consultant Cardiologist, Great Ormond Street Hospital for Children NHS Foundation Trust, London, UK

**James Diviney**
Paediatric Intensive Care Registrar, Great Ormond Street Hospital for Children, London, UK

**Nadine Dobby**
Consultant Anaesthetist, Great Ormond Street Hospital for Children NHS Foundation Trust, London, UK

**Pascale du Pré**
Consultant Paediatric Intensivist, Great Ormond Street Hospital for Children NHS Foundation Trust, London, UK

**Naomi Edmonds**
Paediatric Intensive Care Consultant, Royal London Hospital, London, UK

**Bruce Emerson**
Consultant Anaesthetist, St Andrew's Centre for Plastic Surgery and Burns, Broomfield Hospital, Chelmsford, UK

**Philippa Evans**
Consultant Anaesthetist, Great Ormond Street Hospital for Children NHS Foundation Trust, London, UK

**Elena Fernandez**
Consultant Anaesthetist, Great Ormond Street Hospital for Children NHS Foundation Trust, London, UK

**Michael Frost**
Consultant Anaesthetist, St Andrew's Centre for Plastic Surgery and Burns, Broomfield Hospital, Chelmsford, UK

**Marina George**
Consultant Anaesthetist, Great Ormond Street Hospital for Children NHS Foundation Trust, London, UK

**Jonathan Groome**
Specialty Registrar in Anaesthesia, Great Ormond Street Hospital for Children NHS Foundation Trust, London, UK

**Lucy Hepburn**
Consultant Anaesthetist, Great Ormond Street Hospital for Children NHS Foundation Trust, London, UK

**Jane Herod**
Consultant Anaesthetist, Great Ormond Street Hospital for Children NHS Foundation Trust, London, UK

**Joseph Hussey**
Consultant Anaesthetist, St Andrew's Centre for Plastic Surgery and Burns, Broomfield Hospital, Chelmsford, UK

**Ioannis Ioannou**
Consultant Anaesthetist, Great Ormond Street Hospital for Children NHS Foundation Trust, London, UK

**James Ip**
Consultant Anaesthetist, Great Ormond Street Hospital for Children NHS Foundation Trust, London, UK

**Ian James**
Consultant Anaesthetist, Great Ormond Street Hospital for Children NHS Foundation Trust, London, UK

**Mae Johnson**
Consultant Paediatric Intensivist, Great Ormond Street Hospital for Children NHS Foundation Trust, London, UK

**Helen Laycock**
Consultant Anaesthetist, Great Ormond Street Hospital for Children NHS Foundation Trust, London, UK

**Hannah Lewis**
Consultant Paediatric Anaesthetist, Evelina Children's Hospital, London, UK

**Christie Locke**
Consultant Anaesthetist, East Surrey Hospital, Surrey and Sussex Healthcare NHS Trust, UK

**Daniel Lutman**
Consultant Paediatric Anaesthetist, Children's Acute Transport Service, London, UK

**Louise MacKenzie**
Consultant Anaesthetist, Lister Hospital, London, UK

**Su Mallory**
Consultant Anaesthetist, Great Ormond Street Hospital for Children NHS Foundation Trust, London, UK

**Vaithianadan Mani**
Consultant Anaesthetist, Addenbrookes NHS Trust, Cambridge, UK

**Jon McCormack**
Consultant Anaesthetist, Royal Hospital for Sick Children, NHS Lothian, Edinburgh, UK

**Alice Miskovic**
Consultant Anaesthetist, Great Ormond Street Hospital for Children NHS Foundation Trust, London, UK

**Gema Munoz-Mozas**
Vascular Access Advanced Nurse Practitioner, Lead Vascular Access Nurse, The Royal Marsden Hospital NHS Foundation Trust, London, UK

**Pratheeban Nambyiah**
Consultant Anaesthetist, Great Ormond Street Hospital for Children NHS Foundation Trust, London, UK

**Reema Nandi**
Consultant Anaesthetist, Great Ormond Street Hospital for Children NHS Foundation Trust, London, UK

**Jamuna Navaratnarajah**
Consultant Anaesthetist, Great Ormond Street Hospital for Children NHS Foundation Trust, London, UK

**Breda O'Neill**
Consultant Paediatric Anaesthetist, The Royal London Hospital, London, UK

**Naveen Raj**
Jackson Rees Department of Anaesthesia, Alder Hey Children's NHS Foundation Trust, East Prescot Road, Liverpool, UK

**Ellen Rawlinson**
Consultant Anaesthetist, Great Ormond Street Hospital for Children NHS Foundation Trust, London, UK

**Steve Roberts**
Consultant Anaesthetist, Jackson Rees Department of Anaesthesia, Alder Hey Children's Hospital NHS Foundation Trust, Liverpool, UK

**Ravi Shihurkar**
Paediatric Anaesthesiologist, Great Ormond Street Hospital for Children, London, UK

**Sophie Skellett**
Consultant Paediatric Intensivist, Great Ormond Street Hospital for Children NHS Foundation Trust, London, UK

**Amaki Sogbodjor**
Consultant Anaesthetist, Neurosurgery, Interventional Radiology, General Surgery and Urology, Great Ormond Street Hospital for Children, London, UK

**Emma Stockton**
Consultant Anaesthetist, Great Ormond Street Hospital for Children NHS Foundation Trust, London, UK

**Grant Stuart**
Consultant Anaesthetist, Great Ormond Street Hospital for Children NHS Foundation Trust, London, UK

**Eleanor Walker**
Consultant Anaesthetist, ENT, Urology and Ophthalmology, Great Ormond Street Hospital, London, UK

**Isabeau Walker**
Consultant Anaesthetist, Great Ormond Street Hospital for Children NHS Foundation Trust, London, UK

**Agnes Watson**
Consultant Anaesthetist, St Andrew's Centre for Plastic Surgery and Burns, Broomfield Hospital, Chelmsford, UK

**Hugo Wellesley**
Consultant Anaesthetist, Great Ormond Street Hospital for Children NHS Foundation Trust, London, UK

**Kyrie Wheeler**
Perfusionist, Great Ormond Street Hospital for Children NHS Foundation Trust, London, UK

**Glyn Williams**
Consultant Anaesthetist, Great Ormond Street Hospital for Children NHS Foundation Trust, London, UK

**Valentine Woodham**
Consultant Anaesthetist, Great Ormond Street Hospital for Children NHS Foundation Trust, London, UK

**Jo Wray**
Senior Research Fellow and Health Psychologist, Centre for Outcomes and Experience Research in Children's Health, Illness and Disability (ORCHID), London, UK

# Preface

Children comprise almost a quarter of the population, and many will require general anaesthesia for surgery or an investigative procedure. It is important that the facilities and environment for such procedures are appropriate for children, and those administering anaesthesia are knowledgeable, competent and reliable. It is an oft-repeated adage that the child is not a miniature adult, and nowhere is this truer than in paediatric anaesthesia, where there are significant differences, for instance, in pharmacology, psychology, common clinical conditions and legal issues such as consent. Our intention with this book has been to provide the core knowledge necessary to assist all those involved in anaesthetising children to do so safely and competently. We hope that this text will be particularly useful to trainees aspiring to become specialist paediatric anaesthetists.

We have tried to go further than just covering the core curriculum for training in paediatric anaesthesia. For the clinical chapters, we asked our authors, who are all recognised experts in their specialist areas, to share their experience by outlining in a succinct manner how they manage their patients. It seems to us particularly helpful to read how those who are regularly anaesthetising patients with specific disorders have fine-tuned their practice to minimise problems and achieve good outcomes. We have included additional reading for all chapters. Although we have discussed some of the more common syndromes affecting children, we have not provided a comprehensive list of all the congenital disorders that may be encountered. Many of these are rare, and their salient features can quickly and easily be obtained on the Internet.

We hope that our book will also be useful for anaesthetists who work in the general hospital, especially those who only see children presenting as emergencies. Over the past 20 years or so, a plethora of reports have espoused the benefits of centralisation of paediatric surgery. Subsequent organisational changes have resulted in the transfer of much of this work to specialised centres, particularly for children under four years of age. For many anaesthetists working outside these specialist centres, this has resulted in reduced opportunity to maintain competence and, perhaps of equal importance, confidence in anaesthetising small children, even though over half of all paediatric procedures still take place in district general hospitals. This book is no substitute for regular hands-on experience, but we hope that it will be helpful in providing core knowledge and tips from established experts that can be used to supplement refresher courses and clinical attachments.

We would like to thank those who have helped in developing this book, particularly family and friends who have been neglected during its long gestation. We are also grateful to Cambridge University Press for their patience as the book's post-conceptual age increased.

***James Ip, Grant Stuart, Ian James and Isabeau Walker***

Chapter 1

# Anatomical and Physiological Issues Affecting Anaesthesia in Neonates and Young Children

Pratheeban Nambyiah

## Introduction

The neonatal period (first 28 days after birth, or to 44 weeks postconceptional age) is a time of transition from prenatal to postnatal life. It is characterised by rapid physiological change and developmental plasticity. It is also the time of maximum vulnerability in childhood. Whilst overall infant mortality in England and Wales is low (3.7 per 1,000 live births in 2019), neonatal mortality accounts for 2.8 deaths per 1,000 live births, and this is up from 2.5 in 2014 (driven by the small increase in babies born in extreme prematurity). Anaesthesia at this stage has the potential to cause adverse effects or to alter the neurodevelopmental outcome of the child. Understanding the physiological changes in this period is key to ensuring safe and effective care. Anaesthesia for the premature and ex-premature infant will be considered in more detail in Chapter 19.

## The Development of the Respiratory System

There are five stages of lung development. During the embryonic stage, between three to eight weeks of gestation, the respiratory diverticulum arises as a protrusion of the foregut endoderm. It separates from what will become the oesophagus and forms the trachea and major bronchopulmonary segments.

In the pseudoglandular phase (5–16 weeks), the structure of the bronchial tree is laid down, and all lung elements are added except those involved in gas exchange; this includes the conducting airways, cartilaginous exoskeleton, pulmonary vasculature and diaphragm. The airways are lined with columnar epithelium.

In the canalicular phase (16–26 weeks), the bronchial tree enlarges, and respiratory bronchioles and alveolar ducts are formed. The surrounding mesenchyme (embryonic connective tissue) thins, and the capillary network which will supply the respiratory acini becomes established. The epithelium of the proximal airways differentiates into mucus-producing goblet cells, ciliated cells and basal cells. Distal regions, where the future acini will develop, are lined with cuboidal epithelium with a glycogen-laden cytoplasm. Towards the end of this phase, some terminal sacs develop, and respiration becomes possible. The acinar cuboidal epithelium differentiates into type 1 pneumocytes, which form part of the gas exchange surface, and type 2 pneumocytes, which contain the lamellar bodies that will store phospholipid surfactant for secretion.

The terminal saccular phase (from 26 weeks to birth) sees the continued development of terminal sacs and primitive alveoli. The epithelium thins, and capillaries become closely apposed to the walls of the terminal sacs. Fetal plasma cortisol levels rise in preparation for birth, stimulating alveolar cell differentiation, fluid resorption and surfactant release, which reduces surface tension to prevent airway collapse.

In the alveolar phase (from birth to eight years), the alveolar morphology matures, and there is an exponential rise in their number.

## The Cardiovascular System in Utero

The heart is the first functional organ within the embryo, beginning its work in the fourth week, when the nutritional demands of the fetus can no longer be met by diffusion from the placenta. Initially, it beats as a primitive tube, but loops and folds into a recognisable four-chambered structure by week eight. However, the physiology of the emerging fetal circulation (Figure 1.1) is very different from that of the postnatal

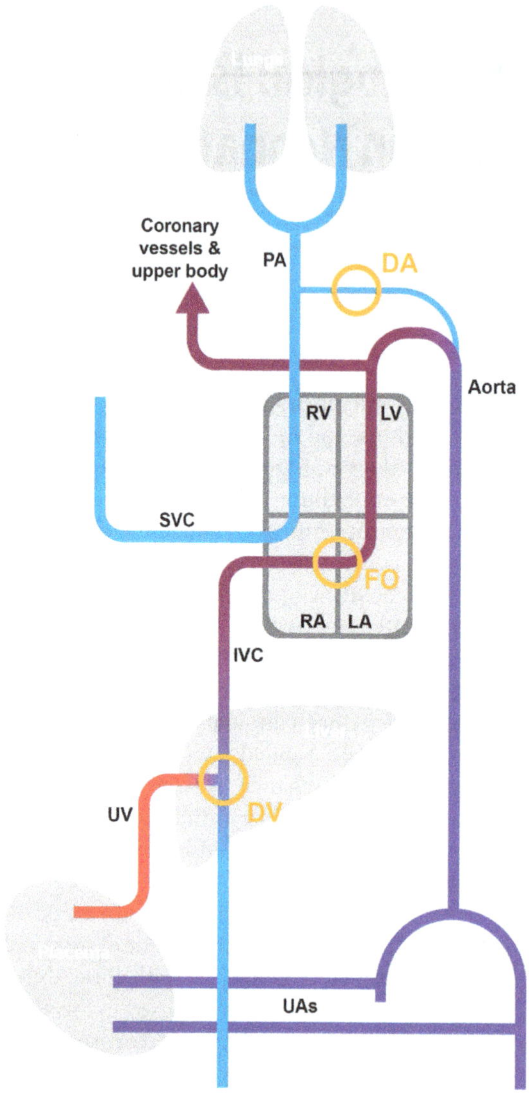


**Figure 1.1** The fetal circulation. In utero supply is dependent on the presence of three shunts: the ductus venosus (DV), between the umbilical vein and inferior vena cava (IVC); the foramen ovale (FO) between the right and left atria; and the ductus arteriosus (DA) between the pulmonary artery and the descending aorta. See the text for full details. Vessels: PA = pulmonary artery; SVC = superior vena cava; UAs = umbilical arteries; UV = umbilical vein. Heart chambers: RA = right atrium; LA = left atrium; RV = right ventricle; LV = left ventricle.

circulation, largely due to the presence of three right-to-left shunts:

- The ductus venosus, between the umbilical vein and inferior vena cava (IVC)
- The foramen ovale between the right and left atria
- The ductus arteriosus between the pulmonary artery and the descending aorta

Taken together, the function of these is to direct oxygenated blood away from organs whose postnatal roles are largely performed by the placenta in prenatal life: the lungs and abdominal organs.

Oxygenated blood from the placenta travels in the umbilical vein. Most passes through the ductus venosus to the IVC, with a small amount supplying the liver via the portal vein. In the IVC, there is now a mixture of oxygenated blood from the placenta and desaturated blood returning from abdominal organs. On entering the right atrium, most of this blood is directed through the foramen ovale into the left atrium, from where it passes into the left ventricle and is pumped into the ascending aorta to supply the coronary vessels and upper body. Deoxygenated blood from the head and upper limbs returns via the superior vena cava (SVC) to the right atrium; this blood is preferentially directed to the right ventricle (RV) and main pulmonary artery. Pulmonary arterioles are tightly constricted due to low levels of oxygen, nitric oxide and prostacyclin $PGI_2$, and pulmonary vascular resistance (PVR) is high. As a consequence, only about 15% of the RV output reaches the lungs. The rest is shunted across the ductus arteriosus to supply the descending aorta, returning to the placenta via the umbilical arteries.

## Cardiorespiratory Adaptation for Birth

At birth, this circulation must transition to one capable of supporting independent life. In most infants, this remarkable process happens within the course of a few hours. Failure of the process can have serious consequences, and stressors early in postnatal life can cause a reversion to the fetal physiology.

Fetal lung fluid is essential to lung development. It distends the lung and provides a stimulus to growth. Inadequate fluid volume leads to lung hypoplasia. However, this fluid must be cleared to allow postnatal respiration. The secretory pulmonary epithelium becomes absorptive towards term. Glucocorticoids and thyroid hormones sensitise the epithelium to β-adrenergic agonists, which mediate increased sodium and water uptake. Catecholamine surges during labour facilitate this process, and there is a modest contribution from mechanical thoracic compression in vaginal birth.

Tactile stimulation and exposure to cold at delivery prompt the neonate's expiratory efforts, mediated via an upregulation in central chemoreceptors and release from placental inhibition. The lungs become aerated, aided by mature surfactant activity and the resultant reduction in alveolar surface tension. Fluid is cleared by expulsion from the trachea. Crying increases end-expiratory airway pressure and helps avoid airways collapse, as well as displacing liquid from the airways into the interstitial space. The increased alveolar volume provides a greater surface area for this resorption. At the same time, there is a dramatic increase in pulmonary blood flow, which helps to drain the interstitial fluid into the microcirculation. This early increase in flow is due to vasodilation of pulmonary arterioles and a rapid fall in PVR, mediated by lung aeration, oxygenation and release of vasoactive agents by the pulmonary endothelium, including nitric oxide and prostacyclin (prostaglandin $PGI_2$). PVR then continues to fall slowly in the first weeks after birth due to involution of smooth muscle in the arteriolar walls.

Pulmonary flow is also promoted by involution of the ductus arteriosus. Immediately after birth, there is a decline in the levels of prostaglandins which promote duct patency ($PGE_1$ and $PGE_2$, produced during intrauterine life by the placenta and by the duct itself) and therefore a reduction of the right to left shunt at the ductus arteriosus. The loss of the low-resistance placental circulation and the resulting increase in systemic vascular resistance (SVR) contribute to this reduction. Constriction of the duct leads to functional closure by day 2 in healthy term infants, and by day 4 in most preterm babies. The increase in pulmonary venous return and left atrial pressure then causes a functional closure of the 'flap valve' of the foramen ovale.

The ductus venosus closes functionally within hours of birth but can be used immediately after birth to provide access to the central circulation via an umbilical venous catheter. In healthy term babies, anatomical closure of the shunts usually occurs within days to weeks, although the foramen ovale may remain 'probe patent' into adult life.

## Managing the Transition from Intrauterine to Extrauterine Life

The transition from intrauterine to extrauterine life may not be smooth, and it can be influenced by clinical interventions. Premature babies may produce inadequate levels of surfactant and are at risk of respiratory distress syndrome (RDS). Antenatal corticosteroids are given to mothers at risk of preterm birth to increase endogenous surfactant, and exogenous surfactant is administered to preterm infants. Surfactant function can be impaired by the presence of blood, meconium and bacteria and also by high glucose concentrations (e.g. in gestational diabetes); RDS may therefore complicate other diseases. For infants who do not breathe adequately at birth, the priority is to establish a patent airway, lung aeration and a functional residual capacity. Intermittent positive pressure ventilation (IPPV) with positive end expiratory pressure (PEEP) may be required, with $FiO_2$ titrated to oxygen saturation. There is growing recognition of the dangers of hyperoxaemia, and 100% oxygen is no longer recommended for initiation of resuscitation. It is associated with increased mortality in term infants and reduced cerebral perfusion in preterm infants.

Recent work has examined the effect of delayed cord clamping (DCC) on cardiovascular parameters and developmental outcomes. In utero, pulmonary venous return makes only a small contribution to left atrial filling, which is largely achieved by the right-to-left shunt across the foramen ovale. This in turn is dependent on flow from the umbilical vein. At birth, cord clamping leads to an immediate drop in left atrial volume, which only recovers once the lung is aerated, PVR drops and pulmonary venous return is established as the source of left atrial filling. DCC (by one to two minutes after birth) provides a transfer of 80–100 ml of blood to the newborn, which helps maintain left atrial volume. DCC is associated with increased birth weight, haemoglobin concentration and iron stores in term babies, and improved cardiovascular stability, decreased need for blood transfusion and lowered incidence of necrotising enterocolitis and intraventricular haemorrhage in preterm infants. There is also an association with improved motor and social neurodevelopmental outcomes, which may be linked to the alleviation of iron deficiency. No mortality benefit has yet been shown, although trials are under way.

Persistence of the fetal shunts into extrauterine life can be pathological or be vital to sustaining the circulation in some congenital cardiac lesions. Patent ductus arteriosus (PDA) may be seen in about 30% of preterm infants, rising to 50% in babies with birth weight $<800$ g. In utero ductal patency is dependent on low fetal arterial oxygen tension and elevated prostaglandin levels. For a healthy infant at birth, reversal of this situation leads to constriction of the smooth muscle of the ductus and a subsequent ischaemic hypoxia, which causes irreversible remodelling of the ductus into the ligamentum arteriosum. Persistently low oxygen tension or elevated prostaglandins, as often seen in preterm infants with respiratory insufficiency, can cause failure of duct constriction. Even where there is some constriction, the hypoxic ischaemia required to cause remodelling does not always occur, meaning that preterm infants can reopen their ductus and revert to a transitional circulation during times of oxygen stress, (including intraoperative stress, as may occur during neonatal surgery). If PVR is sufficiently low, a haemodynamically significant PDA will cause left-to-right shunting and increased pulmonary flow, with worsening respiratory distress and heart failure.

If PVR fails to fall after birth or increases in early neonatal life, then shunting will be right to left. This causes central hypoxaemia when the shunt occurs at the foramen ovale, and systemic hypoxaemia if the shunt occurs at the ductus arteriosus (therefore implying that pulmonary arterial pressures are suprasystemic). This condition is termed persistent pulmonary hypertension of the newborn (PPHN). It may be idiopathic or occur in association with perinatal asphyxia, sepsis, meconium aspiration, or pulmonary hypoplasia (e.g. congenital diaphragmatic hernia). In this setting, continuing hypoxia and acidosis can exacerbate pulmonary vasoconstriction, creating a vicious cycle that can quickly lead to deterioration. Treatment requires management of the underlying pathology (or relief from the precipitating factor during an intraoperative crisis) by:

- Alleviation of elevated PVR with increased $FiO_2$ support
- Pulmonary vasodilator therapy
- Adequate sedation
- Increased systemic pressures to reduce the unfavourable gradient between the pulmonary and systemic circulations

An untreated left-to-right shunt with high pulmonary flows will eventually lead to pulmonary vascular remodelling and a secondary rise in PVR, with subsequent reversal in ductal flow (Eisenmenger's syndrome).

Initial management of a PDA may be medical, with COX inhibitors such as ibuprofen or indomethacin, which block prostaglandin synthesis and hence promote ductal constriction. These methods become less successful with increasing gestational age, in which case transcatheter closure or surgical ligation and division may be required.

Continued ductal patency may be essential in some cardiac conditions (see Chapter 31) to allow flow into either the systemic circulation (e.g. hypoplastic left-heart syndrome or critical coarctation) or to the pulmonary circulation (e.g. pulmonary atresia). In these cases, a prostaglandin infusion may be required to keep the duct open until surgical correction can be performed.

Ventricular remodelling occurs after birth. In utero, the right ventricle pumps 65% of the cardiac output. After birth, the left ventricle becomes dominant, and left-ventricular wall thickness increases to adapt to the rising SVR. In babies with transposition of the great arteries, the left ventricle pumps into the low-resistance pulmonary circulation. These children require an arterial switch procedure in the first weeks of life. If this is delayed, left-ventricular remodelling does not occur, and the left ventricle will be unable to respond to the demands of the systemic circulation.

## Clinical Implications of Newborn Physiology and Anatomy

### Respiratory

Oxygen consumption in neonates, at 6–8 ml $kg^{-1}$ $min^{-1}$, is twice that of adults. Tidal volume is relatively fixed at around 7 ml $kg^{-1}$, but respiratory rate is raised (30–40 per minute), resulting in a high minute ventilation, which accelerates induction and emergence from anaesthesia.

Airway obstruction is a hazard for neonates and infants undergoing anaesthesia. The prominent occiput predisposes to neck flexion. The tongue is large, and together with the soft palate it can easily obstruct the airway by falling against the posterior pharyngeal wall. Loss of pharyngeal tone during anaesthesia exacerbates this situation. The long epiglottis, coupled with a relatively high and anterior larynx, means that a straight blade laryngoscope may offer better visualisation of the laryngeal inlet (although whether it is placed within the vallecula or used to lift the epiglottis directly may be judged on a case-by-case basis by the practitioner). A shoulder roll can help by reducing the neck flexion caused by the large occiput. Traditionally, the infant larynx was held to be conical in shape, with the narrowest portion at the level of the cricoid cartilage. This led to the mantra that cuffed tracheal tubes (TT) were to be avoided in children under eight years old because of the risk of airway oedema and subsequent subglottic stenosis. Recent studies have questioned this view. Some endoscopic assessments of children undergoing anaesthesia suggest that the larynx may in fact be the narrowest portion. However, in vitro studies of autopsy specimens continue to show that the smallest fixed and non-distensible aperture in the upper airway is at cricoid level. Nevertheless, the new generation of high-volume, low-pressure cuffed tubes are widely and safely used now in children down to <3 kg. Uncuffed tubes are associated with leaks, which may lead to inaccurate monitoring of tidal volumes and capnography and potentially inadequate delivery of ventilation. In one large single-centre trial, cuffed tubes were associated with *lower* risks of perioperative laryngospasm and postoperative stridor, whilst another multi-centre trial failed to show a difference in postoperative stridor between cuffed and uncuffed tubes. A recent Cochrane review concluded that there was insufficient evidence to draw definitive conclusions about the advantages of one over the other. If cuffed tubes are used, cuff pressures should be monitored and care taken to avoid over-inflation ($<20$ cm $H_2O$).

The trachea is short, and accidental endobronchial intubation is a common hazard, so the TT position should be checked by auscultation and/or endoscopy. A small TT, when placed out of sight under warm drapes, can soften and kink. The airways are narrow and easily blocked by blood, oedema or secretions. They are also more compliant in neonates and so can be compressed relatively easily. As per Poiseuille's law, airway resistance is inversely proportional to the fourth power of airway radius, so small reductions in airway size can have significant consequences for airflow. Children with laryngo-, tracheo- or bronchomalacia are at particular risk of conducting airways narrowing during expiration, when intrathoracic pressure rises. This risk is raised if expiratory efforts are increased due to airflow obstruction, thus increasing the work of breathing and intrathoracic pressure and reducing airways' diameter further.

The lower airways in infants are also more likely to collapse because of reduced tissue elasticity. Elastic recoil is a property of mature lungs and maintains the patency of small airways through radial attachments between alveoli. In infants, the process of alveolarisation is not yet complete, and these attachments are not mature.

The functional residual capacity (FRC) is the volume remaining in the lungs at the end of a normal expiration. It represents an equilibrium: the point at which the tendency of the lung to recoil inwards is balanced by the tendency of the chest wall to recoil outwards. The infant chest wall is highly compliant and less able to recoil outwards, meaning that FRC is reduced; it also wastes diaphragmatic energy on chest wall deformation. This means that there is a smaller oxygen store available, which, combined with the higher oxygen consumption, means that desaturation occurs quickly if the child becomes apnoeic. The poor elastic properties of both the lung and the chest wall means that closing volume in infants is greater than FRC, with dependent airways closing during expiration in normal tidal breathing. Infants exhibit several adaptations to mitigate this:

- A higher respiratory rate, which allows less time for exhalation down to the equilibrium point
- Laryngeal adduction during exhalation ('auto-PEEP'), which increases airflow resistance (at the expense of raised mean intrathoracic pressure)
- Diaphragmatic tone is maintained during expiration

Several factors combine to reduce the efficiency of neonatal respiration. The thoracic cavity is round rather than dorso-ventrally flattened, and the ribs are soft and horizontally aligned, so the 'bucket handle' action that increases thoracic volume in adults does not occur. The diaphragm is less efficient because of the compliant chest wall, and because it is more horizontally mounted. It also has fewer fatigue-resistant type 1 fibres, so increasing the neonate's susceptibility to respiratory failure.

Gastric insufflation is common after face mask ventilation and may result in diaphragmatic splinting. Decompression with a nasogastric tube will improve respiratory function and reduce the aspiration risk.

In anaesthetised infants, apparatus dead space and resistance should be kept to a minimum to reduce the work of breathing. In neonates, spontaneous ventilation under anaesthesia is best avoided except for very short cases, and pressure support should be employed to supplement efforts. Application of continuous positive airway pressure (CPAP) or PEEP increases lung volumes and maintains FRC, reduces the work of breathing, improves gas exchange and reduces atelectasis.

Lung-protective ventilation strategies should be employed where possible to reduce the risk of ventilator-induced lung injury, which is a risk factor for the development of bronchopulmonary dysplasia. Volutrauma, barotrauma and atelectrauma (injury caused by ventilating inadequately recruited lungs, such that there is shear stress from repeated alveolar collapse and distension) can combine to trigger biotrauma (lung injury caused by the release of inflammatory mediators). Oxygen toxicity via free radical formation is another cause of lung biotrauma. Unrestricted oxygen concentrations also promote atelectasis and decrease FRC, as oxygen is easily absorbed (whereas nitrogen is poorly absorbed). They also increase the rate of retinopathy of prematurity (ROP) in preterm infants. The clinically optimal saturation range for infants is unknown; neither is it known whether saturations on spontaneously breathing babies should be the same as ventilated, or whether infants ventilated on intensive care should be managed differently from those anaesthetised for surgery. The pragmatic practice in our institution is that $FiO_2$ for infants undergoing surgery should be titrated to maintain oxygen saturation in the normal range.

Control of carbon dioxide levels is also important in neonates, and particularly in preterm infants. Hypocapnia has been associated with an increased risk of bronchopulmonary dysplasia (BPD), development of periventricular leukomalacia and intraventricular haemorrhage. Mild hypercapnia appears to be safe, and a permissive hypercapnia strategy (target 6–8 kPa whilst maintaining a normal pH) may help reduce lung injury in mechanically ventilated infants.

## Control of Ventilation

Control of ventilation is immature at birth. Brainstem rhythm-generating centres and peripheral and central chemoreceptors mature to oversee a transition from irregular fetal breathing efforts to continuous respiratory activity capable of maintaining homeostasis. The response to hypoxia is biphasic, with an initial increase in ventilation followed by hypoventilation or apnoea. Hypercapnia leads to an increased minute ventilation in term neonates and children, but this response is attenuated in preterm infants.

Apnoeic episodes are common in neonates, occurring predominantly during REM sleep. Laryngeal reflexes are potentiated and can stimulate prolonged apnoea. Paradoxical breathing (chest and abdominal movements out of synchrony) can be seen in REM sleep because of underdeveloped control of musculature. The risk of apnoeic episodes increases with prematurity, anaemia and exposure to opioids or other respiratory depressants and decreases with increasing age. Term infants are at low risk after 44 weeks postmenstrual age (PMA). For premature neonates, 60 weeks PMA is often taken as the timepoint at which control of ventilation is sufficiently mature to reduce the risk to acceptable levels. Most institutions would not routinely schedule day-case surgery for premature infants before this date. Apnoeas are mostly central, but obstructive and mixed episodes are seen and are more common in preterm infants.

Anaesthetic agents affect both control of ventilation and ventilatory parameters. Inhaled volatiles depress ventilatory drive, tidal volume and minute ventilation, whilst also blunting the response to $CO_2$. Neuromuscular blocking agents and propofol decrease FRC.

## Cardiovascular

Cardiac output is high in neonates (300 ml $kg^{-1}$ $min^{-1}$ vs 60–80 ml $kg^{-1}$ $min^{-1}$ in adults) to meet the increased metabolic demand and oxygen requirement. As in adults, the Frank–Starling mechanism regulates the relationship between myocyte stretch and contractility. However, the ability to increase stroke volume is limited, particularly in preterm infants. Studies show that fluid response in neonates is maintained only to around 1.3 times normal end diastolic volume. Beyond this, preload responsiveness is unlikely, and the risk of pulmonary oedema rises. In addition, immature myocytes do not generate the same contractile force as adult myocytes throughout the entire range of the length-tension curve. It is often said therefore that cardiac output in infants is rate dependent, and whilst this may be an over-simplification, the immature myocardium has limited reserve to increase its output. The neonatal heart is also very sensitive to changes in afterload; increases in systemic or pulmonary vascular resistance can reduce cardiac output.

Neonates are sensitive to the negative inotropic effects of anaesthetic agents and less able to mount a compensatory response. Volatile agents depress contractility and diastolic function by impairing $Ca^{2+}$ flux, and this effect appears to be more pronounced in infants than adults.

Innervation of the heart is functionally immature at birth, and sympathetic tone dominates, resulting in high contractility and high resting heart rate. Parasympathetic tone increases with age, but vagally mediated cardiac reflexes are well developed in infancy and can predispose to bradycardia when stimulated in certain situations. Examples include $CO_2$ insufflation to create a pneumoperitoneum in laparoscopic surgery and the oculocardiac reflex during ophthalmic surgery. Atropine protects against vagally mediated reflexes and was once given routinely as a premedication, but this practice is now uncommon.

## Haematology

At birth, fetal haemoglobin (HbF) forms 70–80% of total haemoglobin. HbF has a higher affinity for oxygen than adult haemoglobin (HbA), ensuring that oxygen is transferred from mother to fetus in the placental circulation. Figure 1.2 displays the oxyhaemoglobin dissociation curves for HbA and HbF and is annotated with generally accepted values. Note that the $P_{50}$ (the value at which haemoglobin is 50% saturated) for HbA is 3.5 kPa but around 2.5 kPa for HbF, indicating the higher affinity of the latter for oxygen. This higher affinity comes at the cost of oxygen dissociation. In the relatively hypoxic environment of the fetal organs, oxygen dissociates readily from HbF and is available for tissue extraction. However, in post-natal life, tissue oxygen extraction occurs between the arterial $PaO_2$ of 13.3 kPa and the venous $PaO_2$ of 5.3 kPa. Under these conditions, the amount of oxygen available for the tissues is significantly

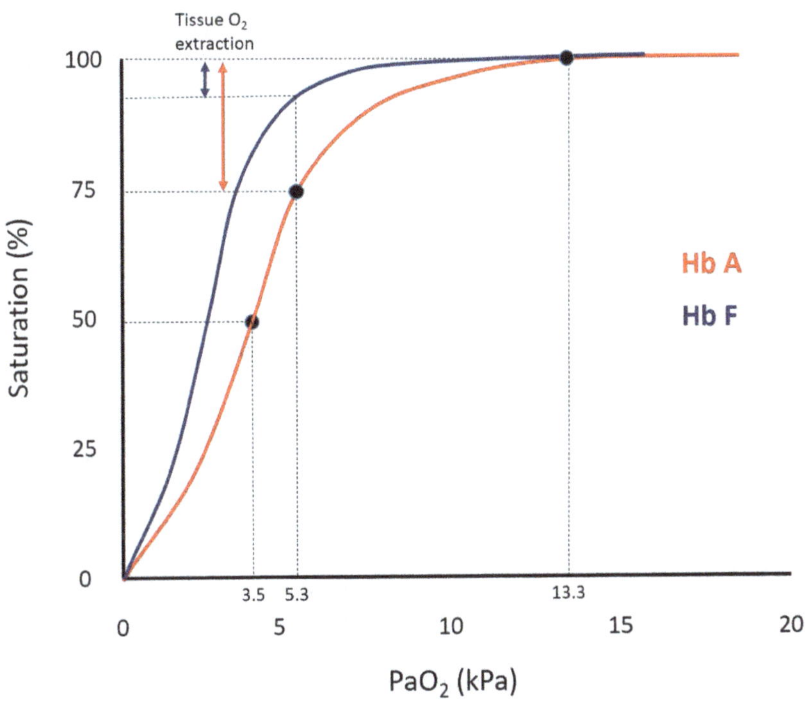


**Figure 1.2** Oxygen-haemoglobin dissociation curves for HbA and HbF haemoglobin molecules, annotated with generally accepted values. Note the P50 values for HbA and HbF are 3.5 and 2.5 respectively, indicating the higher affinity of HbF for oxygen. Tissue oxygen extraction occurs between the arterial value of 13.3 kPa and the venous value of 5.3 kPa. Arrows indicate the difference in tissue oxygen delivery between the two haemoglobin molecules.

greater from the HbA carrier compared to HbF. A high Hb concentration during the neonatal period partially compensates for this – 180–200 g $L^{-1}$ at birth, falling to around 150 g $L^{-1}$ in the first week of life. HbA then quickly becomes the dominant component, reaching over 90% of total haemoglobin in the first weeks of life. At this infant age, tissue oxygen delivery is even more efficient than in adults because of a high cardiac output coupled with increased levels of 2,3-diphosphoglycerate (2,3 DPG), which shift the oxyhaemoglobin dissociation curve further rightwards.

Many infants requiring intensive care will receive a blood transfusion at some point. The British Committee for Standards in Haematology (BCSH) transfusion guidelines for neonates suggests the thresholds given in Table 1.1. These are based on a number of studies and a 2011 Cochrane analysis on the risks and benefits of a liberal versus restrictive transfusion strategy. However, the safe lower limits for neonatal haemoglobin levels remain unknown, and clinical judgement must be exercised, particularly in the perioperative setting, when strict adherence to these guidelines may be inappropriate. As a guide, 4 ml $kg^{-1}$ of packed red blood cells (PRBC) raises the haemoglobin (Hb) level by approximately 10 g $L^{-1}$. Neonates should receive cytomegalovirus (CMV) negative PRBC.

Thrombocytopenia is a common finding in unwell neonates. There is no clear correlation between the severity of thrombocytopenia and major bleeding, and prophylactic platelet transfusions are rarely indicated. Suggested platelet thresholds for transfusion are:

**Table 1.1** BCSH-recommended haemoglobin threshold levels for neonatal top-up transfusions

| Postnatal age | Suggested transfusion threshold Hb (g $L^{-1}$) | | |
|---|---|---|---|
| | Ventilated | On oxygen or CPAP | Off oxygen |
| <24 hr | 120 | 120 | 100 |
| 1–7 days | 120 | 100 | 100 |
| 8–14 days | 100 | 95 | <75–85 depending on clinical situation |
| Day 15 onwards | | 85 | |

- $<20 \times 10^9$ $L^{-1}$ in the absence of bleeding
- $<50 \times 10^9$ $L^{-1}$ if actively bleeding or requiring surgery
- $<100 \times 10^9$ $L^{-1}$ if major bleeding or planned surgery in critical areas (e.g. eye or neurosurgery)

The typical dose is 10–20 ml $kg^{-1}$.

Tests of coagulation in neonates are difficult to interpret because of age-related differences in normal values, and because laboratory reference ranges vary. Vitamin K-dependent clotting factors are low in neonates and preterm infants, and vitamin K prophylaxis is given to reduce the risk of haemorrhagic disease of the newborn.

Fresh frozen plasma or a solvent/detergent-treated pooled human plasma product (e.g. Octaplas®) are indicated for vitamin K deficiency with bleeding, disseminated intravascular coagulation (DIC) with bleeding or coagulation factor deficiencies where no specific factor concentrate is available. The usual dose is 15 ml $kg^{-1}$. There are significant adverse reactions associated with these products, so the expected benefit of transfusion must be balanced against the associated risk.

Cryoprecipitate is indicated for fibrinogen deficiency, at a dose of 5–10 ml $kg^{-1}$. In practice, these products are also used in the management of acute or intraoperative bleeding where surgical control is not possible, and in this setting their use should be guided by laboratory assays. Thromboelastography measures the global viscoelastic properties of blood clot formation and may be a better guide to rational blood product use in the acute setting than conventional tests of coagulation.

## Renal, Hepatic and Metabolic

Renal development begins at 5 weeks gestation, with nephrogenesis commencing at around 9 weeks and being complete by 36 weeks. A functional renin-angiotensin system is present from early in gestation and is crucial for normal renal development. Fetal urine output contributes the majority of the amniotic fluid, which in turn is important for lung development. Renal abnormalities at this stage are associated with pulmonary hypoplasia. Preterm babies have fewer nephrons at birth and more abnormal glomeruli and often display impaired renal function in infancy. In adulthood, there are associations with chronic kidney disease and hypertension.

At birth, antidiuretic hormone (ADH) levels are high and the glomerular filtration rate (GFR) is low, so urine output is low, and sodium and water are conserved. A brisk diuresis then occurs as ADH levels fall. Term infants lose around 10% of their extracellular fluid, with a corresponding loss of sodium. By day 3 in term neonates, distal tubular function becomes more responsive to aldosterone, and sodium conservation increases. An immature urinary concentrating ability means that babies produce large amounts of dilute urine that is isotonic with plasma. They are prone to dehydration if fasted, and renal failure is common in sick infants. Preterm infants have impaired ability to both conserve and excrete sodium, and sodium disturbances are common.

The liver in newborn infants contains only 20% of the adult complement of hepatocytes. Drug-handling systems are immature (see Chapter 2), and in general drug effects are pronounced and prolonged. Dose adjustments must be made for common perioperative drugs, including paracetamol and opioids.

Glucose is the primary energy substrate for the fetus and neonate. Until birth, the fetus is dependent on placental transfer to meet glucose and other metabolic requirements. Glycogenesis and lipogenesis occur in preparation for postnatal life. At birth, a cortisol and catecholamine surge leads to glycogenolysis and hepatic gluconeogenesis to meet neonatal energy requirements whilst enteral feeds are established. As glycogen is depleted, lipolysis yields glycerol and free fatty acids. The former is used for further gluconeogenesis, and the latter as a metabolic substrate either directly or after conversion into ketone bodies. Newborn infants have high metabolic rates but relatively small hepatic stores of substrate and immature gluconeogenic enzyme systems. They are therefore highly susceptible to hypoglycaemia if nutrition is interrupted. Asymptomatic hypoglycaemia may have neurodevelopmental sequalae. The normal range for blood glucose concentrations in neonates is undefined, but the World Health Organisation (WHO) suggests <2.6 mmol $l^{-1}$ as the operational threshold of hypoglycaemia.

Some practical suggestions are given here for the management of glucose and fluid requirements in the term neonate. These may not be applicable in all circumstances; premature infants, those with hypoxic ischaemic encephalopathy, those in renal or cardiac failure or those suffering from critical illness may need further advice from neonatal intensive care unit (NICU) or specialist teams. Fluids should be restricted until the postnatal diuresis has occurred. Excessive fluids may impair cardiorespiratory adaptation and promote PDA, particularly in premature infants. Sodium is usually withheld in the first days of life but is added to maintenance fluids after the postnatal diuresis. Table 1.2 reflects standard practice for maintenance fluids in our NICU.

**Table 1.2** Standard fluid maintenance volumes for the term neonate

| Age | Fluid regime |
|---|---|
| Day 1 | 60 ml $kg^{-1}$ $day^{-1}$ 10% glucose |
| Day 2 | 90 ml $kg^{-1}$ $day^{-1}$ 10% glucose + 0.45% NaCl ± 10 mmol potassium |
| Day 3 | 120 ml $kg^{-1}$ $day^{-1}$ 10% glucose + 0.45% NaCl ± 10 mmol potassium |
| Day 4+ | 150 ml $kg^{-1}$ $day^{-1}$ 10% glucose + 0.45% NaCl ± 10 mmol potassium |

A balanced crystalloid solution containing glucose (e.g. Plasma-Lyte 148 with 5% glucose) may be preferable to hypotonic solutions for perioperative care. Blood sugar should be measured routinely during surgery, and guidelines in our institution are to maintain this between 2.6–8.3 mmol $L^{-1}$. Intraoperative fluid boluses should be from a glucose-free balanced salt solution such as Hartmann's solution.

## Endocrine

Glucocorticoids, thyroid hormones and catecholamines play a vital role in fetal organ maturation. Cortisol is produced in the fetal adrenal glands and provided by placental transfer of maternal cortisol. Before birth, cortisol activates the hypothalamic–pituitary–adrenal (HPA) axis, induces liver enzyme activity and promotes organ maturation in the lung, digestive system and kidneys. It also plays a role in the onset of parturition. Exogenous corticosteroids are given to women at risk of preterm delivery, and these also coordinate the maturation response. Exposure to cortisol alters the lung parenchyma; collagen and elastin fibres increase, and the alveolar septae thin in readiness for gas exchange. Surfactant production is upregulated. Thyroid maturation is driven by a cortisol rise before delivery, leading to increased circulating tri-iodothyronine (T3), which acts synergistically with cortisol to promote maturation in many tissues. The process of lung fluid resorption at birth is dependent on cortisol, T3 and adrenaline. Thyroid hormones play a role in cardiac growth, differentiation and contractility, and, together with catecholamines, prime the cardiovascular response to birth.

## Thermoregulation

Thermoregulation in the neonate is limited and easily overwhelmed by environmental conditions. Thermal energy arises from two major sources: metabolically active tissues (primarily brain) and non-shivering thermogenesis. The latter describes metabolism of brown fat, a specialised store located within the thorax and abdomen, where adenosine triphosphate (ATP) synthesis within mitochondria is uncoupled from respiration. This process is inhibited by volatile anaesthetic agents, and there is a great potential for heat loss due to a high body surface area to weight ratio, increased thermal conductance and increased evaporative heat loss through thin skin. Premature infants are at particular risk and should have minimal handling and exposure to minimise heat loss. Where possible, surgery should be performed on the NICU to mitigate these risks.

## Pain

Neonates, including premature neonates, show well-developed responses to painful stimuli. These responses are not always recognised in clinical practice, resulting in under-treatment of neonatal pain, which can have both short- and longer-term consequences. The former includes potentially deleterious physiological instability such as changes in heart rate and respiration. The latter may include altered pain thresholds and neurocognitive development in later life. In fact, the neonatal period is a time of great neuronal plasticity, and both pain stimuli and administration of exogenous analgesia may have effects on neuronal development.

## Long-Term Effects of Early Exposure to General Anaesthesia

It is increasingly apparent that general anaesthetics have wider effects on the nervous system beyond altering consciousness, and that these effects persist beyond the period of clinical anaesthesia. In fact, it seems unlikely from first principles that anaesthetics *should* have only benign and reversible actions on consciousness. They are thought to act promiscuously on receptor targets such as γ-Aminobutyric acid (GABA), N-methyl-D- aspartate (NMDA) and a variety of other protein channels and are typically given at large concentrations to overcome their lack of selectivity. These targets are widespread and have important roles in neural development and plasticity. It is unsurprising, therefore, that interruption of consciousness at particular timepoints in brain age may be accompanied by other effects on the neuronal architecture, network or function. This has led to a call for anaesthetics to be seen not just as drugs which temporarily interrupt consciousness but as modulators of neural plasticity.

Although there is potential to harness these effects for good, (e.g. modulation of glutamatergic signalling by ketamine is being investigated in the treatment of severe depression), there is also significant public health concern about long-lasting and potentially toxic developmental effects of general anaesthetics. In 1999, ketamine, an NMDA receptor antagonist and widely used general anaesthetic, was shown to induce apoptotic neurodegeneration in the developing rat brain. Further work followed, showing that almost all clinically relevant general anaesthetic agents, including volatile gases, ketamine, nitrous oxide, midazolam and propofol, are associated with this phenomenon. Furthermore, rat pups exposed to commonly used anaesthetic agents also developed persistent impairments in learning and memory. These findings have now been broadly replicated in multiple different organisms, including non-human primates.

The most consistent and robust findings of neuropathology and behavioural impairment have generally come under the following conditions:

- Exposure at particular species-specific developmental windows (for both rodents and non-human primates, this has typically been in postnatal days 1–7)
- Prolonged exposure rather than short episodes (typically for several hours)
- Exposure to combinations of multiple anaesthetic agents rather than to monotherapy

In 2016, the FDA placed an advisory warning on the administration of anaesthesia to children under the age of three or to pregnant women in their third trimester. This has raised concerns amongst both practitioners and patient groups and led to much debate. In most situations where general anaesthesia is contemplated, there are simply no alternatives. Regional and neuraxial techniques block pain pathways without affecting consciousness but can rarely be used as a sole technique in young children. The only drugs in clinical use that have not been consistently shown to cause neurodegeneration in animal models are dexmedetomidine and opioids; neither are generally sufficient to provide anaesthesia on their own. Safely delaying surgery to an older age is rarely an option. Finally, suboptimal anaesthesia and pain may in themselves lead to altered neurodevelopmental trajectories.

Some studies of human children suggest an association between exposure to anaesthesia at a young age and diagnosis of neurodevelopmental disorders, whilst others have failed to demonstrate a correlation. These contradictory findings are not surprising; the challenges encountered in this field are well recognised and have been comprehensively discussed in the literature. Most studies have used retrospective cohorts drawn from historical databases and have found it difficult to separate the effects of anaesthesia from surgery or comorbidity. They encounter use of historical drugs and techniques, heterogeneous dose-exposure relationships and surgical interventions and are hampered by multiple population-specific confounders. The absence of a recognised human phenotype associated with anaesthesia-induced neurotoxicity means that there is no consistency in the use of outcome measures. To date, there have been three large trials with prospective neurodevelopmental testing: the Pediatric Anesthesia and NeuroDevelopment Assessment (PANDA) study, the General Anaesthesia Spinal (GAS) trial and the Mayo Anaesthesia Safety in Kids (MASK) study. These are reassuring to the extent that they suggest that a single short exposure to general anaesthesia in infancy does not lead to measurable differences in the studied primary outcome of global cognitive function in later childhood. However, paediatric anaesthetists should remain cautious. There *were* measurable differences in some parent-reported secondary outcome measures. The MASK study also found that multiple exposures are associated with impaired neurodevelopmental outcomes. Across these three studies, there are no significant associations across the same neurodevelopmental domain, raising questions about why this lack of consistency arises. Finally, neurodevelopmental outcome measures may have poor predictive validity, such that it is difficult to establish the significance of a finding at a particular point in time for a child's future development. The author's preferred position is that there is currently no compelling evidence to prompt immediate changes in clinical practice (beyond the pragmatic consideration of minimising exposure where possible).

Adverse Outcome Pathways (AOPs) are a structured approach to integrating the available information and aiding evidence synthesis. An AOP seeks to build a chain that links the key events, from the initial molecular stressor to the phenotypic change in the organism, with intervening steps at cellular, tissue and organ levels. Such pathways offer a framework for future integrated research in this area and may help to reconcile the pathology seen in basic science models with the uncertain clinical implications in the paediatric-population.

### Key Points

- Early neonatal life is a time of rapid development, adaptation and plasticity.
- The physiological adaptation to postnatal life is complex, and failures in this process underlie many common neonatal presentations.
- Respiratory complications are common in the perioperative period and are mitigated by meticulous preparation, supported ventilation, titrated oxygen concentrations and constant vigilance. Apnoeas in preterm infants are to be expected, and risks are increased with anaemia and with exposure to opioids and other respiratory depressants.
- Cardiovascular reserve is limited, volume-loading has a limited ability to improve stroke volume and anaesthetic agents have a negative inotropic effect.
- BCSH transfusion guidelines for neonates assist the rational management of transfusion requirements, but clinical judgement must always be exercised.

- Organ development is immature, and homeostatic function is impaired. Disorders of fluid, electrolyte and glucose handling are common. Thermoregulation is limited.
- Neonates feel pain, and failure to treat pain is both cruel and may have longer-term developmental implications.
- Anaesthetics do not just impair consciousness. They are implicated in the modulation of neural plasticity, and animal evidence suggests they may affect neurodevelopmental trajectories. However, as yet there is no compelling evidence in children to change current best practice.

## Further Reading


Baum VC, Palmisano BW. The immature heart and anesthesia. *Anesthesiology* 1997; 87(6):1529–48. doi:10.1097/00000542-199712000-00032

Ikonomidou C, Bosch F, Miksa M, et al. Blockade of NMDA receptors and apoptotic neurodegeneration in the developing brain. *Science* 1999; 283(5398):70–4. doi:10.1126/science.283.5398.70

Murphy PJ. The fetal circulation. *Continuing Education in Anaesthesia Critical Care and Pain* 2005; 5(4): 107–12. doi:10.1093/bjaceaccp/mki030

Neumann RP, Ungern-Sternberg BS von. The neonatal lung: physiology and ventilation. *Pediatric Anesthesia* 2014; 24(1):10–21. doi:https://doi.org/10.1111/pan.12280

Riviere D, McKinlay CJD, Bloomfield FH. Adaptation for life after birth: a review of neonatal physiology. *Anaesthesia and Intensive Care Medicine* 2017; 18(2):59–67. doi:10.1016/j.mpaic.2016.11.008

Walkden G, Pickering A, Gill H. Assessing long-term neurodevelopmental outcome following general anesthesia in early childhood: challenges and opportunities. *Anesthesia and Analgesia* 2019; 128(4):681–94. doi:10.1213/ANE.0000000000004052

Waspe J, Chico T, Hansen T. Applying the adverse outcome pathway concept to questions in anaesthetic neurotoxicity. *British Journal of Anaesthesia* 2021; 126(3):1097–102.

Chapter 2

# Pharmacological Issues Affecting Anaesthesia in Neonates and Young Children*

Eleanor Walker

## Introduction

Paediatric patients differ significantly from adults in the way that drugs affect them for several reasons:

- Size: There is a more than 100-fold difference in weight between a premature neonate and a healthy adult, but weight alone is an inadequate indicator of dosage because of changes in body composition.
- Physiology: Developmental changes, particularly during the first few months of life, profoundly affect both the pharmacokinetics and pharmacodynamics of anaesthetic drugs.
- Comorbidities: The range of conditions requiring anaesthesia in children is different. Whilst age- and lifestyle-related conditions may be rare or absent, congenital abnormalities may be more frequent.
  In addition, local/regional anaesthesia and/or sedation are less likely to be used.

This chapter provides a general overview of these considerations, followed by a more detailed discussion of individual drugs commonly used in paediatric anaesthetic practice.

## Size and Paediatric Drug Dosing

Calculating the correct dose of a drug for a neonate or young child invariably involves scaling the dose according to the patient's size. Scaling for size (allometrics) has been based on weight, surface area and power models based on surface area, but no single model is appropriate for all drugs. Figure 2.1 illustrates some of the difficulties of using size models to predict paediatric doses. The variation in the dose of thiopental required to produce sleep in 50% of subjects (ED50) with age is biphasic, which cannot be modelled by a single mathematical function. Power models are not generally practical to use, and any method which entails a complex calculation is more likely to result in errors. Drug doses are much less predictable in infants aged less than one year owing to immaturity of organs and enzyme systems, and reduced doses are frequently required in this age group.

The first years of human life are characterised by rapid growth, differentiation and maturation. In the first six weeks, the birth weight will increase by 50% and double in the first three to four months. By approximately one year of age, the birth weight will have tripled. Over the same period, body length and body surface area increase by 50% and 100% respectively, whilst caloric expenditure increases fourfold. Predictably, these developmental changes lead to significant variation in how neonates, infants and children respond to medications, and age-appropriate adjustments in drug doses are necessary.

## Physiology

Developmental changes, particularly during the first few months of life, profoundly affect both the pharmacokinetics and the pharmacodynamics of anaesthetic drugs.

### Factors Affecting Pharmacokinetics

#### Absorption

Drugs administered by routes other than intravenous must overcome chemical, physical, mechanical and/or biological barriers to achieve their effect. The gastrointestinal tract, skin and pulmonary tree all undergo developmental changes which affect the absorption of drugs across their surfaces and thus their bioavailability. Oral absorption of drugs

* Many thanks to Dr George Meakin, who wrote the first edition of this book chapter, much of the content of which has been used in this revision.

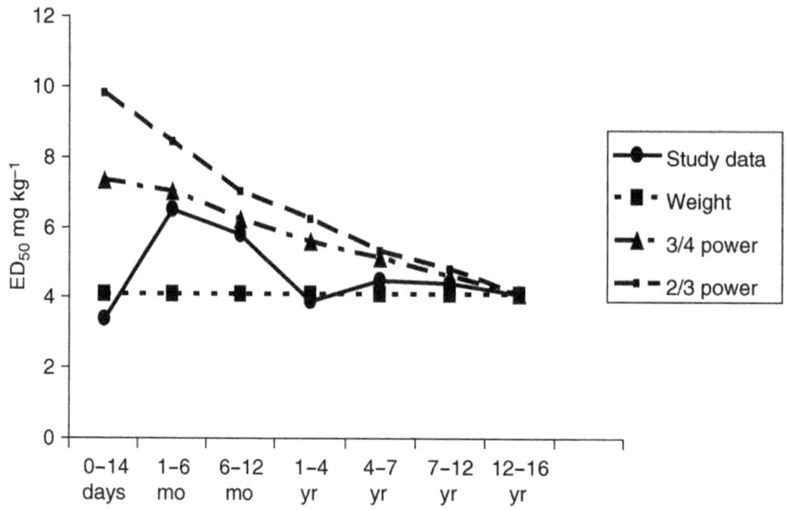


**Figure 2.1** Biphasic variation in the ED50 sleep dose of thiopental with age presented as a solid line. The broken lines represent paediatric doses of thiopental predicted from the adult dose of 4 mg $kg^{-1}$ using one of three size models (weight, 3/4 power and 2/3 power). The weight model predicts the lowest doses, the 2/3 power model the highest; the 3/4 power model predicts doses intermediate between the other two and provides the best fit to the data in children aged one to six months and older.
*Source:* Data taken from Jonmarker C, Westrin P, Larsson S et al. Thiopental requirements for induction of anesthesia in children. *Anesthesiology* 1987; 67:104–7; and Westrin P, Jonmarker C, Werner O. Thiopental requirements for induction of anesthesia in neonates and in infants one to six months of age. *Anesthesiology* 1989; 71:344–6.

is affected by changes in intraluminal pH, biliary function, gastric emptying time and intestinal motility. At birth, gastric pH is roughly neutral, and within 48 hours it decreases to approximately pH3 before returning to neutral over the subsequent 24 hours, where it remains for the following 10 days. It then decreases gradually to reach adult pH values by two years. Differences in intestinal motility at different stages of development influence the gut transit time, resulting in prolonged transit times in neonates compared to older children and adults but faster transit times in infants. The ability of neonates to absorb lipophilic drugs may be altered due to immature biliary function leading to a reduction in the solubility effect of bile.

Few studies have investigated the effects of developmental changes in absorptive function in children; however, the absorption of oral paracetamol has been shown to be significantly lower in the first few days of life. Greater absorption following cutaneous application of a drug in neonates is because of their proportionally higher body surface area and more permeable skin. Percutaneous absorption in preterm infants is inversely related to gestational age, with permeability rates 100–1,000 greater before 30 weeks of gestation compared to term neonates, and only three to four times increased permeability beyond 32 weeks. There is some evidence that the increased permeability in preterm infants is short-lived, lasting only two weeks postnatally even in the most immature infants. Topical use of the local anaesthetic cream EMLA (lidocaine/prilocaine) for pain relief may lead to methaemaglobinaemia in neonates due to higher systemic absorption and an increased susceptibility of fetal haemoglobin to prilocaine.

### Distribution

Distribution of drugs to body compartments, tissues and cells is affected by:

- Body composition (e.g. total body water and fat percentage)
- Cardiac output and regional blood flow
- Protein binding
- Blood–brain barrier

*Body composition:* Total body water accounts for 85–90% of body weight in very immature and preterm infants and their total fat content is only 10–15%. This ratio declines gradually into adulthood, where total body water accounts for 55–60% of body weight. In neonates the extracellular water content is approximately 45% of body weight, whereas in adults it is only 20% (Figure 2.2).

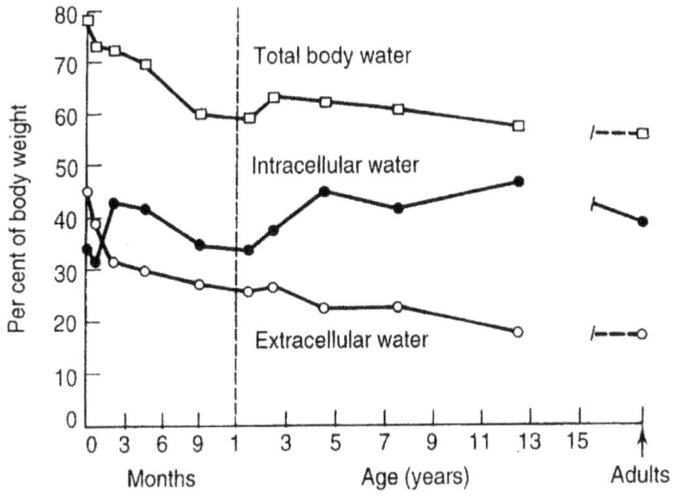


**Figure 2.2** Variation in body water compartments with age.
*Source:* Adapted from Friis-Hansen B. Body water compartments in children: changes during growth and related changes in body composition. *Pediatrics* 1961; 28:169–81.

Higher initial bolus doses (mg $kg^{-1}$) of water-soluble drugs are required to achieve similar plasma concentrations in neonates compared to older children and adults. The effect of age on the distribution of lipophilic drugs in children is less clear. During infancy, the total body fat content increases steadily, which is likely to influence the volume of distribution of lipophilic drugs such as propofol.

*Cardiac output and regional blood flow*: The initial phase of distribution from the central compartment reflects regional blood flow. Redistribution from the brain, heart, liver and kidneys to other relatively well-perfused tissues such as skeletal muscle follows, with much slower distribution to the less perfused tissues, such as fat. These less well-perfused areas become important in relation to long-term drug infusions. Relative organ mass and regional blood flow alter as infants mature. During the neonatal period, blood flow as a proportion of the cardiac output increases to the kidneys and brain, whereas that to the liver decreases. Relative to their body weight the cerebral and hepatic mass in infants is much higher than in adults. Both the increased cardiac output and cerebral perfusion mean that the onset time after intravenous induction is shortened in neonates.

*Protein binding:* Drug distribution is influenced by the concentration of circulating plasma proteins such as albumin and α-1-acid glycoprotein (AAG). Neonates and young infants often display a reduction in both the quantity and the binding affinity of circulating plasma proteins. Plasma albumin concentration approximates adult values by five months and binding capacity by one year of age. Neonates also tend to a metabolic acidosis that alters the ionisation and binding properties of plasma proteins.

*Blood–brain barrier (BBB):* It is thought that BBB permeability to water-soluble drugs changes with maturation; the BBB is less well developed in neonates than older children and is therefore more permeable to partially ionised drugs (e.g. morphine, bupivacaine). Besides passive diffusion, there are specific transport systems within the BBB that mediate active transport. These include the adenosine triphosphate (ATP)–dependent processes that transport opioids such as fentanyl and morphine. Modulation of transporter proteins (e.g. p-glycoprotein) will have a significant influence on brain distribution and onset time as well as the magnitude and duration of analgesic response of opioids.

## Elimination

The main routes of drug elimination are either through metabolism (mainly hepatic) or excretion of the parent compound or its metabolites (mainly renal). Both hepatic metabolism and renal clearance mature in early life.

*Metabolism*: Metabolic processes mainly transform lipid-soluble drugs into water-soluble metabolites, which can be excreted more readily by the kidney. The concentrations and activities of microsomal enzymes are reduced or absent in the newborn. In particular, elements of the mixed oxidase or cytochrome P450 system are less than half as active as in adults and may take from a few weeks to several years to mature. This results in reduced metabolism of many drugs, including barbiturates, diazepam and amide local anaesthetics. Similarly, the ability to form glucuronide conjugates is impaired owing to a reduction in the activity of glucuronyl transferase and uridine diphosphate glucose (UDPG) dehydrogenase. This is of major importance in the metabolism of morphine, which is greatly reduced in the neonate and takes over six months to approach adult levels.

Many drugs are metabolised at extrahepatic sites, frequently by esterases. Studies with neonatal plasma have shown that the rate of hydrolysis of procaine by butyryl-cholinesterase (plasma cholinesterase) is half of that in adults. However, the reduction in butyryl-cholinesterase activity has no effect on the duration of action of suxamethonium in the newborn, which seems to be influenced more by the rapid redistribution of the drug from its site of action.

*Excretion*: Drugs and their metabolites are excreted principally by the kidney, involving glomerular filtration and tubular secretion. Some drugs are simply filtered, in which case their rate of elimination will depend upon the glomerular filtration rate (GFR). GFR is lower in newborns and infants than in adults, and when related to body surface area it achieves adult values at three to five months of age. However, when related to body weight, GFR reaches adult values at one to two weeks, which reflects more accurately the age at which the half-times of unmetabolised drugs approach adult values. Proximal tubular secretion is important for the elimination of some conjugated drugs; it reaches adult levels by about seven months of age.

#### Pharmacodynamics

Developmental pharmacodynamics describes the impact of maturation of biologic systems on responses to drugs. The pharmacodynamic outcomes commonly measured in anaesthesia are pain, neuromuscular blockade and depth of anaesthesia or sedation. Age-related pharmacodynamic variation may be influenced by developmental changes in receptor number, type, affinity and the availability of endogenous ligands. Beyond drug-receptor interactions, drug responses may be significantly impacted by the child's developing physiology. For example, neonates have increased postnatal expression of the μ-opioid receptor, and this, coupled with differences in their tendency to apnoeas, contributes to this age group being more sensitive to morphine. Further examples of pharmacodynamic considerations are covered later in discussions of specific drugs.

#### Comorbidities

The presence of certain congenital abnormalities and syndromes will affect responses to some medications. Patients with genetic conditions affecting organ systems (e.g. heart, liver, kidney) may need to be monitored more closely for adverse reactions. Caution should be taken with the use of specific drugs in patients with liver disease and those at risk of decreased drug clearance. Drugs that may enhance the neuromuscular blocking action of suxamethonium should be noted, including several medications that may be prescribed for patients with genetic disorders. These may include aminoglycoside antibiotics, β-blockers, procainamide, lithium carbonate, glucocorticoids, metoclopramide, terbutaline and monoamine oxidase inhibitors. Those with inherited metabolic disorders and myopathies may be particularly susceptible to certain side effects, and some drugs should be avoided entirely in certain patients (see Chapter 8 for further details).

## Intravenous Anaesthetic Agents

### Propofol

Propofol is the most widely used IV anaesthetic agent and can be used for both induction and maintenance of anaesthesia in infants and children but is less commonly used in neonates. It can also be used for sedation. Propofol has largely replaced thiopental as the intravenous induction agent of choice because of its rapid, clear-headed recovery and antiemetic effect. Propofol also suppresses laryngeal and pharyngeal reflexes, thereby facilitating laryngeal mask airway insertion and tracheal intubation.

The faster and more clear-headed recovery following a single dose of propofol compared with thiopental is due to propofol's shorter distribution half-time and more rapid plasma clearance. The rapid elimination of propofol (plasma clearance approximately six times as fast as thiopental in paediatric studies) reduces the potential for accumulation, making the drug suitable for the maintenance of anaesthesia. Induction and maintenance doses of propofol are greater in children than in adults because the volume of the central compartment is 50% larger and the plasma clearance 25% faster in children. Average induction doses (1.3 × ED50) in unpremedicated patients are as follows:

- Infants: 4 mg $kg^{-1}$
- Children: 3 mg $kg^{-1}$
- Adults: 2 mg $kg^{-1}$

When given with an opioid, the average infusion dose of propofol for maintenance of anaesthesia in children is 0.1–0.2 mg $kg^{-1}$ $min^{-1}$, approximately twice the dose required in adults.

The use of propofol for prolonged sedation (>48 hours) in paediatric intensive care units has been associated with a rare syndrome comprising lipaemia, metabolic acidosis, heart failure, rhabdomyolysis and death. The cause of this syndrome is unknown, but attention has focused mainly on impairment of fatty acid oxidation by propofol as a possible cause. In view of these reports, the drug regulatory authorities of the United Kingdom, Canada and the United States have recommended that propofol should not be used for intensive care sedation of children under 16 years.

## Thiopental

Thiopental is a barbiturate with a rapid onset of action following intravenous administration. In the newborn, plasma protein binding of thiopental is reduced, so that the fraction of unbound drug is almost twice that found in older children and adults. In addition, the elimination half-time is more than three times as long in neonates as in older children; however, as recovery depends primarily on redistribution, the effect of an induction dose is not significantly prolonged.

The usual induction doses of thiopental are:

- Healthy neonates: 4–5 mg $kg^{-1}$
- Infants: 7–8 mg $kg^{-1}$
- Children: 5–6 mg $kg^{-1}$

The lower dose for thiopental in neonates compared with infants may be explained by decreased plasma protein binding, greater penetration of the neonatal brain and increased responsiveness of neonatal receptors.

The increased dose for thiopental in infants and children compared with adults (average dose 4 mg $kg^{-1}$) may be due to the increased cardiac output in younger patients, which should reduce the initial concentration of thiopental arriving at the brain.

## Ketamine

Ketamine is a unique drug with anxiolytic, analgesic, amnesic and dissociative properties and a wide safety margin. As an induction agent, it causes less hypotension than propofol or thiopental and can be used for procedural sedation for children undergoing short, painful or frightening procedures in the emergency department. Ketamine can cause hallucinations, nightmares and other transient psychotic effects; these can be reduced by co-administration of a benzodiazepine such as midazolam.

Neonates and young children require lower doses of ketamine of 1–2 mg $kg^{-1}$ for induction of anaesthesia compared to older children (>12 years) (1–4.5 mg $kg^{-1}$). Ketamine can also be administered via intramuscular injection with neonates requiring a reduced dose of 4 mg $kg^{-1}$ in comparison to infants and older children, where doses of 4–13 mg $kg^{-1}$ are required.

# Sedatives

## Dexmedetomidine

Dexmedetomidine has anxiolytic, sedative and analgesic properties and is notable for its ability to provide sedation without risk of respiratory depression. It was launched in the United Kingdom in 2011, with marketing authorisation for sedation of adult intensive care patients only. However, due to its unique pharmacological profile its clinical use has expanded to unlicensed applications in children. It is the S-enantiomer of the veterinary sedative medetomidine and a highly selective α2-adrenoceptor agonist, and administration is possible via multiple routes (oral, nasal, buccal, IV).

Dexmedetomidine induces sedation that resembles physiological sleep in terms of electroencephalography (EEG). Its use can reduce emergence delirium as well as acute postsurgical pain and opioid requirement. Disadvantages include transient hypertension, hypotension and bradycardia.

Dexmedetomidine can be used as an infusion or as a bolus dose intraoperatively. An infusion is given at a dose of 0.2–0.7 mcg $kg^{-1}$ $hr^{-1}$ and the bolus dose in children is 0.5–1 mcg $kg^{-1}$.

## Midazolam

Midazolam is a water-soluble benzodiazepine associated with profound sedation when high doses are given intravenously or when it is used with certain other drugs. It may be used to provide sedation, anxiolysis and amnesia prior to diagnostic, therapeutic or endoscopic procedures, before induction of anaesthesia or as a sedative agent in mechanically ventilated patients in intensive care. Midazolam is the only benzodiazepine approved by the US Food and Drug Administration (FDA) for use in neonates; in this population, the half-life is much longer (6–12 hours). Severe hypotension has been reported with midazolam in neonates after bolus administration, and this effect appears to be compounded in those also receiving fentanyl. When used as a sedative and analgesic in neonates in intensive care, a loading dose is avoided, and continuous intravenous infusions depending on gestation are recommended:

- <32 weeks' gestation: 30 mcg $kg^{-1}$ $hr^{-1}$ adjusted according to response
- >32 weeks' gestation: 60 mcg $kg^{-1}$ $hr^{-1}$ adjusted according to response
- Dose may be gradually increased up to 150 mcg $kg^{-1}$ $hr^{-1}$

As with older children and adults, neonates can become tolerant to midazolam, thus abrupt withdrawal after prolonged use should be avoided.

# Opioids

Until the late 1980s, the use of opioids was avoided in newborns and young infants because of their increased susceptibility to respiratory depression. However, attitudes changed following the demonstration that neonates mount a significant stress response to surgery which can be modified by opioids.

The susceptibility of newborns to opioid-induced respiratory depression may be due to:

- Increased central nervous system (CNS) penetration by opioids
- Reduced capacity for opioid elimination
- Developmental changes in the relative proportions and affinities of opioid receptors

## Morphine

Morphine remains the drug of choice for the management of severe postoperative pain in infants and children. It is usually administered by continuous infusion or by nurse- or patient-controlled analgesia (NCA/PCA). In view of the long time constant of morphine, a loading dose is required to achieve an effective plasma concentration within a reasonable time.

Following an intravenous injection of morphine, brain uptake is slow owing to poor lipid solubility. Similarly, the decay of CNS concentration is slow as it depends on elimination of the drug by the liver. Conjugation with glucuronide produces both active and inactive metabolites which are excreted by the kidneys. Morphine clearance in neonates is only 25% of that in adults and takes six months to approach adult values. Accordingly, the elimination half-time of morphine is significantly prolonged in young infants. The fraction of protein-bound morphine is similar in all age groups (~20%).

For children and infants aged over six months, a loading dose of 100 mcg $kg^{-1}$ followed by a maintenance infusion rate of 10–30 mcg $kg^{-1}$ $h^{-1}$ should achieve and maintain an adequate target concentration of 10–25 ng $ml^{-1}$.

In newborns, a plasma concentration of morphine of 10–25 ng $ml^{-1}$ should be achieved with a loading dose of 25 mcg $kg^{-1}$ followed by an infusion rate of 5–10 mcg $kg^{-1}$ $h^{-1}$. All infants and children receiving morphine infusions should be monitored with continuous pulse oximetry, and infants aged less than one month should be nursed in a high-dependency unit.

## Fentanyl

Fentanyl is a synthetic opioid with a high lipid solubility that confers increased potency, rapid onset and short duration of action. After a dose of 1–3 mcg $kg^{-1}$, the clinical effects of fentanyl are terminated by redistribution and its duration of action is limited to 20–30 minutes. However, after repeated doses or a continuous infusion, progressive saturation of peripheral compartments occurs, and its effects may last for several hours.

The mean plasma clearance of fentanyl in infants is greater than that in adults, although there is great inter-patient variability due to age and the type of surgery. Fentanyl clearance increases during the first two weeks of life, reflecting rapid maturation of the cytochrome P-450 3A4 enzyme. During the same period, the volume of distribution of fentanyl is two to three times that in adults, and there is a corresponding increase in the half-time of elimination. Accordingly, single doses of fentanyl in neonates should be reduced (e.g. 0.5–1 mcg $kg^{-1}$).

## Remifentanil

Remifentanil is an ultra-short acting, ester-linked synthetic opioid introduced into clinical practice in 1996. Following intravenous infusion, it is rapidly hydrolysed by non-specific blood and tissue esterases to produce a virtually inactive carboxylic acid compound. As remifentanil is not a substrate for butyrylcholinesterase (plasma cholinesterase), its elimination is not affected by a deficiency in this enzyme.

The volume of distribution (Vd) is greatest in infants under two months old and decreases with age, and clearance is more rapid in the younger age groups. Thus, half-life is similar in all age groups (means of 3.4 to 5.7 minutes). The short time constant frequently makes a loading dose unnecessary and facilitates control of the infusion. Unlike other opioids, its duration of action does not increase with increasing dose or duration of infusion, because its volume of distribution is small and its clearance is fast. The usual infusion rate of remifentanil is 0.1–0.5 mcg $kg^{-1}$ $min^{-1}$. Its use in neonatal and infant anaesthesia is associated with a reduction in the requirements for volatile anaesthetic agents, stable cardiovascular conditions and a low incidence of postoperative apnoea.

## Muscle Relaxants

### Suxamethonium

Suxamethonium is the only depolarising neuromuscular blocking drug in clinical use. A unique combination of rapid onset and short duration of action makes it especially useful for emergency tracheal intubation. Elimination depends on hydrolysis by butyrylcholinesterase, hence a deficiency in this enzyme may result in prolonged block.

Studies during thiopental-fentanyl-nitrous oxide anaesthesia showed that the doses of suxamethonium for 90% depression of the twitch response (ED90) in neonates, infants and children were 0.52, 0.61 and 0.35 mg $kg^{-1}$ respectively. These values were all greater than that obtained in a comparable adult study (0.29 mg $kg^{-1}$; see Figure 2.3). It was recommended that neonates and infants should be given 3 mg $kg^{-1}$ and children 2 mg $kg^{-1}$ of suxamethonium for tracheal intubation. The duration of action of these doses was about the same as or less than that produced by 1 mg $kg^{-1}$ in adults (six to eight minutes), reflecting the shorter half-times of suxamethonium in infants and children.

When intravenous access is not available, suxamethonium may be given by intramuscular injection. In this case, doses of 5 mg $kg^{-1}$ for infants and 4 mg $kg^{-1}$ for children produces 85–100% twitch depression. Maximum block will be achieved at 3 to 4 minutes, and full recovery will occur after 15–20 minutes (see Figure 2.3).

The increased dose requirement of suxamethonium in younger patients probably results from its distribution into a larger extracellular fluid (ECF) volume rather than an altered response to the action of the drug at acetylcholine receptors. The unique mode of action of suxamethonium (sustained depolarisation) and its activity at muscarinic acetylcholine receptors are responsible for

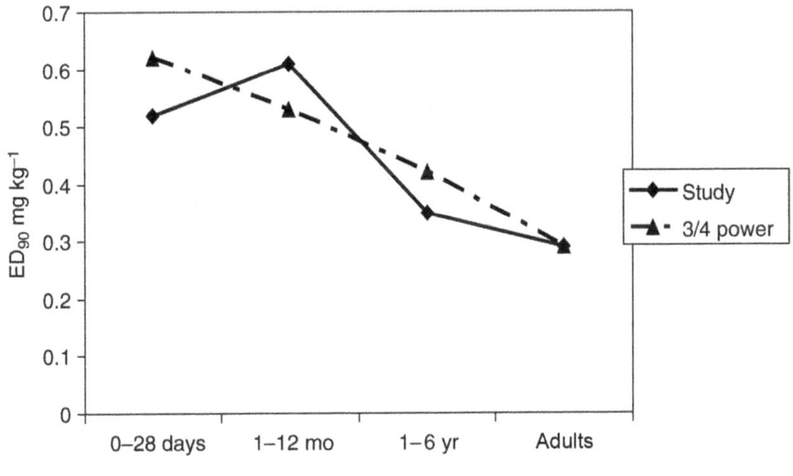


**Figure 2.3** Monophasic variation in the ED90 dose of suxamethonium with age (solid line). The broken line represents paediatric doses of suxamethonium predicted from the adult dose of 0.3 mg $kg^{-1}$ using the 3/4 power size model.
*Source:* Data taken from Meakin GH, McKiernan EP, Morris P et al. Dose-response curves for suxamethonium in neonates, infants and children. *British Journal of Anaesthesia* 1989; 62:655–8; and Smith CE, Donati F, Bevan DR. Dose–response curves for succinylcholine: single versus cumulative techniques. *Anesthesiology* 1988; 69:338–42.

many adverse effects. Of greatest concern have been reports of rare, but often fatal, hyperkalaemic cardiac arrests in boys with undiagnosed muscular dystrophy. As a result of these reports, the FDA recommends that the use of suxamethonium in children should be reserved for emergency intubation and instances where immediate securing of the airway is necessary (e.g. laryngospasm, difficult airway, full stomach) or for intramuscular use when a suitable vein is not available.

### Non-depolarising Neuromuscular Blocking Drugs

Clinical studies in the 1960s and 1970s produced conflicting results about the sensitivity of paediatric patients to non-depolarising neuromuscular blocking drugs (NMBDs). The question was largely resolved in 1982 by a study which demonstrated that the steady-state concentration of tubocurarine corresponding to 50% depression of EMG twitch (Cpss50) in neonates was only one-third of that in adults, whilst that of infants was about one-half. However, when the dose corresponding to 50% depression of EMG twitch (D50) was determined for each patient by multiplying the Cpss50 by the volume of distribution (Vdss), there were no significant differences between the groups (Table 2.1). It was concluded that whilst neonates and infants were more sensitive to tubocurarine in terms of the lower plasma concentration required to produce a given effect, this was countered by an increased volume of distribution (ECF volume), such that the dose did not vary significantly with age. The same appears to be true of other NMBDs.

Experimental data from young rats suggest that the increased sensitivity of the neuromuscular junction of the human neonate and infant to NMBDs is due to a reduction in the release of acetylcholine (ACh) from developing motor nerves. A prejunctional locus for the weakness in neuromuscular transmission in human infants is also consistent with the mature appearance of the motor endplate from 31 weeks gestational age, the absence of fetal acetylcholine receptors (AChRs) after this time and the apparently normal response of the motor endplate to suxamethonium in newborns.

**Table 2.1** Steady state concentration of tubocurarine for 50% depression of EMG twitch ($C_{pss50}$), steady state volume of distribution ($V_{dss}$) and dose for 50% depression of twitch ($D_{50}$) calculated from the other two parameters.

| | $C_{pss50}$ (mcg ml$^{-1}$) | $V_{dss}$ (l kg$^{-1}$) | $D_{50}$ (mcg kg$^{-1}$) |
|---|---|---|---|
| Neonates | 0.18 | 0.74 | 155 |
| Infants | 0.27 | 0.52 | 158 |
| Children | 0.42 | 0.41 | 163 |
| Adults | 0.53 | 0.30 | 152 |

Adapted from Fisher DM, O'Keefe C, Stanski DR *et al.* Pharmacokinetics and pharmacodynamics of D-tubocurarine in infants, children and adults. *Anesthesiology* 1982;**57**:203–8.

### Atracurium

Atracurium is a bis-quaternary benzylquinolinium diester with an intermediate duration of action.

It is metabolised by non-enzymatic cleavage at body temperature and pH (Hofmann elimination) as well as by hydrolysis. Plasma clearance of atracurium is therefore independent of organ function and, when normalised for body weight, is greater in infants than in older children.

When compared during thiopental–nitrous oxide–narcotic anaesthesia, the ED95 of atracurium has been shown to be significantly lower in neonates and infants than in children (119 and 163 vs 195 mcg kg$^{-1}$). Following a standard intubating dose of atracurium 0.5 mg kg$^{-1}$ (~2 × ED95), 95% depression of twitch occurred more rapidly in neonates than in children (0.9 vs 1.4 min), whilst recovery to 10% of control twitch height occurred more rapidly in neonates compared with the other two groups (22.7, 29.7 and 28.6 minutes; for neonates, infants and children respectively). Prompt, predictable recovery in all age groups is a major advantage of atracurium when used for paediatric anaesthesia.

The adverse effects seen with atracurium relate mainly to histamine release. Commonly, this results in a macular rash or erythema along the course of the vein of injection, which may subsequently spread peripherally. Occasionally the rash may be accompanied by more serious histamine effects such as hypotension, tachycardia or bronchospasm. The cardiovascular changes are dose related and usually occur at doses greater than twice the ED95.

### Cisatracurium

Cisatracurium is 1 of 10 stereoisomers that make up the commercially available atracurium mixture. The ED95 of cisatracurium is 45 mcg kg$^{-1}$, therefore it is approximately three times as potent as atracurium. The increased potency of cisatracurium compared with atracurium confers greater specificity of action and fewer histamine-related side effects. The main disadvantage of increased potency is a slower onset of action. Consequently, a dose of ~3 × ED95 of cisatracurium (0.15 mg $kg^{-1}$) is required to produce intubating conditions at two minutes comparable to those obtained with 2 × ED95 of atracurium. Following a dose of cisatracurium 3 × ED95, 25% recovery time was shown to be longer in infants than in children (43 vs 36 minutes), which could have clinical importance in infants undergoing short surgical procedures.

### Vecuronium

Vecuronium is a monoquaternary aminosteroid relaxant of intermediate duration of action, which is largely eliminated unchanged by the liver. As with other non-depolarising relaxants, the variation in effective dose of vecuronium is biphasic with the ED95 in infants being like that in adolescents whilst the maximum effective dose occurs in children aged five to seven years. Significantly, a standard intubating dose of 100 mcg $kg^{-1}$ of vecuronium (~2 × ED95) maintains over 90% neuromuscular blockade for almost an hour in newborns and infants compared with only 18 minutes in children. Vecuronium is therefore a long-acting muscle relaxant in neonates and infants, reflecting its dependence on hepatic function for elimination.

### Rocuronium

Rocuronium is an analogue of vecuronium with a more rapid onset of action, making it a suitable for rapid sequence induction. Rapid onset is the result of reduced potency, which necessitates an increase in dose. When compared during nitrous oxide–opioid anaesthesia, the ED95 of rocuronium was significantly lower in infants than in children (248 vs 396 mcg $kg^{-1}$), whilst the duration of clinical effect following a standard intubating dose of 0.6 mg $kg^{-1}$ (~2 × ED95) was much longer (42 vs 27 minutes). These results confirm that rocuronium, like vecuronium, is longer acting in infants than in children. However, unlike vecuronium, rocuronium retains the characteristics of an intermediate-acting muscle relaxant in infants.

### Antagonism of Non-depolarising Relaxants

Any residual non-depolarising neuromuscular blockade at the end of anaesthesia should be antagonised with a cholinesterase inhibitor. This is especially important in infants because of their reduced respiratory reserve. Neostigmine is the most used agent. In the presence of 10% recovery of twitch height, 35 mcg $kg^{-1}$ of neostigmine has been shown to provide maximal antagonism in both paediatric and adult patients. Recovery after neostigmine was faster in paediatric patients compared with adults. For convenience, a somewhat larger dose of 50 mcg $kg^{-1}$ of neostigmine is usually given, in combination with glycopyrrolate to prevent muscarinic effects.

### Sugammadex

Sugammadex reverses neuromuscular blockade with a mechanism that differs from the commonly used acetylcholinesterase inhibitors like neostigmine. It is a modified gamma-cyclodextrin that selectively binds the aminosteroid muscle relaxants, rocuronium and vecuronium. It forms a complex with the muscle relaxants, which leads to a decrease in the concentration of drug available to bind to the nicotinic receptor in the neuromuscular synapse. Sugammadex is only recommended for routine reversal of rocuronium-induced blockade in children and adolescents over the age of two (dose 2 mg $kg^{-1}$). It is not recommended for use in children and adolescents for recovery after vecuronium or for rapid recovery after any muscle relaxant.

### Inhaled Anaesthetics

The commonly used inhalational agents in paediatric anaesthesia worldwide are halothane, sevoflurane, isoflurane, desflurane and nitrous oxide. Halothane is no longer commercially available in the United Kingdom or the United States but remains on the World Health Organisation's List of Essential Medications for both adults and children. Sevoflurane has mostly replaced halothane as the induction agent of choice in children because of its non-pungent odour, rapid induction characteristics and relative cardiostability.

Uptake and elimination of inhaled anaesthetics occur more rapidly in paediatric patients than in adults, primarily because of an increased level of ventilation in relation to functional residual capacity (FRC) and a corresponding increase in weight-normalised cardiac output. The increased rate of uptake of inhaled anaesthetics in infants correlates with more rapid induction of anaesthesia and earlier development of adverse cardiovascular events.

### Halothane

Halothane is a halogenated alkane with a non-pungent odour, making it suitable for inhalation induction in infants and children. Induction of anaesthesia is rapid owing to its relatively low blood–gas partition coefficient and high potency (Table 2.2). In newborns, the minimum alveolar concentration (MAC) of halothane is 0.9%, but it increases rapidly to a maximum of 1.2% at age one to six months and thereafter declines gradually to 0.8% in the adult. The reduced MAC of halothane in neonates compared with infants may relate to immaturity of the CNS or attenuation of the pain response due to increased plasma concentrations of endorphins. The higher MAC in infants compared with older children and adults may be due to reduced solubility of inhaled anaesthetics in brain tissue owing to an increased water content. Neonates and young infants are more sensitive to the myocardial depressant and vagotonic effects of inhaled anaesthetics than older children.

### Sevoflurane

Sevoflurane is trifluoromethyl isopropyl ether; fluorination decreases solubility in fat and blood, thereby reducing anaesthetic potency whilst increasing the rate of uptake and elimination. Because of its lower blood solubility (Table 2.2), induction and recovery are more rapid with sevoflurane than with halothane.

The MAC of sevoflurane varies with age, being higher in neonates and young children than in adults (Table 2.2). Sevoflurane produces less myocardial depression and bradycardia than halothane; however, significant hypotension may still occur in neonates.

Although an estimated 5% of the inhaled dose of sevoflurane is metabolised producing inorganic fluorides, peak concentrations of fluoride in paediatric studies have not exceeded two-thirds of the suggested nephrotoxic level of 50 mmol $l^{-1}$, and there have been no reported cases of sevoflurane nephrotoxicity.

Emergence agitation is a significant problem with sevoflurane. The reported incidence varies (30–80%), affecting mainly preschool children. Episodes typically last for ~10 minutes during which the child appears to be agitated, restless, combative, frightened and inconsolable. It cannot be attributed solely to pain or rapid emergence from anaesthesia and has been described as a short-lived acute organic mental state of uncertain aetiology. It may be the result of different washout times between excitatory and inhibitory centres in the CNS. Its incidence can be reduced using sedatives and short-acting opioids, e.g. intravenous induction with propofol and administration of 1 mcg $kg^{-1}$ of fentanyl 10 minutes before the end of anaesthesia.

**Table 2.2** Properties of volatile anaesthetics

| | Halothane | Isoflurane | Sevoflurane | Desflurane |
|---|---|---|---|---|
| Odour | Non-pungent petrolic | Pungent ethereal | Non-pungent ethereal | Pungent ethereal |
| Blood–gas coefficient | | | | |
| *Neonates* | 2.1 | 1.2 | 0.7 | – |
| *Adults* | 2.3 | 1.4 | 0.7 | 0.4 |
| MAC (%) | | | | |
| *Neonates* | 0.9 | 1.6 | 3.3 | 9.2 |
| *Adults* | 0.8 | 1.2 | 2.0 | 6.0 |
| Rate of metabolism (%) | 20 | 0.2 | 2.0 | 0.02 |
| Myocardial depression | ++ | + | + | + |
| Peripheral vasodilation | + | ++ | ++ | ++ |
| Respiratory depression | + | ++ | ++ | ++ |

*Source:* Adapted from Meakin G. Neonatal anaesthetic pharmacology. In: Hughes DG, Mather SJ, Wolf AR, eds. *Handbook of Neonatal Anaesthesia*. Saunders. 1996; 18–54.

### Isoflurane

Isoflurane is a halogenated methyl-ethyl ether with irritant properties rendering it unsuitable for inhalational induction. The potency of isoflurane varies with age in a similar manner to that of halothane; the MAC is approximately 1.6% in neonates, 1.9% at age one to six months and thereafter declines gradually to about 1.2% in adults. The MAC of isoflurane is further reduced in premature infants: at 32 weeks gestational age, it is approximately 1.3% whilst at 32–37 weeks it is 1.4%. Equipotent concentrations of isoflurane and halothane produce similar reductions in blood pressure in infants and children, although heart rate and myocardial function are better preserved with isoflurane.

### Desflurane

Desflurane is synthesised by the replacement of the single chlorine atom of isoflurane with fluorine. Like isoflurane, desflurane has a pungent odour making it unsuitable for inhalation induction. However, because of its lower blood solubility (Table 2.2), recovery after desflurane anaesthesia is faster than that after halothane or sevoflurane. The MAC of desflurane varies with age in a way similar to most other volatile anaesthetics, being 9.2% in newborns, 9.9% in infants aged 6–12 months and thereafter declining gradually to 6.0% in adults. The cardiovascular profile of desflurane is like that of halothane; metabolism is negligible, and the drug resists degradation by soda lime. The rapid recovery seen after desflurane may be of special benefit in neonates and ex-premature infants in view of their increased susceptibility to postoperative apnoea and ventilatory depression. Increasing awareness of desflurane's potent greenhouse gas effect (approximately 26 times that of sevoflurane) has led to a recent reduction in its usage.

### Nitrous Oxide

Nitrous oxide is a sweet-smelling, non-irritant, anaesthetic gas with a low blood–gas partition coefficient (0.47) resulting in rapid uptake and elimination. When used as a carrier gas with oxygen, it speeds the uptake and elimination of potent volatile anaesthetics by the second gas effect and reduces their MAC requirement for anaesthesia. The low potency of nitrous oxide may be an added safety factor when the agent is used in neonates who generally tolerate anaesthetics poorly.

In recent years there have been calls for the abandonment of nitrous oxide in routine anaesthesia owing to a greater appreciation of its disadvantages (e.g. potential for delivering a hypoxic mixture, distension of air pockets in the body, increase in intracranial pressure, contribution to greenhouse gas effect). Although paediatric anaesthetists still find nitrous oxide useful for inhalation induction of anaesthesia, its use for maintenance of anaesthesia is declining in line with recent trends in adult anaesthetic practice.

### Local Anaesthetics

Local anaesthetics are commonly used for wound infiltration, perioperative nerve blocks and neuraxial blockade as part of a multimodal approach to analgesia. Drugs of the amino-amide type are used most frequently. Lower concentrations of α-1-acid glycoprotein in young infants increase the amount of unbound local anaesthetic and the potential for CNS and cardiovascular toxicity. Total body clearance is also reduced in young infants because of the limited oxidising capacity of the liver, which, together with an increase in the volume of distribution, leads to a prolonged elimination half-time. Accordingly, the maximum permitted single and infusion doses of local anaesthetics should be reduced in young infants. Bupivacaine is a racemic mixture of R (+) and S (–) enantiomers. Its chief advantage is its long duration of action (e.g. four to six hours after a single epidural injection). For patients aged over six months, the maximum single injection dose (plain or with adrenaline) is 2.5 mg $kg^{-1}$, and the maximum epidural infusion rate is 0.5 mg $kg^{-1}$ $h^{-1}$ for a maximum of 36 hours. In infants aged less than six months, these doses should be halved, and consideration should be given to reducing the rate of infusions by a further one-third after 24 hours as there is evidence of drug accumulation even with the reduced doses.

Bupivacaine toxicity is a particular concern in children since most blocks are carried out under anaesthesia when early signs of impending catastrophe are absent. Demonstration in the 1970s that the S (–) enantiomer of bupivacaine was significantly less cardio-depressant than the R (+) enantiomer led to the development of ropivacaine and levobupivacaine. In view of their wider safety margins, these S (–) enantiomer drugs should be the local anaesthetics of choice for paediatric anaesthetic practice. In comparative trials, ropivacaine, levobupivacaine and bupivacaine were found to be equally effective when given in equal doses and concentrations to children for caudal and epidural analgesia, but ropivacaine and levobupivacaine were associated with less motor block.

## Further Reading

Blumer JL, Reed MD. Principles of neonatal pharmacology. In: Yaffe SJ, Aranda JV, eds. *Neonatal and Pediatric Pharmacology.* Lippincott Williams & Wilkins. 2005; 146–58.

Hansen TG. Developmental paediatric anaesthetic pharmacology. *Anaesthesia and Intensive Care Medicine* 2018; 19:437–43.

Kearns GL, Abdel-Rahman SM, Alander SW, Blowey DL, Leeder JS, Kauffman RE. Developmental pharmacology: drug disposition, action and therapy in infants and children. *New England Journal of Medicine* 2003; 349:1157–67.

Chapter 3

# Developmental Psychology and Communicating with Children and Families

Jo Wray

## Introduction

### Picture the Scene

S is a ten-year old girl with complex heart disease who has been admitted for an interventional cardiac catheterisation. She had coped well with two previous heart operations – albeit when she was much younger – and is familiar with hospitals, so it is assumed that she will cope well this time too. On admission to hospital, she appears relaxed and cheerful, but as the time for her afternoon procedure approaches she becomes increasingly agitated and anxious. Her behaviour changes – she becomes more withdrawn until it is time to go to the anaesthetic room, where she starts crying and screaming, resisting any attempts to calm her down and reassure her. Her mother accompanies her and is also distressed, alternating between calmness and exasperation herself, also in tears, not sure what to do. This has never happened before. As S becomes physically aggressive and increasingly resistant and a 'time out' fails to calm her down, the procedure is cancelled and she is discharged home. She is upset with herself – she knows she needs the procedure and wants another date soon. She is adamant that next time will be different and she will be fine . . . but will she? How can anyone be sure of that?

Hospitals can be frightening places for children, but an awareness of how a child understands and reacts to medical procedures can enable professionals to work with children and families to reduce feelings of anxiety. A child's understanding is linked to their developmental stage rather than their chronological age, and knowledge of the tasks of each stage can help to inform the choice of intervention to reduce anxiety. Incorporating evidence-based psychological strategies into anaesthetic practice, using a developmental framework that takes account of individual child, family and situational factors, can help to reduce preoperative anxiety through fostering resilience and adaptive coping skills.

## Developmental Psychology

There is a vast literature on the study of developmental psychology which clearly cannot be comprehensively covered in a few paragraphs, but a brief overview of some of the key concepts of developmental theory may help to illustrate why children behave in the way they do and how that knowledge can be applied in the hospital setting.

## Developmental Theory

There are a number of theories of child development describing the social, cognitive and emotional changes that occur during childhood. Developmental theories provide an important framework for understanding child development, and one of the most influential is that of Jean Piaget, whose cognitive theory addressed how an individual's thought processes develop. Whilst seemingly obvious to us now, one of Piaget's tenets was that children think differently from adults. Unlike some earlier theorists, Piaget asserted that children are active agents in shaping their own development. Through continual interaction and cognitive adaptation, children become better able to understand and manage their world. Piaget described four stages of development through which children progress, characterised by qualitatively different ways of thinking as they develop an increasing ability to use logic and separate internal realities (e.g. wishes, needs and thoughts) from the outside world (Table 3.1).

Although development is described as occurring in discrete stages, in reality these aspects of development occur as a continuous process. Information is acquired, organised and applied,

**Table 3.1** Stages of cognitive and psychosocial development, corresponding beliefs about illness and translation to the hospitalised child

| Cognitive development | Psychosocial development | Beliefs about illness | Impact on ill/hospitalised child |
|---|---|---|---|
| *Sensorimotor stage: birth–2 years*<br>• Knowledge of the world limited to infant's sensory perceptions and motor activities<br>• Coordinating movement and action is primary focus<br>• As child develops language, they learn that words represent words and objects<br>• Concept of object permanence develops<br>• Extent of understanding is greater than that of verbal expression<br>• As infant develops sense of heightened attachment to caregiver(s), a fear of strangers develops at about 6–9 months | *0–18 months*<br>• Focus is on developing trust due to complete dependency of infant on their carer<br>• Failure to adequately meet physical and emotional needs results in child coming to believe they cannot trust adults, resulting in fear and a view that the world is inconsistent and unpredictable<br>• Successful development of trust results in feeling safe and secure and the formation of a secure attachment with their caregiver(s) | *Birth–2 years*<br>• Very limited understanding of health and illness | *Birth–2 years*<br>• Respond to distraction, play, carer presence<br>• Stranger anxiety and separation anxiety can result in high levels of distress<br>• Can respond to parents' emotions<br>• Can show fear/anger/sadness in response to painful procedures<br>• Interventions should reinforce child–parent bond |
| *Preoperational stage: 2–6 years*<br>• Child learns to use increasingly sophisticated language<br>• Thinking is magical and egocentric, and causality is understood through magic<br>• Become able to distinguish between appearance and reality<br>• Start to develop intuitive reasoning but cannot yet mentally manipulate information<br>• Have difficulties in retelling stories coherently (egocentric speech)<br>• Believe that inanimate objects can think and feel like people do (animism) | *18 months–3 years*<br>• Goal is to develop a sense of autonomy<br>• Failure to successfully complete this stage results in a sense of self-doubt and inadequacy<br>*3–5 years*<br>• Begin to assert some control and take some responsibility for themselves through directing play and other social interactions, leading to development of initiative<br>• May ask many questions to make greater sense of the world | *2–6 years*<br>• *Phenomenism* – cause of illness seen to be external concrete phenomenon that may occur with illness but is temporally and spatially remote; unable to offer explanations of how these events cause illness<br>• *Contagion* – cause of illness is believed to be objects or people near to but not touching child; link between the two may be 'magic' | *2–6 years*<br>• Egocentric nature makes them believe that they have caused their illness or hospitalisation<br>• Noxious events are seen as punishments for bad behaviour; pain confirms this<br>• Important to emphasise that illness is not their fault<br>• Respond well to role play and play therapy – e.g. wearing masks, playing with medical equipment with a toy<br>• Simple concrete language should be used to inform child of what is happening and what they can expect to see, hear, taste and feel |

| | | | |
|---|---|---|---|
| *Concrete operational stage: 7–11 years*<br>• Less egocentric<br>• Start to develop logical thought<br>• Thinking still very concrete but begin to order and organise information and coordinate information from several sources<br>• Can use logic to understand more about the physical world but limited by lack of experience in the range of possibilities that exist in that world<br>• Can use inductive logic (going from a specific experience to a general principle) but struggle using deductive logic | *6–11 years*<br>• Begin to develop sense of pride in their achievements through social interactions<br>• Those who successfully cope with new demands develop feeling of competence, socially and academically<br>• Child who is not encouraged and nurtured doubts their abilities to be successful, resulting in feelings of inferiority | *7–11 years*<br>• Increased ability to differentiate between self and other<br>• *Contamination* – child distinguishes between cause of illness (person, object or action) and how it is effective; illness is contracted through child's body physically touching the person/object or child physically engaging in the action and becoming contaminated<br>• *Internalisation* – illness is perceived to be located in the body, but cause may be external; external cause is linked to internal effect of illness through internalisation – e.g. swallowing | *7–11 years*<br>• Begin to understand that medical treatment will help to make them well<br>• Cannot understand how swallowed tablets or medication ending up in their stomach will help pain elsewhere<br>• May fear surgery as form of mutilation<br>• Anaesthesia may provoke anxiety because of confusion between sleep and death<br>• Require explanations and reassurance<br>• Distraction and relaxation techniques can work, and coping strategies can be taught<br>• Giving some element of choice can increase sense of autonomy and control |
| *Formal operational stage: 11+ years*<br>• Thinking becomes less concrete<br>• Can use logic to solve abstract problems<br>• Able to develop and use hypotheses, develop planning strategies, values and theories and manipulate ideas in their head | *11+ years*<br>• Key attainment is of a sense of self and personal identity, which endures throughout adulthood | *11+ years*<br>• Clear differentiation between self and other<br>• *Physiological* – source and nature of illness are in specific internal physiological structures and functions<br>• *Psychophysiological* – most mature conceptions of illness; awareness that thoughts and feelings can affect how body functions | *11+ years*<br>• Can rationalise sufficiently to contribute to discussions about consent<br>• Fear loss of autonomy and control in hospital setting<br>• Require more sophisticated explanations tailored to their own personal experience<br>• Involvement about treatment choices should be encouraged |

allowing the child to develop increasingly complex ways of interacting with the world. In conjunction with the development of thought processes, other aspects of development such as social, emotional, motor and personality development also occur simultaneously, with each influencing the others. Similar to Piaget, psychologist Lev Vygotsky also believed that children developed through a series of stages, but, in contrast to Piaget's view that children learn through doing, Vygotsky believed that children learn through being shown. He described the importance of knowledgeable adults helping children to explore ideas which are just beyond their current stage of development, thereby bridging the gap between what they know and what they can be taught. Erik Erikson's eight-stage theory of psychosocial development covers the life span and highlights the importance of social interaction and relationships and the conflicts that arise during the different stages, with each stage being concerned with becoming competent in an area of life. An individual achieves a sense of mastery if they succeed in handling a stage well, or, if they manage a stage poorly, they develop a sense of inadequacy in that area of development. Each stage builds on the preceding stages and paves the way for subsequent stages. The first five stages relate to children, from infancy through to adolescence, and during the early stages in particular the interactions between children and their adult carers are critically important (Table 3.1).

## Children's Understanding of Health and Illness

Knowledge about the stages of children's understanding of the causes of illness and its treatment can be helpful in managing children in the hospital environment. An awareness of how children understand health and illness and the misconceptions that they have at different ages is important when trying to explain medical procedures to children or informing them about their condition and its treatment. Simply talking in child-appropriate language is not sufficient – it is also necessary to appreciate what they think about illness and why they think about it in the way that they do (Table 3.1). A frequent assumption is that children with previous experience of illness and hospitalisation will have an increased level of understanding, but this is not necessarily so, and in some cases children will regress behaviourally and emotionally to an earlier stage of development when they are unwell or very anxious.

## Children within a Family

Children usually live within a family structure, and families are important partners in their child's health care. Proponents of a family-centred approach to care recognise the vital role that families play in ensuring the health and well-being of children; parents are seen as experts in their child's care, and they are invited to actively participate in decision-making and the planning and provision of their child's care. Whilst there are many advantages to such an approach, some families may feel that they are expected to input into their child's care at a level which is beyond their expectations or capabilities, and this in itself can increase levels of stress and anxiety. Other approaches whereby the clinical team leads the planning of care and families are expected to comply with those plans may work better for some families but less well for others. Parents usually take on some advocacy role for their children and may have a clear view about what information they want their child to receive. Although many will have talked to their child about a forthcoming hospital visit and need for an operation or procedure, responding positively to the opportunity to meet the anaesthetist and supporting their child to engage in an age-appropriate dialogue with the clinical team, others may adopt a level of gatekeeping in relation to the information their child receives. Some parents may have avoided any discussion with, or in front of, the child about their hospital admission, usually to stop their child from worrying. Occasionally parents may have misled their child entirely about their hospital visit, and when the child realises this there can be a loss of trust. In situations where a child is clearly unaware of what is going on but is old enough to be given some information, discussions with parents should focus on the need to explain in an age-appropriate way why the child has come to hospital and what will happen. Some parents may find it challenging to give the information themselves and will welcome the support to enable this; others may still be resistant to allowing their child to be told. Whilst this may be a difficult situation that needs handling sensitively, it is usually unadvisable to perpetuate a situation where a child is given no information or deliberately misinformed.

In some instances, parents' own anxieties or personal experiences can influence their interactions with clinical staff, and they can transmit these anxieties to their child. For example, a parent may describe their child as being needle-phobic when it is actually they who (also) have the phobia. Exploring parents' concerns in such situations is important but also serves to highlight the importance of talking directly to children themselves when appropriate and involving them in decision-making in partnership with parents. Moreover, parents' perceptions of their child's feelings may not be an accurate reflection of how the child actually feels, particularly in the case of older children.

Finally, family factors and cultural influences can significantly impact how children experience illness. In our increasingly multi-cultural society, it is important to recognise racial, ethnic, socio-economic and cultural diversity as well as the diversity in beliefs about health and parenting practices in relation to health. Families may have a myriad of complex issues to deal with, of which their child's health is just one, and an awareness of, and respect for, what else is happening in a family's life can increase the likelihood of care being provided in a way that is acceptable to them.

## Communicating with Parents

Parents often experience high levels of anxiety when their child is unwell or requiring surgery and will often look for reassurance from the professionals caring for their child. They may seek further opinions about their child's treatment and prognosis in an attempt to make the most informed decisions they can as advocates for their child. Providing parents with appropriate information at each stage of their child's treatment and checking that parents have correctly understood what they have been told is crucial, as is recognising that parents' own anxiety can impact their ability to absorb information. Parents need a comprehensive and accurate account of the anaesthetic process, what will happen and why and what measures will be taken to keep their child safe. More complex procedures may require more time to explain, and if parents are to provide informed consent for their child's surgery it is vital that they have this time. Parents need reassurance that their child's well-being is the priority of the medical team and that there will always be someone with their child, they will be kept as pain-free as possible and as soon as they can be with their child they will be allowed to be so. Parents will usually accompany their child to the anaesthetic room to reduce separation anxiety, but it is essential that they understand their role, the importance of them staying calm to help their child stay calm and the need for them to leave when they are asked to. Special consideration needs to be given to those parents who do not speak English, with trained interpreters available to ensure understanding about what will happen to their child. Similarly, parents with a learning disability may need additional time, support and/or other reasonable adjustments during the preoperative visit or in the anaesthetic room.

## Communicating with Children

Effective communication between clinicians and children is essential if good care is to be provided. Understanding what children know, what else they want and need to know and what their hopes or fears are about their treatment all contribute to this goal. Whilst it is often quicker to focus on communicating with parents to gather information and review treatment plans, discussions which are exclusively with parents will prevent the anaesthetist from building rapport with the child – which is important both for the initial meeting but also later in the anaesthetic room. Children may have existing fears and misconceptions about their forthcoming treatment which are already compromising their ability to interact positively with unfamiliar clinical staff, so it is crucial that the anaesthetist creates an atmosphere that is calm, unhurried, non-threatening and engenders trust.

## The Environment

The setting in which medical teams meet children and their families is important. Providing an environment in which children feel relaxed and at ease makes it much more likely that they will accept and interact with people they have not met before. Ensuring that the appearance of the physical space is welcoming and non-threatening, without medical equipment which may be frightening but with appropriate decoration, child-sized furniture and age-appropriate activities, helps to reassure a child who may already be anxious. Other considerations include privacy, low noise levels and separate facilities to see an older child or adolescent on their own if indicated. Appearance of the anaesthetist is also important – some children may be fearful of a stranger in theatre scrubs whilst others may not realise that the friendly person they met at the preoperative clinic or earlier on the ward who was wearing ordinary clothes is the same person who is now dressed in scrubs in the anaesthetic room. Talking to children about what is going to happen should also include some information about what people will be wearing and what the anaesthetic room itself looks like.

## Non-verbal Communication

Non-verbal communication is something that we all use, intentionally and unintentionally, and even very young children are able to pick up and respond to non-verbal cues. First impressions are important – facial expressions and gestures, making eye contact and appearing confident before even speaking to the child all matter. Children want people to look at them when they are talking to them. It is also helpful to be at the same physical level as the child – sitting on the floor with them or bending down so as not to be standing over them.

The child's body language provides clues about how they are feeling and how cooperative they might be with subsequent procedures. A child who refuses to make eye-contact, is fiddling with their fingers or a toy or is particularly clingy and hiding behind a parent is likely to be less tolerant of anaesthetic procedures than the child who has been responsive, interacting directly and making eye contact.

## Verbal Communication

Verbal communication is not just about the language used – even very young children can pick up on the tone, character and speed of speech, so speaking in a calm and friendly manner is important. Language needs to be age appropriate, avoiding medical jargon and complicated explanations, and checking what a child has understood should also be part of the conversation. Some strategies for communicating with children are outlined in Table 3.2.

**Table 3.2** Strategies for communicating with children

- Tell the child and parent who you are and your role.
- Speak in a quiet, calm, reassuring voice.
- Make eye-contact – children want staff to look at them when they are talking to them.
- Do not rush or make the child feel there is not enough time for them to share their feelings.
- Do not stand above them – get down to their eye level.
- Ensure any frightening medical equipment is out of sight.
- Use age/developmentally appropriate language.
- Identify beforehand how the child communicates and whether or not they have any particular issues with communication.
- Ensure that if a child uses alternative methods of communication – e.g. signing, symbols – these are available.
- If you do not have the necessary skills, ensure there is someone available to facilitate meaningful communication.
- Do not use words that may make the child more anxious.
- Periodically check the child's understanding.
- Give the child opportunities to ask questions.
- Be honest and open.
- Give choice if possible and appropriate to increase the child's sense of control.
- Always value the child's feelings – never let them think that their feelings are unimportant or irrelevant.
- Do not tease or laugh at the child or be patronising or condescending.
- Be aware of non-verbal cues – both the child's and your own.
- Provide the opportunity to see a young person without their parents present if appropriate.

## Providing Explanations and Information

It is not always easy to gauge how much information and explanation to offer a child about anaesthesia and the procedures and risks involved. Each communication should be tailored to the needs of the individual child and the specific situation – explanations should be comprehensive, honest, accurate, reassuring and appropriate to their age and level of understanding. Consideration should be given to any special needs the child may have, including learning disabilities, communication disorders, sensory impairments and mental health difficulties and how these may impact their ability to receive and process information, as well as the timing of information provision in terms of elective versus emergency procedures.

## Information for Children to Access at Home

It is often useful if some preparation has begun before the hospital visit. Children should receive information that is meaningful and relevant to them, and any information should be age-appropriate, accurate, appealing and accessible. Consideration should also be given to information in different languages for children who do not speak English. Many hospitals now provide excellent written information on their websites, and there are guides produced by organisations such as the Royal College of Anaesthetists and the British Psychological Society. Hospitals increasingly have virtual hospital tours on their websites that enable children to develop a degree of familiarisation with the hospital before arrival. Some of the age-appropriate virtual tour apps also include the anaesthetic room and a virtual reality doctor, nurse and anaesthetist who explain what happens when a child needs an anaesthetic and the equipment that will be used. Children and their families may be introduced to these more specific apps at a preoperative visit and can then view the app again before they are admitted for their procedure.

## Behavioural Approaches

For many children, age-appropriate explanations may not be sufficient to enable them to cooperate with induction of anaesthesia. Whilst the presence of parents to provide reassurance and avoid separation anxiety is important, play specialists and psychosocial team members have a range of strategies to reduce anxiety. For example, play specialists can help to prepare children for anaesthesia by demystifying some of the equipment and procedures – the preschool child who has pretended to give their favourite toy an anaesthetic and been allowed to play with the mask may be more tolerant of a mask themselves in the anaesthetic room. Distraction techniques can also be very effective, using books, tablets, game consoles or activities such as blowing bubbles. More recently, use of virtual reality has been used as an immersion technique in an imagined environment (distraction) or a real-world environment such as the anaesthetic room which provides familiarisation through preparation and an opportunity for rehearsal of coping strategies. Guided imagery in conjunction with relaxation is also a powerful tool that some children find helpful for reducing anxiety, whereby a child is guided to use their imagination to create positive images whilst maintaining a state of relaxation. All of these techniques depend on the development of rapport and trust.

## The Highly Anxious Child: Recognising Anxiety

Despite everyone's best efforts, there will always be the child who refuses to cooperate with anaesthesia induction. In most cases, this will be a manifestation of extreme anxiety and may be predictable in advance, enabling a sedative premedication to be given to facilitate a calm induction. Some children may demonstrate anxiety overtly by their behaviour – such as being withdrawn, tearful, uncommunicative – or they may verbally express their anxiety. Others may refuse to cooperate from the outset with any interventions – even the simpler ones such as putting on a hospital gown. In some instances, parents may report that their children who are seemingly calm in the hospital environment have been exhibiting signs of anxiety at home such as disturbed sleep, changed eating patterns or expressing high levels of concern. There is a wealth of evidence indicating that high levels of preoperative anxiety can lead not only to a more difficult anaesthetic induction but also to adverse emotional and behavioural sequelae postoperatively such as sleep disturbance, separation anxiety, enuresis and temper tantrums. Whilst these changes are usually transient, they may persist for up to 12 months. The incidence of such sequelae is greatest in preschool children but can happen at any age. Early identification of such children will enable appropriate psychological and/or sedative premedication interventions to be implemented.

## Lack of Cooperation in the Anaesthetic Room

In situations where a child refuses to allow anaesthetic induction despite preparation, behavioural techniques and/or premedication, there are a number of options available to the anaesthetist, depending on the developmental and chronological age of the child, the urgency of the planned surgery and the views of the parents/caregivers:

- Very young children who are clearly unable to rationalise or assent to the process but who can be safely held by their parents can often be rapidly induced by an inhalational technique, although it is important to have good engagement with the parents so they are able to work with the anaesthetist to facilitate this calmly and safely.
- For older children who can express their refusal, it is clearly not appropriate to carry out a forced inhalation, as this would require a degree of restraint. If the anaesthetic is being given for an elective procedure, a 'time-out' should be given to enable the distressed child to become calmer or, if the child has changed their mind, an opportunity to talk about the reasons for their decision. At this stage, options include negotiation about the mode of induction, offering sedative premedication if it has not already been given, engaging other behavioural techniques or postponing the procedure to another day to allow more time for discussion and preparation.
- Physical restraint or forced induction are acceptable only in exceptional circumstances such as when life-saving emergency surgery is being refused.

## Children with Special Needs

It is estimated that 2.5% of children in the United Kingdom have a learning disability. Compared to those without, children with a learning disability are more likely to need health care interventions and are at increased risk for developing challenging psychiatric disorders and behaviours. Communication impairments may limit the child's ability to express physical and emotional feelings, which can result in behaviours that are difficult to manage. It is common for children with a learning disability to find the process of anaesthesia particularly difficult.

A number of strategies and reasonable adjustments can be implemented to improve the experience of children with special needs, such as placing them first on the operating list to minimise waiting and fasting times, understanding their routine and keeping to this as much as possible, providing the right space on the ward for the individual child that takes into account factors such as sensitivity to light or noise and using premedication judiciously.

Working with parents before admission to proactively gather information about the child's individual requirements can help to improve the admission and anaesthetic room experience. Many children will have a health passport which provides useful information about their usual level of function, any particular physical or mental health difficulties and how they communicate. Such children often have complex health needs requiring multiple interventions, and knowledge of their previous experience(s) is useful. Advance planning with the multidisciplinary team and the family about all aspects of the proposed hospital admission is key.

Children with learning disabilities and/or language and communication disorders may use forms of augmentative and alternative communication (AAC). These are methods of communication such as gestures, picture boards, symbols and voice output communication aids. Using inclusive communication methods helps to inform, involve and empower children to make choices and decisions – for example, a child may be able to indicate 'yes' or 'no' and therefore contribute to discussions in which they can have a choice, such as options for anaesthesia induction. AAC methods can help children understand the unfamiliar procedures associated with hospital treatment, such as using a symbol system to create a timeline of a hospital visit, where each step in the process is represented by a symbol which is used as a prompt and a form of explanation (Figure 3.1).

Children with autistic spectrum disorders (ASD) may present a particular challenge in terms of communication. They often struggle with the loss of their usual, often rigid, routine and may become very agitated in noisy, open waiting areas. They may struggle to interact with strangers and resist being touched or examined. Different approaches may be necessary to help them understand what will happen and what is expected of them. In general, children with ASD respond best to communication techniques that help them to learn *how* to manage a hospital visit, such as social stories which give details of the social situation, social cues and expected behaviour. Virtual reality can also be particularly helpful for familiarisation with the anaesthetic room.

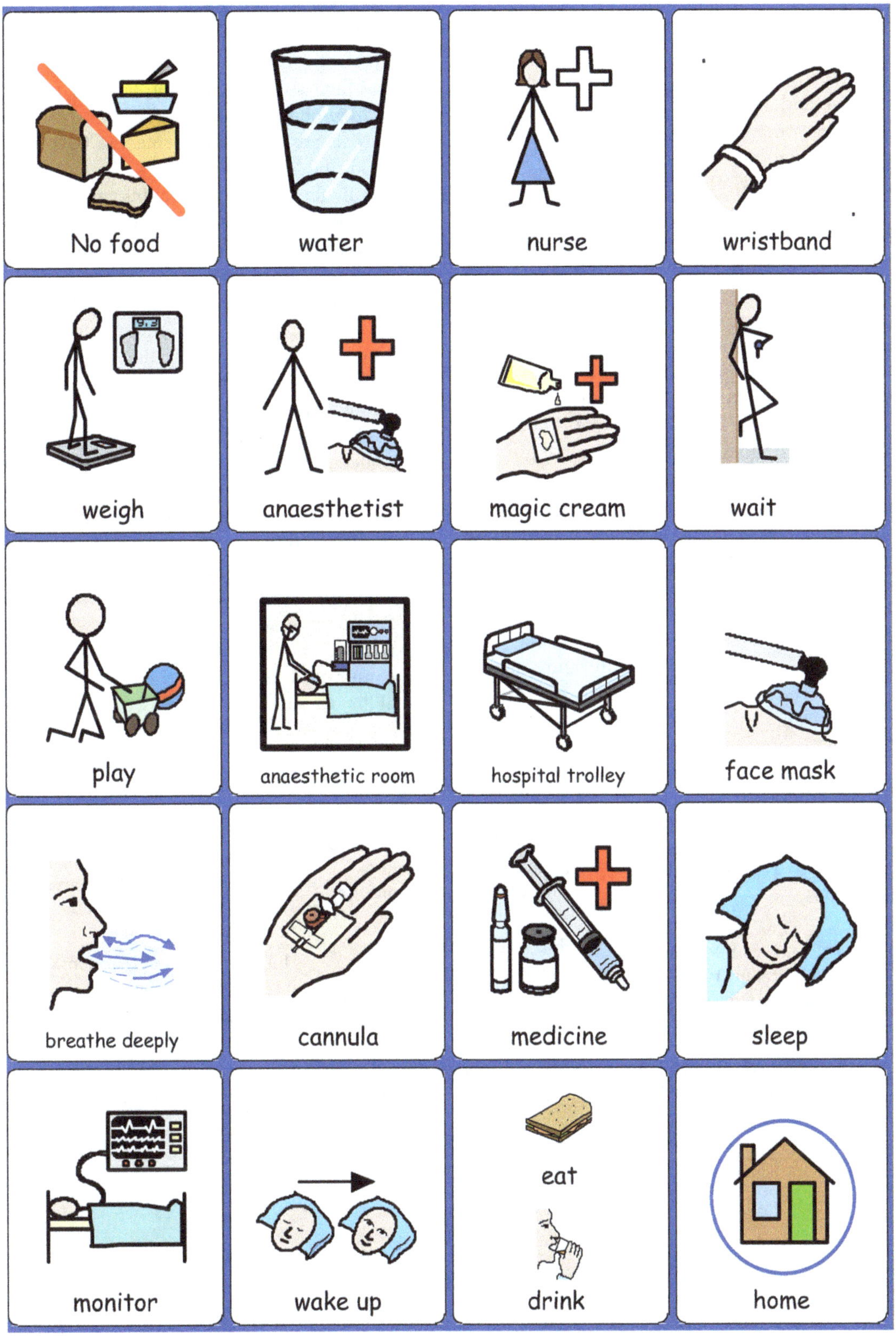
No food
water
nurse
wristband
weigh
anaesthetist
magic cream
wait
play
anaesthetic room
hospital trolley
face mask
breathe deeply
cannula
medicine
sleep
monitor
wake up
eat
drink
home

**Figure 3.1** An example of a symbol system, used to create a timeline of a hospital visit.
*Source:* Used with permission from Widgit Symbols © Widgit Software. 2002–2011 www.widgit.com.

## Finally …

So what happened to S? She was referred for specialist input from the psychologist and play specialist and was taught guided imagery and relaxation strategies. She had another preoperative visit at which the anaesthetist explained what would happen, reassuring her about pain relief, waking up after the procedure and not being on her own at any time. The psychologist also met with her mother to help her work through her own anxiety. On the day of the procedure, her mother and the play specialist accompanied her to the anaesthetic room. Her mother provided effective support, and S was able to use the rehearsed guided imagery techniques. Overall, the induction was calm and uneventful. The learning from this experience highlighted the importance of firstly not making assumptions based on a child's previous experience; secondly, the need for child-centred, age-appropriate communication, which is not only about giving information but also about exploring understanding and any concerns a child may have; and thirdly, the need to work with and engage parents to be effective sources of support to their children.

### Key Points

- Efficient communication with children and their families is central to the delivery of high-quality anaesthetic care.
- Parents are important partners in their child's health care.
- Family factors and cultural influences can significantly impact how children experience illness and their responses to medical interventions.
- Children require age and developmentally appropriate information and explanations.
- Good preoperative preparation may reduce adverse postoperative emotional and behavioural sequelae.
- Gathering information, assessing understanding and avoiding assumptions are as important as providing information.
- Behavioural and psychological techniques may help to reduce anxiety and promote cooperation.
- Children with special needs may need a flexible approach, including using augmentative and alternative communication methods to ensure their ability to interact is maximised.

## Further Reading

Cyna AM, Andrew MI, Tan SG. Communication skills for the anaesthetist. *Anaesthesia* 2009; 64:658–65.

Manyande A, Cyna AM, Yip P, Chooi C, Middleton P. Non-pharmacological interventions for assisting the induction of anaesthesia in children. *Cochrane Database of Systematic Reviews* 2015 July 14;(7):CD006447. doi: 10.1002/14651858.CD006447

Packer MJ. *Child Development: Understanding a Cultural Perspective*. Sage. 2017.

Royal College of Anaesthetists patient information series: www.youranaesthetic.info

Smith L, Callery P. Children's accounts of their pre-operative information needs. *Journal of Clinical Nursing* 2005;14:230–8.

West N, Christopher N, Stratton K, Görges M, Brown Z. Reducing preoperative anxiety with child life preparation prior to intravenous induction of anesthesia: a randomized controlled trial. *Paediatric Anaesthesia* 2020 February;30 (2):168–80. doi: 10.1111/pan.13802

Information about Makaton: www.makaton.org

Information about symbol resources: www.widgit.com

General information on AAC: www.communicationmatters.org.uk

Chapter

4

# The Law and Paediatric Anaesthesia

## Consent, Refusal, Restraint and Research

Hugo Wellesley

## Introduction

A nine-year-old boy is listed for circumcision. You preassess him on the paediatric day ward. He appears nervous but cooperative. He is tearful as you collect him from reception, but he walks to the anaesthetic room with his mother. He refuses to accept either inhalational induction or insertion of a cannula, or indeed to get on the trolley. His mother is insistent that you proceed. Would you continue, and if so, how?

This chapter aims to give you a legal and ethical framework on which to base your approach to such clinical problems. It relates to practice in the United Kingdom (UK). There are differences between the law in England and Wales and the law in either Scotland or Northern Ireland.

## Consent

### Self-Determination

Self-determination with respect to one's body is a fundamental human right. From the 1960s, the rights of those under 18 to self-determination have been progressively recognised and protected in law. Medical examinations, treatments and investigations all represent intrusion of bodily integrity and as such require consent from the child or their guardian. Only in limited circumstances can a doctor proceed without it. Consent may be expressed or implied, and it can be written, verbal or even non-verbal. For consent to be valid, the person giving consent must be capable of taking that particular decision, be acting voluntarily and be provided with enough information to make an informed decision.

Consent serves several purposes. It recognises the individual's rights of autonomy and self-determination. It demonstrates cooperation and belief in a treatment modality, which in itself is integral to the success of many treatments. It also offers some protection to the medical practitioner where disputes arise.

### Battery

Failure to obtain consent can result in an action for battery (a criminal case) or a claim of negligence (a civil lawsuit). It can also result in disciplinary action for the professional concerned from their regulatory body. An action for battery arises where the defendant has been touched and for which there has been no consent, either expressed or implied. No actual physical harm need arise, and the intentions of the perpetrator are irrelevant. An action of battery can be pursued where a doctor has proceeded in the face of a refusal to a procedure or has undertaken an additional procedure unconnected to the one for which consent was obtained. In order to avoid an action of battery, a doctor needs only to explain the 'broad nature' of the procedure that is proposed – this is a much lower standard than that required to avoid a claim of negligence, as well as the standard required of doctors by the General Medical Council (GMC).

### Negligence

In an action based on negligence, on the other hand, the plaintiff must prove causation. The plaintiff must show that the defendant proceeded without valid consent, and that this *caused* the injury for which they are seeking damages. The court must be satisfied that the patient would not have given their consent had they been properly informed of what was to be done. Where a patient has consented to a procedure but the doctor failed to mention a complication that the patient subsequently suffered, there is a basis for a claim in negligence. The negligence refers to the failure to inform rather than the way in which the procedure was performed.

## Minors 16–18 Years

Anyone under the age of 18 is legally a minor; however, the rules regarding consent differ between those who are under 16 and those who are 16 or 17 years old. Sixteen- and 17-year-olds are presumed to be competent. This is referred to as the presumptive test of competence and is defined by the Family Law Reform Act 1969 in England and Wales or the Age of Legal Capacity (Scotland) Act 1991. For those who are felt might not be competent, the onus is on the treating doctor to demonstrate that they are not competent, for which there is a two-stage test, as laid out in the Mental Capacity Act 2005:

(1) Does the patient have a disturbance in the functioning of the mind or brain?
(2) Is the patient unable to understand the information relevant to the decision, retain that information and then use or weigh that information to make a decision at the particular time that it needs to be made?

The child must be provided with all the support they need to maximise their ability to fulfil the requirements of capacity; if it is decided that the child lacks capacity, then someone with parental responsibility can give consent for the child.

## Minors under 16 Years: Gillick Competence

Below the age of 16 years, a minor can give valid consent themselves if they demonstrate Gillick competence. This test of competence is derived from the case of *Gillick v West Norfolk & Wisbech AHA* (1985) and requires the child to be able to demonstrate competence (whereas it should be presumed for the 16- and 17-year-olds). The Gillick case set a precedent that permitted children of sufficient maturity to seek contraceptive advice without the knowledge of their parents but was subsequently applied more generally to allow children who fulfilled the criteria to consent to other forms of medical treatment. The age at which Gillick competence can be demonstrated will depend on the child and the complexity of the treatment or procedure. Where a Gillick-competent child requests non-disclosure to their parents, their confidentiality must be respected, although it is good practice to encourage children to involve their parents.

In order to demonstrate Gillick competence, the child should understand that there is a choice to be made and demonstrate a willingness to make it. The child should be able to understand the nature of the proposed treatment and the risks involved. They should appreciate what the effects of non-treatment might be. It is important that the child can retain the information long enough to come to a decision.

## Assent to Treatment

The term 'assent' is sometimes used to describe an agreement by the child to participate with a degree of explanation and understanding appropriate to their age and development but falling short of fully valid consent. It is a term borrowed from the United States and does not have a legal basis in the United Kingdom but is nevertheless sometimes used to refer to a child's willingness to participate. It does not replace the need for full consent from someone who is able to give it.

## Parental Responsibility

Where the child does not have the capacity to give consent, it must be sought from someone with parental responsibility (PR). In most situations, the law only requires consent from one person with PR; however, it is good practice to involve all relevant parties. One important exception is for circumcision, where consent from everyone with PR is required (usually this means both parents). As a rule, you should be very wary of proceeding with any treatment if you are aware that someone with PR actually objects.

The following people have parental responsibility:

- The child's mother
- The child's father, if married to the mother at the time of conception (for births registered in Scotland) or at the time of birth (in the rest of the United Kingdom)
- If unmarried at conception or birth, the child's father can obtain PR by one of the following means:
  - If the couple subsequently marry
  - By being recorded on the child's birth certificate: for all children in Northern Ireland, and for children registered after 1 December 2003 in England and Wales, or after 4 May 2006 in Scotland (this can be the date of the original registration or a subsequent re-registration). For children

born outside the United Kingdom, the rules of the country of residence apply.
  - By making a parental responsibility agreement with the mother (this must be registered with a court)
  - By court order
- Adoptive parents
- A court-appointed guardian
- A testamentary guardian (i.e. one appointed in a person's will) if no one with PR survives the testator
- A person awarded a residence order
- A local authority designated in a care order (except where the child is being 'accommodated' or in 'voluntary care' – see Section 20 of the Children Act)
- A person or authority holding an emergency protection order for that child

Since 2009, both parents, regardless of gender, can have their names on the birth certificate, giving them both parental rights. Parents do not lose PR if they divorce, even if a parent has no contact with the child. Grandparents, stepparents, and foster parents do not have parental responsibility unless it has been specifically arranged through a parental responsibility agreement (registered with the court) or a court order. For children born under surrogacy arrangements, the surrogate mother has PR (along with her husband, if she is married) until the intended parents either adopt the child or obtain a parental order from a court (under the Human Fertilisation and Embryology Act 1990).

Parents have parental responsibility in order to give them the legal power to make decisions to safeguard and promote their child's health, welfare and development. Parental rights only exist to enable them to fulfil their responsibilities. These rights can therefore be challenged if it is felt that the parents are not acting to promote their child's interests.

It may be that those with PR do not themselves have the capacity to consent on behalf of the child owing to mental illness or special needs, in which case legal advice should be sought.

## Emergency Treatment

In the situation where no one is able to give valid consent, it is lawful to provide emergency treatment in the absence of consent on the basis that it is in the child's best interests. Assessment of best interests should be based on the physical, emotional, social, cultural and psychological needs of the individual. The views of and the effect on other family members may need to be considered. Evidence of the effectiveness of the proposed treatment, risks of treatment and of delaying or withholding treatment must be taken into account. Where possible, treatments that maximise the patient's future choices should be offered so the child can exercise their autonomy when they do attain competence. It is not necessarily the case that any treatment that prolongs life is in a child's best interests.

## Refusal of Treatment

Although it might seem logical that someone who is competent to consent to treatment should also be competent to refuse treatment, this will not always be the case. Treatment is only proposed where it is felt to be in a child's best interest, so refusal of that treatment will usually be considered to be against their best interests. A refusal therefore requires a greater level of understanding, and there remain circumstances in which a decision by a competent minor can be overridden if it is in their best interests.

A court clearly can do this. There are also judgements that state that parents can do this; however, these predate the introduction of the Human Rights Act 1998, and there is a risk that accepting the consent of a parent in the face of a competent child's refusal could be found to have breached the child's rights. It has therefore been recommended by the Department of Health that 'it would be prudent to obtain a court declaration or decision if faced with a competent child or young person who is refusing treatment, to determine if it is lawful to treat the child'. The Mental Capacity Act 2005 Code of Practice also recommends a similar approach in the case of a disagreement between a 16- or 17-year-old with capacity who is refusing treatment to which a parent wants to consent.

It could be argued that children require a greater level of understanding than is asked of adults. The case of *Re E* in 1990 demonstrates this point. The patient was 15 years old and a Jehovah's Witness, as were his parents. He was suffering from leukaemia. The case arose when he and his parents refused a treatment regimen that offered a high chance of cure but involved blood transfusions, in favour of a less successful treatment avoiding the use of blood products. Although impressed with his level of understanding and conviction to his faith, the judge declared that he did not adequately appreciate the pain and distress that would arise nor the effect on his family. Moreover, he felt the details were too distressing to even contemplate telling the boy. The court was unwilling to arm him with the information to allow him to make an informed choice. The ruling resulted in the boy receiving blood transfusions as part of his treatment. He continued to voice his objection until he reached adulthood, when he refused further blood transfusions and died.

## Advance Directives, Living Wills

Although advanced care planning is encouraged for children with life-limiting illnesses, advance directives and living wills are not legally binding.

## Obtaining Consent

The responsibility for seeking a patient's consent lies with the doctor undertaking the procedure. This task can be delegated to someone else provided that individual is suitably trained and qualified and has sufficient knowledge of the proposed procedure.

## Legal and Professional Standards

The most pertinent legal case in this area is *Montgomery vs Lanarkshire Health Board* [2015] UKSC 11. This involved a woman (Mrs Montgomery) who had gestational diabetes and her son who had a very difficult vaginal delivery complicated by shoulder dystocia, which resulted in his developing a brachial plexus injury and severe cerebral palsy. The Supreme Court found that she had not been adequately informed of the risks of a vaginal delivery and had not been offered a caesarean section as an alternative. The court stated that a doctor should warn of all 'material risks'. It went on to define these as the risks to which a 'reasonable person in the patient's position would be likely to attach significance' and also the risks to which the 'doctor is or should reasonably be aware that the particular patient would attach significance'.

The GMC publishes guidance on consent which all doctors are professionally bound to follow. These are also cited in legal judgements and used to assess doctors' actions, so in effect they also become legally binding. Interestingly, the GMC intervened in the *Montgomery* case on behalf of Mrs Montgomery.

These guidelines were updated in 2020 and apply to consent for treating children as well as adults. They should be read in conjunction with the GMC's *0–18 Years: Guidance for All Doctors*. They emphasise the importance of a 'meaningful dialogue' with patients rather than just giving them lists of benefits and risks. The guidance states that the following information should be shared with patients:

- Recognised risks of harm that you believe anyone in the patient's position would want to know
- The effect of the patient's individual clinical circumstances on the probability of a benefit or harm occurring
- Risks of harm and potential benefits that the patient would consider significant for any reason
- Any risk of serious harm, however unlikely it is to occur
- Expected harms, including common side effects, and what to do if they occur

There is therefore a high degree of agreement between the legal standard as described in *Montgomery* and the GMC's standards.

## Documentation of Consent

There is no legal requirement for a signed consent form except for living organ donation and fertility treatment. A signed consent form serves as a record that a discussion took place, but it is not proof of valid consent. Where a competent child has given consent, their signature alone is sufficient. When obtaining consent for anaesthesia, this can be verbal, but you should always carefully document the consent and the discussions that have informed it.

The question of who takes written consent for radiological investigations under general anaesthesia has been the subject of debate. It has been argued that the risk associated with anaesthesia is greater than the risk of the investigation; however, the risk of anaesthesia can only be taken into context when one understands how the information the scan provides will help the child, what the alternatives to having that investigation are and the implications of not having the scan. These can only be imparted by the clinician or team requesting the test.

## Court Orders

If agreement between a child, their parents and the medical team cannot be reached within a reasonable time period, then it may be necessary to ask the court to intervene. This typically happens in cases involving withdrawal of life-sustaining treatment. Second opinions should be sought in situations involving serious disagreement, and increasingly there is a move to try formal mediation before referral to the court. The courts have the power to consent to treatment on behalf of a minor when they consider that treatment to be in the child's best interests. However, no child, parent or court has the power to force a doctor to perform a procedure that the doctor does not feel is clinically justified.

Cases can also be referred to the court when parents disagree amongst themselves about what to do, particularly for certain procedures such as organ donation, sterilisation or circumcision.

# Restraint

The Department of Health defines restraint as 'the positive application of force with the intention of overpowering the child'. Restraint implies a restriction of liberty or freedom of movement, and so constitutes a breach of an individual's autonomy. Restraint also breaches the Human Rights Act Articles 3, 5 and 9 and therefore needs to be justified. Justification for restraint in limited circumstances can be argued on the principles of beneficence and non-maleficence, but it needs to be in the overall best interests of the child.

## Restraint in Anaesthesia Practice

It is common for a child to demonstrate varying degrees of resistance to aspects of medical management. The causes may be many and include a wariness of strangers, unfamiliar settings, anxiety, frustration, phobia or a genuine refusal. Management in the setting of surgery and anaesthesia is made more difficult because the anaesthetist will often not have a pre-existing relationship with the child, preoperative fasting results in distress to the child and the process can involve separation from their parents. Decisions as to whether to proceed often have to be made in a very narrow time frame. It is important to try to interpret the child's behaviour in light of their developmental age. In addition to the views of the child, consideration must also be given to the urgency of the procedure, the presence of valid consent from someone with parental responsibility and the consequences of not proceeding or delaying treatment. Proceeding with treatment against the child's wishes may be legal but may require either physical and/or pharmacological restraint and may have unwanted psychological sequelae, even if it is done as considerately as possible. This risk must be taken into account when assessing whether or not the procedure is still in the child's best interests.

Using restraint or force to impose a treatment on an unwilling patient is in practice very difficult and fortunately rarely necessary. With sufficient time and explanation, most children will accept and cooperate with treatment. Most of the medical literature regarding restraint appears in relation to psychiatry and some articles relating to dentistry for those with special needs.

The Royal College of Nursing has guidance on the appropriate use of restraint. This guidance uses the term 'clinical holding', which is defined as the use of limited force to hold a child still to enable a health care procedure. According to these guidelines, it should be clear who is deciding what is in the child's best interests, and there should be an effective mechanism for staff who disagree to be heard. Where clinical holding might be required, staff should:

- Carefully consider whether the procedure is really necessary and explore alternatives to holding
- Anticipate and prevent the need for holding by giving the child information, encouragement, distraction, analgesia and, if necessary, sedation
- Obtain the child's express agreement in all but the very youngest children and, for any procedure which is not a true emergency, seek parental consent
- Pause prior to a procedure to discuss with the child and their parents what will happen and what people's roles will be
- Ensure that any holding that is used is the least restrictive option required and is used for the minimum amount of time

- Ensure parental presence and involvement if they wish to be present and involved
- Explain parents' roles in supporting their child and provide support for them during and after the procedure
- Comfort the child where it hasn't been possible to obtain their agreement, and explain clearly why it was necessary to hold them still
- Ensure clear documentation afterwards

The degree of force used should not be excessive and should be in proportion to the perceived benefit. Inappropriate use of restraint may result in criminal charges, action in civil law or prosecution under health and safety legislation.

## Research in Children

Society as a whole benefits from quality research. However, the extent to which individuals should be subjected to risks for the good of others, especially where those individuals lack the ability to consent, is a difficult ethical dilemma. The Nuremberg Code of 1947 suggests that those who cannot express their views should be excluded from research. There is a strong argument, however, that excluding children from research is unjust because it breaches their right to the best attainable health care. Therapeutic research can be in a child's best interests, but non-therapeutic research is harder to justify. However, if the purpose of research is ultimately to improve diagnosis and treatment of patients, then not to allow children to participate in research is to deny the paediatric population advances in clinical management.

## Professional Guidance for Research Involving Children

The Royal College of Paediatrics and Child Health (RCPCH) has guidance for research involving children. It recognises that many diseases are unique to children, and that response to treatment differs from that in adults, making research involving children vital. Children should, therefore, 'be offered the opportunity to participate in research, and have their care *assured by research*'. It also states that research that is of 'no benefit to that child (non-therapeutic research) is not necessarily either unethical or illegal'.

All trials must be approved by a research ethics committee, and studies involving particularly vulnerable groups (such as children with life-threatening illnesses) should be reviewed by a research ethics committee with appropriate knowledge and experience. As always, voluntary informed consent is essential, and it must be emphasised to the patient and family that they are free to withdraw at any time without care being affected. When consent has been obtained from the parents, the agreement of school-age children should also be requested by researchers. A parent cannot override a Gillick-competent child's refusal to consent for non-therapeutic research.

## Levels of Risk

It is generally accepted that a lower degree of risk is acceptable for children subjected to research compared with adults. There is little consensus, however, as to how to define acceptable risk.

Minimal risk describes procedures such as non-invasive urine sampling or using blood or tissue taken as part of management of a clinical condition.

Low risk describes procedures that cause brief pain, emotional distress or small bruises such as blood sampling. Low-risk procedures are unlikely to be considered acceptable if there is no benefit to the child. However, if the child shows altruism and on careful explanation is willing to accept this discomfort, then it may be reasonable to proceed.

High-risk invasive procedures may only be justifiable for research when the procedure is part of diagnosis or treatment intended to benefit the child subject.

## Clinical Scenario

Returning to the opening clinical example of the nine-year-old boy listed for circumcision, one approach would be to remove the child from the stressful environment or alternatively remove all the unnecessary staff from the room so it appears less threatening. Ascertain whether the child is anxious about a particular aspect of the procedure, such as insertion of the cannula, or fundamentally does not want the operation. It can be very helpful to involve the surgeon who may already have a rapport with the child from a previous clinic appointment. It is also an opportunity to establish with the child how strong the indication for surgery is. It may be that his symptoms have subsided and that he is rightfully questioning the need for surgery. If he is fearful of a particular element of the procedure but in agreement with the need for surgery, returning to the ward for an anxiolytic premedication might be an acceptable way to proceed. An alternative to this would be to postpone surgery to allow a play therapist or clinical psychologist to work with the child. This would have the advantage of hopefully arming the child with coping strategies to deal with similar stressful situations in the future. If the child consistently disagrees with there being a need for surgery, then restraint, whether it be chemical or physical, is inappropriate and the child should be reviewed in clinic.

### Key Points

- A child below the age of 16 can give consent if they demonstrate Gillick competence.
- Once a child is 16, they should be presumed to be competent to consent to medical treatment.
- Discussions with patients and families should include those risks and benefits that anyone in their position would want to know and also those risks and benefits you are able to ascertain that they would consider significant for any reason.
- The use of restraint should be avoided if possible and, where it is used, needs to be justified and in the child's best interests.
- Research involving children is vital but poses unique ethical challenges. Given the right conditions, both therapeutic and non-therapeutic research can be ethical and legal.

## Further Reading

Association of Paediatric Anaesthetists of Great Britain and Ireland. APA Hot Topic 18: Should the anaesthetist obtain consent when a child undergoes an MRI scan? Available at: www.apagbi.org.uk/professionals/education-and-training/apa-hot-topics. Accessed 18 May 2021

British Medical Association (BMA). *Consent, Rights and Choices in Healthcare for Children and Young People*. BMA Books. 2001

BMA. *Parental Responsibility*. BMA. 2008

General Medical Council (GMC). *0–18 Years: Guidance for All Doctors*. GMC. 2018.

GMC. *Decision Making and Consent*. GMC. 2020.

Modi N, Vohra J, Preston J. Guidance on clinical research involving infants, children and young people: an update for researchers and research ethics committees. *Archives of Disease in Childhood* 2014; 99:887–91.

Royal College of Nursing. *Restrictive Physical Interventions and the Clinical Holding of Children and Young People*. RCN. 2019

Yentis S, Hartle A, Barker I, et al. AAGBI: Consent for anaesthesia. *Anaesthesia* 2017; 72:93–105.

Chapter 5

# Safeguarding Children and Its Implications for the Anaesthetist

Pascale du Pré

Child protection and safeguarding children are integral to good medical practice.

Safeguarding is a broad concept and includes all actions that are taken to promote the welfare of children and protect them from harm. Safeguarding means:

- Protecting children from abuse and maltreatment
- Preventing harm to children's health or development
- Ensuring children grow up with the provision of safe and effective care
- Taking action to enable all children and young people to have the best outcomes

Child protection is part of the safeguarding process. It focuses on protecting individual children identified as suffering or likely to suffer significant harm. This includes child protection procedures which detail how to respond to concerns about a child.

## Role of the Anaesthetist

Child maltreatment/abuse is not an uncommon problem. All National Health Service (NHS) and independent hospitals treating children should have safeguarding and child protection strategies in place. They must also ensure that all staff are adequately trained to identify the child at risk and deal with the situation appropriately. Anaesthetists need to be trained to a level commensurate with their level of responsibility and involvement with children. Anaesthetists should be aware of both national and local child protection policies:

- To act in the best interests of the child, which are always paramount
- To be aware of the child's rights to be protected
- To respect the rights of the child to confidentiality
- To contact a senior paediatrician for explicit advice or support when required (on-call consultant paediatrician, named or designated doctor/nurse)
- Where appropriate, to contribute to reports describing child protection/safeguarding concerns to relevant professionals, including social care
- To be aware of local child protection mechanisms
- To clearly document findings in association with paediatric colleagues
- To be aware of the rights of those with parental responsibility

In the United Kingdom, all practitioners should follow the principles of the Children Acts 1989 and 2004 and the 2014 Children and Families Act. These state that the welfare of children is paramount and that they are generally best looked after within their families, with their parents playing a full part in their lives, unless compulsory intervention in family life is necessary.

In this chapter, a child is defined as anyone who has not yet reached their 18th birthday.

The fact that an individual has reached 16 years of age, is living independently or is in further education, is a member of the armed forces or is in hospital or in custody does not change their status or entitlements to services or protection. 'Children', therefore, means 'children and young people' throughout this chapter. It's important to recognise that everyone who comes into contact with children and families has a role to play.

Anaesthetists need to be fully aware of safeguarding processes. Some examples where they may be involved include:

- When a baby or child is admitted as an emergency for resuscitation or surgery and the cause of the presenting illness is unclear, e.g. severe head injury
- When a baby or child is admitted for investigation of safeguarding concerns, such as when a child protection plan is in place

- When the baby or child is admitted for urgent or elective surgery and coincidental suspicious signs are noted that may be the result of abuse or neglect
- When a child, parent or carer discloses concerns that prompt a suspicion that there may be maltreatment or abuse within a family. In practice this is rarely reported to the anaesthetist but may be to another member of the theatre team so knowledge how to deal with this is important.

Growing numbers of young people are presenting to the acute hospital setting with self-harm and self-poisoning. Repeat attendances are common and a challenge. It is important to consider and discuss children with perplexing presentations or fabricated or induced illness with colleagues within the multi-disciplinary team. Consideration should be given to the drivers for childhood distress as these are often linked with deprivation, abuse, neglect, bullying or other adverse childhood experiences. Safeguarding concerns should be considered and discussed, if present, and responded to appropriately. The focus must be on the potential harm to the child rather than the perceived severity or type of caregiver motivations, actions and behaviours. In particular, one should always bear in mind that abuse does not need to be intentional on the part of the caregiver for it to constitute maltreatment.

## High-Risk Groups

There are particular high-risk groups of children who are more vulnerable to abuse and neglect. This can be by nature of their socioeconomic, physical or mental health or because of pre-existing disability that makes them more vulnerable to all types of maltreatment. Child maltreatment occurs in all sectors of society and in all age groups.

It is worth considering the following high-risk groups in particular. These include children and young people who are:

- Looked after children (LAC)
- Refugee and unaccompanied children
- Children and young people with physical or intellectual disability

## Looked after Children (LAC)

The Royal College of Paediatrics and Child Health reports that more than 93,000 children in the United Kingdom are in care, 70,000 in England. This term typically denotes children whose welfare is the responsibility of the state and therefore generally directly involves social care. Most are taken into care over fears of abuse or neglect. They are vulnerable to health inequalities and exhibit significantly higher rates of mental health issues, emotional disorders (anxiety and depression), hyperactivity and autistic spectrum disorder conditions.

This diverse group includes children under foster care and those in residential homes, though exact definitions vary between the four nations. It also includes unaccompanied asylum seekers and those accommodated compulsorily for their own protection or those around them (e.g. under the criminal justice system). Young people who have been under the care of the local authority for the period of 13 weeks that spans their 16th birthday are termed 'care leavers' and are also at higher risk of maltreatment.

## What Is 'Abuse'?

Somebody may abuse or neglect a child by inflicting harm or by failing to act to prevent harm. Children may be abused by an adult or adults or another child or children. All are forms of maltreatment.

The broad types of maltreatment include physical, emotional and sexual abuse as well as neglect. It is not uncommon for several forms of maltreatment to coexist. Children may be vulnerable to neglect and abuse or exploitation from within their family and from individuals they come across in their day-to-day lives. Additional threats can include exploitation by criminal gangs and organised crime groups, trafficking, online abuse, sexual exploitation, female genital mutilation and the influences of extremism leading to radicalisation.

## Physical Abuse

This form of abuse may involve hitting, shaking, throwing, poisoning, burning or scalding, drowning, suffocating or otherwise causing physical harm to a child. Physical harm may also be caused when a parent or carer fabricates the symptoms of, or deliberately induces, illness in a child.

## Emotional Abuse

Working Together to Safeguard Children 2015 defines emotional abuse as the persistent emotional maltreatment of a child such as to cause severe and persistent adverse effects on the child's emotional development. It may involve conveying to a child that they are worthless or unloved, inadequate, or valued only insofar as they meet the needs of another person. It may include not giving the child opportunities to express their views, deliberately silencing them or 'making fun' of what they say or how they communicate. It may feature age or developmentally inappropriate expectations being imposed on children. It may involve seeing or hearing the ill-treatment of another. It may involve serious bullying (including cyber bullying) causing children frequently to feel frightened or in danger or the exploitation or corruption of children. Some level of emotional abuse is involved in all types of maltreatment of a child, though it may occur in isolation.

## Online Abuse

Online abuse is any type of abuse that happens on the internet. It can happen across any device that's connected to the web, such as computers, tablets and mobile phones. It can happen anywhere online, including social media, text messages and messaging apps, emails, online chats, online gaming and live-streaming sites.

Children can be at risk of online abuse from people they know or from strangers. It might be part of other abuse which is taking place offline, like bullying or grooming. Or the abuse might only happen online.

## Sexual Abuse

Involves forcing or enticing a child or young person to take part in sexual activities, not necessarily involving a high level of violence, whether or not the child is aware of what is happening. The activities may involve physical contact, including assault by penetration (for example, rape or oral sex) or non-penetrative acts such as masturbation, kissing, rubbing and touching the outside of clothing. They may also include non-contact activities, such as involving children in looking at or in the production of sexual images, watching sexual activities, encouraging children to behave in sexually inappropriate ways or grooming a child in preparation for abuse. Sexual abuse is not solely perpetrated by adult males. Women can also commit acts of sexual abuse, as can other children.

## Grooming

Grooming is when someone builds an emotional connection with a child to gain their trust for the purposes of sexual abuse, sexual exploitation or trafficking. Children and young people can be groomed online or face to face, by a stranger or by someone they know – for example a family member, friend or professional.

## Child Sexual Exploitation

Child sexual exploitation is a form of child sexual abuse. It occurs where an individual or group takes advantage of an imbalance of power to coerce, manipulate or deceive a child or young person under the age of 18 into sexual activity either in exchange for something the victim needs or wants and/or for the financial advantage or increased status of the perpetrator or facilitator. The victim may have been sexually exploited even if the sexual activity appears consensual. Child sexual exploitation does not always involve physical contact.

## Female Genital Mutilation (FGM)

The World Health Organisation (WHO) defines FGM as 'all procedures that involve partial or total removal of the external female genitalia, or other injury to the female genital organs for non-medical reasons'. FGM is recognised internationally as a violation of the human rights of girls and women. It is nearly always carried out on minors and is a violation of the rights of children. FGM has been illegal in the United Kingdom since 1985. In 2003 it also became illegal to take a British national or permanent resident overseas for FGM procedures to be carried out, or to help someone trying to do this. A mandatory reporting duty for FGM came into force on 31 October 2015 and requires regulated health and social care professionals and teachers to report to the police known cases of FGM in those under 18. Most professionals will only visually identify FGM as a secondary result of undertaking another action, when they are informed by a girl under 18 that an act of FGM has been carried out on her, or if they observe physical signs which appear to show that an act of FGM has been carried out on a girl under 18 and they have no reason to believe that the act was necessary for the girl's physical or mental health or for purposes connected with labour or birth.

## Neglect

Neglect has been defined in Working Together to Safeguard Children 2015 as 'the persistent failure to meet a child's basic physical and/or psychological needs, likely to result in the serious impairment of the child's health or development'. Neglect may occur during pregnancy as a result of maternal substance abuse. Once a child is born, neglect may involve a parent or carer failing to:

- Provide adequate food, clothing and shelter (including exclusion from home or abandonment)
- Protect a child from physical and emotional harm or danger
- Ensure adequate supervision (including the use of inadequate caregivers)
- Ensure access to appropriate medical care or treatment

It may also include neglect of, or unresponsiveness to, a child's basic emotional needs.

## Radicalisation

Radicalisation is the process through which a person comes to support or be involved in extremist beliefs or behaviour. This goes beyond terrorism, and those who seek to promote these beliefs target the vulnerable – including the young – by seeking to sow division between communities on the basis of race, faith or denomination. They may justify discrimination towards women and girls, persuade others that minorities are inferior or argue against the primacy of democracy and the rule of law in our society.

Whatever the form of abuse or neglect, practitioners should put the needs of children first when determining what action to take.

## Child Trafficking

Child trafficking is defined by the United Nations as the 'recruitment, transportation, transfer, harbouring or receipt' of a child for the purpose of exploitation. In adults, the definition of trafficking also requires the threat or use of force or other forms of coercion. Child trafficking recognises that a child cannot give informed consent to their own exploitation, so protection applies even if a child agrees to travel or complies with their predicament.

## What to Do When Concerns Arise

Anaesthetists may encounter abused children during resuscitation or the care of a sick or injured child, during routine perioperative care, preoperative assessment or (rarely) in the context of an ongoing consultation such as might occur in a pain clinic. The Royal College of Anaesthetists (RCoA), the Association of Paediatric Anaesthetists of Great Britain and Ireland (APAGBI) and the Royal College of Paediatrics and Child Health (RCPCH) have developed a flowchart to guide anaesthetists in the operating theatre if they have child protection concerns (Figure 5.1).

## The Referral Process

Anaesthetic trainees and staff or associate specialist anaesthetists are generally advised to discuss safeguarding matters initially with a consultant anaesthetic colleague. Thereafter, it may be necessary to involve a senior paediatrician for advice or support or, when available, with the nominated or designated safeguarding consultant or nominated senior nurse. The emphasis should be on good communication using non-threatening terms. Unless there is risk of immediate, serious harm to the child's health or life, caregivers can be informed about the need to share information between different professionals involved in the child's life. Choice of language is important – it is helpful to think and speak about this in terms of getting a 'second opinion'.

The views of the child or young person should always be sought where possible. The anaesthetist will rarely make detailed follow-up enquiries, but anyone working with children should see and speak to the child, listen to what they say and take their views seriously. The role of the child health professional is to work with children and their families collaboratively when deciding how to support their needs. Special provision such as the use of play therapists or interpreters should be put in place to support conversations with children who have communication difficulties, unaccompanied children, refugees and those children who are victims of modern slavery and/or trafficking, where language difficulties may add additional complexities.

Anyone who has concerns about a child's welfare can make a referral to the local authority children's social care and should do so promptly if there is a concern that the child is suffering

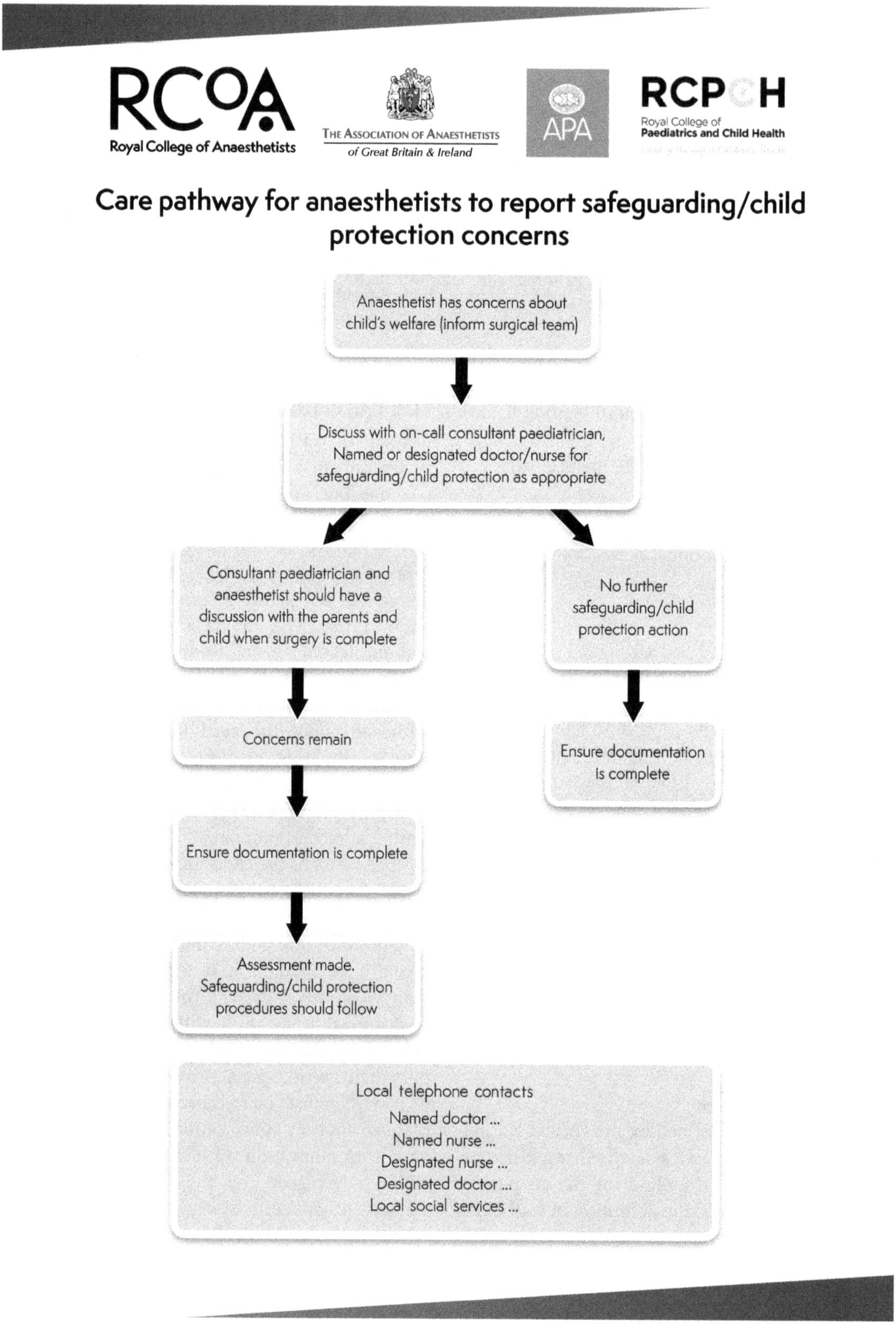


**Figure 5.1** Flowchart explaining what should be done to safeguard children in the operating theatre.
*Source*: Produced jointly by the RCoA, RCPC and APA in 2007 and updated in 2014.

significant harm or is likely to do so. For anaesthetists, this will generally be in association with paediatric colleagues. Practitioners who make a referral should always follow up their concerns if they are not satisfied with the response.

A comprehensive record of any discussions held should be kept throughout, including decisions made, in line with standard safeguarding practice. Anaesthetists may be asked to add a note if they witnessed particular behaviours or had conversations that revealed abuse. In all instances, it is important to stick with fact and not stray into 'opinion'. This will include the circumstances surrounding the initial identification or disclosure of abuse and details of any safeguarding actions that were taken. The organisation's designated safeguarding lead must be updated as appropriate.

If practitioners have concerns that a child may be a potential victim of modern slavery or human trafficking, then a referral should be made to the National Referral Mechanism, as soon as possible.

In England, a local authority social worker should acknowledge receipt to the referrer within *one working day* of a referral being received and *make a decision* about next steps and the type of response required. This will include determining whether:

- The child requires immediate protection and urgent action is required
- The child is in need and should be assessed under Section 17 of the Children Act 1989
- There is reasonable cause to suspect that the child is suffering or likely to suffer significant harm, and whether enquiries must be made and the child assessed under Section 47 of the Children Act 1989
- Any services are required by the child and family and what type of services
- Further specialist assessments are required to help the local authority to decide what further action to take
- To see the child as soon as possible if the decision is made that the referral requires further assessment

Similar but not identical processes are in place in the four UK nations (see 'Further Reading').

## When a Child Dies

In England, investigation of all child deaths follows a standardised path that includes immediate decision-making and notifications and a decision as to whether there is a need for a joint agency response. A designated rapid response team gathers information for unexpected deaths or, when otherwise required, to assist investigation and information gathering. A joint meeting will be convened at which professionals involved in the care of the child will be invited to attend.

These processes are described by the NHS England Child Death Review Statutory and Operational Guidance (2018) and are to be followed after the death of any child under the age of 18 who normally resides in England. This includes the death of any live born baby where a death certificate has been issued, but does not include stillbirths, late fetal loss or terminations of pregnancy. It builds on the statutory requirements set out in Working Together to Safeguard Children (2018) and clarifies how individual professionals and organisations across all sectors involved in the child death review should contribute to reviews. The process is designed to capture the expertise of professionals who were involved in the care of the child through the systematic collection of data to inform local and national learning via the Child Death Overview Process (CDOP) and National Child Mortality Database (NCMD). Child death review meetings need to be flexible and proportionate but must be held for all child deaths, not just unexpected deaths.

A set of notifications need to be made to the Child Death Overview Panel (CDOP) via a series of Notification Forms. A standardised dataset is collected for all children who die for the purposes of the NHS England National Child Mortality Database (NCMD).

## Joint Agency Response (JAR)

This is multi-agency response which will be triggered if the death is due to external causes, when the death is sudden and there is no immediate apparent cause, when the death occurs in custody, where initial circumstances raise suspicions that the death may not have been natural and in the case of stillbirths where no health professional was in attendance.

A Joint Agency Response meeting is held within 48 hours of the death. A JAR should also be triggered if a child is brought into hospital in a moribund state, successfully resuscitated but then expected to die. This is a common scenario in paediatric intensive care units, where the JAR should be initiated at the point of presentation in order to enable an accurate history of events to be taken, and if necessary so that a scene of collapse visit takes place.

## Child Death Review Meeting (CDRM)

The Child Death Review Meeting is a multi-professional meeting where all matters relating to an individual child's death are discussed by professionals directly involved in the care of that child during life. The meeting is held within the hospital where the child died and chaired by a paediatrician with designated time in their job plan. The meeting should take place within three months of the child's death or as soon as results of investigations are available, for example postmortem examination. The guidance advocates that attempts are made to engage with other professionals, for example the paramedic, the local paediatrician and the local team, which might include an anaesthetist if relevant. In every case, an analysis form is completed and sent to the relevant child death overview panel.

The aim of the child death review process is to put bereaved families at the centre of the review process. A key worker is allocated to the family to make sure their questions are brought to the CDRM and so that their questions can be answered sensitively. This role is in addition to usual bereavement support services. The key worker is nominated by the lead paediatrician to act as the named point of contact throughout the process of the child death review.

## Child Death Overview Panel Meeting (CDOP)

The statutory responsibilities of the CDOP are set out in Working Together to Safeguard Children (2018). The panel is required to conduct an anonymised secondary review of each child death. Meetings are attended by senior representatives across health, police, social services and other agencies as well as paediatricians.

The aim of the CDOP review is to:

- Identify the cause of death
- Provide support to families. Families should have an identified key worker to act as named point of contact throughout the process of the child death review.
- Identify modifiable/contributory factors
- Ensure statutory obligations are met
- Learn lessons that can be applied to promote the health and well-being of other children.

NHS England has published guidance for the bereaved 'When A Child Dies' (2007) as a guide for parents and carers, setting out the steps that follow the death of a child.

## Medical Examiner

A new medical examiner system has been rolled out across England and Wales to provide greater scrutiny of deaths.

Medical examiners are senior medical doctors who are contracted for a number of sessions a week to undertake medical examiner duties outside of their usual clinical duties. They are trained in the legal and clinical elements of death certification processes.

The national network of medical examiners was recommended by the Shipman Inquiry 2002–2005, the Mid-Staffordshire NHS Foundation Trust Public Enquiry 2013 and the Report of the Morecambe Bay Investigation 2015. In October 2017, Lord O'Shaughnessy, Parliamentary Under Secretary of State for Health, announced that a national system of medical examiners would be introduced in April 2019.

The purpose of the medical examiner system is to:

- Provide greater safeguards for the public by ensuring proper scrutiny of all non-coronial deaths
- Ensure the appropriate direction of deaths to the coroner
- Provide a better service for the bereaved and an opportunity for them to raise any concerns to a doctor not involved in the care of the deceased
- Improve the quality of death certification
- Improve the quality of mortality data

The system will also offer a point of contact for bereaved families to raise concerns about the care provided prior to the death of a loved one.

**Key Points**

When considering safeguarding in children it is essential:

- To act in the best interests of the child, which are always paramount

- To be aware of the child's rights to be protected
- To respect the rights of the child to confidentiality
- To contact a paediatrician with experience of child protection for advice (on-call paediatrician for child protection, named or designated doctor/nurse)
- Where appropriate, to report child protection/safeguarding concerns to relevant professionals including social care
- To be aware of local child protection mechanisms
- To be aware of the statutory processes for reviewing deaths of children

## Further Reading


Child Death Review England. Statutory and operational guidance for clinical commissioning groups +and local authorities as child death review partners. Available at: www.gov.uk/government/publications/child-death-review-statutory-and-operational-guidance-england. Accessed 10 May 2021.

Creighton SM, Hodes D. Female genital mutilation: what every paediatrician should know. *Archives of Disease in Childhood* 2016; 101:267–71. Accessed 10 May 2021.

Department for Education. *The Protection of Children in England: A Progress Report. Lord Laming.* The Stationery Office Limited. 2009. Available at: www.gov.uk/government/publications/the-protection-of-children-in-england-a-progress-report. Accessed 10 May 2021.

Department of Health England E-learning for Health. Safeguarding children and young people, level 2 and 3. Available at: www.e-lfh.org.uk/programmes/safeguarding-children/. Accessed 10 May 2021.

Department of Health Northern Ireland. Co-operating to safeguard children and young people in Northern Ireland. 2017. Available at: www.health-ni.gov.uk/publications/co-operating-safeguard-children-and-young-people-northern-ireland. Accessed 14 March 2024.

General Medical Council. 0–18 years: guidance for doctors. 2007. Available at: www.gmc-uk.org/ethical-guidance/ethical-guidance-for-doctors/0-18-years. Accessed 14 March 2024.

General Medical Council. Protecting children and young people. The responsibilities of all doctors. 2012. Available at: www.gmc-uk.org/ethical-guidance/ethical-guidance-for-doctors/protecting-children-and-young-people. Accessed 14 March 2024.

HM Government. Working Together to Safeguard Children. Statutory guidance on inter-agency working to safeguard and promote the welfare of children. 2018. Available at: www.gov.uk/government/publications/working-together-to-safeguard-children–2. Accessed 14 March 2024.

National Guidance for Child Protection in Scotland 2014. 2014. Available at: www.gov.scot/publications/national-guidance-child-protection-scotland/. Accessed 10 May 2021.

National Institute for Health and Clinical Excellence. When to suspect child maltreatment in under 18s. (Guideline 89). 2009, last updated October 2017. Available at: www.nice.org.uk/guidance/cg89/evidence/full-guideline-pdf-243694625. Accessed 14 March 2024.

National Society for the Prevention of Cruelty to Children (NSPCC). Learning, Child Protection System in the UK. Available at: https://learning.nspcc.org.uk/child-protection-system. Accessed 14 March 2024.

NHS England. When a child dies: a guide for parents and carers. 2018. Available at: www.lullabytrust.org.uk/wp-content/uploads/parent-leaflet-child-death-review.pdf. Accessed 14 March 2024.

Royal College of Anaesthetists, SafeguardingPlus. Available at: www.rcoa.ac.uk/safety-standards-quality/guidance-resources/safeguarding-ethics-consent/child-protection. Accessed 10 May 2021.

Royal College of Paediatrics and Child Health. Child Protection Portal. Available at: https://childprotection.rcpch.ac.uk/. Accessed 14 March 2024.

Scottish Government. A guide to getting it right for every child. Available at: www.gov.scot/policies/girfec/. Accessed 10 May 2021.

Wales Safeguarding Procedures, Children and young people at risk of harm. Available at: www.safeguarding.wales/chi. Accessed 10 May 2021.

Chapter 6

# Paediatric Anaesthesia in Non-specialist Centres

Samantha Black and Louise MacKenzie

## Introduction

There has been a trend to centralisation of paediatric services in the United Kingdom over the last 30 years. According to the Office for National Statistics (ONS), in 2019 there were 12.7 million children under the age of 16 in the United Kingdom. However, the specialist care for these children and young people is provided by only 27 specialist centres. Centralisation has reduced the volumes of paediatric surgery in the district hospitals, reducing confidence and experience, and has increased the waiting times for children to access elective surgery. Centralisation of children's services has in turn also led to a significant shift in the delivery of non-specialist, low-complexity elective surgery to tertiary centres, increasing pressures on specialist resources, beds and productivity. In many cases, these children could be treated locally as day cases. Children are often transferred to a tertiary centre when earlier care closer to home would be a better option, for example, for appendicectomy or treatment of testicular torsion. This chapter will describe the importance of multidisciplinary networks of care and outline how to provide high-quality services for children in a non-specialist centre.

## Background: Paediatric Surgery in Non-specialist Centres

The overarching principle for children's surgery is that children are treated safely, as close to home as possible, in an environment that is suitable to their needs. Concerns about outcomes in paediatric surgery in the United Kingdom led to the 1989 National Confidential Enquiry into Perioperative Deaths (NCEPOD) and the recommendation that surgeons and anaesthetists should not undertake occasional paediatric practice. This in turn led to the centralisation of children's surgery, a trend that has continued in the United Kingdom over the last three decades. The recent Anaesthesia Practice in Children Observational Trial (APRICOT) study highlighted a lower incidence of severe critical events during anaesthesia in children from UK hospitals compared to a non-UK cohort of patients, partly attributed to more experienced dedicated paediatric anaesthetists managing higher-risk patients in the United Kingdom.

A recent review of paediatric surgical services by NHS England and NHS Improvement highlighted the need to release capacity in specialist centres, to increase the use of day surgery, make hospital environments safer and more child friendly, reduce the variation in the delivery of paediatric surgery at individual hospitals and improve the care of children requiring emergency surgery. The report identified whole system change was required to develop networks through a coordinated approach for children to access both specialist and non-specialist care. Strong leadership and good relationships between management and clinicians are key to this process.

Ideally, clinicians in non-specialist centres should be trained to provide care for less complex cases, whilst children with complex conditions or that require specialised surgery are treated in specialist centres with access to appropriate expertise and facilities. General paediatric surgery, ENT, orthopaedics and ophthalmology form the bulk of elective surgery that can be delivered in the district general hospital (DGH). There needs to be support and continual training for surgeons, anaesthetists, paediatricians and paediatric nurses to improve confidence to undertake the work locally, and networks should ensure the right workforce and resources are available. Care should be child and family centred and as close to home as possible. Some specialist hospitals can provide an outreach service to deliver non-specialised elective surgery locally.

## Regional Networks

Networks bring together hospitals and commissioners within a region to work collaboratively to deliver services, ensuring children can be treated safely as close to home as possible, with referral pathways designed for surgery and critical care agreed between specialist and non-specialist hospitals in the network.

A network is led by a clinical director and manager with representation from hospitals across the region and patient groups. There should be a clear governance infrastructure. The working groups are accountable to the commissioning body, and there are key performance targets to work towards based on national recommendations.

Working groups and services include, for example, elective and emergency paediatric surgery pathways and models of care, critical care pathways and retrieval pathways. Most children's services should be provided locally, but at times transfer of children to specialist centres is needed, and within the network there should be robust arrangements and standards for this.

The aim of networks is to ensure a reduction in the variation of treatment, improve access to treatment no matter where you live in the region, standardise clinical management and upskill and train staff across the network.

Tertiary centres can support the DGHs in the network through development of clinical guidelines, educational competency frameworks and training opportunities and outreach training, ideally based on cases that have been transferred, particularly if there have been any untoward events.

## Surgery and Procedures in a Non-specialist Centre

Day-case surgery is often preferred for children having elective surgery, especially in a DGH providing that the child is ASA 1 or 2 and the surgical procedure is straightforward with low risk of post-operative complications. When managing a paediatric service within a DGH, it is crucial that standards be maintained at the same level as in a specialist centre. The Royal College of Anaesthetists Guidelines for the Provision of Paediatric Anaesthetic Services 2020 made the following recommendations for day-case surgery:

- Day-case surgery should be delivered to the same standard as inpatient care. Additional measures to promote early discharge, for example scheduling younger patients early in the day allowing time for recovery and discharge and management and prevention of postoperative pain and nausea, are vital.
- The type of surgery provided in each hospital is linked to the skills and competency of the staff.
- Ideally patients should be managed in a dedicated paediatric unit, on a dedicated theatre list or have specific paediatric time allocated if using shared adult facilities.
- An experienced anaesthetist appropriately trained in paediatrics is present for the cases/theatre list (paediatric anaesthetic services should always be consultant led).
- The lower age limit for children will depend on the facilities, patient condition and staff experience. Ex-premature infants should not be considered until at least 60 weeks postmenstrual age.
- Good preoperative information should be provided.
- Clear discharge criteria should be available and documented, along with clear discharge advice for parents/carers and analgesic requirements for when at home.

The Royal College of Anaesthetists (RCOA) curriculum 2010 states that all certificate of completion of training (CCT) holders (and equivalent) should be competent in the perioperative care of children aged three years and over after successfully completing their higher-level training. With the upcoming changes in the anaesthetic curriculum in 2022, this will be reduced to children aged over 12 months. It is expected that all anaesthetists who may be exposed to paediatric emergencies (even those without regular elective paediatric lists) maintain their competence and confidence in paediatrics via continuing professional development (CPD), simulation and visits to specialist centres.

Surgery can either be performed by visiting specialist paediatric surgeons (usually from a specialist centre) or by adult surgeons who have expertise in paediatric surgery. Currently, the paediatric surgical training pathway is a six-year programme starting from ST3 recruitment, following core surgical training; these surgeons will undertake the Fellowship of Royal Colleges of Surgery (FRCS) in paediatric surgery. There may also be clinicians who have previously undergone adult surgical training but are proficient in paediatric surgery given their personal experience and case exposure. Regardless, all individuals are expected to undergo regular CPD to ensure their skills are maintained. One of the challenges faced by DGHs is how to ensure that there is appropriate surgical on-call cover for emergency procedures.

Anaesthetic services are provided to a wide range of surgical specialties in the DGH, including ENT, dental, urology, general, ophthalmology and orthopaedics (see Table 6.1).

It is not only the surgical procedure that determines whether the case should be performed in a DGH. Factors that may influence the decision include:

- Very young age. Protocols must clearly define the minimum age of patients that can be treated; this may vary between different hospitals. Generally, all patients less than 12 months are referred to specialist centres, but there is varying practice for children aged one to two years. Younger children have an increased risk of perioperative respiratory complications, and so the accepted age thresholds depend on the skills, training and environment of each hospital. Infants and younger children will also tend to require more complex types of surgery, and therefore the numbers passing through a DGH will be fewer.
- Existing comorbidities
- Lack of professional experience and skills (surgical, anaesthetic or nursing), and health care infrastructure in place

**Table 6.1** Common surgical procedures undertaken in the DGH

| Specialty | Procedure |
|---|---|
| General | Herniotomy (umbilical/ inguinal)<br>Orchidopexy for undescended testes<br>Circumcision<br>Minor soft tissue abnormalities<br>*Testicular torsion*<br>*Appendicectomy* |
| ENT | Tonsillectomy<br>Adenoidectomy<br>Grommet insertion<br>Examinations under anaesthetic |
| Oral and maxilla-facial surgery | Extractions<br>Orthodontics<br>*Dental trauma*<br>*Closure of lacerations* |
| Ophthalmology | Strabismus surgery<br>Tear duct obstruction surgery |
| Orthopaedics and trauma | *Open reduction internal fixation (ORIF)*<br>*Manipulation under anaesthesia (MUA)* |

Note: Italics indicate emergency procedures.

Ideally, there should be a clear referral pathway within the regional paediatric surgery network and clearly defined parameters as to which patients should be referred to the specialist centre for their surgery.

Anaesthesia services may also be needed in remote non-theatre environments, for instance for radiology (CT or MRI scan). Depending on the age or condition of the patient, this may require a general anaesthetic. Not all MRI scanners will be set up to provide care for patients under general anaesthetic, so it is important to be aware of the equipment available at these sites (e.g. MRI-compatible anaesthetic machine and equipment).

Vascular access can be difficult for paediatric patients, given their smaller size and challenges with cooperation. Anaesthetists may be asked to assist with difficult access. The provision of ultrasound training to other health care professionals, can reduce the burden of out of hours access requests. Long-term intravascular (IV) access is preferable for patients who require prolonged IV medication, therefore it can benefit patients to have a peripherally inserted central catheter (PICC) line service in a DGH utilising specialist nurses or anaesthetists, although these services are not yet well established in UK hospitals.

In some instances, the anaesthetic team may be requested to provide sedation for patients undergoing procedures in the emergency department (ED). If there is a safe environment with appropriate monitoring and trained staff available, then this can avoid the need for the patient to be booked onto the theatre emergency list and consequently reduce the length of hospital stay. A local protocol will determine the drugs, equipment, team and monitoring that should be used to ensure a safe sedation.

## Preassessment for Elective Paediatric Surgery

Most of the paediatric surgery in fit and healthy ASA 1 or 2 children is for minor procedures and can be carried out on a day-case basis. Preassessment can ensure paediatric surgery/anaesthesia is carried out at the most appropriate time, in the correct environment and by the best team.

All patients should be seen at a preassessment clinic to ensure health screening, optimisation of medical conditions, risk assessment and psychological preparation prior to the day of surgery and to assess suitability for local surgery or the potential for referral to a specialist centre. This will increase surgical list efficiency and reduce last-minute cancellations. It improves patient and parent satisfaction, reduces anxiety, helps both parent and child to know what to expect and provides an opportunity to ask questions or express any concerns they might have.

Some children might be under the care of a paediatrician locally for conditions such as diabetes or asthma and might need a referral for a review and medication plan for the day of surgery before undergoing the procedure and anaesthesia. Other children might be under the care of a specialist at a tertiary centre for conditions such as cardiac disease, ex-prematurity or genetic syndromes and may need assessment of the stability of the condition before embarking on surgery locally. An identification of increased risk in such children may indicate a need for the non-complex surgery to be undertaken at a specialist centre.

Preassessment is an opportunity to provide advice on lifestyle issues such as nutrition, smoking in the household and exercise, although currently there are no national standards or referral pathways, and much will depend on your services locally.

A nurse-led service is safe and cost effective. There should be locally agreed and developed preoperative policies and guidelines (for example, when to order preoperative investigations or when to refer to an anaesthetist – usually the paediatric anaesthetic lead and/or paediatric anaesthetists with an interest in preassessment). The preassessment nurses should have appropriate paediatric experience and training. Each hospital requires a written local definition of the type of procedures and age thresholds for elective surgery that they can conduct at their centre.

A preassessment service should be face to face, but telephone or virtual assessment can be part of the service for selected patients. The assessment should be guided by a standardised proforma and include at a minimum:

- Complete birth history including prematurity
- Congenital or acquired disease, with focus on the airway, cardiovascular system, respiratory systems (for example obstructive sleep apnoea), endocrine (diabetes), metabolic, neuromuscular, haematological (anaemia, coagulopathy) or any other relevant physiological system
- Family history of anaesthetic problems, for instance malignant hyperpyrexia or suxamethonium apnoea
- Drug history
- Special educational needs
- Social history, including any safeguarding concerns
- Sickle cell status in at-risk populations
- Observations: weight, height, temperature, saturations, heart rate, blood pressure
- Airway assessment (as per local protocol/ proforma)
- The need for a perioperative anxiety management plan

Medical concerns picked up by the nurse may require further examination by a consultant paediatric anaesthetist, for example, examination of the cardiorespiratory system or further airway assessment.

Most children are ASA 1 or 2 and will not need investigations. Investigations undertaken need to be reviewed by a consultant paediatric anaesthetist.

The use of local anaesthesia, regional anaesthesia, sedation or general anaesthesia should be explained to the parent/carer and child as part of informed consent, and the perioperative benefits and risks should be discussed timeously before the procedure.

## Creating a Child-Friendly Experience

Delivering care locally/close to home where possible improves the patient and parent experience.

Children have different emotional and physical needs than adults, and the perioperative process can be stressful for families. Medical encounters can be significant events in a child's life, no matter how small we think the procedure is. Long-lasting effects can arise from the use of 'nocebo talk' and negative expressions, and it is important to guide colleagues and trainees who usually work with adults. For instance, the phrase 'sharp scratch coming' prior to cannulation may potentially induce anxiety and fear of pain.

Most children will be anxious when presenting for an anaesthetic. There may be fears about pain, unfamiliar surroundings, separation from parents, loss of control/autonomy and fear of the unknown. Such anxiety can lead to increased postoperative pain, nausea and vomiting, prolonged recovery time and behavioural disturbance.

Well-managed procedural care, optimising the psychological well-being of the child, can have significant long-term benefits for a child's health. Some methods are summarised in Table 6.2.

All locations where children are treated (preassessment, ward, theatres) should be child friendly and create a welcoming environment. These areas should be physically separate from those with adult patients. There should be play spaces and equipment available, and they should meet the needs of children with physical disabilities. Parents/carers should be able to be present with their child when they wake up in recovery areas.

The use age-appropriate materials such as leaflets and videos can help prepare children and their families for their procedure. More recently we have seen the development of apps and the use of virtual reality to deliver such information. The 'little journey' app (https://littlejourney.health) is utilised by NHS hospitals in the United Kingdom, providing age-appropriate information for patients and their families about their hospital visit and anaesthetic. The app is fully interactive, providing virtual reality tours with animated characters of the chosen hospital, along with games, meditative coping exercises and breathing techniques. It also includes details of fasting guidelines and perioperative information specific to each hospital and can be used in the upcoming weeks to prepare a child for their operation. Hospital tours can be offered to provide familiarity with the paediatric ward and theatres. These are usually conducted by the preassessment nurse as part of the child's preassessment journey. Play specialists and distraction aids should be available to complement this journey and help prepare the child for their admission.

**Table 6.2** Methods to reduce preoperative anxiety in children

| | |
|---|---|
| Preoperative preparation | Printed information, hospital tour, play therapy, clear management plan |
| Parental preparation | Coaching |
| Parental presence | At induction of anaesthesia and in the recovery room |
| Behavioural intervention | Play therapy, storytelling, distraction, guided imagery (a relaxation technique that draws on the ability to visualise), hypnosis |
| Pharmacological | Midazolam, topical anaesthesia |

It is important to involve children as much as possible and respect their autonomy. Providing choices or allowing them to wear their own clothes to theatre can help to reduce anxiety.

Extremely anxious children should be scheduled to be first on the operating list, and particular attention should be paid to their fears/dislikes and likes to help improve their experience.

Prolonged fasting times and incorrect timing of topical local anaesthetic before cannulation can lead to an increase in anxiety and a poor experience. Some children may need to see an anaesthetist in advance of the day of surgery to create an individualised anaesthetic plan, including the potential use of premedication. Hypnotic and relaxation techniques are becoming more recognised as part of the treatment plan (see Chapter 3).

## Paediatric Acute Pain Management in a DGH

Pain protocols should be in place for common elective surgical procedures performed in the DGH for managing and treating simple surgical emergencies in children (e.g. reduction of fractures, appendicectomy) and for medical emergencies such as sickle cell crisis. Paediatric validated age-appropriate pain scoring tools along with escalation plans should be available. Most procedures in a DGH are carried out as day-case procedures, so careful planning of discharge analgesia is vital and should follow a local standardised protocol. Pain can persist for many days after certain procedures, for example tonsillectomy, and patients should be discharged with clear advice such as taking regular paracetamol and ibuprofen (if the patient has no allergies) for up to one week postoperatively. Children are at greater risk of drug and dosing errors, particularly in an 'adult' setting. Local systems should be in place to minimise such errors, with multidisciplinary learning from any events that may occur.

DGH's usually have a smaller paediatric caseload compared to specialist centres, and the acute pain service is likely to be provided by the adult pain team who liaise with paediatricians, emergency physicians and the paediatric anaesthetic team. Strict local protocols and guidance is therefore paramount.

Analgesic regimens will follow a multimodal approach based on the WHO analgesic ladder. It's important not to forget the importance of local anaesthetic use, especially in elective day cases. This can take the form of wound infiltration or regional blocks. It is important that adult-trained surgeons and nurses are aware of the toxic doses of local anaesthetics when using local infiltration. A common procedure performed as a day case is circumcision; this causes significant postoperative pain, and a caudal or penile block is ideal in these cases. Complex analgesia techniques such as epidural infusion or continuous wound infiltration catheters are not generally suitable for the non-specialist centre.

Analgesia such as ketamine may be used in the ED for management of fractures, for example, and adherence to local paediatric guidance regarding dosing and monitoring is vital. There should also be local guidance on techniques such as morphine patient-controlled analgesia or nurse-controlled analgesia, especially for children with sickle cell disease or in cases of orthopaedic trauma.

## Medical and Surgical Transfers to a Specialist Centre

Decisions concerning which patients should be transferred for emergency surgery should not fall to the expertise and skills of individual team members on duty that day, as such variability could impact on patient outcomes. Ideally, these decisions should be made in advance within the network, with standardised protocols describing when and where patients should be referred to when they arrive at a non-specialist centre with an acute surgical problem that cannot be managed locally. A decision to transfer will be based on the complexity of the surgery required, the age and comorbidities and the clinical condition of the child.

In certain circumstances, a child may need to be stabilised or managed locally, for instance a time-critical surgical emergency or if the patient is critically unwell/injured. It is vital that staff are prepared and the environment equipped for this scenario with local protocols in place. A close working relationship with the tertiary centre is essential, with regular training opportunities utilising simulated paediatric resuscitation scenarios within multidisciplinary teams to improve confidence.

These events may be very infrequent for staff in a smaller DGH. Education and training within the paediatric network are a vital tool to make sure that skills and confidence of staff in the non-specialist centres are maintained. Anaesthetic trainees may be a useful resource in an acute situation due to their experience obtained rotating to specialist centres. Provision of easily accessible guidelines, checklists and a standardised kit can greatly aid staff during these stressful and time-pressured scenarios.

A child may sometimes require short-term admission to the local adult intensive care unit in cases where they are expected to recover quickly (e.g. perioperative anaphylaxis) or whilst awaiting the arrival of the paediatric retrieval team from the specialist centre. The intensive care team should work closely with the paediatricians and anaesthetists and must ensure the appropriate equipment and skills are available. Different teams' expertise may of use in difficult aspects of care in these scenarios. For example, if a medically unwell neonate presents in the emergency department with difficult intravenous access, the neonatal team, if available, may be best placed to assist in gaining access. Similarly, a neonatologist may be skilled at intubation of neonates, but a trained anaesthetist is likely to be the best person to manage the airway of an older child in an emergency, even if their practice is predominantly adult.

The paramedics usually provide a pre-alert when a critically unwell child is to arrive in the emergency department, allowing time for the on-call paediatric emergency team to gather and prepare. An effective use of time prior to the patient arriving is to allocate roles to individuals within the team (e.g. the anaesthetic team to maintain the patient's airway, a paediatrician to establish IV access) and to calculate the appropriate doses of drugs and sizes of equipment that may be required. Using web applications can be immensely useful to reduce error when attempting to recall formulae or drug doses in extremely pressurised situations.

Commonly the senior ED doctor will become the 'leader' of the emergency and will use advanced paediatric life support principals to guide immediate resuscitation and treatment of the child. Clear and concise communication is required by all members of the team, and particular attention should be paid to ensuring that all tasks be allocated to named individuals, and the receiving person should confirm when the task has been performed (i.e. closed-loop communication).

Another key role within the multidisciplinary team is the liaison to the child's parents or guardians. An experienced paediatric or ED nurse may be best suited to this role.

The establishment of paediatric critical care networks has led to the evolution of specialist paediatric intensive care transport teams that are available to both retrieve patients from non-specialist centres as well as offer telephone advice on the immediate management of these patients. The retrieval teams will usually manage the transfer of these patients; however, it may be necessary for the local team (usually an anaesthetist) to transfer in time-critical scenarios, such as acute neurosurgical emergencies or major trauma. In this situation, a calm and methodical approach to the transfer and use of checklists optimises safety for the patient. Standardising equipment between transferring and receiving centres will also reduce errors. One way that this can be ensured is to provide 'transfer trolleys' in local emergency departments and paediatric wards so that when a patient is acutely unwell, this sealed trolley can be opened, and all the necessary equipment is available. This includes a range of airway equipment (including laryngoscopes, blades, tracheal tubes, oral/nasal airways, lubricating jelly, tube ties) in the top drawer (labelled 'A'). Subsequent drawers are labelled 'B' containing all the breathing equipment, 'C' for circulation and 'D' for disability. Transfer trolleys should ensure that items that are commonly difficult to find (e.g. capnography monitoring block) are easily to locate. This setup is standardised across all hospitals within a particular critical care network, so that familiarity with equipment by members of staff who may rotate around several hospitals within a region is increased.

## Keeping Up to Date in a Non-specialist Hospital

Completion of specialist training in anaesthesia in the United Kingdom should enable consultants to provide anaesthesia to children without any major comorbidity from the age three. Many anaesthetists complete advanced training in paediatric anaesthesia and are thus equipped to deliver a regular paediatric elective list in a non-specialist hospital (e.g. paediatric general surgery or ENT surgery). Paediatric anaesthetists in the DGH face the challenge of maintaining an adequate caseload and of retaining their skills in managing sick children if they are on an on-call rota and they do not anaesthetise children regularly.

Getting it right first time (GIRFT) is a quality-improvement initiative funded by the Department of Health and jointly overseen by NHS England and NHS Improvement. The reports seek to create improvements in patient safety, patient experience and operational efficiency in hospitals. The aim of the GIRFT paediatric group is to ensure that clinicians in DGHs continue to be trained and maintain skills to provide the less complex paediatric care locally for families via a network approach and to support training/competencies and maintenance of skills, including paediatric resuscitation. The recommendation is for surgeons and anaesthetists to maintain competence through delivery of regular paediatric lists, joining their colleagues as supernumerary on lists and continuing professional development activities for appraisal and revalidation.

Many DGH anaesthetists arrange to attend regular paediatric lists at their regional specialist centre to further develop and update knowledge and skills. It is hoped that a certificate of honorary practice will be developed in due course to facilitate this process. All anaesthetists providing elective or emergency care in paediatric anaesthesia must undertake the minimum of level 2 training in safeguarding/child protection as part of their annual mandatory training at trust level, along with annual updates in paediatric life support. Multidisciplinary paediatric simulation training should also be used to maintain competencies and skills. APAGBI offers a 'linkman scheme' that provides regular meetings and opportunities for collaboration for paediatric anaesthetists, especially in DGHs. Many regions also provide local networks to support education in paediatric anaesthesia in DGHs, often linked to their specialist centre.

At a local level, each department should identify a lead paediatric anaesthetist who is responsible for oversight of the paediatric anaesthetic service. This will include ensuring there are up-to-date guidelines and policies for both elective and emergency anaesthesia; teaching and training of anaesthetic trainees, nurses and operating department practitioners (ODPs); ensuring the local standards are maintained (e.g. equipment, pain management, sedation and resuscitation); and leading on paediatric anaesthetic audit, quality improvement, research and safety.

## Research and National Audits

Undertaking research in paediatric anaesthesia in a DGH can be a daunting prospect as historically the focus has been on service delivery. However, many hospitals have research opportunities available, usually with teams looking for National Institute for Health Research portfolio trials and national audits to take part in. Organisations conducting and being part of research tend to improve their standards and provide better care for their patients and have better patient outcomes.

In the United Kingdom, the Paediatric Anaesthesia Trainee Research Network undertakes multi-centre research and audit projects, supported by the APAGBI (for instance, the recent PEACHY project looking into the effect of obesity on perioperative complications in paediatric patients undergoing anaesthesia). Other perioperative national research projects in paediatrics can be found through networks such as the perioperative medicine clinical trials network (POM-CTN). The Health Service Research Centre's first paediatric initiative is under way (jointly delivered in collaboration with the APAGBI and the British Association of Paediatric Surgery). The Children's Acute Surgical Abdomen Programme (CASAP) is a prospective observational cohort study aiming to characterise the type and quality of care being delivered to children undergoing urgent/emergency abdominal surgery. Many of this study's recruits will be patients undergoing appendicectomy in DGHs.

### Key Points

- Most paediatric surgery carried out is for minor procedures in fit and healthy children and can be performed as day-case procedures. A large quantity of this work is performed in non-specialist hospitals.
- Children and families need to be able to access high-quality services as close to home as possible.
- Delivering care locally or close to home where safe and possible can add to the patient and parent experience.
- A non-specialist centre should have provisions and local guidance for treating and managing simple surgical emergencies in the paediatric population, along with the ability to resuscitate and stabilise critically ill children of all ages before transfer to a tertiary specialist centre for either critical care or surgery.
- Continual education and training within regional networks are vital in maintaining skills and confidence of staff in non-specialist centres.
- Standardisation of care along with protocols are helpful for the anaesthetic management, analgesic management, pre assessment and critical transfer of children in a non-specialist centre.

## Further Reading

Campling EA, Devlin HB, Lunn JN. The report of the National Confidential Enquiry into Perioperative Deaths 1989. 1989. Available at: www.ncepod.org.uk/1989report/Full%20Report%201989.pdf. Accessed 16 May 2021.

Engelhardt T, Ayansina D, Bell GT et al. Incidence of severe critical events in paediatric anaesthesia in the United Kingdom: secondary analysis of the anaesthesia practice in children observational trial (APRICOT study). *Anaesthesia* 2019; 74:300–11.

Getting it Right First Time. Reports. Available at: www.gettingitrightfirsttime.co.uk/girft-reports/. Accessed 14 March 2024.

NHS England and NHS Improvement. Paediatric critical care and surgery in children review. 2019. Available at: www

.england.nhs.uk/wp-content/uploads/2019/11/paediatric-critical-care-and-surgery-in-children-review-summary-report-nov-2019.pdf. Accessed 14 March 2024.

Rollins AM. Working together for the sick or injured child: the Tanner Report. *Anaesthesia* 2006; 61:1135–7.

Royal College of Anaesthetists. Chapter 10: guidelines for the provision of paediatric anaesthesia services. 2020. Available at: www.rcoa.ac.uk/gpas/chapter-10. Accessed 21 April 2024.

Royal College of Surgeons of England. Ensuring the provision of general paediatric surgery in the district general hospital. 2010. Available at: www.rcseng.ac.uk/library-and-publications/rcs-publications/docs/ensuring-the-provision-of-general-paediatric-surgery-in-the-district-general-hospital/. Accessed 21 April 2024.

Chapter 7

# Preoperative Assessment for Paediatric Anaesthesia

## Considerations for Common Medical Conditions and Risk

Pamela Cupples

## Introduction

Preoperative assessment is an essential part of paediatric anaesthesia. Whilst every child will be seen on the day of their procedure by the responsible anaesthetic team, there is broad acceptance that anaesthetic preoperative assessment (APOA), in advance of the admission, is the optimal standard of care.

The purpose of APOA is to:

- Ensure that the child is medically optimised in advance of their admission
- Identify specific anaesthetic issues, such as difficult airway, previous anaesthetic complications, genetic conditions such as malignant hyperpyrexia or suxamethonium apnoea
- Liaise with the relevant medical teams for those with complex comorbidities to ensure that their expertise and knowledge of the patient is incorporated into the plan for admission, such as endocrine, metabolism and haematology
- Identify high-risk patients, for whom a perioperative multidisciplinary team meeting (MDT) should be convened to consider whether surgery is appropriate and if so to agree on the perioperative plan, including ceilings of care
- Order appropriate investigations – this will be guided by the child's medication, the underlying comorbidities and the type of surgery the child is having
- Prepare the child and the family and explain the specifics of the anaesthetic process, including:
    - Discussion around induction techniques
    - Options for premedication if required, and support for the induction process such as distraction techniques and play therapists
    - Pain management and the options available – regional and opioid-based techniques
    - The recovery process
- Discuss side effects and risks of anaesthesia
- Disseminate information leaflets to support discussion and understanding
- Allow the child and family time to ask questions and explain to the anaesthetic team what is important to them
- Provide contact details should they wish to discuss any part of the anaesthetic again in advance of the admission

APOA services have been shown to:

- Reduce cancellations on the day of surgery and improve theatre efficiency
- Reduce complication rates and mortality
- Improve patient experience and reduce perioperative anxiety

The delivery of an APOA service is reliant on a hybrid model of medical and nursing assessments. Specialist APOA nurses are effective at preoperative screening and are an integral part of the team. Anaesthetic consultants must always support nurse-led clinics. The Association of Paediatric Anaesthetists of Great Britain and Ireland (APAGBI) guidance document on the running of preoperative assessment clinics helps guide the development and running of paediatric APOA services.

Paediatric APOA differs from adults in several key areas:

- The interview will be with both the child and the parent, as young children will be unable to give a detailed history.
- Older children and adolescents should be encouraged to give a history, but this will need

to be supported by a joint discussion with the parent/carer.

- Gillick competent children should ideally make consent decisions for themselves, supported by their parent/carer.
- There is significant anxiety and stress for the family in dealing with children for surgery. You are not only looking after the child but the parent and carer too.
- Comorbidities are more likely due to congenital disorders, prematurity or acute illness.

## APOA Process

### Clinical Evaluation

A detailed review of the medical notes is essential to identify comorbidities, their physiological implications and the indication for surgery. If the child has had previous anaesthetics, these charts should be reviewed if possible, noting the level of anxiety at induction, the need for premedication and induction technique. An assessment of the airway and how it has been managed should be documented, together with any intraoperative complications. The child's current medication and history of allergies should also be reviewed and documented.

The review of the notes should then be combined with an interview to confirm the medical history and allow a physical assessment of the child.

### Interview

The interview process helps to develop a rapport with the child and parent and to explain the anaesthetist's role during the child's admission. A systematic approach to assessment is essential to ensure that nothing is overlooked. A detailed antenatal and neonatal history is important when infants present for surgery. Time spent in NICU, the need for respiratory support and any ongoing respiratory requirements, such as oxygen therapy or non-invasive ventilation, should be documented.

The child's physiological status should be assessed and documented along with objective measurements such as echocardiography (ECHO) and lung function testing where indicated.

If this is the patient's first general anaesthetic (GA), asking about any family history of problems under GA will help to identify those at risk of malignant hyperpyrexia and suxamethonium apnoea. If the child has had previous anaesthetics, it is an opportunity to understand how successful the induction was and what, if anything, can be improved upon, such as distraction techniques, play therapy or premedication.

Medication history should be captured as part of the assessment, including recently stopped drugs that may have anaesthetic relevance, such as steroid therapy or herbal medicines. This should include any allergies the patient may have and their significance, including whether the child carries an adrenaline auto-injector, such as EpiPen®.

Recent laboratory tests should be documented along with the child's vaccination history. Adolescents should also be questioned about smoking and drinking habits and the possibility of pregnancy. Due to the sensitive nature of this questioning, it may be prudent to do this confidentially.

A key part of the interview is a discussion about the anaesthetic process itself, including induction techniques, invasive monitoring if required, approaches to analgesia, need for intraoperative blood transfusion, as well as recovery and postoperative care. This is particularly important for children having major surgery who may require an elective admission to critical care.

### Side Effects and Risks

No assessment is complete without a discussion about side effects and risks of general anaesthesia. Information leaflets can provide a useful adjunct to these discussions; these may outline the admission process, the general anaesthetic, analgesic techniques and side effects and risks. These discussions need to occur well in advance of the admission to allow the family and the patient time to consider the information, ask questions and agree the perioperative plan.

Common side effects such as postoperative nausea and vomiting (PONV), sore throat, behavioural changes and emergence delirium need to be discussed with the family as part of the preoperative assessment. Minor cuts to the lips and tongue and the potential of dental damage may also be mentioned.

New General Medical Council (GMC) guidance has highlighted that communication with families should be clear and consistent even when the risks of serious harm and death are extremely rare.

There are no validated clinical risk scoring tools that are used in paediatric anaesthesia. Data rely on published audits from different paediatric centres to inform the speciality about the incidence of morbidity and mortality.

The National Audit Projects (NAPs) have helped to inform our discussions around anaphylaxis and accidental awareness. The risk of perioperative anaphylaxis has been quantified as 1:10,000. The risk of accidental awareness during general anaesthesia is quoted as 1:60,000 (NAP 5); whilst rare, when it does occur it is not usually associated with pain or distress.

In due course, the completion of the UK NAP 7 audit into perioperative cardiac arrest will be completed and will inform the specialty of the incidence of cardiac arrest during GA.

The risk of a child dying during a general anaesthetic is rare (1:10,000) and more commonly seen in neonates and those with significant comorbidity, particularly congenital heart disease and pulmonary hypertension. In the fit and healthy child presenting for elective surgery, the risk of dying under GA is quoted as being between 1:100,000 and 1:1,000,000.

## Jehovah's Witnesses (JW)

There are approximately 8.5 million Jehovah's Witnesses worldwide, and 150,000 live in the United Kingdom and Ireland. It is an essential part of the anaesthetic assessment for any child of a JW to have detailed discussions about the surgery and the risks of requiring a blood or blood product transfusion.

The discussions should take the form of an MDT. It should include the responsible surgeon, anaesthetist and senior haematologist with input from the hospital liaison committee and hospital legal team if required. The purpose of the MDT is to:

- Clarify the reason for the proposed surgery and what blood or blood products may be required
- Discuss alternatives to blood transfusion, including cell salvage
- Explain what the risks of blood transfusion are and the consequences of withholding transfusion in the face of life-threatening haemorrhage
- Consult with the family to understand what they will consent to

In the elective setting, if the parents refuse to give consent and it is deemed unsafe to operate without the option to give blood, then a second opinion can be sought. The family may be happy to give consent with some caveats. As long as the team feels it can safely work within these caveats, the case can proceed. It is essential that the family feel that their beliefs are being respected, and that the team will do everything to avoid transfusion where possible. The discussion and the agreed plan need to be documented clearly in the notes.

The team must always work in the best interests of the child, and if blood transfusion is deemed to be lifesaving, it can be done even if parents refuse. Legislation varies between countries, but in England and Wales, a special issue order under Section 8 of The Children's Act 1989 can be obtained from the High Court. They can issue an order providing legal permission for treatment in the face of parental refusal. In an urgent or dynamic situation, blood should be given to minimise the threat to life or to prevent lasting disability whilst such an application is made. Seeking the opinion and agreement of another senior colleague and documenting this in the notes is advised. The hospital's legal team can be helpful in this setting.

## Vaccinations

Immunisation is not a contraindication to GA in healthy children scheduled for elective surgery. Historically, there have been concerns around anaesthesia influencing the efficacy and safety of vaccines or the inflammatory response to vaccines being mistaken for an acute infection. The guidance for non-immunocompromised children is:

- A minimum delay of 48 hours is advised for inactivated vaccines.
- No delay is required for children having a live attenuated vaccine, but there is a small risk of the child developing a fever in the weeks following the vaccination, which may coincide with the admission. This will require assessment at the time to decide if this is vaccine related or due to another cause.
- Children can be safely vaccinated following a GA, providing they have made a full recovery.

## Physical Examination

All children presenting for GA should have the following observations performed:

- Heart rate, oxygen saturation, respiratory rate, temperature
- Blood pressure in children over three and those under three with known hypertensive comorbidity
- Height and weight

In an emergency setting, obtaining an accurate weight may be difficult, and clinicians will need to use a formula to estimate the child's weight. Examples include:

- The Advanced Paediatric Life Support (APLS) formula:
  weight (kg) = 2 × (age + 4)
- Luscombe formula:
  weight (kg) = (3 × age) + 7
- Modified Australian BG method:
  weight (kg) = (2 × age) + 10

All estimates may be inaccurate, but the APLS formula is now felt to be a significant underestimate, and there is a move towards using the Luscombe or the Modified Australian BG method. An accurate weight should be obtained as soon as clinically appropriate.

The respiratory and cardiovascular systems should be examined and the airway assessed according to the Mallampati classification if possible. Any restriction of neck movement should also be assessed. Examination will depend on the age and cooperation of the child. Cormack and Lehane grade of laryngoscopy may be obtained from previous anaesthetic records. The state of the child's teeth should be noted, including the position of any loose teeth or braces. Known or anticipated difficult venous access should be noted.

## Investigations

Preoperative investigations will depend on the child's comorbidities, current medication, and the surgery they are having. Routine investigations, such as full blood count or urea and electrolytes, are not required in the otherwise healthy child presenting for minor routine surgery. Neonates less than 60 weeks postconceptual age are at increased risk of apnoea following GA, and this risk is increased in those neonates who are also anaemic. In this setting, a full blood count to assess the haemoglobin level is prudent.

Whilst testing for sickle cell anaemia is routine for babies born in the United Kingdom, it is essential to check the status of children from racial groups at increased risk of sickle cell anaemia. The sickle cell solubility test (Sickledex) can rapidly identify the presence of haemoglobin S (HbS) in a blood sample, but it does not distinguish between sickle cell trait (SCT) and disease (SCD). Furthermore, this test is not reliable when HbS levels are below 15–20%, so it is not suited for newborn screening. In the case of a positive test, more detailed haemoglobinopathy testing is required.

Chest X-rays, sleep studies, spirometry and echocardiograms should be ordered based on the child's associated comorbidities.

## Heart Murmurs

Incidental heart murmurs are commonly picked up during a preoperative assessment. The challenge is differentiating innocent murmurs from those that are deemed to be pathological. Less than 1% of children with an incidental murmur have an underlying cardiac condition.

Most children with congenital heart disease (CHD) are diagnosed either antenatally during routine scanning or within the first three months of life. Some conditions can be asymptomatic, so all infants less than one year of age who have a murmur identified should be referred to a cardiologist.

A detailed history should be taken, and children with the following symptoms suggestive of an underlying cardiac condition warrant further investigation:

- Failure to thrive
- Recurrent respiratory tract infection
- Tachypnoea
- Cyanosis
- Pallor/mottling
- Sweating
- Difficulty with feeding
- Syncope or chest pain
- Reduced exercise tolerance
- Family history of sudden death

There should be a high index of suspicion of underlying cardiac disease in the following groups:

- Trisomy 21
- CHARGE syndrome (coloboma of the eye, heart defects, atresia of the choanae,

retardation of growth and/or development, genital and/or urinary abnormalities, ear abnormalities and deafness)
- VACTERL association (vertebral, anal, cardiac, tracheal-oesophageal fistula (TOF), renal, limb)
- Turner syndrome
- DiGeorge syndrome

The challenge is identifying those who require referral to cardiology before anaesthesia. Innocent murmurs are usually:

- Soft murmurs in early systole sometimes described as musical, blowing or vibratory
- Not associated with a pre-cordial thrill
- Variable with changes in posture
- Not associated with increased mortality or morbidity under general anaesthesia

Pathological murmurs are often:

- Pansystolic, late systole or in diastole
- Harsh quality
- Associated with thrills
- Present in clinically symptomatic patients

Children with innocent murmurs should have an electrocardiogram (ECG), looking for signs of ventricular hypertrophy. Children with critical aortic stenosis and hypertrophic obstructive cardiomyopathy (HOCM) can be clinically asymptomatic. ECG features of ventricular hypertrophy include:

- RVH: R-wave in V1 >1.75 mV (<5 yr) or R-wave in V1 >1.25 mV (5–12 yr) or upright T-wave
- LVH: R-wave in V5 or V6 > 4 mV

An asymptomatic child over one year old with an innocent murmur (i.e. venous hum or soft, early systolic with no thrill) and a normal ECG can proceed with surgery and be referred for investigation after the operation. If there is any doubt about the nature of a murmur, transthoracic echocardiography is a non-invasive and straightforward way to resolve the matter in most cases.

The algorithm shown in Figure 7.1 can help in the preoperative assessment of children presenting with incidental murmurs.

## Respiratory Tract Infections

Children will experience between six and eight upper respiratory tract infections (URTI) per year. Of these, 95% will be caused by one of the 200 viruses known to cause coryzal symptoms (cough, nasal congestion and discharge, sore throat and sneezing). Rhinovirus is responsible for 30–40% of these infections.

Due to airway hyperreactivity, there is an increased risk of perioperative complications for two to six weeks following an URTI. This is thought to be due to inflammatory mediators (histamine, interleukin, bradykinin), viral neuraminidases inhibiting the muscarinic M2 receptor and increased tachykinin levels due to viral inhibition of endopeptidases. These postulated mechanisms all promote airway hyperreactivity and bronchoconstriction.

Children who have or are recovering from a recent URTI are thus at increased risk of perioperative respiratory adverse events (PRAE) such as:

- Laryngospasm
- Bronchospasm
- Oxygen desaturation
- Coughing and breath holding
- Atelectasis and pneumonia

In the APOA setting, it is important to take a complete history and to consider other causes for coryzal symptoms such as:

- Croup
- Bronchiolitis
- Pneumonia
- Influenza
- Inhaled foreign body
- Gastro-oesophageal reflux disease (GORD)
- Allergic rhinitis

There are additional independent risk factors for adverse respiratory events in children who have a URTI:

- Ex-premature baby
- <1 year of age
- Asthma or atopy
- Living in a house with a smoker
- Copious secretions
- Airway surgery
- History of snoring

Despite these complications, the evidence would suggest that the majority can be managed safely without any long-term sequelae.

The decision to proceed with or postpone surgery in a child with an active or recent URTI

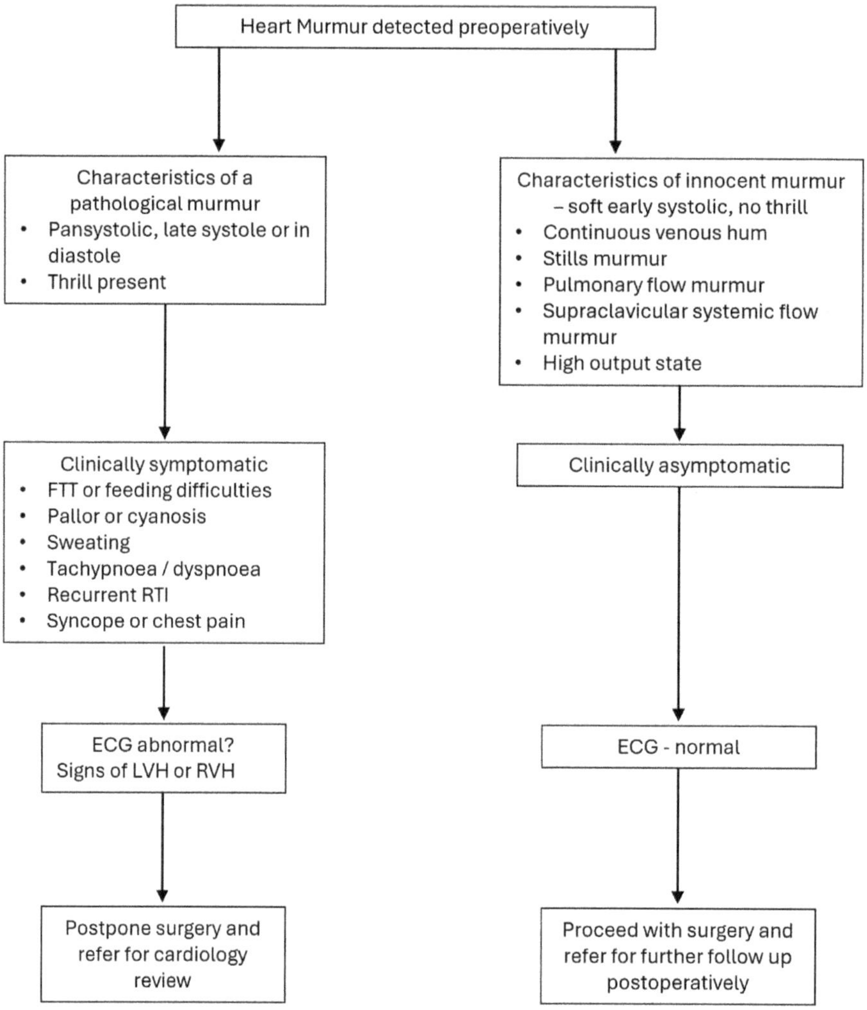


**Figure 7.1** Heart murmur algorithm.

requires an individualised approach, which takes into account:

- Detailed history and examination of the child
- Independent risk factors
- Comorbidities
- Type of surgery

Children who have minimal symptoms, such as isolated clear runny nose or dry cough, who are apyrexial and constitutionally well should proceed with the planned admission. Cancellation should be considered in children who show signs of a more severe URTI:

- A clinically unwell or lethargic child
- Pyrexia, with a temp >38°C
- Copious purulent secretions
- Associated risk factors, as detailed previously
- Complex comorbidities
- Major surgery

Those children with signs of a moderate or severe URTI (green nasal discharge, wet cough and pyrexia >38°C) should be postponed for two weeks and re-evaluated. Providing they have made a full recovery, they can then be re-scheduled.

In the case of croup, bronchiolitis and lower RTI, the procedure should be delayed for six weeks. If the surgery is deemed to be urgent, then a discussion with the surgical team is required to discuss clinical concerns and agree on what time frame would be in the child's best interest.

Additional investigations should only be considered on an individual basis. Routine blood

**Table 7.1** Premedication

| Drug | Dose | Onset | Additional comments |
|---|---|---|---|
| Midazolam | 0.5 mg $kg^{-1}$ oral<br>Max. dose 20 mg<br><br>0.3 mg $kg^{-1}$ buccal<br>Max. dose 10 mg | 30 min | Anxiolytic, amnesic<br>Bitter taste so may need to be disguised in flavoured juice<br>Occasional paradoxical excitation |
| Clonidine | 0.3 mg $kg^{-1}$ oral | 45–60 min | Colourless and tasteless<br>Caution in cardiovascular disease/ instability |
| Ketamine | 3 mg $kg^{-1}$ oral combined with oral midazolam | 10–15 min | |
| Dexmedetomidine | 2 µg $kg^{-1}$ (range 1–4 µg $kg^{-1}$) intranasal or buccal | 25 min | |
| Temazepam | 10 mg used in adolescent age group | 60 min | |

inflammatory markers and chest X-ray (CXR) may be normal in the face of a severe viral URTI.

## Premedication

Perioperative anxiety can be a challenge for the anaesthetic team and cause significant distress for the child and their parent. It is associated with adverse outcomes, including behavioural changes, emergence delirium and enuresis.

The management of perioperative anxiety starts with the APOA. The main concerns are explored and addressed through reassurance and explanation. Several specific strategies can be employed ahead of the admission:

- Information leaflets, videos and the use of hospital and operating theatre tours
- Play therapists
- Psychology in severe cases of perioperative anxiety

Despite a detailed discussion, anxiety on the day of the procedure needs to be anticipated and managed. Play therapists can be extremely helpful, as may:

- Distraction techniques – videos, books, toys, blowing bubbles
- Hypnosis and breathing techniques
- Keeping the anaesthetic room environment calm and quiet, altering the ambient light, playing music and limiting the number of health care professionals present

Even when the aforementioned techniques are used, some children will still require premedication (see Table 7.1). This is more common in:

- Children <4 years of age
- Children requiring multiple GAs
- Children who have had previous traumatic experience
- Children with learning difficulties

Planning for premedication should be discussed with the parent and the child. They should understand the range of responses with the particular drug prescribed and the anticipated time to optimal effect. Once administered, the child should be monitored closely by skilled staff, and resuscitation equipment must be close to hand, such as suction, oxygen, and self-inflating bag-valve-mask.

Sedative premedication may not be appropriate in some clinical conditions:

- Anticipated difficult airway
- Obstructive sleep apnoea (OSA)
- Risk of gastric aspiration
- Obtunded conscious level / raised intracranial pressure
- Acute systemic illness

Other drugs that may be required in the preoperative setting are:

- Topical local anaesthetic agents to facilitate cannulation:
  - 4% tetracaine gel, e.g. Ametop®, effective within 30–45 minutes

- 2.5% prilocaine and 2.5% lidocaine cream, effective after one hour of application and giving up to 120 minutes of topical anaesthesia, e.g. EMLA® or Nulbia®
- Ethyl chloride spray, e.g. Cryogesic®, which causes a reduction in skin sensation within a few seconds of application and lasts for approximately one minute

- Analgesics: ibuprofen and paracetamol can be given orally 30 minutes before GA
- Antimuscarinics may be given before airway surgery
- $H_2$ receptor antagonists, which are rarely given in the paediatric setting but can be used in those at risk of aspiration

## Fasting

In 2018 the APAGBI published a consensus statement, endorsed by many national paediatric anaesthetic societies, to support a change in the fasting guidance for clear fluids from two hours to one hour. The evidence supporting this change includes:

- A two-hour fast is usually significantly longer in practice, commonly six to seven hours and in some cases 15 hours.
- There is increased incidence of thirst, hunger and anxiety with longer fasting times.
- Patients exhibit better behaviour when allowed clear fluids up to one hour before surgery.
- There is less behavioural and metabolic derangement.
- Stomach volumes are low with clear fluids given up to one hour before anaesthesia.

The current guidance is:

- Clear fluids (max 3 ml $kg^{-1}$) can be given up to one hour prior to surgery
- Breast milk up to four hours
- Solid foods and formula milk up to six hours

It is important to remember that there is delayed gastric emptying in a trauma patient, which will be compounded by the use of opioids. In the trauma setting, the gastric contents and volume will be determined by the time between the last food taken before the injury took place. It is prudent to consider an induction technique that allows for the full stomach.

## Prevention of Perioperative Deep Venous Thrombosis (DVT)

The incidence of DVT in children is thought to be 0.05–0.14 per 10,000 of the paediatric population. In hospitalised children, the incidence is higher, quoted as 5–8 per 10,000 admissions. DVT is associated with increased morbidity and mortality, mainly due to the development of pulmonary embolism.

There are two peaks in the incidence of DVT; children <2 years of age, usually associated with central venous access, and adolescents over 13 years of age.

All children over 13 years or >40 kg presenting for surgery should have a DVT risk assessment. Eighty per cent of children developing a DVT will have at least one associated risk factor:

- Immobility
- Obesity
- Malignancy
- Infection
- Presence of central venous catheter: risk for femoral > subclavian > internal jugular lines
- Acquired and congenital thrombophilia
- Sickle cell anaemia
- Oestrogen-containing oral contraceptive pill (OCP)

## Prophylaxis

Immobility is a risk factor for DVT, so early mobilisation should be encouraged when appropriate. Dehydration should be avoided, and any reversible risks factors reduced where possible. Central venous lines should be removed at the earliest opportunity.

Anti-embolic stockings and intermittent pneumatic compression devices should be used in children over 13 years of age or those weighing >40 kg having surgery lasting >1 hour.

The use of thromboprophylaxis with low molecular weight heparin (LMWH) will depend on the number of associated risk factors the child has balanced against the bleeding risk during the surgical procedure. LMWH used in the perioperative period include:

- Enoxaparin
    - 0.75 mg $kg^{-1}$ every 12 hours in children <5 kg
    - 0.5 mg $kg^{-1}$ every 12 hours in children >5 kg

- Dalteparin
  - 75 IU $kg^{-1}$ every 12 hours, in children <5 kg
  - 50 IU $kg^{-1}$ every 12 hours, in children >5 kg

The anti-coagulated child must be monitored closely whilst on LMWH using anti-factor Xa levels. The placement, removal or repositioning of an epidural catheter should occur at least 12 hours after administering standard prophylactic LMWH doses. The care of children on LMWH requires coordinated care with surgeons, anaesthetists, the pain team and haematology.

## Common Medical Conditions of Childhood

Anaesthetists involved in the care of children must have comprehensive knowledge of common medical conditions found in childhood and their impact on anaesthesia. Collaboration between local hospitals and tertiary centres supports anaesthetists delivering paediatric anaesthesia in district general hospitals.

### Obstructive Sleep Apnoea (OSA)

Sleep-disordered breathing describes a spectrum of conditions, ranging from primary snoring through upper-airway resistance syndrome to OSA. OSA is the most serious condition, with the highest associated incidence of perioperative morbidity and mortality. OSA has a prevalence of 1–4% compared to snoring, which is 20%.

Patients with OSA have repeated episodes of airway obstruction and arousal from sleep. In contrast, those with primary snoring do not have apnoea, hypopnoea or gas exchange abnormalities due to compensatory neuromuscular mechanisms to maintain airway patency.

Several conditions can be associated with OSA:

- Adenotonsillar hypertrophy
- Craniofacial abnormalities
- Hypotonia
- Obesity
- Retrognathia and micrognathia
- Midface hypoplasia
- Macroglossia and glossoptosis
- Genetic conditions

It is worth noting that in conditions such as Down syndrome, mucopolysaccharidosis and achondroplasia, there may be airway obstruction at multiple levels.

Untreated OSA can lead to chronic hypoxia, hypercapnia and respiratory acidosis, leading to pulmonary hypertension and cor pulmonale. Chronic hypoxia is an independent risk factor for right-ventricular hypertrophy.

A detailed history may identify signs and symptoms of OSA:

- Snoring or gasping
- Paradoxical breathing
- Apnoea or cyanosis
- Laboured breathing during sleep
- Daytime somnolence
- Headaches
- Poor performance at school
- Enuresis
- Behavioural changes

A child with a history suggestive of OSA may need further diagnostic investigations such as a sleep study, for example polysomnography (PSG), which is the gold standard for the diagnosis and quantitative description of OSA. PSG continuously monitors physiological variables during different sleep phases and can differentiate primary snoring from OSA. It will also provide a more complete description of obstructive events occurring during sleep. Some patients, especially those with neuromuscular conditions, may display a mixed picture of both central and obstructive sleep apnoea.

Apnoea is defined as a decrease in flow by more than 90% for two breaths or more. Hypopnoea is defined as a decrease in flow by more than 50% coupled with a 3% decrease in oxygen saturation or electroencephalographic evidence of arousal.

The apnoea/hypopnoea index (AHI) quantifies the number of apnoeas or hypopnoeas occurring during one hour of sleep and helps to classify the grade of OSA.

Mild OSA has one to five episodes per hour, moderate OSA is 6–10 per hour and severe is >10 per hour.

PSG is expensive and not readily available, so that overnight oximetry may be used instead. It has high specificity but low sensitivity for the diagnosis of OSA. The McGill Oximetry Scoring System measures the number of clusters of oxygen desaturations. A child with severe OSA would have three or more desaturations to <90%. In addition, the oxygen saturation nadir and the ETCO2 gives valuable information about the severity of the OSA.

Children with severe OSA and chronic hypoxia are at significant risk of PHT, RVH and cor pulmonale, and this will require investigation with ECG and ECHO.

The ideal GA for children with OSA is sedative and opioid sparing; they are sensitive to opioids, so the dose will need to be reduced and titrated carefully. Regional anaesthesia should be used when appropriate. Such children are at increased risk of airway obstruction and oxygen desaturation at induction and emergence. The anaesthetist must be prepared for this and be able to safely intervene with airway adjuncts. Those children with OSA and airway anatomy that would raise concerns of a potential difficult intubation require careful planning and preparation.

The immediate postoperative period is also a critical time where they may show signs of ongoing airway obstruction and desaturation. Those children on continuous positive airway pressure (CPAP) or bilevel positive airway pressure (BIPAP) at night should bring their non-invasive ventilators as they may need to be used in the immediate postoperative period.

Day surgery should be avoided due to the risk of postoperative airway obstruction, and overnight monitoring will be required in a ward environment able to manage children on non-invasive ventilation.

## Asthma

Asthma is characterised by reversible airway obstruction, inflammation and bronchial hyper-reactivity; it is associated with an increased risk of perioperative morbidity and mortality due to bronchospasm and hypoxia. Its incidence is increasing worldwide. Despite the additional risk, severe bronchospasm is relatively rare in asthmatics undergoing GA. Most well-controlled asthmatics can be anaesthetised safely.

Asthma is more commonly seen in atopic children, mediated via IgE hypersensitivity. It may also be seen in ex-premature children with a history of intermittent positive pressure ventilation (IPPV), children exposed to passive smoking and other environmental factors.

Not all wheezing is asthmatic; in some children it may be due to post-viral wheeze or tracheobronchomalacia. These groups are at risk of airway hyperreactivity and of developing bronchospasm under GA.

A thorough preoperative assessment is an essential part of preparing an asthmatic child for elective surgery. A detailed history is required to assess how well controlled the child is, focusing on:

- Symptoms: wheeze, usually polyphonic; nocturnal cough causing sleep disturbance; signs of shortness of breath
- Frequency of acute episodes: whether infrequent and short-lived or frequent requiring admission to hospital
- Triggers such as changes in temperature, exercise, animals and URTI
- Effectiveness of current medication
- Compliance with medication
- Who oversees the management: general practitioner (GP) led or under specialist care
- Hospital admissions requiring intubation, ventilation and admission to the paediatric intensive care unit (PICU)
- A recent course of oral steroids to manage exacerbations

Asthmatic children presenting for elective surgery should be medically optimised, and if this is not the case, surgery should be deferred if possible.

### Investigations

Children under five years of age will not have a formal diagnosis of asthma but will be medically managed with inhalers. Some of these children will not have asthma but will have post-viral wheeze, which will get better with time.

A formal diagnosis requires children over the age of five to engage with testing such as spirometry, FeNO and the bronchodilator reversibility test.

### Perioperative Management

There should be meticulous attention to preoperative assessment and medical optimisation. Continuation of medications in the perioperative period is essential with the avoidance of triggers. Despite comprehensive preparation, acute bronchospasm can occur, and the anaesthetist must have a plan to manage this.

Bronchospasm is more likely at induction, during airway management or at extubation. Vagal stimulation during endoscopy, with peritoneal or visceral stretching, or suctioning of the airway can also trigger bronchospasm.

Initial signs include reduced lung compliance with a rising $ETCO_2$ and a characteristic obstructive pattern on the capnograph tracing. Hypoxia may ensue without appropriate treatment.

Management of intraoperative bronchospasm includes:

- Use 100% inspired oxygen.
- Address reversible causes (e.g. endobronchial intubation or carinal irritation).
- Deepen anaesthesia using a volatile agent.
- Administer a short-acting βeta 2 agonist such as salbutamol or ipratropium bromide, either as a metered dose inhaler via an airway adaptor or as a nebuliser.
- Give IV salbutamol 5–15 mcg $kg^{-1}$ or aminophylline 5mg $kg^{-1}$ over 10–15 minutes.
- Use magnesium sulphate IV 40 mg $kg^{-1}$ as a bronchodilator and anti-arrhythmic.
- Administer hydrocortisone 4 mg $kg^{-1}$ IV.
- Resistant bronchospasm may require IV adrenaline 1 mcg $kg^{-1}$.
- Ventilation strategies should include a slow respiratory rate, with a longer expiratory time to allow for increased airway resistance.
- Higher airway pressures will be required, but the balance should be a peak pressure to deliver an adequate tidal volume to allow oxygenation and tolerating moderate hypercapnia.
- Placement of an arterial line may be required as there will be a discrepancy between $ETCO_2$ and $PaCO_2$.

It is important to remember the potential adverse cardiovascular effects of many of these treatments.

Non-asthmatic causes of bronchospasm should also be excluded, such as anaphylaxis or aspiration of gastric contents or foreign body.

## Cystic Fibrosis (CF)

CF is a multi-system autosomal recessive disease with an incidence of 1:2,500, mainly affecting the exocrine glands. It is prevalent in Western Europe, and the UK carrier rate is 1:25. CF is caused by a mutation in a single gene coding for the cystic fibrosis transmembrane regulator (CFTR), which is located on the long arm of chromosome 7. The genetic defect causing CF was first identified in 1989; more than 2,000 mutations of this gene have now been identified.

The CFTR is a chloride channel located at the apical border of the epithelial cells lining most exocrine glands. Disruption in the chloride channel adversely affects the $Na^+/Cl^-$ balance, causing mucus to be viscid and difficult to clear in children with CF.

Since 2007 there has been national neonatal screening for CF, such that most cases are identified early. Despite this, some cases are still not detected until later life. Carrier testing is available as well as antenatal testing.

CF can present in the neonate as bowel obstruction due to meconium ileus. Other presentations include recurrent respiratory tract infections, failure to thrive and malabsorption.

CF is a multi-system disease, but the effects on the respiratory system tend to be the most significant. Progressive lung disease occurs due to reduced clearance of viscid mucus producing patchy atelectasis. Cycles of inflammation and infection follow with associated chronic hypoxia. The lungs become chronically colonised with pathogens, which include Pseudomonas aeruginosa, Staphylococcus aureus, Haemophilus influenzae, Stenotrophomonas maltophilia, Burkholderia cepacia and Aspergillus. CF patients develop chronic airway obstruction and bronchiectasis. End-stage progression leads to pulmonary hypertension, cor pulmonale and death.

The exocrine function of the pancreas is reduced, and pancreatic duct obstruction leads to reduced absorption of essential vitamins. CF patients require lifelong pancreatic enzyme replacement therapy to maintain normal nutrition. Endocrine function is also affected, and CF-related diabetes (CFRD) may occur in adolescence. Other important sequelae of CF include liver disease, including biliary cirrhosis and portal hypertension; infertility; nasal polyps; and osteoporosis.

Treatment aims to minimise respiratory infections, optimise the patient's nutritional status, slow the disease process and offer symptom control.

Children with CF require carefully planned admission for any elective surgery. This should include a recent medical review by the CF team and recent investigations detailing the child's current medical state (full blood count [FBC], coagulation screen, urea and electrolytes [U&Es], liver function tests, blood glucose, CXR, arterial blood gas [ABG] and spirometry).

Before admission, the frequency of chest physio should be increased in anticipation of the admission, and all nebulised medication should be continued in the immediate preoperative period. Respiratory complications are the biggest concern and should be anticipated. Surgical and anaesthetic decisions should be taken to reduce respiratory complications wherever possible. For example, laparoscopic surgery is preferable to open surgery since it will reduce pain and diaphragmatic splinting. Short surgical procedures are tolerated best.

### Anaesthetic Considerations

A detailed APOA is required ahead of elective surgery. Surgery may need to be postponed if there are concerns about intercurrent respiratory infection. Perioperative physiotherapy is essential to help with mucus clearance and minimise the risks of respiratory tract infection in the perioperative period. Oxygen therapy will be required postoperatively, and this should be humidified to help with mucus clearance. Airway management will depend on the length and type of planned surgery. Intubation is tolerated and allows access to toileting of the airway and tighter control on ventilation during the surgical procedure. Postoperatively, these children will generally require an overnight stay and may require admission to PICU depending on their preoperative respiratory status. Those with CFRD will require a perioperative plan detailing how to manage their diabetes. Glycaemic control can be challenging due to steroid medication and potential intercurrent infection.

## Bronchopulmonary Dysplasia (BPD)

This chronic lung disease is one of the most common long-term sequelae of premature birth. Advances in the care of premature babies have significantly improved the course of this condition, including:

- Surfactant
- Antenatal steroids
- Lung-protective ventilation strategies

Babies at risk of developing BPD are usually born between 24–28 weeks gestation. Due to advances in the care of premature babies, the clinical course of 'new' BPD is one of mild respiratory distress syndrome (RDS) with a continued need for supplemental oxygen. There are consistent signs of arrested lung development with a simplified alveolar structure and dysmorphic capillaries. 'New' BPD is classified as mild, moderate or severe depending on the baby's gestational age, their continued need for oxygen beyond 36 weeks and their need for positive pressure ventilator support.

Babies and children with BPD presenting for GA may have sequelae of long-term ventilation, such as tracheobronchomalacia, subglottic stenosis and airway granulomas, and are at risk of:

- Ongoing airway reactivity and obstruction
- Oxygen desaturation
- High peak airway pressures during ventilation and higher $PaCO_2$

They are also at risk of pulmonary hypertension (PHT); this carries a high morbidity and mortality rate under GA and should be actively excluded. Infants requiring continuing ventilatory support, a high oxygen requirement, high $PaCO_2$, cyanotic episodes and failure to thrive are at particular risk of PHT.

The assessment needs to detail the respiratory support required when in NICU (type of ventilatory support, duration, etc.) their current level of ventilatory support and ongoing oxygen requirement. Where there are concerns about PHT, ECG and echocardiography will be necessary.

Patients with BPD may also require regular steroid inhalers and diuretics. Those on diuretics must have hypokalaemia excluded. Those on long-term steroids may require perioperative steroid cover.

## Diabetes Mellitus (DM)

DM is one of the most common metabolic disorders, with approximately 96,000 children under 15 years of age developing type 1 DM annually worldwide. Type 1 DM accounts for 90% of new diagnoses, with type 2 accounting for the remainder. The incidence of DM is increasing annually, and the increase in type 2 DM is associated with rising obesity levels.

The gold standard of care for children with DM is an intensive insulin regime, with differential substitution of basal and prandial insulin aiming to achieve optimal metabolic control. Tight glycaemic control reduces rates of acute and long-term complications.

There are several different diabetic regimes which use a combination of ultra-short-, short- and long-acting insulins to mimic normal physiological insulin release, as closely as possible (see Table 7.2).

**Table 7.2** Types of insulins used in management of type 1 DM

| | | Onset (h) | Peak (h) | Duration (h) |
|---|---|---|---|---|
| Ultra-short | Novorapid®<br>Humalog®<br>Glulisine | <0.5 | 1 | 3–4 |
| Short acting | Actrapid®<br>Humulin S® | 0.5–1 | 2–6 | 3–8 |
| Long acting | Insulatard®<br>Glargine<br>Determine | 3–4<br>2–4<br>2–4 | 4–12<br>None<br>None | 10–20<br>20–24<br>12–18 |
| Mixed | Novomix 30® | 0.5 | 2–6 | 8–10 |

Examples of commonly used insulin regimes include:

- Basal bolus/multiple dose insulin (MDI) regime
- Twice daily insulin – biphasic premixed insulin
- Three times daily dosing
- Continuous subcutaneous insulin infusion (CSII)

All diabetic children need a thorough APOA, which should include a history of their diabetic control, including the frequency of episodes of hypoglycaemia, how they present symptomatically and if diabetic ketoacidosis (DKA) has been a feature of their disease. Preoperative investigations should include FBC, U&E, glucose, HbA1C and urinary glucose/ketones.

Essential perioperative planning includes:

- Multidisciplinary care with preoperative assessment and input from the diabetic team can ensure good perioperative glycaemic control.
- First on the list will help to minimise the risk of excessive fasting.
- Insulin control around the perioperative period will be determined by length of surgery and anticipated time to re-establishing oral intake.
- PONV should be actively managed to give the best chance of returning to normal diet and insulin regime as quickly as possible.
- A multimodal approach to analgesia using regional techniques can minimise the need for opioids, which may increase the chance of PONV.
- Any sign of intercurrent infection should be reviewed and surgery postponed if appropriate.

Each hospital should have a guidance document for the management of the diabetic child presenting for surgery. The principles of the protocol are:

- Avoiding hypoglycaemia and DKA
- Minimising fasting times
- Recognising that children will still require insulin even when fasting
- Ensuring that the child is first on the list if possible
- Maintaining blood glucose at 5–10 mmol $l^{-1}$
- Instigating active treatment if blood glucose is <5 or >14 mmol $l^{-1}$
- Checking blood glucose hourly or more frequently if glycaemic control is difficult
- Checking blood or urine for ketones

## Minor Surgery Guidance

Diabetic children having minor surgery, which is expected to last <90 minutes with no delays to returning to eating and drinking and low risk of PONV, have the following approach to their perioperative insulin:

- Those on MDI take their normal basal dose of insulin.
- Those on an SCII continue on the pump throughout the admission.

Blood glucose must be monitored regularly and a bolus dose of insulin is given if blood sugar is >14 mmol $l^{-1}$. Children are encouraged to eat and drink after surgery and are given their normal dose of rapid-acting insulin with their first postoperative meal. Children who are managed with twice-daily insulin cannot be managed in the same way for minor surgery and are required to follow the guidance for major surgery.

### Major Surgery Guidance

Diabetic children on MDI or twice-daily insulin having planned major surgery stop their normal basal insulin dose before surgery and commence on a variable rate insulin infusion (VRII) along with maintenance fluids (5% dextrose/0.45% saline/0.15% KCl) at the same time (see Table 7.3). Those on an SCII should have the pump stopped two hours prior to surgery and have a VRII started at the same time as the pump is stopped. Blood glucose should be checked hourly and the VRII altered according to the child's blood glucose result.

In an emergency setting, it is important to contact the diabetic team to guide perioperative management. DKA can present with signs of an acute abdomen, so DKA must be excluded; if present, treatment should follow the DKA protocol. Emergency surgery should be delayed until hypovolaemia and electrolyte deficit has been corrected. The management and rehydration of a child with DKA need to be done carefully and slowly with isotonic fluids.

## Adrenal Insufficiency (AI)

Many children presenting for surgery will have adrenal insufficiency due to primary, secondary or tertiary causes, as detailed in Table 7.4.

These children are at increased risk of adrenal crisis in the perioperative period. Any child at risk of adrenal insufficiency needs a detailed history identifying the cause of the AI and their regular management regime when the child is well. If the child has had an adrenal crisis, this should be documented, detailing the background and management. Children with AI will have a rescue regime, which they follow when they are unwell, as in sickness, infection or trauma. Any admission should be made in close consultation with the child's endocrinologist.

The following key points should be adhered to:

- The plan should be medically optimised and discussed with the endocrine team to agree on the perioperative steroid plan.
- Test preoperative FBC, U&Es and blood glucose.
- Regular steroid medication should continue uninterrupted.

**Table 7.3** VRII regime (50 units of actrapid insulin in 50 mls of 0.9% saline to give a concentration of 1 u $ml^{-1}$)[a]

| Blood glucose mmol $l^{-1}$ | Insulin infusion rate units $kg^{-1}$ $h^{-1}$ |
|---|---|
| <4 mmol $l^{-1}$ | 0.01 |
| 4–6.9 mmol $l^{-1}$ | 0.02 |
| 7–8.9 mmol $l^{-1}$ | 0.03 |
| 9–12 mmol $l^{-1}$ | 0.04 |
| >12 mmol $l^{-1}$ | 0.05 |

*Note:* [a] The infusion regime needs to be monitored closely and may need altering in the setting of severely ill children or those on steroid medication. Do not stop the infusion if the blood glucose is <4 mmol $l^{-1}$, as this will cause rebound hyperglycaemia. The insulin rate should be reduced further and the glucose infusion increased to return blood glucose to normal level.

**Table 7.4** Classification of adrenal insufficiency

| Classification of adrenal insufficiency (AI) | Underlying causes |
|---|---|
| Primary AI | Abnormalities of the adrenal gland<br>Most common cause in childhood being congenital adrenal hyperplasia (CAH)<br>Incidence 1:8–10,000 |
| Secondary AI | Abnormalities of the hypothalamus +/– pituitary, e.g. congenital disorders of the hypothalamus +/– pituitary or acquired as a consequence of brain tumour |
| Tertiary AI | Long-term treatment with glucocorticoids with suppression of the hypothalamic–pituitary–adrenal axis – any child taking more than 10–15 mg $m^{-2}$ hydrocortisone equivalent per day for more than a month regardless of the route of administration.<br>Asthma, juvenile chronic arthritis, renal disease, inflammatory bowel disease (IBD), Duchenne muscular dystrophy (DMD) |

- The patient should be first on the list to minimise dehydration.
- Administer IV bolus of hydrocortisone 2 mg $kg^{-1}$ at induction. Major cases can be followed by either a hydrocortisone infusion or four-hourly boluses of hydrocortisone (see 'Further Reading').
- Particular attention should be given to glycaemic control.
- Dexamethasone has no mineralocorticoid action.

CAH is a group of autosomal recessive disorders characterised by abnormal cortisol synthesis. Consequently, children with CAH will have absent cortisol production, elevated levels of ACTH and abnormal production of androgen and mineralocorticoid hormones. Children with CAH require lifelong treatment with glucocorticoids and, depending on the cause of their CAH, mineralocorticoid may also be required. Glucocorticoids replace the deficient cortisol but also help to suppress excess androgen production (see Table 7.5).

The primary goal of treating classical CAH is to reduce the excess androgen production and replace deficient hormones. Proper treatment with the correct dosage of these hormones is crucial in preventing adrenal crisis and virilisation.

Deficiency of 21-hydroxylase is the most common cause of CAH and is responsible for 95% of all CAH cases. The remaining 5% of cases of CAH are caused by other essential enzymes required in cortisol biosynthesis such as 11-beta–hydroxylase. CAH can be classified into classical CAH and non-classical CAH.

Classical CAH due to 21-hydroxylase deficiency can be subdivided into two groups. In the salt-losing form (accounting for 75% of classic CAH), not only is there absent cortisol production but also reduced production of aldosterone, with associated problems with fluid and salt regulation. A concomitant increase in androgen production can present with over-virilisation and ambiguous genitalia in females born with CAH. The simple virilising group accounts for 25% of classic CAH and does not have deficient aldosterone production, so there is normal regulation of fluid and salts.

Children with CAH are at risk of adrenal crisis, electrolyte abnormalities and altered glycaemic control. Stressors such as intercurrent infection or surgery can increase their requirements of these essential hormones. All children with CAH will have a rescue regime for steroid replacement during periods of increased demand and should be reviewed preoperatively by their endocrine team, which can advise on the best perioperative management of their steroid requirements. Normal steroid medication should not be interrupted preoperatively, and they will require additional steroid cover at induction, usually 2 mg $kg^{-1}$ of IV hydrocortisone, repeated every four hours. Some children will require a hydrocortisone infusion. All children with classical CAH should be reviewed preoperatively to ensure that their endocrine team is aware of the planned surgery and can advise on the best perioperative management of their steroid requirements.

The AAGBI has published comprehensive guidance on the management of adults and children requiring glucocorticoids in the perioperative period. See 'Further Reading'.

**Table 7.5** Glucocorticoids and their equivalent doses

| 1 mg of prednisolone is equivalent to: | |
|---|---|
| Dexamethasone | 150 mcg |
| Betamethasone | 150 mcg |
| Methylprednisolone | 800 mcg |
| Triamcinolone | 800 mcg |
| Deflazacort | 1.2 mg |
| Hydrocortisone | 4 mg |

## Obesity

Childhood obesity is a major health concern, with one in three children in the United Kingdom being obese by the age of nine. The WHO has estimated that in 2019 38 million children under 5 and more than 340 million children and adolescents aged between 5 and 19 were overweight or obese.

In most cases, obesity is preventable, stemming from excessive calorie intake and physical inactivity. Secondary causes, linked to genetic syndromes such as Prader–Willi, endocrine or neurological disorders or medication related, are rare but important to exclude.

### Defining Obesity in Childhood

The simple application of BMI (kg $m^{-2}$) in isolation to define obesity in children can be misleading as growth is highly variable, particularly in young children. WHO gender-specific body mass index (BMI) growth charts are considered the gold standard for defining obesity in childhood. In children under five, obesity is defined as having a BMI >3 standard deviation (SD) above the median; in older children, obesity is defined as having a BMI >2 SD above the median. The WHO growth charts may also be used to determine the ideal body weight (IBW) for that child, which may be helpful for perioperative drug dosing.

Children who are obese have an increased perioperative risk due to a higher incidence of:

- Hypertension
- OSA and PHT
- Asthma
- Insulin dependent type 2 DM
- GORD

Preoperative assessment should identify and investigate these associated risk factors. Investigations should include:

- Blood pressure (BP) and ECG
- FBC, U&Es, cholesterol and blood glucose
- Sleep study
- ECHO
- IBW calculation

If GORD is a significant problem, appropriate medications should be commenced in advance.

Preoperative consideration must be given to the theatre environment, including the weight limit of the theatre table and having manual handling equipment available. Careful positioning is very important to minimise the risk of pressure sores and nerve injury.

It is well recognised that obese children are at increased risk of perioperative respiratory complications, including laryngospasm, bronchospasm and oxygen desaturation due to reduced FRC, forced vital capacity (FVC) and lung compliance. The abnormal respiratory mechanics are accentuated in the supine position when the abdominal contents exert greater pressure on the diaphragm. Mask ventilation can be difficult, and an oral or nasal airway adjunct may be necessary. Where possible, all obese children should be preoxygenated, and it is generally considered safer to intubate obese children, even for short surgical procedures.

Drug administration can be problematic, as obesity results in variations in the pharmacokinetics and pharmacodynamics of many drugs. Obesity increases the volume of distribution, particularly for lipophilic drugs, and can alter drug clearance and elimination half-life. Renal clearance is higher in obesity, increasing linearly with lean body weight (LBW) rather than total body weight (TBW).

Consequently, there are recommendations for some drugs to be administered according to TBW, such as succinylcholine, whilst others such as propofol, rocuronium and morphine may be more appropriately based on IBW or LBW:

$$LBW = IBW + 0.3\ x\ (TBW - IBW)$$

However, very few studies have been undertaken on obesity-related pharmacokinetic changes in children, and these recommendations are largely extrapolated from adult studies.

In practice, most anaesthetic drugs can be administered titrated to effect, which will usually be less than a TBW dose. In an emergency, succinylcholine should be administered at a dose of 1mg $kg^{-1}$.

# Haemoglobinopathies

## Sickle Cell Anaemia

SCD is a congenital haemoglobinopathy caused by a mutation on chromosome 11. This mutation results in an amino acid substitution on the beta-globin subunit leading to the formation of HbS. HbS is unstable and can precipitate out of solution when in the deoxygenated state forming the classical sickle or curved red cell. SCD is most commonly found in Africa, Southeast Asia, the Middle East and parts of the Mediterranean. The heterozygous state is protective against *Plasmodium falciparum*, and the distribution of SCD closely matches the distribution of malaria worldwide.

Since 2006, all newborns in the United Kingdom have been tested for SCD as part of their neonatal blood spot screening. The incidence of SCD in England in 2021 was 1:2,000 live births.

SCD has an autosomal recessive pattern of inheritance. Those that are heterozygous have SCT and produce both HbA and HbS. The proportion of HbS is approximately 30–40%. Those with SCT have a more benign disease and only show signs of sickling when under extreme physiological conditions, for example when their oxygen saturations are approximately 40% or during cooling for cardiopulmonary bypass surgery.

The homozygous state (HbSS) has almost 100% HbS, which is a serious life-limiting condition associated with:

- Chronic haemolytic anaemia, due to a reduced red cell life span in SCD of 12 days (versus 120 days for normal red cells)
- Vaso-occlusive disease affecting particularly the bones, extremities, bowel and lungs
- End organ failure
- Severe pain
- Premature death

Sickling in patients with HbSS can be triggered by hypoxia, hypothermia, infection and dehydration.

Surgery in patients with SCD requires meticulous planning, optimisation and input from haematology from the beginning. Clinical history should include the number of acute crises, their triggers and how they were managed, treatment to date and a detailed transfusion history. End organ disease should be investigated appropriately and documented (see Table 7.6).

Patients with SCD will be on folic acid due to the high cell turnover rate. They should be vaccinated against *Strep pneumoniae, Neisseria meningitides,* Hepatitis B, *Haemophilus influenza* Type B; they may be on a penicillin to reduce the chance of infection with pneumococcus. Hydroxycarbamide is used to increase the levels of HbF, which reduces the episodes of sickling and the need for transfusion. Those on hydroxycarbamide may be at risk of neutropenia, so this should be considered as part of the preoperative investigations.

Baseline investigations should include:

- FBC, U&Es and liver function tests (LFTs)
- Hb electrophoresis to quantify the percentage of HbS
- Crossmatch and antibody screening
- CXR
- Echocardiogram
- Spirometry to assess lung function
- Neurological assessment if there is a history of stroke – transcranial Doppler or MRI may be recommended

Patients with SCD are at risk of sickling in the perioperative period. Preoperative exchange transfusion may be indicated, depending on the type of surgery and Hb level. If undertaken, it should be done well in advance, overseen by haematology, aiming for a Hb of 100 g $l^{-1}$ and a HbSS of <30%. To avoid hyperviscosity, the Hb should not increase by more than 40 g $l^{-1}$ in a single transfusion.

Principles of perioperative care for those with SCD include the following:

- Avoid hypovolaemia – consider admitting the night before for IV fluids, encourage oral fluids until one hour before surgery.

**Table 7.6** Clinical impact of SCD

| End organ | Impact of SCD |
|---|---|
| Cardiac | Cardiomegaly and congestive cardiac failure due to anaemia and pulmonary hypertension |
| Respiratory | Multiple pulmonary infarcts leading to pulmonary hypertension<br>Acute chest syndrome<br>OSA |
| Gastrointestinal | Splenomegaly with splenic sequestration and acute drops on haematocrit and platelets<br>Functional asplenism with risk of infection<br>Gallstones<br>Hepatic enlargement but usually with maintained hepatic function |
| Central nervous system (CNS) | Increased incidence of transient ischemic attack (TIA), thrombotic and haemorrhagic stroke |
| Renal | Renal impairment and painful priapism |
| Infections | Prone to infections<br>Parvovirus leading to hypoplastic crisis |
| Bones | Avascular necrosis<br>Extramedullary haematopoiesis – frontal bossing, enlarged maxilla with potential for difficulty in managing the airway |
| Haematology | Bone marrow failure<br>Haemolytic anaemia, hypoplastic anaemia |

- Maintain oxygenation – this may require supplemental oxygen to maintain $SpO_2$ > 95% postoperatively.
- Maintain normocarbia and avoid respiratory acidosis.
- Avoid hypothermia and acidosis.
- Avoid using vasoconstrictors.
- Minimise use of tourniquets (as explained in the following text).

The use of tourniquets is controversial, with concern around ischaemia of the limb distal to the tourniquet and sickling due to acidosis and release of vaso-active substrates when the tourniquet is released. The decision to not use a tourniquet needs to be weighed against the risk of sickling triggered by significant blood loss from major surgery. If a tourniquet is used, the limb must be fully exsanguinated, and there needs to be meticulous attention to the patient's acid/basis status and volume status. As always, the tourniquet time should be minimised.

Analgesia should be multimodal, using regional techniques where appropriate to minimise opioid use. If using opioids, the patient must be monitored to ensure they are well oxygenated, receiving supplemental oxygen if required. Patients with SCD having major or emergency surgery or those with significant end organ disease, such as significant OSA or PHT, are best looked after in a critical care setting.

## Thalassaemia

This is a group of hereditary anaemias, which are caused by defective synthesis of the alpha chain (alpha thalassaemia) or the beta chain (beta thalassaemia) of haemoglobin.

Beta thalassaemia is due to deletion or mutations in the HBB gene located on chromosome 11. The worldwide prevalence of symptomatic beta thalassaemia is thought to be 1:100,000. It is most commonly seen in the Middle East, Southeast Asia, India and China.

There are three forms of beta thalassaemia, depending on the inheritance: beta thalassaemia minor (or trait), intermedia and major. Children who are heterozygous for beta thalassaemia are said to have beta thalassaemia minor or trait and are either asymptomatic or show very mild anaemia. Those with homozygous inheritance have beta thalassaemia major, also known as Cooley's anaemia. In the most severe form, children present with microcytic, hypochromic anaemia and signs of extramedullary haematopoiesis. Treatment depends on the severity of the anaemia but may include oral supplementation with folic acid or regular blood transfusions combined with oral chelating agents.

Alpha thalassaemia is prevalent in Southeast Asia with an incidence of 1:10,000 compared to an incidence in Northern Europe of 1:1,000,000. Those who are heterozygous for the condition have alpha thalassaemia trait and can be asymptomatic or have very mild anaemia. Those who are homozygous exhibit a more severe phenotype, featuring a microcytic, hypochromic anaemia that may require blood transfusions and other supportive measures.

Children with thalassaemia require preoperative investigations to assess the extent of the disease. Those with severe phenotypes who require regular blood transfusions are at risk of iron overload, so an assessment of their cardiac status, including an ECHO, will be required preoperatively. Extramedullary hematopoiesis may lead to facial changes due to medullary hyperplasia, and this may make laryngoscopy more difficult.

## Glucose-6-Phosphate Dehydrogenase (G6PD) Deficiency

Glucose-6-phosphate dehydrogenase (G6PD) is a housekeeping enzyme expressed in all cells where it catalyses the first step in the pentose phosphate pathway. In red blood cells, this is the sole pathway for the production of NADPH, which is required to maintain glutathione in a reduced state. Failure of this process impairs the ability of the red cell to deal with oxidative stress, which may lead to haemolytic episodes and anaemia that can be severe and, in some cases, fatal.

G6PDd is the most common red blood cell (RBC) enzymopathy in humans, with a global prevalence of 400 million people. There are nearly 200 mutations identified, but a few mutations account for most cases. The most common is the Mediterranean variant, followed by the African (G6PDd – A), Indian and Southeast Asian variants.

The magnitude of enzyme deficiency determines the severity of disease: Class I variants have severe enzyme deficiency with chronic non-spherocytic haemolytic anaemia (<10% residual enzyme activity), Class II variants also have severe enzyme deficiency (<10% residual enzyme activity) but with intermittent acute haemolysis and Class III variants have moderate enzyme deficiency (10–60% residual enzyme activity) with intermittent acute haemolysis. Class IV and V variants are of no clinical significance – Class IV has no enzyme deficiency, and Class V has increased enzyme activity.

Perioperative care is determined by the type of deficiency the patient has. Patients with G6PD deficiency should not have elective surgery during a haemolytic episode or in the presence of intercurrent infection, which is known to be a potential trigger. Preoperative blood tests should include FBC, LFTs, reticulocyte count, lactate dehydrogenase (LDH) and haptoglobins.

Potential triggers of oxidative stress should be minimised. Measures include avoiding dehydration due to excessive fasting and addressing perioperative anxiety. Intraoperative temperature and glycaemic control should be monitored closely. It is important to be aware of other triggers in this patient group, such as:

- Fava beans
- Dapsones
- Antimalarials, such as primaquine
- Methylene blue
- Nitrofurantoin
- Quinolones, such as ciprofloxacin
- Sulphonamides, such as co-trimoxazole

## Coagulation Disorders

Whilst relatively rare, congenital disorders of coagulation may pose challenges in the perioperative period. Haematology advice should be sought where appropriate.

Von Willebrand disease (VWD) is the most common congenital coagulation disorder. It is caused by a qualitative or quantitative deficiency of von Willebrand factor (VWF), required for platelet aggregation and adhesion. VWF also helps maintain the levels of factor VIII as it acts as a carrier for this factor and in doing so reduces factor VIII clearance.

The incidence is 1:100, with the vast majority of those afflicted being asymptomatic. It is only clinically significant in 1:10,000 patients. VWD has variable autosomal inheritance (dominant or recessive) depending on the subtype. Type 1 VWD is a mild form of the disease due to qualitative deficiency of VWD, type 2 has several subtypes and there is both qualitative and quantitative reduction in VWF. Type 3 is the most severe form as there is no VWF.

Perioperative management depends on the type of VWD. Desmopressin (1-desamino-8-D-arginine vasopressin, DDAVP) works by stimulating the release of VWF and can be used in VWD type 1. Type 3 VWD requires replacement of VWF and factor VIII, with the addition of platelet transfusion if bleeding persists despite replacement of these factors.

Haemophilia can be classified as haemophilia type A, B or C depending on the deficiency of factors VIII, IX or XI, respectively. Haemophilia type A and B are inherited as X-linked recessive disorders, so males are affected, whilst females are carriers. The incidence of haemophilia A is 1:5,000–10,000. Haemophilia B is rarer with an incidence of 1:35,000–50,000.

In the perioperative period, children with haemophilia require replacement of the deficient factor VIII or IX. They should also be assessed for the presence of inhibitors to factor VIII, and if they are present, treatment with recombinant activated factor VII (rFVIIa) or factor VIII inhibitor bypassing activity (FEIBA) may be required.

Preoperatively, patients with inherited coagulation disorders need:

- Detailed history of the underlying condition, type of coagulation disorder and its severity
- History of previous bleeding episodes and their management
- Response to DDAVP, factors VIII and IX
- baseline bloods – FBC, coagulation screen, factor assay, fibrinogen level
- An MDT approach with involvement from haematology, surgery and anaesthesia
- A perioperative plan detailing the management of the coagulation disorder – use of DDAVP, tranexamic acid, recombinant factors or plasma

## Epilepsy

Epilepsy is the most common neurological condition of childhood, with an incidence of 0.5–1% of the paediatric population. The incidence is highest in the first year of life and 1:150 children will be diagnosed before the age of 10. The incidence appears to be declining in high-income countries.

Primary or idiopathic epilepsy has a genetic predisposition with a 1.5–3% risk with paternal inheritance and a 3–9% risk with maternal inheritance. Secondary epilepsy is due to pre-, peri- and postnatal causes. Prenatal causes of epilepsy include inborn errors of metabolism and chromosomal abnormalities, such as trisomy 21. Prenatal infections and congenital malformations such as tuberous sclerosis and neurofibromatosis can also be a cause.

Perinatal causes include hypoglycaemia, hypocalcaemia, hypoxic ischaemia events and intraventricular haemorrhage, which are more commonly found in premature babies. Postnatal events such as infections, including meningitis, cerebral abscess, trauma due to non-accidental injury, or malignancy, can all cause the development of epilepsy.

Seizures can be either partial (focal) or generalised. Partial seizures can show motor, sensory or autonomic characteristics depending on the region of the cerebral cortex from which they originate. In a generalised seizure, there is bilateral symmetrical electrical activity with associated generalised muscle contractions. Seizures are defined as simple when there is no loss of consciousness and complex when consciousness is lost. Infantile spasm, myoclonic seizures and benign partial seizures are very specific to the paediatric population.

Children with epilepsy will be on anti-epileptic drugs (AEDs). The type of drug will depend on the type of seizure, frequency, age of child and side effect profile of the AED. AEDs have significant drug interactions and side effects. Commonly used AEDs such as phenytoin and carbamazepine are hepatic enzyme inducers. Some are also hepatotoxic and can cause thrombocytopenia and platelet abnormalities, such as sodium valproate and carbamazepine. It is therefore important to understand the side effect profile of the AEDs the child is on and check this preoperatively.

Several anaesthetic agents produce epileptiform EEG activity (sevoflurane) or are proconvulsant (ketamine and alfentanil). Ketamine and alfentanil should be avoided, but sevoflurane can be used despite the epileptiform activity that is part of the pharmacological profile.

Children with epilepsy should have a detailed history and examination focusing on:

- Type of seizures, triggers, frequency and duration
- How well controlled the seizures are
- What AEDs the child is currently on – what side effects, if any, has the child had
- What rescue medication the family has and how often is this being given to the child

In the elective setting, the child's seizures should be optimally controlled, but this may not be possible in the child presenting with multiple drug-resistant seizures. Continuing medication in the perioperative period is essential. If there is any anticipated delay to returning to oral intake, then a parenteral form of the AED should be started with the guidance of the neurology team.

A ketogenic diet which is high in fat and low in protein and carbohydrate is used in children with intractable epilepsy or those who struggle with the side effects of AEDs. There are several important issues to consider:

- Avoid IV fluid containing glucose as this may precipitate a relapse in seizure control.
- Neonates and ex-prems are at risk of hypoglycaemia – in this setting, IV glucose should be used and closely monitored to maintain blood glucose within normal limits.
- Monitor the blood sugar perioperatively and aim to keep the glucose level between 3–4 mmol $l^{-1}$.
- Avoid Ringer's lactate as this can compound a metabolic acidosis.
- Urinary ketones should be monitored and kept in the range of 8–16 mmol $l^{-1}$.
- Acid-base status should be monitored regularly along with the blood glucose level.

## Cerebral Palsy (CP)

CP is the most common motor disorder in children. It describes a diverse group of permanent neurological disorders characterised by varying degrees of sensory, motor or intellectual impairment.

The incidence of cerebral palsy (2:1000 live births) has changed little over the past 30–40 years despite improvements in antenatal care. This has been attributed to increased survival rates in premature babies who have a significantly higher incidence (10–50 times higher) of CP. Eighty per cent of cases develop antenatally, and 20% develop postnatally in the first two years of life. In 30% of cases, no significant abnormality can be identified.

The classification is based on a description of the resting muscle tone – spastic, (accounting for

**Table 7.7** Summary of clinical issues with the child with CP

| Affected system | Clinical Issues |
| --- | --- |
| Respiratory | Scoliosis with restrictive lung disease – pulmonary hypertension and cor pulmonale at the extreme<br>Respiratory impairment due to chronic aspiration and weak respiratory muscles<br>Chronic lung disease (CLD) due to neonatal RDS<br>Reduced cough |
| Cardiovascular | Difficult to assess exercise tolerance due to limited mobility |
| Gastrointestinal | Poor nutrition due to reduced ability to chew and swallow – combination of oro-motor dysfunction and pseudobulbar palsies<br>Unsafe swallow<br>GORD<br>Malnutrition with anaemia and electrolyte abnormalities |
| Temperature control | Large surface area to body mass, underweight, reduced subcutaneous fat, thin skin and atrophic muscles |
| Musculoskeletal | Spasticity, contractures leading to deformity and dislocation<br>Pain and issues with mobilising and or sitting and positioning are commonplace |

80% of children with CP) dyskinetic, ataxic and mixed. The Gross Motor Function Classification System (GMFCS) is used to characterise different levels of function with the emphasis on the child's ability rather than their disability. A child with GMFCS level 1 can walk unaided and has gross motor skills but will have issues with speed, balance and coordination. At the other end of the scale, a child with GMFCS level 5 will be wheelchair dependent and have issues with anti-gravity control of the head and trunk.

It is important to remember that in the most severe form, CP can have a wide-reaching impact on the patient's neurological, musculoskeletal, gastrointestinal, respiratory and urological function. The patient needs to be medically optimised with careful consideration of the child's physiological status.

## Preoperative Considerations

Assessing the child's intellectual and cognitive level is an essential part of the preparation. This ensures that they have as much input to the process as possible. The child's parents or carers will be invaluable in the perioperative period as they usually have expert knowledge of the child's chronic medical conditions and how best to communicate with them. Children with CP can have significant deformities such as scoliosis and limb deformities, and the parents or carers will be able to guide positioning and support of the child.

Table 7.7 summarises the key clinical issues that should be reviewed and considered. Many children with CP will be on several drugs, including anti-epileptics, antispasmodics, antisialogues, analgesics, proton pump inhibitors/antacids and antibiotics. It is important that these medications are continued in the perioperative period to avoid acute withdrawal, which can present with worsening seizure control or muscle spasms.

Anxiety in the perioperative period can be an issue due to the child being unable to communicate easily or because of previous bad experiences. Sedative premedication needs to be used with caution in CP patients with significant hypotonia.

Preoperative investigations need to be considered as many CP patients have significant comorbidity. Recent blood tests including FBC and U&E, are usually required. Other investigations, such as CXR and more detailed assessment of respiratory status, should be considered where appropriate.

Analgesia is a key consideration. A multimodal approach including regional techniques should be used where appropriate. The impact of opioids on the respiratory system should be considered, incorporating appropriate monitoring and titration to effect. Postoperative spasms can be an issue in children with CP and require anti-spasmodics such as diazepam or midazolam to avoid the cycles of spasm precipitating pain. A careful balance is required to reduce pain and muscle spasms without compromising respiratory function.

## Renal Failure

The UK Renal Registry (UKRR), in its 22nd annual report, quotes the incidence of children requiring long-term treatment for kidney failure as nine in every 1 million of the UK's child population. The majority are aged between 12 and 16 years. In 50% of cases, there is an abnormality of the structure of the kidneys and urinary tract that has been there since birth, such as renal agenesis. Other causes include glomerular disorders and inherited/familial conditions, such as Alport syndrome or polycystic kidney disease (PKD).

There are five stages of chronic kidney disease (CKD). Children in stage 1 have a normal glomerular filtration rate (GFR; normal >90 ml $min^{-1}$ per 1.73 $m^2$) but have evidence of kidney damage, such as proteinuria. Those in stage 5 are in established renal failure and have a GFR of <15 or are on a form of dialysis.

CKD is a multisystem disease. Children in CKD stages I–III are generally asymptomatic, with symptoms evolving as renal function declines.

Children presenting with CKD or chronic renal failure (CRF) require a detailed history and assessment, specifically addressing:

- The underlying cause of CRF
- Whether the child is anuric and at risk of fluid overload or oliguric and at risk of hypovolaemia
- Their normal fluid balance – 'dry' and 'wet' weight
- Current management, such as peritoneal or haemodialysis and any complications of these treatments to date
- Suitability for transplantation
- Cardiovascular complications – hypertension, left-ventricular hypertrophy (LVH), uraemic pericarditis, uraemic cardiomyopathy, congestive cardiac failure (CCF) and pulmonary oedema
- Pleural effusions and diaphragmatic splinting in those on peritoneal dialysis
- Peripheral and autonomic neuropathy
- Altered biochemistry – hyperkalaemia and risk of dysrhythmia and arrest, hypocalcaemia
- Metabolic acidosis
- Gastrointestinal disease – uraemic induced anorexia and gastroparesis and delayed gastric emptying
- Normochromic, normocytic anaemia due to reduced erythropoietin production and uraemic bone marrow suppression
- Whether the condition is part of a syndrome, in which case other aspects of the disease need to be considered
- The psychological impact of chronic disease

Preoperative investigations should include FBC, coagulation screen, U&Es, GFR, ECG and ECHO +/– CXR.

## Perioperative Considerations

Nephrologists are central to the perioperative care of these children. All normal medication should be continued. The fluid status of the child and the timing of the last haemodialysis (HD) sessions is important. Ideally, surgery should wait for four to six hours after dialysis to allow fluid shifts to settle and take into consideration the use of heparin during HD. In an emergency setting, HD can be done with minimal or no heparin to expedite surgery postdialysis. Premedication with antacids should be considered as well as anxiolytics.

Induction should consider the potential of delayed gastric emptying, so a modified rapid sequence induction may be required. Alterations in pharmacokinetics need to be recognised and drug dosing altered accordingly. Vascular access can be challenging, and central venous access may be required. It is prudent to avoid, if possible, vascular access at the wrist or elbow of the non-dominant hand as arteriovenous fistulas may be required for HD.

**Key Points**

- APOA in advance of admission is the standard of care.
- Side effects and risks need to be discussed in advance and supported by written or electronic information leaflets.
- Perioperative MDTs should be held to discuss high-risk patients and agree on ceilings of care.
- A new murmur which is heard in systole, pansystolic or early diastole, associated with clinical signs or ventricular hypertrophy confirmed on ECG, requires a cardiology review prior to a general anaesthetic.
- Children can drink water up to one hour before GA.

- Poorly controlled asthmatics who have had a recent URTI are at increased risk of bronchospasm, and elective surgery should be deferred.
- Infants with BPD are at increased risk of airway hyperreactivity and PHT in extreme cases.
- Acute illness can precipitate DKA and can have a similar presentation to an acute abdomen. Ketoacidosis should be excluded.
- Coagulation disorders require specific management of the underlying condition.
- The prevalence of obesity is increasing, and comorbidities associated with obesity can present in adolescence.
- Epileptics on a ketogenic diet should avoid dextrose containing IV fluids and should have close monitoring of the blood glucose, which should be kept between 3–4 mmol $l^{-1}$.

## Further Reading

Association of Paediatric Anaesthetists of Great Britain and Ireland (APAGBI). Guidelines on the peri-operative management of patients with sickle cell disease. *Anaesthesia* 2021; 76(6):805–17. https://doi.org/10.1111/anae.15349.

AAGBI. Preassessment services for children undergoing surgery or procedures. Spring 2022. Available at: www.apagbi.org.uk/sites/default/files/2022-05/Best%20Practice_Preassessment%20standards%20in%20Children%20%202022%20-%20Published.pdf. Accessed 21 April 2024.

Haché M, Sun LS, Gadi G et al. Outcomes from Wake Up Safe, the pediatric anesthesia quality improvement initiative. *Paediatric Anaesthesia* 2020; 30 (12):1348–54.

International Society for Pediatric and Adolescent Diabetes. 2018. ISPAD clinical practice consensus guidelines. Available at: www.ispad.org/general/custom.asp?page=ISPADGuidelines2018. Accessed 21 April 2024.

Masaracchia MM, Lee M, Dalesio NM. Obesity in childhood. *BJA Education* 2022; 22(5):168–75. https://doi.org/10.1016/j.bjae.2021.12.003.

Morgan J, Checketts M, Arana A et al. Prevention of perioperative venous thromboembolism in pediatric patients: guidelines from the Association of Paediatric Anaesthetists of Great Britain and Ireland (APAGBI). *Paediatric Anaesthesia* 2018; 28(5):382–91.

National Institute for Health and Care Excellence Asthma. 2021. Diagnosis, monitoring and chronic asthma management. Available at: Asthma: diagnosis, monitoring and chronic asthma management - PubMed (nih.gov). Accessed 21 April 2024.

Thomas M, Morrison C, Newton R, Schindler E. Consensus statement on clear fluids fasting for elective pediatric general anesthesia. *Paediatric Anaesthesia* 2018; 28(5):411–4. https://doi.org/10.1111/pan.13370.

Chapter 8

# Congenital and Inherited Disorders Affecting Anaesthesia in Children

Nargis Ahmad

## Introduction

Children with congenital anomalies or inherited metabolic disorders can present a challenge to the paediatric anaesthetist. An encyclopaedic knowledge of these conditions, however desirable, is unrealistic for most practising paediatric anaesthetists. For some of these rare disorders, the evidence base is limited to single case reports or small series describing the conduct of anaesthesia. This synopsis will outline general principles and include some of the more common conditions. For the rarer anomalies, the reader should consult a more comprehensive text or one of the web-based resources, such as UpToDate®, Orphan Anesthesia and the Online Mendelian Inheritance in Man® database accessible via the National Center for Biotechnology Information (NCBI) website.

## General Points

The classification of many conditions has its basis in phenotypes with inheritance patterns observed and described. Great progress has been made in understanding the genetic basis of many congenital anomalies, and it is clear that phenotypic and genetic heterogeneity are common.

## Preoperative Assessment

A systematic approach to preoperative assessment provides a useful filter to identify aspects of relevance to anaesthesia. Any involvement of the airway, the cardiovascular and respiratory system merit close scrutiny. In some conditions, there may be endocrine or metabolic issues that need to be considered, such as glucose and steroid management. Limb abnormalities or fragile skin require careful assessment for potential sites for vascular access and also for protection of skin and joints during positioning.

Many conditions are associated with dysmorphic features, abnormal growth parameters, developmental delay and learning disability. These should be identified during the preoperative assessment. The behavioural implications of any congenital or inherited disorder should always be considered preoperatively. Some conditions are associated with seizures, in which case it is important to note the nature of the seizures and how well these are controlled.

The family will often provide a wealth of useful information about their child. Families may have accessed web-based resources extensively and have joined condition-specific support groups. It is not uncommon for them to be more knowledgeable about the syndrome and its ramifications than non-specialist clinical staff. Some of these children undergo a number of surgical procedures; previous anaesthetic records should always be reviewed.

## Airway

Airway assessment can help predict whether difficulty in airway management, direct laryngoscopy and intubation may be encountered. Assessment should include consideration of the nasal passages; mouth opening; oropharynx, including palate, tongue, maxilla, mandible and mandibular space; temporomandibular joint; and cervical spine.

Some disorders distort the normal anatomy of the bones and soft tissues associated with the airway. Some examples follow:

- Maxillary hypoplasia, such as Apert syndrome (a syndrome with associated craniosynostosis)
- Mandibular hypoplasia, such as Pierre Robin sequence
- Mandibular and maxillary hypoplasia, such as Treacher–Collins syndrome
- Hemifacial microsomia, for example Goldenhar syndrome

- Mucopolysaccharidoses (MPS) with thickened, stiff, abnormal soft tissues
- Macroglossia, such as Beckwith–Wiedemann syndrome and Down syndrome (Trisomy 21)

Potential challenges that may arise include the following:

- Face masks may be difficult to fit.
- The upper airway may be crowded and prone to obstruction on induction of anaesthesia.
- Mouth opening may be limited.
- Oral airways may be difficult to insert.
- Nasal passages may be too small for a nasopharyngeal airway.
- Laryngoscopy and intubation may be very difficult.
- Cleft palate may also be present, compounding any difficulty with laryngoscopy.

The impact of growth, development, medical and surgical treatment should be considered during the assessment. The natural history of some conditions is such that some airways tend to improve with age, as with Pierre Robin sequence, but may worsen in others, such as MPS.

A history of sleep disordered breathing may be suggestive of obstructive apnoea (OSA). This is usually during sleep but in rare cases may occur when awake.

## Cervical Spine

The craniocervical junction (CCJ) is the site of a wide range of developmental and acquired anomalies in children. The CCJ may be compromised by:

- Deformity
- Instability
- Compression

*Deformity* may arise as a result of distortion of normal anatomy or anomalous vertebral segmentation. Anomalous segmentation often coexists with craniovertebral anomalies such as craniosynostosis and disorders of branchial arch development. For example, cervical hemivertebrae are a feature of Goldenhar syndrome. In Klippel–Feil syndrome, fusion of cervical vertebrae results in a short neck with very limited mobility, this can lead to difficulty with laryngoscopy and intubation.

*Instability* of the CCJ may occur at the occipito-atlanto and atlanto-axial joints. Anomalies of the odontoid process leading to atlanto-axial instability are well recognised in Trisomy 21, Morquio syndrome (MPS IV), Hurler syndrome (MPS I) and Klippel–Feil syndrome. Excessive movement of the neck can contribute to cervical spine injury. Airway manoeuvres and patient positioning are times of great vulnerability during general anaesthesia.

*Compression* of the cervicomedullary junction is a feature of some of the MPS syndromes when tissue infiltration leads to stenosis of the cervical canal. Cervical cord compression is also a common feature of achondroplasia.

## Breathing

Respiratory muscle and bulbar weakness are features of myopathic conditions, and chronic aspiration and recurrent infections are common. Generalised hypotonia may be present in neuromuscular disorders, and some conditions are associated with kyphoscoliosis, which may progressively limit respiration. Limited respiratory reserve may be masked by a low level of activity in patients, such as in wheelchair-dependent children.

## Cardiovascular

Many congenital syndromes have an associated cardiac lesion. In older patients, it is most likely that this will have been repaired or palliated. The implications for anaesthesia in the presence of a cardiac lesion are dealt with in Chapter 33. Particular care should be taken in patients with Williams syndrome, who may have a range of cardiovascular anomalies, including supra-aortic valvar stenosis and pulmonary stenosis, and who may also have coronary artery involvement. Other noteworthy groups are patients with cardiomyopathy, such as those with Duchenne muscular dystrophy, Pompe disease or disorders of fatty acid metabolism. A comprehensive cardiovascular workup is essential prior to anaesthesia. This should include quantitative echocardiographic assessment of cardiac function.

## Endocrine, Metabolic and Renal Systems

Patients who have been on long-term steroids may need additional steroid administration to cover surgical stress. This is particularly important in adrenogenital syndrome. Careful management of glucose homeostasis is essential in children with glycogen storage disorders (e.g. von Gierke,

Pompe, Cori, Andersen, McArdle) and Beckwith–Wiedemann syndrome. It is important that fasting time is kept to a minimum, and it may be necessary to start an infusion of glucose before anaesthesia. In conditions where renal dysfunction is an associated factor, careful attention should be paid to fluid management and to the use of drugs that rely on the kidney for excretion.

## Skin, Bone and Joint Disorders

Great care must be taken with positioning in patients with fixed joint deformities, or where there is abnormal joint laxity, as in Marfan syndrome. As noted earlier, some patients have a fixed or potentially unstable cervical spine which must be handled and positioned carefully. Similar considerations apply to patients with fragile bones, such as those with osteogenesis imperfecta. In Ehlers–Danlos syndrome, abnormal collagen leads not only to joint laxity but also to extremely fragile skin and other tissues. It can be difficult to site and secure intravenous access. Epidermolysis bullosa (EB) is a syndrome in which management of skin and mucosal surfaces is particularly challenging. EB is discussed in more detail in the section 'Epidermolysis Bullosa (EB)'.

## Some Specific Syndromes

### Trisomy 21

This is one of the most common congenital syndromes, occurring in approximately one in 600–700 live births; 95% are trisomy 21 and 2% are mosaic. The incidence increases with advancing maternal age. The characteristic phenotype includes features of low-set ears, up-slanting eyes, a small nose, large tongue, brachycephaly, short neck, clinodactyly, a single palmar crease and a varying degree of intellectual impairment.

The large tongue and a narrow nasopharynx result in a tendency to upper airway obstruction. Sleep disordered breathing and OSA are common. Laryngo-tracheo-bronchial pathology, such as subglottic stenosis and tracheomalacia, may be present. Other associated features of relevance to anaesthesia include a significant incidence of occipito-atlanto-axial instability, and hence careful manipulation of the head and neck is important during intubation and subsequent positioning. A history of recurrent chest infections should raise concern about pulmonary aspiration secondary to cervical cord compression and should prompt radiological investigation of the cervical spine.

Forty to fifty per cent have congenital heart disease, most commonly an atrial or ventricular septal defect, frequently as part of an endocardial cushion defect. Duodenal atresia may occur. Children with Trisomy 21 may be moderately hypotonic and can be hypothyroid; they also have an increased risk of leukaemia.

### Epidermolysis Bullosa (EB)

This is a group of disorders characterised by mechanical fragility of the epidermis and mucous membranes which separate readily from the underlying tissues. The patient is at risk of formation of bullae and non-healing wounds with trivial trauma, particularly on exposure to shearing forces. Three major types of EB are recognised: simplex, junctional and dystrophic. In the severe forms, such as recessive dystrophic EB, recurrent skin damage and scarring of the fingers and toes lead to pseudosyndactyly and severe contractures, so-called mitten hands. Scarring of the corners of the mouth leads to progressive microstomia, and oropharyngeal mucosal scarring leads to fixation of the tongue within the mouth. There is frequently very poor dentition, and oesophageal strictures are common. Laryngeal involvement has been reported with the Herlitz subtype of junctional EB and one of the variants of simplex EB (Dowling–Meara subtype). Cardiomyopathy has also been reported, but this is rare.

These patients usually present for repair of their fused digits, oesophageal dilation and dental restoration. They are a particularly challenging group and must be treated with great care. Surgical procedures should only be undertaken in specialist units where there is ward-based nursing expertise. Patients are often colonised with methicillin resistant *Staphylococcus aureus* (MRSA).

### Anaesthesia for Children with EB

Careful handling is essential for these patients. Friction and sliding during transfer must be avoided, and adhesive tapes should not be used. Pure liquid paraffin sprays (Emollin®) can be used to lubricate face masks and gloved hands. Intravenous lines should be secured with a non-adhesive dressing. Silicon-based products suitable for use are available, such as Mepiform®, Siltape®

and Mepitac®. Arterial and central lines, if required, should be sutured in. Gel should be used to cover the eyes. These patients can lose heat rapidly; a warm theatre environment is helpful.

### Airway Management

Careful airway assessment is imperative to assess limitation of mouth opening and degree of neck movement. All airway equipment, including the face mask, airway and laryngoscope, should be generously lubricated with paraffin spray, jelly or vaseline gauze. Vaseline gauze should be placed under the chin where the anaesthetist places their fingers. The immobility of the tongue may keep the airway from obstructing and avoid the need for adjuncts such as oropharyngeal airways; these should be well lubricated and carefully used when needed. Laryngoscopy and intubation can be difficult because of limited mouth opening, which tends to get worse with increasing age. Although involvement of the larynx is possible, tracheal intubation does not usually appear to cause laryngeal or tracheal bullae and is generally considered safe. Nasal intubation may be preferable for extensive dental work, but whichever route is used it is essential that great care is taken to avoid sliding or shearing forces. The tube can be secured with ribbon gauze or clingfilm. A well-lubricated supraglottic airway device (SGA) may be used with caution.

### Monitoring

Small ECG electrodes can be secured with non-adhesive silicon dressings, as with intravenous lines, or with clingfilm. Clip-on oximeter probes should be used.

Blood pressure cuffs can be used safely as they do not produce a shearing force, but the limb should be well padded.

### Postoperative Care

Effective postoperative analgesia is essential as it will reduce the likelihood of restlessness and agitation during emergence from anaesthesia. Intravenous analgesia may be the most effective route. Regional analgesia, single dose or by continuous infusion, has been utilised successfully and will be useful in some patients. The increasing use of ultrasound to improve the success rate of regional nerve blockade may be beneficial. Many patients have difficulty with oral medications, and rectal analgesia may be helpful.

## Inborn Errors of Metabolism

An overview of the more common inborn errors of metabolism is shown in Table 8.1. The signs and symptoms of inherited metabolic disease (IMD) arise as a consequence of a failure of one or more steps within a metabolic process. In essence, they result in one or more of the following:

- Accumulation of substrate
- Accumulation of metabolite
- Deficiency of normal product of metabolic pathway
- General metabolic derangement, such as acidosis

The inherited disorders of metabolism are a diverse group. They may present with acute encephalopathy, seizures or hypotonia or as a movement disorder. Hypoglycaemia or a metabolic acidosis may also be the first presentation. Myopathy is not uncommon.

Broad principles of anaesthetic management of patients with IMD include:

- Assessment of the patient and the severity of the IMD, the natural history of the condition, the nature of any treatment and the effect of that treatment.
- Assessment of any organ dysfunction.
- Avoidance of prolonged fasting and maintenance of hydration.
- Close monitoring of glucose and acid-base state.
- Maintaining metabolic homeostasis perioperatively. The aim is usually to prevent or limit metabolism via the abnormal metabolic pathway, for example avoidance of catabolism and provision of glucose during fasting.
- Consideration of strategies to correct severe acidosis, such as haemodialysis and avoidance of lactate-containing fluids.
- Prevention of the accumulation of blood in the stomach. The protein content of blood can trigger acute decompensation in many IMDs, especially those involving amino acid metabolism.
- Attention to temperature regulation. Hypothermia can trigger a metabolic crisis in some conditions.

Close collaboration with relevant IMD specialists is advised.

**Table 8.1** Overview of inherited metabolic disorders

| Classification | Example | Anaesthetic considerations |
| --- | --- | --- |
| Disorders of amino acid metabolism | Phenylketonuria (PKU)<br>Homocystinuria | Seizures – maintain special diet. Marfanoid, thrombosis risk high – maintain hydration, thrombosis prophylaxis. |
| | Maple syrup urine disease (MSUD) | Hypotonic, hypoglycaemia, seizures. |
| Urea cycle disorders | Carbamyl phosphate synthase deficiency | Hyperammonaemia and encephalopathy. Avoid catabolism and dehydration during fasting. Maintain high-carbohydrate, low-protein diet. Avoid blood in the stomach (protein load). Infusion of substrate to optimise non-urea cycles for nitrogen removal is often necessary; specialist advice should be taken. |
| Disorders of organic acid metabolism | Methylmalonic acidaemia, propionic acidaemia | Hypoglycaemia, ketoacidosis, hyperammonaemia. Maintain normoglycaemia, hydration and acid-base status. Restrict protein. |
| Disorders of carbohydrate metabolism | Glycogen storage diseases, e.g. von Gierke, Pompe, Cori, Andersen, McArdle. | Minimise fasting, maintain normoglycaemia and acid-base homeostasis. Avoid lactate-containing fluid.<br>Pompe may have hypertrophic cardiomyopathy. Approximately 6% risk of arrythmias, cardiac arrest and death. |
| | Galactosaemia | Hepatic dysfunction. |
| Lysosomal storage disorders | MPS | High-risk airway, cervical spine, cardiac complications. Seizures. |
| | Lipidoses, e.g. Tay–Sachs, Fabry, Niemann–Pick | Lysosomal accumulation of sphingolipid substrates, hepatomegaly, developmental delay. |
| Disorders of fatty acid oxidation | Medium chain acyl–CoA dehydrogenase deficiency | Minimise fasting, give glucose infusion, maintain acid–base homeostasis. |
| Mitochondrial disorders | Genetic and phenotypic heterogenous group with reduced capacity for oxidative phosphorylation | Myopathic, often with cardiomyopathy and neurodevelopmental delay. Avoid prolonged propofol infusion, avoid lactate containing fluid, maintain normoglycaemia. May have disordered control of respiration. |
| Peroxisomal disorders | Zellweger syndrome | Hypotonia, hepatic and renal impairment, chronic respiratory dysfunction. Associated with congenital heart disease. |

## Mucopolysaccharidoses

MPS are a group of inherited lysosomal storage disorders.

Abnormal sequestration of partially degraded glycosaminoglycans results in a progressive multisystem disease with organomegaly, visual, auditory and intellectual deficits, airway abnormalities, cardiovascular impairment, joint and bony deformities and characteristic coarse facial features. Patients with MPS present a very high risk for anaesthesia, although this risk can be reduced by early treatment.

Treatment options now include haematopoietic stem cell transplantation and recombinant enzyme replacement therapy. Stem cell transplantation halts progression of these diseases and reduces hepatosplenomegaly, joint stiffness, OSA, facial dysmorphism, heart disease, hydrocephalus and hearing loss. Skeletal and ocular abnormalities are not corrected, and neurological outcomes remain poor. Enzyme replacement therapy may be of benefit in MPS I, II, IVA and VI.

## Anaesthesia for Children with MPS

Behavioural problems are common, but sedative premedication should be used with extreme caution. Preoperative assessment should include thorough clinical evaluation of the cardiac and respiratory systems. Cardiomyopathy, valvular heart disease and coronary artery disease may be present. A recent echocardiogram should be reviewed. Active respiratory tract infection is a contraindication to elective surgery. Close postoperative monitoring is essential.

## Airway Management

There can be multi-level airway involvement. Historically the overall incidence of airway difficulties in untreated children with MPS is 25%, with failure to intubate occurring in 8% of MPS cases (rising to 54% and 23% respectively in Hurler's syndrome). Successful early treatment with stem cell transplantation and enzyme replacement therapy and the evolution of airway technologies, such as videolaryngoscopy, has changed airway management with a reduction in the incidence of airway complications. Contributory factors include:

- Airway tissue deposition of glycosaminoglycans
- A short and sometimes unstable neck
- Poor joint mobility including the cervical spine and temporo-mandibular joints
- Macroglossia
- Micrognathia

Previous anaesthetic records should be reviewed, but as all of these factors get worse with age, a difficult airway must always be expected. Careful preparation and planning, including the full range of difficult airway adjuncts, is essential. Preoperative sleep studies may be required as OSA is often present.

Cervical spine instability most often occurs in MPS I (Hurler) and IV (Morquio). Specialist consultation and radiological studies may be indicated. In Morquio syndrome, potential cervical myelopathy secondary to canal stenosis should be evaluated with magnetic resonance (MR) imaging. Neck manipulation should be avoided. Manual inline stabilisation is recommended.

The use of an anti-sialagogue may be helpful. As a result of tissue distortion, face masks may not fit well, oral airways may worsen airway obstruction and nasopharyngeal airways may be difficult to place. An SGA can be particularly useful, and its use as a conduit for intubation is well described. Fibreoptic intubation may be necessary, in which case it is important to anticipate that the correct size tracheal tube may be smaller than that expected. Airway obstruction following tracheal extubation can lead to pulmonary oedema. Awake extubation is advised, and dexamethasone may be helpful.

## Malignant Hyperthermia Susceptibility (MHS)

MHS is a progressive life-threatening hyperthermic reaction occurring during general anaesthesia. It is a genetic disorder of skeletal muscle calcium regulation in which uncontrolled skeletal muscle hypermetabolism, triggered by volatile agents alone or in conjunction with suxamethonium, leads to a life-threatening state known as malignant hyperthermia (MH). The triggering substances release calcium stores from the sarcoplasmic reticulum, causing muscle contracture, glycogenolysis, adenosine triphosphate (ATP) consumption and heat production. Oxygen demand soon outstrips supply, and ATP stores are depleted, leading to lactic acidosis and rhabdomyolysis. If treated promptly, most patients recover, although there remains a mortality rate of around 4%. Diagnostic services for suspected MH in the United Kingdom and Ireland are provided by the MH Investigation Unit in Leeds. This specialist unit provides a screening service, advice to patients and a 'hotline' for health care professionals and also conducts research.

## Who Is at Risk?

The highest reported incidence of MH occurs in paediatric populations. The inheritance of mutations in three genes account for most patients with MH susceptibility. De novo mutations do arise. The majority of mutations are found within the RYR1 gene on chromosome 19 that encodes the skeletal muscle ryanodine receptor type I protein.

Inheritance is in an autosomal dominant pattern, so all closely related members of a family in which

MH has occurred must be considered susceptible. Progress in genetic analysis has greatly enhanced the understanding of MHS and has a promising role in diagnosis. Unfortunately, MHS cannot reliably be excluded by a genetic test as MH has a high level of locus heterogeneity and not all RYR1 variants have been completely evaluated. For new cases or for those with a family history, the gold standard for diagnosis is a muscle biopsy and in vitro contracture test (IVCT). The sample size required is such that muscle biopsies are not performed on children less than 10–12 years old (30 kg).

MHS patients will usually have a normal phenotype, but many myopathic disorders are associated with RYR1 pathogenic variants and have been linked with MH susceptibility. Mutations of the CACNA1S (alpha 1 subunit of the voltage-gated calcium channel gene) or STAC3 (a component of excitation-contraction coupling gene) may also confer MHS.

## Myopathic Disorder Genetic Associations

**RYR1**

- King Denborough
- Central core
- Multi-minicore
- Congenital myopathy with cones and rods
- Idiopathic hyperCKaemia (CK creatinine kinase)
- Nemaline rod myopathy
- Periodic paralysis
- Congenital fibre type disproportion (CFTD)
- Centronuclear myopathy
- Heat- or exercise-induced rhabdomyolysis

**CACNA1S**

- Periodic paralysis
- CFTD
- Multi-minicore

**STAC3**

- Native American myopathy

For any patient with a known RYR1, CACNA1S or STAC3 mutation, MHS must be assumed. If a condition has a phenotype with a range of different underlying genetic aetiologies (e.g. CFTD, periodic paralysis, nemaline rod myopathy) and genetic analysis has confirmed the underlying abnormal gene is not one of the RYR1, CACNA1S or STAC3 genes, then MHS is not present. This information may not always be available, in which case MHS must be assumed.

## Anaesthesia for Children with MHS

The Association of Anaesthetists Malignant Hyperthermia Guideline provides comprehensive guidance. It is important to be aware that a previous history of uneventful anaesthesia does not exclude risk. If MHS is suspected, all volatile agents and suxamethonium should be avoided. The anaesthetic machine should have vaporisers removed, and it is usual to flush the machine and circuits with oxygen for about 30 minutes prior to use to remove residual traces of volatile agent. The precise duration of circuit flushing should be available from each anaesthetic machine manufacturer. A target of 5 ppm is regarded as the maximum safe concentration of inhalation agent. Propofol, opioids, benzodiazepines, nitrous oxide, local anaesthetics and barbiturates can all be used as part of a trigger-free technique. In addition to usual minimal monitoring, it is essential to include core temperature. Dantrolene should be readily available.

## Recognition and Management of MH

### Recognition

At the start of an episode of MH, the patients may exhibit generalised muscle spasm, often first noticed as masseter spasm. Patients then usually develop:

- Unexplained hypercapnia
- Unexplained tachycardia
- Hyperthermia, classically rising >1°C every five minutes
- Hypoxaemia, acidosis and hyperkalaemia
- Myoglobinuria and elevated plasma creatine kinase

### Management

- Immediately eliminate the agent by removal of the vaporiser and administration of 100% oxygen at maximum flow.
- Increase minute ventilation to 2–3 × normal.
- Place activated charcoal filters on the inspiratory and expiratory limbs of the circuit.
- Administer dantrolene sodium 2–3 mg $kg^{-1}$; this may need to be repeated in doses of 1 mg $kg^{-1}$ to a maximum of 10 mg $kg^{-1}$.
- Commence active body cooling, ice packs and cold lavage.
- If surgery cannot be stopped, maintenance of anaesthesia should continue with intravenous agents.

- Treat any acidosis, hyperkalaemia, arrhythmias, myoglobinuria, disseminated intravascular coagulation (DIC) and compartment syndrome.

In due course, the family should be counselled and the patient referred for further investigation.

## Anaesthesia-Induced Rhabdomyolysis (AIR)

AIR is a distinct entity from MHS, although some common features exist. AIR has occurred in children with abnormalities of the dystrophin-glycoprotein complex of the sarcolemma. Children with muscular dystrophies and some myopathies may be at risk when exposed to suxamethonium and volatile anaesthetic agents. Rhabdomyolysis and hyperkalaemia are the main features and can lead to cardiac arrest. Intravenous anaesthesia should be used, although brief exposure to volatile agents has been tolerated to facilitate placement of an intravenous cannula when awake intravenous access has failed.

## Muscular Dystrophy

The muscular dystrophies (MD) are a group of X-linked genetic disorders in which there is absent or abnormal dystrophin, leading to muscle weakness and atrophy. DMD is the most common and severe form, with an incidence of 1 in 3,500 males. Diagnosis is often at the age of around three to five years. Becker MD is a milder form which does not usually present until the teenage years.

Patients with DMD experience progressive degeneration and fibrosis of all muscle types with onset from the age of about three years. It is rapidly progressive, and patients are frequently wheelchair bound by adolescence. Life expectancy has increased with advances in supportive therapies and use of steroids.

## Anaesthesia for Children with MD

MD patients are especially at risk during and after general anaesthesia. The presence of the following should be sought:

- Restrictive lung disease, from respiratory muscle weakness and scoliosis
- Dilated cardiomyopathy (DCM), which is common, although the patient's history may not always reveal symptoms if they are inactive
- Rhythm disturbances, due to fibrosis of the conduction system

Multidisciplinary assessment is essential prior to elective surgery. Lung function tests, sleep studies and echocardiography are regularly undertaken as part of the management of these patients. Cardiorespiratory review should be organised prior to surgery with a current set of investigations. Full assessment may necessitate admission prior to surgery to optimise respiratory function. Non-invasive ventilation (NPPV) may need to be started prior to surgery and continue afterwards.

Perioperative steroid replacement should be used in all patients who have been on steroids in the previous six months. As described earlier, patients with muscular dystrophies are at risk of AIR and hence rhabdomyolysis and hyperkalaemia. Suxamethonium is contraindicated, and there should be minimal exposure to volatile anaesthetic agents. Total intravenous anaesthesia (TIVA) is ideal; use of a range of intravenous agents has been described. Non-depolarising muscle relaxants exhibit altered pharmacokinetics, and their use should be monitored with nerve stimulation. Gastrointestinal smooth muscle is affected in DMD, so gastric stasis may occur.

Postoperative respiratory support for patients with DMD must be available. The postoperative period is a particularly challenging phase of the care of these patients; management on a paediatric intensive care unit (PICU) will be required for all but the most minor surgery. Lung function tests have been used for predicting respiratory insufficiency postoperatively but there is no clear correlation, and the clinical assessment of an experienced anaesthetist is a better guide.

### Key Points

- Many congenital disorders have an associated airway or cardiac abnormality.
- Children with mucopolysaccharidoses are high-risk cases for anaesthesia. They can present major airway difficulties and may have an unstable cervical spine.
- Children with muscular dystrophies and myotonias are not generally at risk of malignant hyperthermia but are at risk of hyperkalaemia and rhabdomyolysis if exposed to suxamethonium or volatile agents.

## Further Reading


Gray RM. Anesthesia-induced rhabdomyolysis or malignant hyperthermia: is defining the crisis important? *Paediatric Anaesthesia* 2017; 27(5):490–3.

Hack HA, Walker RWM, Gardiner P. Anaesthetic implications of the changing management of patients with mucopolysaccharidosis. *Anaesthesia and Intensive Care* 2016; 44(6):660–8.

Hopkins PM, Girard T, Dalay S et al. Malignant hyperthermia 2020: Guideline from the Association of Anaesthetists. *Anaesthesia* 2021; 76(5):655–64. https://doi.org/10.1111/anae.15317.

Litman RS, Griggs SM, Dowling JJ, Riazi S. Malignant hyperthermia susceptibility and related diseases. *Anesthesiology*. 2018; 128(1):159–67.

National Center for Biolotechnology Information. OMIM. Available at: www.ncbi.nlm.nih.gov/omim.

Niezgoda J, Morgan PG. Anesthetic considerations in patients with mitochondrial defects. *Paediatric Anaesthesia* 2013; 23(9):785–93.

Orphan Anesthesia. Available at: www.orphananesthesia.eu/en/.

Walker R et al. Anaesthesia and airway management in mucopolysaccharidosis. *Journal of Inherited Metabolic Disease* 2013; 36(2):211–9.

Chapter 9

# Day-Case Anaesthesia in Children*

Jonathan Groome and Christie Locke

## Introduction

Most children undergoing elective surgery or diagnostic procedures are discharged home on the same day. The development of day surgery was primarily driven by the need to reduce cost and improve utilisation of resources, but there are benefits for children as day-case surgery limits the separation of an otherwise healthy child from their home and family environment. Children with chronic or complex health care needs also benefit as day-case surgery reduces the time spent in hospital and risk of hospital acquired infections. Successful day-case surgery works well both in a specialist paediatric setting and at the local district hospital. It requires the anaesthetist to work as part of a multidisciplinary team and to use techniques to minimise perioperative morbidity, particularly postoperative nausea and vomiting (PONV) and pain.

## Standards for Day-Case Surgery and Anaesthesia

A high-quality paediatric day-case service requires clear organisational leadership, staffing, facilities and information for parents based on the guidance and standards set by the Department of Health and professional bodies. Current standards and guidelines on the delivery of day-case surgery and anaesthesia from different organisations all highlight the following principles:

- Admission should be planned in an integrated way to include preadmission, admission and postadmission periods. Multidisciplinary involvement is essential.
- Infants, children and young people should not be cared for in the same location as adults.
- Medical, nursing and all other staff must have received specific training and be skilled in working with children and their families. This includes training in child protection.
- A staff member with an advanced paediatric life support qualification or an anaesthetist with paediatric competencies should be immediately available in the day surgical unit.
- Parents, caregivers and patients should be given age-appropriate, timely information about what to expect in the pre-, peri- and postoperative period.

Many day units are freestanding or organised as separate units within a larger hospital. In a non-specialist hospital, it is important to foster child-centred care, and in the day unit this may be achieved by reserving dedicated sessions for children. Staff should have the appropriate skills and experience in paediatric day-case surgery and should not be required to look after children of higher acuity (or adult patients) at the same time.

It is important that anaesthetists who care for children are appropriately trained and work within their competency. In day surgery units (DSU) where paediatric surgery occurs, a paediatrician must be available to assist with the management of unwell children or any safeguarding concerns. The delivery of some of these standards is challenging, particularly with respect to training in child protection and paediatric resuscitation and access to paediatric acute pain management teams. The Royal College of Anaesthetists has recognised this in training; it supports local competency-based resuscitation training programs and has developed a specific paediatric anaesthesia e-learning module concerning the management of children in the perioperative period, common operations and safeguarding.

* Many thanks to Dr Peter A. Stoddart, who wrote the first of this book chapter, much of the content of which has been used in this revised update.

# Organisation: Patient Selection and Preparation

## Patient Selection

Historically, the Department of Health (DOH) set a target to achieve more than 75% of elective surgery as day-case care, and whilst this target still exists, it is usually surpassed thanks to the uptake of minimally invasive techniques. The DOH publication 'Day Surgery: Operational Guide' suggests that the default question should be, 'Is there any justification for admitting this case as an inpatient?' rather than, 'Is this patient suitable for day surgery?' This change in emphasis has increased the proportion of children undergoing day-case procedures. Careful patient selection is fundamental to safe, efficient day-case services. Procedures regularly undertaken as day cases are listed in Table 9.1.

Clear exclusions for day surgery in children include:

- Major invasive operations
- Surgery associated with significant physiological derangement or prolonged postoperative pain
- Children needing specialist nursing or nutritional care that cannot be provided at home

Many patients are excluded because of their age, prematurity, coexisting medical conditions, previous anaesthetic problems or social circumstances. Children should be discharged home to an environment where they will receive at least the same level of care they would have by remaining in hospital. Typical exclusions are listed in Table 9.2; however, tertiary paediatric centres are now performing increasingly complex procedures as day cases. Some exclusions are relative, and decisions may have to be made on a case-by-case basis after discussion with an anaesthetist.

The lower age limit for day surgery depends on the individual unit. A tertiary paediatric centre may accept healthy term neonates >44 weeks postmenstrual age for minor day-case procedures. For children born <37 weeks gestational age (ex-premature), a lower limit of <60 weeks postmenstrual age is standard. Many district hospitals have a six- or 12-month minimum age limit because of their infrequent experience with younger infants.

**Table 9.1** Common day-case surgery and procedures

**General**
- Excision of minor lumps and bumps including lymph nodes
- Herniotomy
- Excision of hydrocoele
- Umbilical hernia repair

**Urology**
- Circumcision
- Orchidopexy
- Cystoscopy including removal of ureteric stents
- Minor hypospadias

**ENT**
- Adenotonsillectomy
- Myringotomy
- Diagnostic microlaryngoscopy
- Removal of foreign body
- Nose manipulation under anaesthetic (MUA)

**Dental**
- Extraction
- Conservation

**Ophthalmic**
- Strabismus/ptosis correction
- Examination under anaesthetic
- Tear duct probing

**Orthopaedic**
- Botox injections
- Change of plaster
- Arthroscopy
- Removal of metalwork

**Plastic**
- Dressing changes, removal of sutures
- Excision of skin lesions
- Laser therapy
- Pinnaplasty

**Medical**
- Diagnostic cardiac catheterisation
- Bone marrow sampling
- Lumbar puncture and intrathecal cytotoxics
- Radiotherapy
- MRI, CT scan

The inclusion of tonsillectomy as a day-case procedure was historically controversial in the United Kingdom owing to concerns about post-operative haemorrhage, pain control, obstructive sleep apnoea (OSA) and PONV. Most centres now routinely undertake this procedure using well-defined day-case tonsillectomy guidelines for anaesthesia, surgery and postoperative care

**Table 9.2** Common exclusions for day-case surgery

**Surgical**
- Open cavity surgery involving cranium, thorax or abdomen
- Associated with significant or prolonged pain
- Requirement for specialist nursing, e.g. risk of compartment syndrome
- Prolonged procedure >90 min
- Airway surgery, e.g. laryngeal papillomas
- Risk of significant postoperative haemorrhage

**Patient**
- Prematurity with post-conceptual age <60 weeks
- Poorly controlled systemic disease, e.g. epilepsy, asthma, metabolic disease and diabetes
- Acute viral or bacterial respiratory infection
- Severe obstructive sleep apnoea
- Complex congenital cardiac disease
- Sickle cell disease
- Neuromuscular disease, e.g. Duchenne muscular dystrophy

**Social**
- Parents unable to cope with additional sick child
- Single parent with poor local support
- Lack of telephone
- Inadequate transport home
- Prolonged journey home, e.g. greater than 1 hour

delivered by an experienced consultant-led team. Surgery should be performed in the morning so that children can remain in hospital for at least six hours to ensure that they are pain-free, drinking and not bleeding before discharge home. Children with severe OSA undergoing tonsillectomy should not be managed as a day case. In 2019, in response to a significant increase in tertiary referrals for children with tonsillar hypertrophy requiring tonsillectomy, the British Association for Paediatric Otolaryngology (BAPO), ENT UK, the Royal College of Anaesthetists (RCoA) and the Association of Paediatric Anaesthetists of Great Britain and Ireland (APAGBI) released a consensus statement relating to tonsillectomy in children. They recommended that children >2 years (corresponding weight 12 kg) with no high-risk factors or extremes of BMI could be treated in a secondary centre. This recommendation is reduced to >1 year (corresponding weight 10 kg) if the centre had paediatric high-dependency unit (HDU) facilities. Community follow-up and communication with the general practitioner is essential for all day cases, particularly for children undergoing day-case tonsillectomy.

## Preadmission Preparation

Good organisation and planning by the admission clerks, ward nurses, play therapists, theatre staff, surgeons and anaesthetists are essential to ensure the smooth running of a unit that is welcoming and friendly and minimises potential upset to the child and their family. Adequate preparation for the family is required, with clear written information about what to expect, what to bring and what to do on the day, especially in terms of fasting guidelines and routine medication. An example is shown in Figure 9.1. For the child, information may be presented in the form of a story or interactive book, DVD or internet material. The RCoA and APAGBI have published an excellent series of patient information leaflets and videos for children and young people of different ages and in different languages: www.rcoa.ac.uk/patient-information/patient-information-resources/information-children-parents-carers.

Nurse-led assessment using a preadmission screening questionnaire should be used to identify any potential problems that need to be discussed or assessed by a senior anaesthetist preoperatively and to prevent unexpected cancellations on the day. Preadmission assessment may be carried out at initial booking, on the phone using standardised questionnaires or during a visit to the day unit to meet the nurses and play specialists, and to see the ward and possibly the recovery unit. Many families find this particularly beneficial, and such preoperative visits have been shown to reduce anxiety on admission. Some units offer families visits on a weekend in the form of a Saturday Club. Fit and healthy ASA 1 or 2 children do not need any preanaesthetic screening investigations except for a sickle cell test for those at risk.

All children must be seen on the day of admission by the surgeon (or paediatrician for medical procedures) and anaesthetist to confirm that the procedure is still required, that the child remains fit for anaesthesia and to finalise consent.

After admission to the day unit, children are encouraged to play, read, draw, watch TV/DVDs or play video games to pass the time prior to anaesthesia. In some units, children come to the induction room in their own clothes or nightwear. It is

## What to bring

A favourite toy or comforter

Gaming device, books etc for older children

A special bottle or beaker

Comfortable loose clothing or pyjamas—please bring a change of clothes and avoid metal fastenings (your child may wear a gown to theatre)

Any medication or inhalers your child needs/ uses.

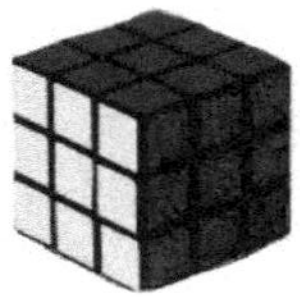

## Preparation

It is important to prepare your child for their surgery– it is helpful to briefly explain why they are coming. Reassure them that you will be there all the time and will go home together.

Children are encouraged to make use of the play room where there are toys, puzzles and games. Our play specialists help to make your child's stay as relaxed as possible. If you feel your child would benefit from a session with our play specialist's prior to admission—please contact Janine on the number below.

## Contact us

If you have any queries please do not hesitate to contact us.

One team Children's Unit

# Outwood Day Surgery

Please call at 6am on the morning of your child's surgery to confirm there is a bed available

**Figure 9.1** Written guidelines to prepare families for day surgery.

An appointment has been made for your child to have day case surgery on the children's ward.

Please bring your child to the ward at the time stated on your letter. It is important that you arrive on time so your child can be assessed by the team before surgery starts.

Please make arrangements to be here all day in case your child is later in the list or needs to stay for a longer period of time after their procedure.

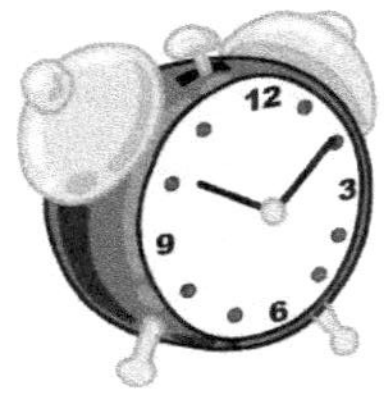

## Where to find us

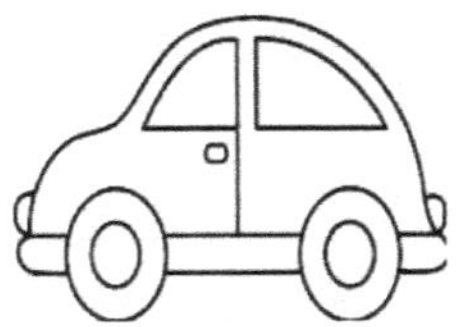

The day surgery unit is part of Outwood children's ward. This is situated on the first floor of the hospital near the east entrance.

There is a car park on site and we will provide you with a ticket to reduce the price of the car park if you are here for the day.

## About the day

When you arrive, you will meet the nurse that will be caring for your child whilst in hospital. If you have any questions the nurse will be able to answer them.

You will then be seen by a surgeon who will go through the procedure and ask you to sign the consent form to confirm you are happy to proceed. An anaesthetist will then see your child and give you information about the anaesthetic that will be used.

The day surgery unit if often quite busy therefore it would help us if your child was accompanied by a maximum of 2 adults, if you have other children please arrange for them to be looked after for the day.

## Fasting

Please make sure you follow the fasting instructions—it is very important before your child has an operation. If your child does not follow these directions it could result in their operation being delayed or cancelled.

**For admission in the morning**

The last time they can have food or formula milk is 6 hours before surgery. This is often the night before however could be up until 0230.

If your child is breast fed they may be fed until 0430

**Clear fluids are allowed until 0730**. Please encourage your child to drink clear fluids until the time allowed. If they are later in the surgery list they may be given a small drink of clear fluids once seen by theanaesthetist.

**For admission in the afternoon**

Your child can have breakfast in the morning– before 0730. (we suggest waking them to have this). They cannot have any food or formula milk after 0730.

If your child is breast fed they may be fed until 0930

**Clear fluids are allowed until 1230**. Please encourage your child to drink clear fluids until the time allowed. If they are later in the surgery list they

## Clear Fluids

Clear fluids are;

- Water
- Dilute squash
- Black tea/ coffee

**NO fizzy drinks, fruit juice or chewing gum**

**Figure 9.1** *(cont.)*

standard UK practice for one or two parents to accompany the child to the anaesthetic room and to remain with them until after induction of anaesthesia. This usually avoids the need for preoperative sedation. However, this may be stressful for the parents; they should understand their role and what to expect, and a member of staff must accompany them. Parents are also encouraged to collect the child from the recovery room as soon as the child is awake. In certain situations, for instance as occurred during the coronavirus pandemic, the number of parents that can accompany the child to theatre and recovery may be restricted.

## Day Surgery and the Child with a Cold

The decision to proceed or cancel the child with an upper respiratory tract infection (URTI) should be made by a senior anaesthetist. Runny nose and low-grade fever are common symptoms and are reported in 20–30% of children presenting for day surgery, especially ENT surgery.

URTI may produce airway hyperreactivity resulting in increased adverse perioperative respiratory events such as laryngospasm, bronchospasm, breath holding and oxygen desaturation.

Surgery should be postponed in the child who is fractious, clearly unwell or pyrexial (temperature >37.5°C) or has clinical signs on chest auscultation.

Most children with URTI are well and otherwise asymptomatic with a simple rhinitis, so delay may not be required. The decision to postpone must rest with the anaesthetist and will be guided by their experience and expertise. Parental smoking, presence of airway anomaly, history of snoring, prematurity and asthma in a child have all been identified as risk factors for perioperative airway complications. Airway surgery is an independent risk factor for adverse respiratory events in children with URTI. There is also an increased incidence of respiratory complications in children under one year and in those cared for by less experienced anaesthetists.

Children who have surgery cancelled because of an URTI should have surgery rebooked at least two weeks later to allow airway hyperreactivity to recover.

## Anaesthesia Techniques

Planning and attention to detail improve outcomes in the perioperative period, and the use of protocols and guidelines can assist in this aim.

**Table 9.3** An example of a perioperative analgesia regimen

| |
|---|
| **Premedication** |
| Paracetamol 20 mg $kg^{-1}$ |
| Ametop/EMLA both hands |
| **Perioperative analgesia** |
| Fentanyl 1–3 mcg $kg^{-1}$ IV |
| Diclofenac 1 mg $kg^{-1}$ PR |
| **Postoperative analgesia** |
| Paracetamol 15 mg $kg^{-1}$ 6 hourly |
| Ibuprofen 10 mg $kg^{-1}$ 8 hourly |

These can include premedication guidelines or postoperative analgesic protocols as in Table 9.3.

## Premedication

Sedative premedication may be needed even if the child and family are well prepared, particularly for children with procedural anxiety, behavioural problems or poor past experiences.

Benzodiazepines (midazolam or temazepam) and $\alpha_2$-adrenoreceptor agonists (clonidine and dexmedetomidine) are the most used agents. Midazolam given as an oral dose of 0.5 mg $kg^{-1}$ (max 20 mg) is suitable for ages 1 month to 18 years (onset 30–45 minutes, duration 45–60 minutes). Its bitter taste can be masked with fruit cordials/syrups. Buccal midazolam at a dose of 0.2–0.3 mg $kg^{-1}$ (max 10 mg) can be given to children aged six months to 18 years (onset 10–20 minutes, duration 30–45 minutes). Midazolam may sometimes cause paradoxical excitation and poor emergence, particularly in preschool children. This may be because midazolam blocks explicit memory but not implicit memory (the memory of being anxious). Midazolam premedication may also be responsible for anxiety and prolonged behavioural changes after discharge. For older children (aged 12–18 years) oral temazepam tablets (10–20 mg) are good options (onset 60 minutes, duration 120–240 minutes).

Clonidine can be given orally, buccal or intranasal at a dose of 2–4 mcg $kg^{-1}$ (max dose of 150 mcg) with an onset of 45–60 minutes. Dexmedetomidine can be given via the oral, buccal or intranasal route at a dose of 1–4 mcg $kg^{-1}$ (max dose of 200 mcg) with a faster onset of 25 minutes. They are both good options for children who have experienced paradoxical excitation with midazolam and can also be combined with midazolam for children where premedication has previously failed. Alpha-2 adrenoreceptor agonists can cause hypotension and bradycardia, so caution must be used when administering them to children with cardiovascular instability.

Caution should be taken when premedicating patients with known difficult airway, metabolic, hepatic, renal or respiratory failure and those at risk of aspiration.

The pain of cannulation for induction of anaesthesia is greatly reduced by topical anaesthesia with local anaesthetic creams or ethyl chloride spray. There are several local anaesthetic creams available for use preoperatively:

- EMLA®. This was the first widely used local anaesthetic cream. It is a 5% eutectic mixture of lidocaine and prilocaine. It needs to be applied for an hour prior to cannulation and often causes vasoconstriction of the surrounding vessels.
- Ametop®. This is a 4% gel of tetracaine that produces topical anaesthesia for venepuncture in about 45 minutes that lasts up to four to six hours after removal. Some children develop associated erythema and skin oedema that may obscure the vein.
- LMX 4®. This is a new liposomal preparation of 4% lidocaine that is effective 30 minutes after application but may also cause erythema and skin oedema.

## Induction of Anaesthesia

Many older children prefer intravenous induction. Venepuncture is better tolerated in a young child if they are sitting on their parent's knee whilst distracted with a familiar comfort toy, blanket, video games or tablet. An inhalational induction with sevoflurane in oxygen or starting with nitrous oxide in oxygen may be preferred in small infants with difficult venous access or at the request of an older child. Inhalation induction may be combined with directed imagery and hypnotic relaxation techniques. Experienced anaesthetic teams are adaptable and use any or a combination of these induction techniques depending on the child and their preferences.

The ideal anaesthetic for painful procedures is achieved by combining general anaesthesia with a local anaesthetic block and/or non-opioid analgesia using paracetamol and a NSAID. Propofol 3–5 mg $kg^{-1}$ is the intravenous induction agent of choice, as it suppresses upper airway reflexes, thereby aiding insertion of a supraglottic airway device (SAD) or a tracheal tube if required. Pain on injection can be reduced with the newer preparations and a small dose of lidocaine 0.2 mg $kg^{-1}$. The antiemetic and recovery properties of propofol are particularly useful in a day-case setting.

## Maintenance of Anaesthesia

Maintenance is achieved either with an inhalational agent or total intravenous anaesthesia using a target-controlled infusion of propofol, sometimes with remifentanil, with meticulous flushing of any indwelling lines after use. The choice of volatile is governed by cost, environmental impact and airway irritability. Compared with isoflurane, the newer agents sevoflurane and desflurane allow rapid awakening but not necessarily earlier discharge from recovery. Both may be associated with agitation on emergence, although this is less common in children who have good analgesia. Emergence delirium in recovery can be treated with a judicious dose of fentanyl 0.5 mcg $kg^{-1}$. Desflurane is an airway irritant, particularly in children with asthma, and is best avoided if the child has had a recent URTI. Recent evidence highlighting desflurane as a potent greenhouse gas with a warming potential 25–40 times more than that of carbon dioxide is leading to a reduction in its use. Total intravenous anaesthesia (TIVA) has a much lower environmental impact and is particularly useful in cases where there is a high risk of emesis, such as in pinnaplasty or strabismus surgery.

## Airway Management

Very short procedures, such as bone marrow sampling or lumbar puncture for chemotherapy, may be managed with simple mask anaesthesia. Anaesthesia for most body surface surgery may be administered with the child breathing spontaneously through a SAD. There are many different types of supraglottic airways in use, with second-generation devices incorporating bite blocks and gastric channels. A flexible reinforced SAD is useful for head and neck surgery, including tonsillectomy or strabismus surgery.

Tracheal intubation is not usually required for day surgery but is not contraindicated, provided the correct size tube is selected and inserted and removed atraumatically. The intubation technique depends on the personal preference of the anaesthetist, some using deep sevoflurane or propofol anaesthesia for intubation, followed by either controlled or spontaneous ventilation. Non-depolarising neuromuscular blocking agents may also be used; 0.5 mg $kg^{-1}$ atracurium can be reversed after 20 minutes with 0.05 mg $kg^{-1}$ neostigmine and 0.01 mg $kg^{-1}$ glycopyrrolate. The use of aminosteroid-based agents such as vecuronium and rocuronium may increase with the greater availability of sugammadex, as this offers reversal of any depth of neuromuscular block with minimal side effects. The current high cost of sugammadex precludes the routine use of this drug. Suxamethonium has many minor and some rare life-threatening side effects, so routine use is avoided in current day-case anaesthesia practice.

## Analgesia

Good pain control and a low incidence of PONV are fundamental to high-quality day-case anaesthesia. Nursing staff must be trained and empowered to routinely monitor, record and treat pain. Long-acting opioids should be avoided, and even fentanyl can increase the risk of emesis, although low doses may avoid poor emergence in recovery.

Paracetamol is usually used in combination with an NSAID and provides good pain relief with minimal side effects. Oral preoperative administration is convenient as most children have good experience of these analgesics and anti-pyretics at home, and they are cheaper and less impactful on the environment when compared to intravenous drugs. NSAIDs, ibuprofen 5–10 mg $kg^{-1}$ PO or diclofenac 1–1.5 mg $kg^{-1}$ PO, PR or IV are well tolerated and frequently used. Recognised contra-indications and side effects must be considered when prescribing, for example in leukaemia patients with thrombocytopenia or children with a family history of aspirin-induced asthma. NSAIDs can be used safely for most non-aspirin-sensitive asthmatic children.

Following reports of several deaths occurring outside of the hospital environment in North America, codeine is no longer used in any children under 12 or for children under 18 who undergo removal of tonsils or adenoids due to sleep apnoea. Alternative analgesics include tramadol (licensed for children over 12) or oral morphine. To facilitate day surgery and discharge, some hospital pharmacies will dispense a limited number of doses of low-dose oral morphine for children >10 kg.

Local anaesthetic blocks are the mainstay of postoperative analgesic management, especially for infra-umbilical surgery. All children's anaesthetists should be practised at both caudal and simple nerve blocks, such as penile and ilioinguinal/iliohypogastric blocks. The addition of clonidine 2 mcg $kg^{-1}$ will increase the duration of caudal bupivacaine with minimal additional side effects. Caudal blocks alter both motor and proprioceptive function in the legs and are probably best reserved for non-ambulatory infants, as older children may find these side effects troublesome. Peripheral nerve and fascial blocks, such as rectus sheath or transversus abdominis plane (TAP) blocks, are associated with lower risk of major complications compared with neuroaxial blocks and act for much longer than simple wound infiltration.

Several studies have demonstrated high success rates of ultrasound-guided blocks using low volumes of local anaesthetic compared with the traditional surface landmark techniques, and ultrasound is routinely used in many centres (see Chapter 15). Low-volume blocks minimise dose requirements of local anaesthetic and improve safety. Specific nerve blocks for limb surgery, such as femoral or sciatic/popliteal blocks, may also be performed using ultrasound guidance or, less commonly, peripheral nerve stimulators. These blocks produce excellent analgesia but also an associated motor block, so if used for day-case procedures, parents must be given explicit advice about mobilisation and to avoid the risk of the child developing pressure sores. Parents should also be given clear advice about starting supplemental oral analgesia postoperatively to cope with the loss of pain relief at home when a local anaesthetic block wears off.

## Postoperative Nausea and Vomiting

In adult practice, PONV after day surgery may result in unplanned admissions, but this is less of a problem in paediatric practice. Routine antiemetic administration is not indicated for young children but should be targeted to high-risk patients, namely those with one or more risk factors for PONV:

- History of PONV or motion sickness
- Older children, particularly adolescent girls
- Children undergoing strabismus surgery, pinnaplasty or adenotonsillectomy
- Children who have received perioperative opioids

Ondansetron 0.15 mg $kg^{-1}$ IV or PO appears to be the most efficacious drug for the prevention of PONV, either alone, or in high-risk children combined with dexamethasone up to 0.15 mg $kg^{-1}$ IV. Dexamethasone appears to be particularly effective for preventing late onset POV (>6 hours). Dexamethasone should be avoided in those at risk of tumour lysis or uncontrolled diabetes, in which case droperidol 20 mcg $kg^{-1}$ is a useful third line drug in the absence of contraindications (such as prolonged QT syndrome).

Dehydration and early fluid intake may provoke PONV. Children should be encouraged to drink clear fluids until one hour preoperatively. Intraoperative intravenous fluids, at least 10 ml $kg^{-1}$ Hartmann's solution, should be given if they have not had a drink or are undergoing anaesthesia for longer than 30 minutes. After surgery, making children drink before discharge will increase the risk of vomiting, but they should be encouraged to drink if they are thirsty. Avoiding inhalational agents by using TIVA should be considered for patients at high risk of PONV. Non-pharmacological techniques such as acupressure have a role with compliant children.

## Discharge after Surgery

Before discharge, the child must have returned to their pre-anaesthetic state, be pain-free and have a clear plan for postoperative pain relief. They should be encouraged to drink and have a light snack before leaving. The time for discharge varies with the child and the procedure undertaken. Most children are ready to leave between 1.5 and 3 hours after returning to the ward.

A benchmark of fewer than 3% of patients should need overnight admission because of an unforeseen surgical complication (typically bleeding) or anaesthetic complication (typically prolonged PONV or poor pain control). The management of unexpected admission needs a clear plan to be in place, particularly if the day unit is separate from an inpatient paediatric unit.

## Care at Home

Parents should be given clear advice about pain relief at home. This is simplified if analgesic combinations are dispensed pre-packed from the day-case unit. The parents should be given both verbal and written postoperative advice concerning analgesic management and wound care, such as bathing, return to school, sporting activities and the possibility of time-limited behavioural and sleep changes. The surgeon and anaesthetist should review the patient postoperatively, or if discharge is nurse led, agreed protocols should be used. A discharge letter for the general practitioner and community nurse should be given to the parents to ensure good communication with the primary health care team. A contact telephone number for parents to seek further advice is essential, and many units routinely contact families within 24/48 hours for further support and feedback.

A successful day-case anaesthetic service is dependent on a multitude of often simple but interrelated issues, such as good local anaesthetic blocks, avoiding tight bandaging for pinnaplasty to reduce PONV or ensuring the child brings in (and takes home!) their favourite toy to reduce stress and anxiety in the anaesthetic room. Regular multidisciplinary audit and review of outcomes including patient, parent and staff satisfaction are therefore prerequisites for continued development.

### Key Points

- Paediatric day-case care is beneficial from both a cost and efficiency point of view and reduces disruption for the child and family.
- Child-centred care pathways are needed, with good organisation and clear information and instructions for families.
- Simple uncomplicated general anaesthesia with supplemental local analgesia is required to provide good pain control and low risk of emesis.
- Plans for unexpected admission, a written discharge summary and guidance for postprocedural symptom control with a telephone contact number are needed.
- Multiple guidelines and standards have been written. Regular patient satisfaction surveys and audit of quality and safety of care should be conducted using these standards.

## Further Reading


Association of Paediatric Anaesthetists of Great Britain and Ireland. Guidelines on the prevention of postoperative vomiting in children. Revised 2016. www.apagbi.org.uk/sites/default/files/inlinefiles/2016%20APA%20POV%20Guideline-2.pdf. Accessed 30 April 2021.

Bailey, R., Ahuja, M., Bartholomew, M. et al. Guidelines for day-case surgery 2019: guidelines from the Association of Anaesthetists and the British Association of Day Surgery. *Anaesthesia* 2019; 74, 778–92. doi:10.1111/anae.14639.

Children's Surgical Forum, Royal College of Surgeons. Standards for children's surgery. 2013. Available at: www.rcseng.ac.uk/-/media/files/rcs/library-and-publications/non-journal-publications/rcs_standards_for_childrens_surgery_2013.pdf. Accessed 31 March 2021.

Combined Working Party of the British Association for Paediatric Otolaryngology (BAPO), ENT UK, the Royal College of Anaesthetists (RCOA) and the Association of Paediatric Anaesthetists of Great Britain and Ireland (APAGBI). Safe delivery of paediatric ENT surgery in the UK: a national strategy. Available at: www.entuk.org/sites/default/files/files/Safe%20Delivery%20Paediatric%20ENT.pdf. Accessed 2 April 2021.

Royal College of Anaesthetists. e-Learning anaesthesia (e-LA), module 4b, paediatrics. Available at: www.e-lfh.org.uk/programmes/anaesthesia/. Accessed 31 March 2021.

Royal College of Anaesthetists. Guidelines for the provision of paediatric services. 2020. In Guidelines for the provision of anaesthesia services. Available at: https://rcoa.ac.uk/gpas/chapter-10. Accessed 31 March 2021.

Royal College of Anaesthetists. Guidelines for the provision of anaesthesia for day surgery. 2021. In Guidelines for the provision of anaesthesia services. Available at: www.rcoa.ac.uk/sites/default/files/documents/2021-03/GPAS-2021-06-DAYSURGERY.pdf. Accessed 31 March 2021.

Royal College of Anaesthetists, Association of Paediatric Anaesthesia and the Royal College of Paediatric and Child Health. Guidance for the administration of codeine and alternative opioid analgesics in children. November 2013. Available at: www.apagbi.org.uk/sites/default/files/paragraphs/files/Codeine_Nov2013.pdf. Accessed 2 April 2021.

Royal College of Nursing. Day surgery for children and young people. 2020. Available at: www.rcn.org.uk/professional-development/publications/rcn-guidance-day-surgery-for-children-and-young-people-pub-009330. Accessed 31 March 2021.

Chapter 10

# General Principles of Safe Anaesthesia in Children*

Emma Stockton and David de Beer

## Introduction

Patient safety is the avoidance of unintended or unexpected harm to people during the provision of health care. Anaesthetists have been leaders in patient safety for decades. In the United Kingdom, wholesale reform of children's surgical delivery was undertaken after review of paediatric surgical outcomes in the 1990s, and in cardiac surgery, after an anaesthetist noted poor patient outcomes in children undergoing the arterial switch operation (see Kennedy 1996 in 'Further Reading').

Safety related to anaesthesia extends from institutional considerations through to preassessment, risk stratification, conduct of anaesthesia and postoperative care to safe discharge. It is too simplistic to see it as only limited to the operative period. This misses the bigger picture regarding keeping children safe. Anaesthetists providing care for children should be satisfied that the entire pathway provides the best possible outcomes for children in a holistic way. Patient safety can be improved by:

- Building psychologically safe teams
- Learning from when things go wrong (Safety II) and near misses, with the emphasis on prevention and system change rather than blame
- Learning from when things go right (Safety II)

Children comprise a quarter of the world's population, and many will require anaesthesia at some time during childhood. Most children undergoing surgery are fit and healthy. In the United Kingdom, approximately 40% of cases are undertaken in non-specialist district general hospitals. There are many situations where children require 'specialised paediatric anaesthesia', for instance neonates and infants, those undergoing complex surgery or those with significant comorbidity. At the time of writing, the first paediatric 'Getting It Right First Time' (GIRFT) report has highlighted unwarranted variation in the delivery of paediatric surgery. This is likely to result in further centralisation of services, especially for neonates and infants. It is essential that wherever children are cared for, staff are appropriately trained, there is suitable equipment and the child is in an environment that is child- and family-friendly. Ideally, specialist and non-specialist centres should work closely together in clinical networks to provide comprehensive services for children. Regular clinical attachments and joint meetings should help to foster links and enable non-specialist anaesthetists to maintain their skills. There is clearly a tension between centralising provision of paediatric care and maintaining skills in teams of non-specialists.

Guidance on the provision of appropriate anaesthetic services for children has been published (see 'Further Reading'). The main principles include:

- Children should be separated from and not treated alongside adults undergoing surgery. The specific needs of adolescents and young people should be recognised.
- Anaesthesia should be undertaken or overseen by staff who have undergone appropriate training and maintain regular paediatric practice. The anaesthetic assistant, recovery and ward staff must possess specific paediatric skills.
- Staff should undergo regular paediatric resuscitation training.
- There should be acute pain services for children.
- There should be neonatal, high-dependency and intensive care services as determined by

* Many thanks to Dr Ian James, who wrote the first edition of this book chapter, much of the content of which has been used in this revision.

the nature of the surgery undertaken in that hospital.
- Where a child presents to a non-specialist centre with a life-threatening condition, and it is not feasible to transfer the child, the most senior appropriately experienced anaesthetist available should care for that child.
- Guidelines for the management of common emergencies in children, including resuscitation, anaphylaxis and management of the head injured child should be readily available.
- Wherever possible, parents (or carers) should be involved in care and decisions about the child.

# Risks of Anaesthesia

## Mortality

General anaesthesia in children without comorbidity undergoing elective surgery is very safe, with a risk of death as a direct result of anaesthesia being 1:100,000 to one in a million. It is difficult to determine the risk of death for an individual child undergoing anaesthesia, as this must be put in the context of their preoperative state and the surgery they are undergoing.

In a large North American survey, the most common cause of perioperative cardiac arrest was cardiovascular, most likely due to hypovolaemia from blood loss or hyperkalaemia from transfusion of stored blood. Respiratory causes were the next most frequent cause, most commonly airway obstruction in recovery due to laryngospasm. Equipment-related cardiac arrest occurred mainly due to vascular injury from central venous lines. Medication-associated cardiac arrest is less frequent since the decline in halothane use. Children at greatest risk of perioperative cardiac arrest and mortality due to anaesthesia are those with heart disease, or pulmonary hypertension, and those under one year of age, with the highest-risk group being neonates undergoing cardiac surgery. Where there is increased risk due to comorbidity or anticipated anaesthetic or surgical difficulty, it is essential that this is discussed with the patient where relevant, parents or carers and documented in the medical records.

## Morbidity

There are some common events and risks for children and young people undergoing anaesthesia for routine surgery. The risks will vary between individuals, the anaesthetic technique used and the nature of the surgery. They can be categorised as being:

- Very common (>1:10) – agitation on waking (mainly one to six years of age); sore throat; nausea and vomiting (particularly in older children); temporary changes in behaviour, such as anxiety, sleep problems, bedwetting
- Common (1:10–1:100) – minor lip or tongue injury, discomfort at injection site
- Uncommon (1:100–1:1,000) – respiratory problems requiring treatment, skin damage (mainly in longer procedures)
- Rare (1:1,000–1:10,000) – need for unplanned intensive care (higher risk in children under one year, especially neonates), corneal abrasion, damage to teeth
- Very rare (1:10,000–1:100,000 or more) – anaphylaxis (1:40,000), awareness (1:60,000), death as a direct result of anaesthesia (1:100,000–1:million), long-term disability (<1:100,000)

Awareness may occur more commonly in children than adults, although fortunately children rarely develop symptoms of posttraumatic stress disorder. Risk factors for awareness appear to be intubation (greater stimulation) and the use of nitrous oxide (possibly associated with use of a lower concentration of inhaled volatile agent).

In the Anaesthesia Practice in Children Observational Trial (APRICOT), the overall incidence of perioperative severe critical events in the UK cohort was found to be 3.3% (cf. 5.2% overall). Cardiovascular instability (1.3%), comprising hypotension, arrhythmias and bleeding, followed by laryngospasm (1.1%), were the most frequent critical events. Postanaesthetic stridor, bronchospasm and aspiration were the next most common. It is now incumbent on anaesthetists to explicitly discuss risks of all procedures that are associated with an anaesthetic. This includes regional blocks, central and arterial lines. We have limited data about how to quantify these risks for individual children, though it is probable that neonates and smaller infants are at greater risk of line-related morbidity such as clots and limb damage.

Occasionally parents may ask whether anaesthetics, especially repeated anaesthetics, can have a detrimental effect on their child's development. In the past decade, concerns have been raised from animal studies suggesting that anaesthetic agents that function as NMDA antagonists or GABA agonists cause neuroapoptosis in the immature mammalian brain. This led to concerns about general anaesthesia in preterm and newborn infants. There is currently insufficient information to suggest that this is a problem in humans. Recent studies suggest that there are no adverse long-term effects on the brain of a single short anaesthetic in young children, but some have suggested that multiple anaesthetics before the age of four years may be associated with learning difficulties, although this is not proven. The consensus of experts is that it is unethical and harmful to deny anaesthesia to neonates and small infants if they require it, and there is no reason to change clinical practice at present. If surgery is required, children should be given an anaesthetic. The uncertainty provides a clear opportunity not to perform unnecessary surgery!

## Preparation for Theatre

It is essential that all children undergo anaesthesia assessment prior to coming to theatre (see Sury et al. 2015 in 'Further Reading'). As well as determining comorbidity and establishing fitness for anaesthesia, this provides an opportunity to discuss the anaesthesia plan and associated risks. The need for premedication will depend on the perceived state of anxiety of the child, the preference of the anaesthetist and the type of surgery being undertaken. Parents may be able to offer advice on their child's likely behaviour, but it is not uncommon for a child to appear calm and unperturbed during the preoperative visit yet become extremely distressed and uncooperative on arrival in the anaesthetic room. If premedication and/or topical analgesia are required, it is important to get the timing of its administration right. The most common premedication is midazolam via the buccal or oral route. Occasionally the children who would most benefit from anxiolysis either refuse or spit it out. Intranasal dexmedetomidine is an alternative but may take over 60 minutes to take full effect. Children must be in a suitable, non-stimulating environment to maximise the effect of any premedication given.

For topical analgesia, tetracaine 4% gel (Ametop®) and lidocaine 4% cream (LMX 4®) work within 45 minutes, whilst EMLA® takes an hour to be effective. Ethyl chloride spray can make the skin less sensitive for a few minutes and is favoured by some older children but is flammable and should be used with caution in environments with a lot of electrical equipment.

There is increasing recognition that restraining children to undertake unpleasant procedures is psychologically harmful. This long-term view should be considered when dealing with a premedication failure. It may be preferable to delay surgery and build long-term trust with health care professionals than to pursue anaesthesia using physical restraint. For some anxious children, it can be beneficial to insert a cannula on the ward prior to their transfer to theatre.

If the procedure is being undertaken in a theatre that is not regularly used for children, the anaesthetist must take particular care to ensure that the appropriate equipment for a child is available and is in working order. This includes ensuring the appropriate ventilator settings. For most children, this will be pressure-controlled ventilation, and the default settings for volume-controlled ventilation suitable for an adult may cause harm in smaller children. Theatre temperature may need to be increased if an infant or small child is to be operated on. Children can lose heat rapidly, and warming equipment should be available for all children. Warming equipment can be very effective and should never be used without monitoring core temperature.

All children must be weighed accurately before theatre as all drug and fluid prescriptions are weight-based. In children with a high BMI, lean body weight (LBW) should be calculated, as this may be required to calculate some drug doses. Drugs and fluids should be drawn up and prepared carefully, using appropriately sized syringes and giving sets.

## Parental Presence during Induction

Parental presence during induction can be extremely helpful, and at the authors' institution both parents/carers are allowed to remain with the child until they are asleep. Exceptions include infants and children with a difficult airway and those who are very small or sick, when it is preferable to ask the parents/carers to leave prior to induction. Many studies have shown that parental presence leads to a reduction in both the child's and parents' anxiety. For small children, induction is often undertaken in the parent's arms or with them sitting on their lap. Both parents and children overwhelmingly support parental presence at induction, although some parents may find the experience upsetting. It is important to explain to parents what to expect and give them the option of not being present should they not wish to be.

For children who are particularly anxious, it may be less distressing if they are allowed to come to theatre in their normal clothes. For adolescent children, anxieties about modesty should be anticipated; they too may feel more comfortable if not compelled to wear a revealing theatre gown. Hair clips and other accessories, if still in place, can be removed once the child or young person is asleep.

## WHO Surgical Safety Checklist

The WHO Surgical Safety Checklist (SSC) was designed to prevent communication failures and reduce readily avoidable surgical complications. Whilst the physical act of 'ticking a box' may not necessarily prevent all adverse events, the checklist is a framework on which the correct attitudes and behaviours towards teamwork and communication can be encouraged. The Surgical Safety Checklist should be used for all cases commencing with a team brief to ensure that all team members are acquainted, that all are clear what surgeries are to be performed and that any special equipment that may be needed is available. Figure 10.1 shows the standard routine at the authors' institution.

## Wrong-Sided Nerve Blocks

Contributory factors to the performance of a wrong-sided nerve block include:

- Distraction in the anaesthetic room
- Prolonged period between the WHO SSC 'sign-in' and performance of the nerve block
- Covering up of the surgical mark to keep the patient warm
- Repositioning of the patient or where blocks are performed infrequently

To reduce the risk of wrong-site anaesthetic nerve blocks occurring, a 'Stop before You Block' check was introduced in the United Kingdom by the Safe Anaesthesia Liaison Group (SALG) and Regional Anaesthesia UK (RA-UK). The check is recommended after the WHO SSC 'sign-in' and before the insertion of the block needle for unilateral regional blocks. The check should be performed by the anaesthetist and anaesthetic assistant and includes visualisation of the surgical arrow indicating site of surgery and double-checking the consent form for operative site. More recently, SALG and RA-UK have published an updated national standard operating procedure, 'Prep, Stop, Block', which enhances the message of 'Stop Before You Block', with the 'stop' moment occurring just before needle insertion.

## Induction

The choice of intravenous or gas induction is determined by the preference of the child, parent and anaesthetist, although the lack of suitable veins may dictate an inhalational induction. As awareness of climate change increases, departments and individual practitioners may wish to move towards more intravenous inductions. Where appropriate, the child should be given the choice. Many children are frightened of needles, whilst others may have previous experience of a gas induction and not want to repeat it. Some children, of course, want neither, and it can sometimes be challenging to proceed without some form of therapeutic restraint or protective holding. Having the parent present to assist can be helpful.

Sevoflurane is the most common means of gaseous induction. There is no 'correct' or 'best' means of using it. For some children, a gradual increase of the vapour works well; for others, moving rapidly to or starting at 8% is preferable. Nitrous oxide speeds up induction, and initial sedation with nitrous oxide and oxygen may make acceptance of a face mask easier.

Some children will tolerate a mask relatively easily, others less so. Applying a mask forcibly to a small child is oppressive and can lead to a more challenging induction at the time and at future surgery. It is often easier and less threatening to use a cupped hand as a 'mask', holding it close to the nose and mouth. At the authors' institution, a range of flavoured lip balms are stocked in each theatre. Children are encouraged to apply their favourite lip balm to the interior of the mask to increase compliance.

The most used intravenous induction agent is propofol, although this can be very painful on administration, especially when given through small veins. Higher doses (3–5 mg $kg^{-1}$) are needed in small children compared to adults. Thiopentone (5–7 mg $kg^{-1}$) is seldom used these days but remains a useful alternative, as it is not associated with pain on injection.

## Airway Management

Many small infants partially obstruct during induction of anaesthesia, and the insertion of an oropharyngeal airway may be beneficial if the

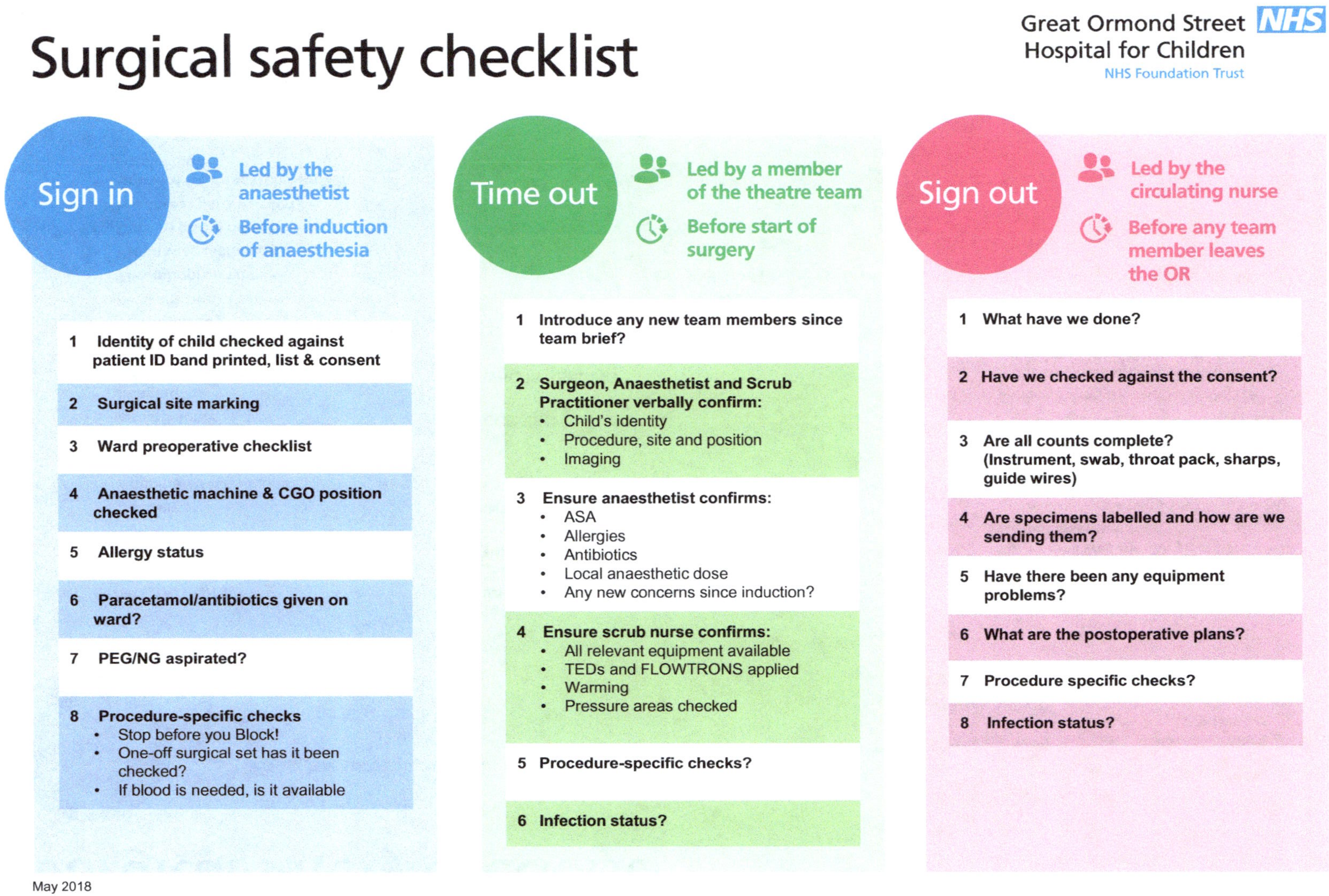

Surgical safety checklist
Great Ormond Street Hospital for Children
NHS
NHS Foundation Trust
Sign in
Led by the anaesthetist
Before induction of anaesthesia
1 Identity of child checked against patient ID band printed, list & consent
2 Surgical site marking
3 Ward preoperative checklist
4 Anaesthetic machine & CGO position checked
5 Allergy status
6 Paracetamol/antibiotics given on ward?
7 PEG/NG aspirated?
8 Procedure-specific checks
• Stop before you Block!
• One-off surgical set has it been checked?
• If blood is needed, is it available
Time out
Led by a member of the theatre team
Before start of surgery
1 Introduce any new team members since team brief?
2 Surgeon, Anaesthetist and Scrub Practitioner verbally confirm:
• Child's identity
• Procedure, site and position
• Imaging
3 Ensure anaesthetist confirms:
• ASA
• Allergies
• Antibiotics
• Local anaesthetic dose
• Any new concerns since induction?
4 Ensure scrub nurse confirms:
• All relevant equipment available
• TEDs and FLOWTRONS applied
• Warming
• Pressure areas checked
5 Procedure-specific checks?
6 Infection status?
Sign out
Led by the circulating nurse
Before any team member leaves the OR
1 What have we done?
2 Have we checked against the consent?
3 Are all counts complete? (Instrument, swab, throat pack, sharps, guide wires)
4 Are specimens labelled and how are we sending them?
5 Have there been any equipment problems?
6 What are the postoperative plans?
7 Procedure specific checks?
8 Infection status?
May 2018


**Figure 10.1** Surgical safety checklist.

# Surgical safety checklist

Great Ormond Street Hospital for Children
NHS Foundation Trust
NHS

## Team brief

Led by the surgeon, nurse or anaesthetist

Before starting the list

**1 INTRODUCTIONS**

**2 REVIEW EACH CASE ON THE LIST:**

- **Concerns**
- **Anticipated blood loss**
  - Where is the blood?
- **Any special equipment, loan sets or one off sets?**
- **Imaging**
- **Infection status?**
- **Surgical Site Infection Bundle**
  - Antibiotics?
  - Warming?
- **Thromboprophylaxis?**
- **Pregnancy testing?**
- **Can we give a drink?**
- **Is a throat pack needed?**
- **Consent for Research Study if applicable?**

**3 WHO IS SCRUBBING/OPERATING?**

**4 ANY STAFFING/TIME ISSUES?**

**5. ANY OUTSIDE ISSUES?**

- e.g. ICU beds

**6 CONFIRM LIST ORDER**

**7 WHO IS SENDING?**

## Team debrief

Led by the surgeon, nurse or anaesthetist

At the end of the list

**1 REVIEW THE PRINTED LIST:**

- **How well was the Surgical Safety Checklist done today?**
- **What worked well today? If relevant complete a praise form.**
- **Were there any staffing, equipment or prosthesis issues?**
- **What could improve for next time?**
- **Were there any avoidable delays?**
- **Did any incidents occur which require a Datix? If yes who will complete the Datix form?**

May 2018

**Figure 10.1** *(cont.)*

obstruction is not relieved by repositioning of the airway. Airway management will depend on the type of surgery. Tracheal tubes are secured with adhesive tape, and it is important to ensure this does not stick to the mucosa of the lips. In small infants, the skin can be fragile, and tape should be removed with care at the end of surgery. It is very easy to inflate the stomach with air when ventilating a small child by face mask. This can impede ventilation, and a nasogastric tube should be inserted to deflate the stomach if this occurs.

It is common practice to extubate neonates and infants fully 'awake', when their airway reflexes have returned, and they are breathing regularly. For some older infants who are breathing spontaneously, it may be appropriate to perform a 'deep' extubation, but this will usually require the minimum alveolar concentration (MAC) of the volatile agent to be around 1.5. Extubating an infant between these two extremes can lead to breath-holding or laryngospasm.

## Laryngospasm

Perioperative laryngospasm is a life-threatening complication that occurs more commonly in children than in adults, particularly in small infants. In the APRICOT study, laryngospasm was one of the most frequent respiratory complications (0.2–6.7%). It most frequently occurs during induction or immediately after extubation, sometimes with no apparent precipitating cause. Often it is due to the airway being stimulated too early during induction or the tracheal tube being removed too early at the end of surgery. Blood or secretions at the larynx can also precipitate laryngospasm.

Partial laryngospasm is characterised by a high-pitched inspiratory noise with increased respiratory effort but minimal visible sign of airflow. If laryngospasm is complete, there will be no airflow or noise. Its effective management requires early recognition and prompt and aggressive treatment, as hypoxia can rapidly ensue. Management of laryngospasm involves the following actions:

- Remove the laryngospasm stimulus.
- Apply CPAP with high-flow 100% oxygen via a tight-fitting face mask (the reservoir bag should be 'tight').
- Apply jaw thrust and small rapid breaths, avoiding gastric inflation if possible.
- Alert the anaesthetic assistant, who should prepare the appropriate intubation equipment and tracheal tube as quickly as possible.
- Ensure the oximeter and electrocardiogram (ECG) remain attached.
- If the laryngospasm does not resolve rapidly, consider deepening anaesthesia with propofol (1 mg $kg^{-1}$).
- If there is still no improvement (14% of cases in the APRICOT study), administer suxamethonium 1 mg $kg^{-1}$ IV and atropine 20 mcg $kg^{-1}$ and ventilate by hand; it may not be necessary to intubate. Suxamethonium 4 mg $kg^{-1}$ IM may be used if the IV cannula has been displaced at the end of surgery.
- Consider passing a nasogastric tube after laryngospasm has resolved.

Laryngospasm will usually settle without the need for intervention other than the application of continuous positive airway pressure (CPAP) with high-flow oxygen. Occasionally, at the end of surgery, it may be difficult to break the laryngospasm, and it may be necessary to re-institute anaesthesia, re-intubate and leave the tracheal tube in place until the patient is fully awake. Negative pressure pulmonary oedema may occur in young people after severe laryngospasm.

## Rapid Sequence Induction

In theory, classic rapid sequence induction (RSI) should be used in all children at risk of regurgitation and aspiration. This includes those requiring emergency surgery who may not be appropriately fasted, particularly those with proximal bowel obstruction, and in the child with posttonsillectomy haemorrhage who may have a stomach full of blood. However, there are practical limitations that make classic RSI difficult in infants and usually inappropriate:

- Attempts to pre-oxygenate a frightened and uncooperative small child may be counterproductive.
- It is not always possible to obtain venous access in small infants to administer an intravenous induction agent and a rapidly acting muscle relaxant. Inhalational induction may therefore be necessary.
- The high oxygen consumption seen in infants leads rapidly to hypoxia if ventilation is avoided before intubation.

- The cricoid ring is higher. Cricoid pressure can make intubation more difficult and may not actually 'obstruct' the oesophagus effectively.

For these reasons, many experienced paediatric anaesthetists will adopt a pragmatic approach in small infants with a potentially full stomach and will gently ventilate whilst waiting for the muscle relaxant to work, with gently applied cricoid pressure. Rocuronium 1 mg $kg^{-1}$ is the standard muscle relaxant, but as apnoea is not a fundamental component of this 'controlled RSI', many will use a slower, non-depolarising agent such as atracurium. Suxamethonium is rarely used these days. For the older child, a classic RSI can be utilised.

## Teeth

For children in the middle of orthodontic treatment, it is important to establish whether their braces are fixed or can be removed. It is also very important to establish whether a child has any loose deciduous teeth. If very loose, it may be necessary to remove a tooth after induction to prevent it being dislodged and lost or inhaled during airway manipulation. This possibility should be explained to the parents during the preoperative visit. The tooth must be kept safe and handed to the parents after the procedure.

Occasionally a permanent tooth may be unintentionally avulsed during airway manipulation. It is important to be aware that this can be successfully salvaged if acted upon immediately. There is a 30-minute golden window for this, and a guideline such as that in Figure 10.2 should be followed.

## Intravenous Lines

These should be well secured and preferably visible throughout the procedure. It is surprisingly easy for extravasation to occur in small infants, especially if fluid boluses are given rapidly under high pressure. When a child arrives in theatre with an IV line already in situ, it must be inspected carefully and tested prior to being used for induction. The skin over the cannula tip should be visible, and this will necessitate the removal of any dressings that may have been applied to prevent the child displacing the cannula. Pain on injection of saline should give rise to suspicion that the line has 'tissued', although it may also be due to phlebitis in a long-standing line. It is not always possible, of course, for IV lines to be visible throughout the procedure. Before the child is covered with drapes, it is important to ensure the line is working well. Many cannulae in children are placed over or near wrist and ankle joints, and ease of injection can be very positional. This must be resolved before the child is covered. If a line becomes more difficult to inject into or if fluids slow down during the procedure, the possibility of extravasation should be considered and the site inspected. Clear drapes mitigate against undetected extravasation but are not always readily available.

At the end of the operation, all IV lines must be flushed with saline to avoid the possibility of flushing of residual drugs into the circulation later. There have been several reports to National Reporting and Learning Service in England of harm due to flushing of residual anaesthetic drugs in IV cannulae in children. It is the responsibility of the anaesthetist to make sure that residual anaesthetic agents in IV lines are cleared prior to the child leaving their care.

## Extravasation

There are some drugs that can cause severe tissue injury in the event of extravasation and in some cases can lead to skin necrosis and nerve or tendon injury. Severe injury may necessitate later surgical release of contractures and skin grafting. Tissue damage may occur due to extravasation of cytotoxic drugs, hyperosmolar substances, highly acid or alkaline solutions, drugs formulated in alcohol or polyethylene glycol or vasoconstrictor drugs (causing local ischaemia). Occasionally damage may occur due to high-volume extravasation causing mechanical tissue ischaemia. Drugs most likely to cause problems during anaesthesia include:

- X-ray contrast media
- Thiopentone
- Ketamine
- Atracurium
- Sodium bicarbonate
- Magnesium sulphate 20%
- Calcium chloride or gluconate
- Vasoactive drugs
- Glucose >10%

Established treatment protocols for extravasation injury must be readily available. Immediate management involves minimising the concentration of the drug at the site of extravasation by stopping the injection and aspirating as much of the drug as possible from the cannula. Where there has been significant leakage of a tissue-damaging drug,

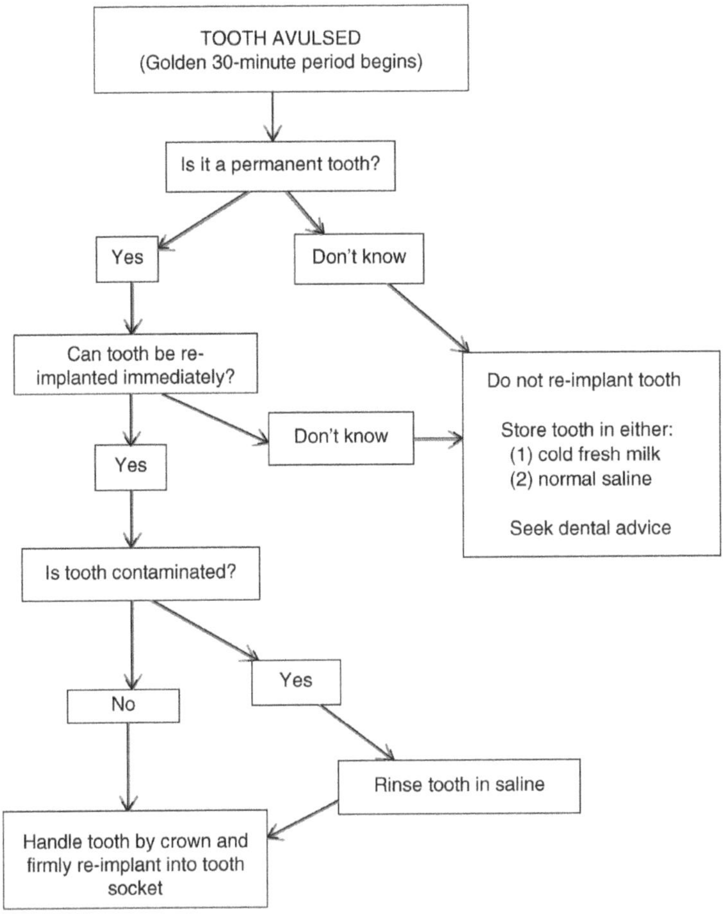


**Figure 10.2** Management of avulsed tooth during general anaesthesia.
From Soneji B, Forde K, Mason C, Dental Department, Great Ormond Street Hospital NHS Foundation Trust.

saline washout should be performed. This involves making multiple skin incisions around the site of extravasation. Saline is then injected through one or more of the incisions with a blunt needle to flush extravasated drug out through the other puncture sites. It may be necessary to obtain input from the plastic surgery service.

## Positioning

This will be dictated largely by the surgical procedure, and most cases will be supine. The head should not be rotated beyond 65°, particularly in paralysed children, as this can lead to C1–2 facet dislocation. This atlanto-axial rotary subluxation can occur in children because of ligamentous laxity, poorly developed cervical musculature, horizontally orientated facet joints and wedge-shaped cervical vertebrae. The head should be supported in a gel ring to prevent abnormal rotation.

Care should be taken to ensure that all pressure points are well padded, particularly when the patient is in the prone or lateral position. Care must be taken to protect the eyes when the patient is prone. If the arms are extended above the head, which may be necessary in some radiological investigations, they should be supported in such a way that there is no tension at the shoulder to avoid the possibility of a brachial plexus injury.

## Acute Major Anaphylaxis during Anaesthesia

Anaphylaxis is a severe life-threatening generalised or systemic hypersensitivity reaction. The reported incidence of perioperative anaphylaxis is one in 10,000, with an incidence of 2.7 per 100,000 in children (NAP6). Clinical presentation includes:

- Pharyngeal or laryngeal oedema
- Acute severe bronchospasm
- Hypotension
- Tachycardia
- Skin/mucosal changes

Unlike in adults, bronchospasm and/or high airway pressures are the commonest presentation (National Audio Project 6, NAP6) in children, and a change in ventilatory parameters is often the first indication to alert the anaesthetist. Severe bronchospasm, with difficulty ventilating the lungs, will lead to a rapid fall in oxygen saturation. In severe cases, it can be exceedingly difficult to ventilate the lungs, and end-tidal $CO_2$ may rise due to hypoventilation. A fall in end-tidal $CO_2$ may be seen if the bronchospasm is so severe that there is little alveolar ventilation. Hypotension may occur rapidly, and bradycardia is more common than in adults (18% vs 12.6%, NAP6).

The most likely causes of a drug-induced anaphylactic reaction in a child are antibiotics (penicillin or cephalosporins), lidocaine, radiological contrast media and latex. Due to the small number of cases reported in children, NAP 6 was not able to make any firm conclusions concerning the risk rates with different drugs, but atracurium, cefuroxime, suxamethonium, aprotinin and cryoprecipitate were all implicated. Reaction to muscle relaxants does not appear to be as common in children as in adults, possibly because they are used less frequently than in adults (24.7% vs 47%, NAP6).

The treatment of a severe anaphylactic reaction is summarised in Box 10.1. Adrenaline is the cornerstone of treatment and should be administered early. Where the treatment has been prolonged, or infusions of adrenaline or noradrenaline have been necessary, the patient should be admitted to a high-dependency or intensive care unit for postoperative monitoring.

Even in cases where the situation is resolved promptly, the patient should remain in hospital overnight, as in up to 20% of cases there can be a biphasic reaction with recurrence of symptoms up to 12 hours later.

Full documentation of the episode is essential. As soon as the patient has stabilised, blood

**Box 10.1** **Emergency management of severe anaphylaxis.**

- Discontinue suspected agent and maintain anaesthesia
- Call for help. Stop or do not start non-essential surgery
- Give 100% oxygen and ensure adequate ventilation (intubate if necessary)
- Give adrenaline bolus, 1 mcg $kg^{-1}$ i.v. (0.1 ml $kg^{-1}$ of 1:**100,000**)
  [1:**100,000** solution made by diluting 1 ml of 1:**10,000** up to 10 ml]
- Repeat adrenaline bolus as necessary for resistant hypotension or bronchospasm; start continuous infusion if multiple boluses required
- Give rapid i.v. crystalloid bolus, 10–20 ml $kg^{-1}$ (Hartmann's solution of similar) and repeat until hypotension resolved
- CPR if necessary

*For adrenaline resistant bronchospasm*

- Salbutamol 5–15 mcg $kg^{-1}$ i.v. over 5 min or
- Aminophylline 5 mg $kg^{-1}$ i.v. over 20 min

*For resistant hypotension*

- Start noradrenaline infusion 0.05–0.5 mcg $kg^{-1}$ $min^{-1}$

**AFTER** initial resuscitation, consider

| | | |
|---|---|---|
| • Hydrocortisone | 4 mg $kg^{-1}$ i.v. | |
| • Chlorphenamine | 6 months | 250 mcg $kg^{-1}$ i.v. |
| | 6 m–6 y | 2.5 mg |
| | 6–12 y | 5 mg |
| | >12 y | 10 mg |

- Check blood gas and treat acidosis if present
- Check coagulation and treat as appropriate
- Take clotted blood sample for serum tryptase as soon as patient is stable. Plan for repeat sample at 1–2 hours and > 24 hours
- Plan transfer of patient to an appropriate critical care area

samples for mast-cell tryptase (5 ml into a plain tube) should be taken as these will help to determine whether there was mast-cell degranulation. Peak levels occur between 1 and 2 hours, and repeat samples should be taken at 1, 2, 4 and 12 hours to document the reaction. The immunology service should be contacted to investigate the patient further.

## Latex Allergy

A substantial number of patients and medical staff have developed sensitivity, and in some cases an allergy, to latex. All departments should have a protocol for managing such patients, the most important measure being establishing a latex-free environment. This should be standard in UK operating theatres, with all supplies being latex-free. Powdered latex gloves are previously thought to have caused most aerosolised latex particles. These are no longer available in National Health Service (NHS) hospitals.

Patients should be highlighted on the theatre list and consideration given to placing them first. Any latex products should be removed from the theatre – usually latex gloves. Patients at high risk for serious reactions fall into three groups:

(1) Those with a history of latex anaphylaxis, confirmed by positive antibody testing
(2) Those with a history of allergy to latex, with urticaria, eye swelling, central dermatitis or bronchospasm
(3) Those with no previous reaction, but who have:
   - Spina bifida
   - Genito-urinary anomalies
   - Multiple surgical procedures
   - Documented reactions to IV drugs

There appears to be cross-sensitivity to peanuts and to some fruits such as kiwi, banana or avocado, so allergy to these should raise an index of suspicion. Previous recommendations for premedication of latex-sensitive patients with steroids, antihistamine and $H_2$-receptor antagonists are no longer advised, as this does not prevent a reaction, nor does it affect the severity of a reaction.

Departments should have clearly documented protocols in the operating theatres and recovery areas detailing what equipment is latex-safe and what should be avoided. Latex-free anaesthetic equipment is now widely available. When drawing up drugs, care should be taken to ensure all bungs are latex free – the vast majority are. Should a severe reaction occur, management is as for acute major anaphylaxis.

## Recovery

It is important to provide a thorough handover to the recovery room or intensive care staff at the end of the procedure. This should include details of intraoperative analgesia, antiemetics and antibiotics that have been given or charted for postoperative administration, any airway or venous access difficulties that have been encountered and any other adverse events. If topical anaesthesia has been applied to the larynx, it is important to advise when the patient can drink. We usually advise that this should be at least two hours after the larynx was sprayed. A simple aide-memoire such as that shown in Figure 10.3 works well in ensuring that no vital information is missed. Recovery handover is another important stop point to check that all intravenous lines have been adequately flushed with saline to avoid later inadvertent administration of residual anaesthetic agents.

## Emergence Delirium

Behavioural disturbance during early emergence from anaesthesia, usually involving agitation, hyperactivity with flailing movements, inconsolable crying and disorientation, has been recognised for many years, and a Paediatric Anaesthesia Emergence Delirium (PAED) scale has been developed. It is particularly common in preschool children and appears to be more common following the use of sevoflurane and desflurane. The use of total intravenous anaesthesia (TIVA) with propofol reduces the risk of emergence delirium. It can be very distressing to recovery staff and to parents who witness it and usually assume their child is in pain. However, it appears to be unrelated to postoperative pain as it can occur in non-painful procedures such as radiological investigations. There is still no clear understanding of the aetiology of emergence delirium and consequently no widely accepted prophylactic strategy. Midazolam does not appear to prevent it, whether given as premedication or during anaesthesia. Some studies have shown that propofol, fentanyl, ketamine, clonidine and dexmedetomidine may be effective. Emergence delirium usually resolves over a period of 10–15 minutes, but when a

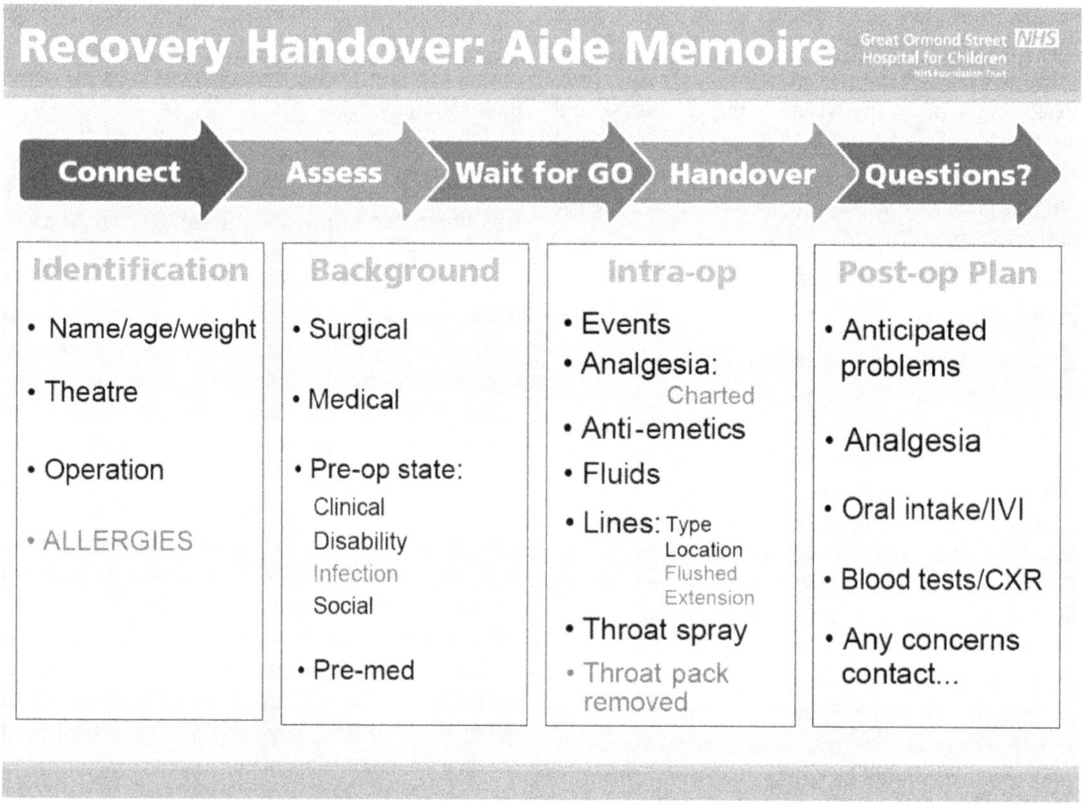


**Figure 10.3** Recovery handover aide-memoire.
Department of Anaesthesia, GOSH, Updated November 2020.

child is very agitated it can be ameliorated with a 0.5–1 mg $kg^{-1}$ bolus of propofol.

## Areas for Future Development

Paediatric anaesthesia appears safe when undertaken in well-planned, appropriately resourced environments. Despite this snapshot, observational studies have shown surprisingly high rates of severe critical events. Additionally, good outcomes of anaesthesia should extend to include psychosocial well-being and avoidance of hospital induced phobias.

As electronic anaesthetic recording becomes a standard of care, opportunities for contemporaneous big data to understand safety risks should become reality.

Areas for quality improvement include standardisation of serious critical event definitions; increased reporting; development of evidence-based protocols for management of serious critical events; development and rational use of paediatric perioperative risk assessment scores; implementation of current best practice in provision of competent paediatric anaesthesia services in Europe; development of specific training in the management of severe perioperative critical events; and implementation of systems for ensuring maintenance of skills.

## Further Reading

Bhanaker SM, Ramamoorthy C, Geiduschek JM et al. Anesthesia-related cardiac arrest in children: update from the pediatric perioperative cardiac arrest registry. *Anesthesia & Analgesia* 2007; 105:344–50.

Dahmani S, Stany I, Brasher C et al. Pharmacological prevention of sevoflurane- and desflurane-related emergence agitation in children: a meta-analysis of published studies. *British Journal of Anaesthesia* 2010; 104: 216–23.

Davidson AJ, Smith KR, Bkusse van Oud-Alblas HT et al. Awareness in children: a secondary analysis of five APRICOT GIRFT cohort studies. *Anaesthesia* 2011; 66:446–54.

Hollnagel E, Wears RL, Braithwaite J. From Safety-I to Safety-II:

A White Paper. The Resilient Health Care Net: Published simultaneously by the University of Southern Denmark, University of Florida, USA, and Macquarie University, Australia. 2015. Available at: www.england.nhs.uk/signuptosafety/wp-content/uploads/sites/16/2015/10/safety-1-safety-2-whte-papr.pdf. Accessed 13 March 24.

Kennedy I. Learning from Bristol. The Report of the Public Enquiry into Children's Heart Surgery at the Bristol Royal Infirmary 1984–1995. 2001.

Available at: www.bristol-inquiry.org.uk/final_report/the_report.pdf. Accessed 13 March 2024.

Lake C, Beecroft CL. Extravasation injuries and accidental intra-arterial injection. *Continuing Education in Anaesthesia Critical Care & Pain* 2010; 10:109–13.

Morris K, Fortune PM. Paediatric Critical Care. GIRFT Programme National Speciality Report 2022. 2022. Available at: https://gettingitrightfirsttime.co.uk/medical_specialties/paediatric-critical-care/. Accessed 13 March 2024.

National Health Service. Workstream: 'Getting It Right First Time'. Available at https://gettingitrightfirsttime.co.uk/workstreams/#surgical. Accessed 13 March 24.

Rappaport B, Mellon RD, Simone A, Woodcock J. Defining safe use of anesthesia in children. *New England Journal of Medicine* 2011; 364:1387–90.

Royal College of Anaesthetists. Guidance on the provision of paediatric anaesthesia services 2010. 2010. Available at: www.rcoa.ac.uk/node/714. Accessed 14 August 2012.

SmartTots (Strategies for Mitigating Anesthesia-Related Neurotoxicity in Tots). Available at: www.smarttots.org. Accessed 16 August 2012.

Sury MR, Arumainathan R, Belhaj AM, MacG Palmer JH, Cook TM, Pandit JJ. The state of UK pediatric anesthesia: a survey of National Health Service activity. *Paediatric Anaesthesia* 2015; 25 (11):1085–92. DOI: 10.1111/pan.12753.

van der Griend BF, Lister NA, McKenzie IM et al. Postoperative mortality in children after 101,885 anesthetics at a tertiary pediatric hospital. *Anesthesia & Analgesia* 2011; 112:1440–7.

Chapter

# 11 Equipment and Monitoring in Paediatric Anaesthesia

Ravi Shihurkar and Philippa Evans

## Introduction

It is important that correct equipment and monitoring are available to provide safe anaesthesia for children. Equipment and monitoring specifications need to consider the anatomical and physiological differences between adults and children, particularly in relation to infants and young children. It is also imperative to conduct inventory checks at regular intervals to ensure the whole range of sizes is available for use. Recent developments have amplified the role of mobile platforms to deliver remote assessments and point-of-care interventions.

## Airway Equipment

### Face Masks

Inhalational induction of anaesthesia is commonly performed in paediatric practice. It is important that face masks are acceptable to the child. Ideally, they should be constructed from clear plastic and have a soft rim. Some manufacturers produce scented masks to make them more attractive to children (applying scented lip balms to the inside of masks will have a similar effect).

Paediatric face masks exist in a range of sizes. The appropriate size should be used so that the face mask sits comfortably over the mouth and nose, pressure on the eyes is avoided and there is a good seal and minimal dead space. Commonly used masks are teardrop-shaped with inflatable seals; round masks are often useful for infants and neonates due to their relative micrognathia. A well-designed face mask facilitates the appropriate technique for maintaining the airway ('chin lift' or 'jaw thrust').

### Oropharyngeal Airways

Infants and young children have a relatively large tongue, and airway obstruction tends to occur early during induction of anaesthesia as airway tone is lost. This may be overcome with simple manoeuvres such as the application of continuous positive airway pressure (CPAP) via the breathing circuit, by a jaw thrust manoeuvre or by the insertion of an oropharyngeal airway once anaesthesia has been deepened. Oropharyngeal airways are available in sizes 000 to 4. The correct size is selected by placing the airway against the side of the mouth; the airway should reach from the angle of the mandible to the centre of the incisors or from the tragus of the ear to the corner of the mouth (see Figure 11.1). Too large an airway will protrude from the mouth and be ineffective; one that is too small may cause obstruction by pushing the tongue back or from the tragus of the ear to the corner of the mouth.

### Nasopharyngeal Airways

Nasopharyngeal airways (NPA) are well tolerated in the awake child and may be useful in a variety of circumstances:

- Children with congenital abnormalities associated with midface hypoplasia (e.g. Apert and Crouzon syndrome) or severe micrognathia (e.g. Pierre Robin sequence)
- Airway management under anaesthesia, such as to avoid problems with poor mouth opening or loose teeth and to aid fibreoptic intubation (FOI)
- Postoperatively to relieve obstruction at the palato-pharyngeal junction, such as posttonsillectomy in children with severe obstructive sleep apnoea (OSA) or palate repair in children with severe micrognathia

The length of the NPA should be such that it can be fixed securely to the face whilst the tip should just protrude from behind the soft palate. Nasopharyngeal airways are commercially available for all ages but have the disadvantage of being of fixed length. Alternatively, an NPA of specific length can be constructed from a cut tracheal tube

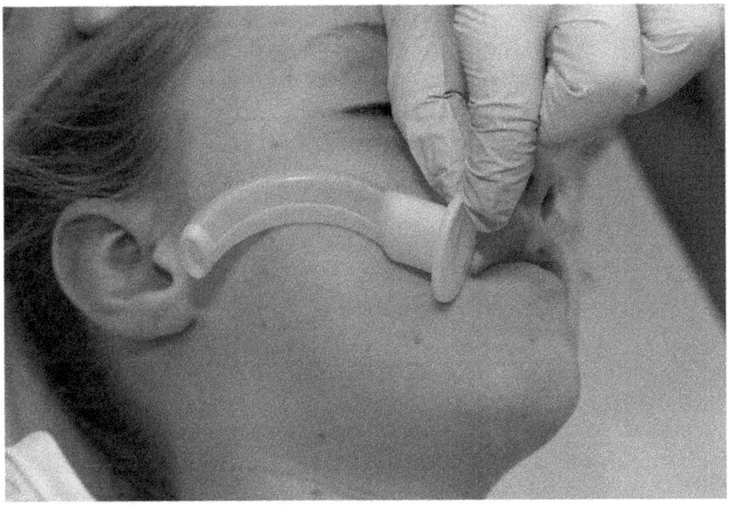

**Figure 11.1** Sizing an oral airway – from the tragus of the ear to the corner of the mouth.

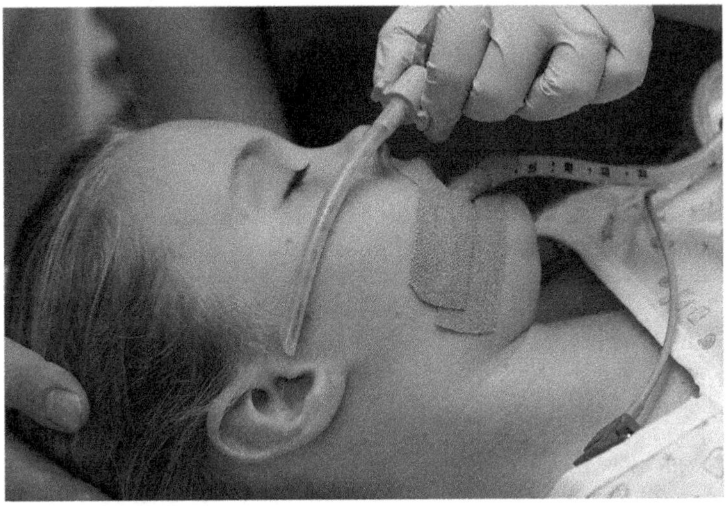

**Figure 11.2** Sizing a nasopharyngeal airway – from the tip of the nose to the tragus of the ear.

(TT), the same size or one size smaller than the age-appropriate TT for intubation. Ideally, a flanged TT connector is used to secure the NPA to the face. It is important that the NPA is neither too long, as it will protrude from the nose or cause laryngeal irritation and coughing, nor too short, as it will be ineffective in relieving airway obstruction at the palato-pharyngeal junction. The length should be approximately the distance from the tip of the nose to the tragus of the ear (see Figure 11.2). For some patients, the NPA can be cut to length under direct vision at the end of surgery. It is important that the length of the NPA is recorded and that the NPA is suctioned to this depth regularly, particularly in postoperative patients. For children needing an NPA to maintain patent upper airway, a spare NPA should be immediately available at the bedside in case of blockage with secretions or blood.

## Supraglottic Airways

Paediatric supraglottic airways (SGAs) are sized according to patient weight (see Table 11.1). The classic paediatric laryngeal mask airway (LMA) was not specifically designed for use in children but is merely a scaled-down version of the adult LMA. This has implications for its use in the paediatric population.

Single-use SGAs are used widely and are available in paediatric sizes 1–3. There is a learning curve when using the SGA in children. The complication rate is inversely proportional to patient size; displacement and airway obstruction occur

**Table 11.1** Supraglottic airway sizes

| Supraglottic airway size | Patient weight (kg) |
|---|---|
| 1 | <5 |
| 1.5 | 5–10 |
| 2 | 10–20 |
| 2.5 | 20–30 |
| 3 | 30–50 |

most frequently with the size 1 and 1.5 SGAs. The SGA has an important role in the management of the difficult paediatric airway (see Chapter 22), and the size 1 SGA has a role in neonatal resuscitation. In infants, airway obstruction may occur if the SGA pushes the large floppy epiglottis down to obstruct the laryngeal inlet. Difficulty can be encountered when using the traditional adult technique for SGA insertion in children. This may be due to adenotonsillar hypertrophy in older children or due to the epiglottis impinging on the SGA grille. Different techniques for SGA insertion and removal have been described. The SGA can be inserted partially inflated against the lateral side of the tongue and gently advanced until resistance from the tonsil is met, and then moved back into the midline. Alternatively, a rotational technique may be used where the SGA is inserted 'back-to-front', with the cuff facing the palate and turned through 180° once the hypopharynx is reached. The rotational and lateral techniques are both associated with high success rates for insertion in children less than six years of age.

Cuff inflation after insertion of SGAs may be according to the manufacturer's guidelines for volume and cuff pressure (<60 cmH2O) or by clinical endpoints such as forward movement of the SGA and ability to ventilate with a good seal. The use of a cuff pressure monitor has been recommended to avoid hyperinflation of the cuff and improve the overall positioning of the SGA (often at lower cuff inflation volumes than suggested by manufacturers). There is no consensus for the optimal timing for removal of SGAs in children. However, young children have reactive airways and show rapid emergence from anaesthesia. They may be more liable to develop laryngospasm if removal is delayed, and many practitioners prefer to remove the SGA whilst the patient is still deeply anaesthetised.

Flexible SGAs are available in size 2 and above. They have a non-kinking flexometallic tube that is longer and has a smaller internal diameter than in the standard LMA. This increases airway resistance and may increase the work of breathing if used with spontaneous breathing in longer cases. Flexible and preformed SGAs (e.g. AMBU®) permit the breathing circuit to be connected away from the operative area on the face (e.g. ophthalmic, dental, facial procedures).

The Pro-Seal LMA™ is available from size 1.5. It has a modified cuff that has been specifically designed for children. The LMA has an additional lumen running from the tip in parallel with the main airway that acts as an oesophageal drainage tube. This allows passive drainage of gastric contents and minimises gastric insufflation during positive pressure ventilation. The drainage tube also provides a route for nasogastric tube insertion and may prevent the epiglottis from obstructing the mask aperture. There is a high success rate for first insertion and overall high success rate for insertion in children. iGel® and LMA Supreme® have shown similar efficacy and ease of use in paediatric patients.

Whichever type of supraglottic device is used, displacement is common in children, particularly during patient transfer. The risk of displacement may be reduced by robust fixation of the device using an adhesive tape together with disconnection from the anaesthetic circuit during patient positioning.

## Tracheal Tubes

The traditional teaching to use uncuffed TTs in children under the age of 8 years stems from a conical model of the subglottic airway; the narrowest part of the airway was thought to be at the level of cricoid cartilage, which is the only cartilage forming a complete ring around the airway. This concept has evolved as more imaging data have become available. The paediatric airway is now believed to be ellipsoidal in the subglottic area, with the anteroposterior diameter larger than the transverse. This shape becomes circular at the level of cricoid cartilage.

This realisation coupled with improvements in TT technology have made cuffed tubes desirable for the following reasons:

- Better likelihood of selection of the correct size tube at the first intubation; avoids potential trauma associated with multiple intubations
- Reduces risk of aspiration

**Table 11.2** Uncuffed tracheal tube sizes

| Age | Internal diameter (mm) | Fixation length (cm) | |
|---|---|---|---|
| | | Oral ETT | Nasal ETT |
| Neonate (3 kg) | 3.0–3.5 | 10–10.5 | 12 |
| 6 months (6 kg) | 4.0 | 11.5–12.5 | 13 |
| 1 year (10 kg) | 4.5 | 13–13.5 | 15 |
| > 1 year | (Age in years/4) + 4.5 | (Age in years/2) + 12 | (Age in years/2) + 15 |

- Allows accurate measurement of $ETCO_2$; facilitates low-flow anaesthesia and reduces environmental pollution and costs
- More effective ventilation in children with poor lung compliance

However, in the absence of an international standard for tracheal tube marking or for the position or length of the cuff of a tracheal tube, there is great variability between manufacturers in the design of cuffed paediatric TTs. Ideally a TT with a high-volume, low-pressure cuff should be used, and care should be taken that the correct size TT is chosen; that the cuff is inflated in the mid-trachea, not in the subglottic region or between the vocal cords (nor to obstruct the right-upper lobe bronchus); and that the minimum cuff inflation pressure is used to seal the TT. The cuff pressure should be monitored and should not exceed 20 $cmH_2O$.

The ideal size of TT is one that will fit snugly to allow ventilation without excessive leak and prevent aspiration whilst avoiding pressure on the tracheal mucosa, particularly in the vulnerable subglottic area. Traditionally, this has been achieved by ensuring that there is a small audible leak around the TT at 20 $cmH_2O$ inflation pressure. Damage to the underlying mucosa can result in airway oedema and post-extubation stridor or, in the most serious cases, mucosal ulceration and necrosis leading to acquired subglottic stenosis. The formula for the selection of the correct size and length of TTs is based on age. These formulae are merely a guide, and TTs half a size smaller and larger than the tube selected should always be available. The formulae are less reliable in children under the age of one year (see Table 11.2). The formula for sizing cuffed TTs is shown in Table 11.3.

Careful selection and placement of an appropriate TT, whether cuffed or not, is important in minimising airway injury. It should be remembered that all TTs can be associated with airway trauma. It is our practice to use uncut TTs so that the tube connector can be seen, and the head can be placed to one side so that the TT will not kink. Some practitioners place an oropharyngeal airway along the side of the TT to provide some stability to the smaller TTs, which are more liable to kink. Once in place, it is important that the TT is fixed securely in position. There are many suitable methods. We use two pieces of adhesive tape cut into a 'trouser shape' to secure the TT. One 'trouser leg' of each piece should be attached to the TT, with the other 'leg' attached to the upper or lower lip (see Figure 11.3). It is important to make sure the tape is clear of the lip mucosa. Various proprietary tube holders/tube fixation devices are available for neonates. The reader must become familiar with the recommended method of securing and releasing tracheal tubes from the specific device used in their workplace.

**Table 11.3** Cuffed tracheal tube sizes

| Age | Internal diameter of ETT (mm) |
|---|---|
| Neonate (3 kg) | 2.5–3.0 |
| 6 months (6 kg) | 3.0–3.5 |
| 1 year (10 kg) | 3.5–4.0 |
| >1 years | (Age in years/4) + 3.5 |

## Polar (RAE) Tracheal Tube

RAE tubes are useful in head and neck surgery, and are named after their inventors, Ring, Adair and Elwin. They are manufactured in a preformed shape, either 'south facing' for oral intubation for cleft surgery or tonsillectomy, or 'north facing' for nasal intubation for dental or maxillofacial surgery. The lengths of the intraoral or intranasal

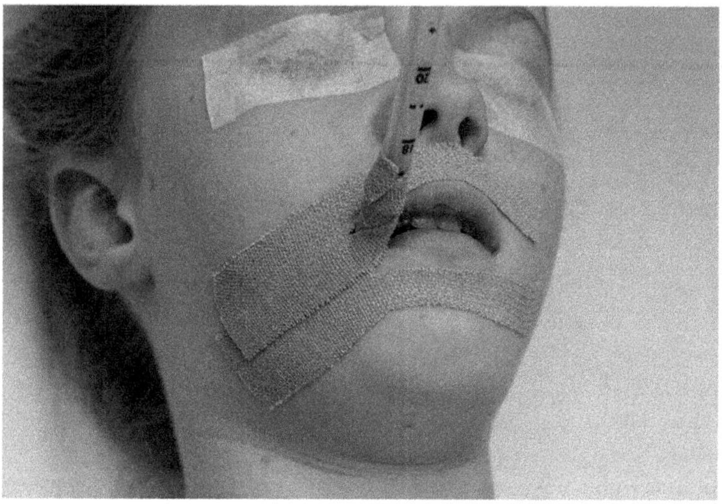

**Figure 11.3** Fixation of a tracheal tube. Two pieces of adhesive tape cut into a 'trouser shape'. One 'trouser leg' is attached to either the upper lip or the lower lip and the other end to the TT. An oropharyngeal airway can be inserted along the side of the TT to improve stability.

sections are fixed. If these proportions are too long, there is a risk of endobronchial intubation. There is currently no international standard for the length of preformed tracheal tubes, and different manufacturers produce tubes of different lengths. Difficulties may also be encountered in a child with failure to thrive where the larynx will be the age-appropriate size, but the child will be small for their age. The length of preformed tubes should therefore be checked after insertion by careful auscultation for bilateral breath sounds, and if necessary, the tube should be withdrawn. If using an oral preformed tube, a dental roll taped to the chin under the curve of the tube may be useful to fix the tube at the correct length. Note that extension of the head and neck reduces the length of the tube in the trachea; flexion of the neck will push the tube down towards the carina. Whatever design of tube is used, the position of the tube should be checked carefully after intubation, and again after repositioning for surgery.

## Armoured Tracheal Tubes

These tubes are indicated in neurosurgery, for surgery in the prone position and in cases where the head position is changed during surgery. A metallic spiral in the wall of the tube provides increased flexibility and reduces the chance of kinking. This increased flexibility may necessitate the use of an introducer or stylet for intubation. They have a greater external diameter than standard TTs, and a tube size half a size smaller than anticipated should be used. Although these tubes do not kink on bending, irreversible narrowing of internal diameter may occur if the patient bites on them, as may happen during reversal. Adequate depth of anaesthesia should be ensured to prevent this situation, or a bite block may be considered whilst waking the patient up.

## Cole Tracheal Tube

These tubes have a wide intraoral section that narrows to the appropriate size distally to pass through the vocal cords. The wider portion affords them more stability than the equivalent size of TT and makes them easier to manipulate. They are popular in neonatal units and are useful in airway rescue when inducing infants with suspected subglottic pathology. The shouldered portion sits against the vocal cords thus reducing the risk of endobronchial intubation. However, the wide portion of the Cole TT must not be allowed to move against or through the vocal cords, as this may lead to vocal cord injury or subglottic stenosis, and for this reason they are not recommended for prolonged periods of intubation.

## Double-Lumen Tracheal Tubes (DLT)

DLTs are used in adults to facilitate single-lung ventilation for a variety of thoracic procedures, including video-assisted thoracoscopic surgery. The smallest commercially available DLTs are 26 Fr gauge, which is roughly equivalent in external diameter to a size 6.5 mm TT. DLTs are therefore only suitable for children from the age of 8–10 years upwards. They are available as left- or right-sided DLTs, referring to which main bronchus is intubated. When used, left-sided DLTs are preferred to avoid the bronchial cuff occluding the right upper lobe bronchus.

If one lung ventilation is required in smaller children, infants or neonates, an appropriate-size TT may be advanced into the main bronchus. Alternatively, a bronchial blocker or Fogarty catheter is placed by the side of a single lumen TT. Cuff position is ascertained with bronchoscopy before inflating it. Utmost care needs to be taken to avoid displacement and overinflation of bronchial cuff.

## Tracheostomy Tubes

Paediatric tracheostomy tubes are available from various manufacturers, with each detailing unique features with respect to material, dimensions, MRI compatibility, extensions, cuff variations, ergonomics, flange shapes, adjustable flange, etc (see Table 11.4). It is vital to ensure that spare tracheostomy tubes (of same make/size and of a size smaller) and adjuncts (suction apparatus with catheters, tracheal dilator, tube securing kit, scissors) are immediately available at all times. The reason for tracheostomy, upper airway patency and emergency care notes should be made clearly visible at the patient's bedspace. Surgeons often place stay sutures in paediatric trachea during first tracheostomy insertion to facilitate quick re-insertion of a new tube in case of accidental extubation. Other adjuncts include heat and humidity exchangers and speaking valves.

# Laryngoscopes and Blades

## Straight Laryngoscope Blades

Straight laryngoscope blades are useful in infants up to about six months of age. Infants have a relatively large tongue, the larynx is relatively cephalad and the epiglottis is long and floppy and may be angled into the lumen of the airway to cover the laryngeal inlet. This combination of factors may make it difficult to visualise the laryngeal inlet by conventional laryngoscopy (i.e. indirect elevation of the epiglottis with the tip of the laryngoscope blade placed in the vallecula above the epiglottis). The straight blade takes up less space in the mouth and allows the epiglottis to be lifted directly to reveal the glottic opening. Two different techniques have been described to visualise the larynx in infants: the laryngoscope blade is slid underneath the epiglottis and the tip of the blade lifted so that the glottis is exposed; or the laryngoscope blade is deliberately advanced into the oesophagus and then, with the tip lifted anteriorly, withdrawn slowly until the larynx drops into view. Both techniques bring the blade into direct contact with the undersurface of the epiglottis, which may cause intense vagal stimulation.

**Table 11.4** Paediatric tracheostomy tubes used in the United Kingdom

| | Variants | Material | ID (mm) | Cuff features | MRI compatibility | Notes |
|---|---|---|---|---|---|---|
| Portex Bivona® | Neonatal (smaller shaft)<br>Paediatric (longer shaft) | Siliconised PVC with wire coil | 2.5–5.5 | Uncuffed and cuffed: Aire-Cuf® (air) TTS™ (water) Fome-Cuf® (foam) | Incompatible (MRI conditional version available) | Available in V & straight flanges; Flextend™ offers long external shaft |
| | Hyperflex™ (adjustable flange) | Stainless steel coil | | | Incompatible | Replace with customised fixed flange tube ASAP |
| Shiley™ | Neonatal (Neo) | Opaque thermosensitive PVC | 3.0–4.5 | Uncuffed only | Compatible | PVC is stiffer & easier to railroad over suction catheters |
| | Standard Paediatric (Ped) | | 3.0–5.5 | Uncuffed and cuffed (standard and long lengths) | | |
| | Paediatric Long (PDL) | | 5.0–6.5 | | | |

Notes: ID: internal diameter; MRI: magnetic resonance imaging; PVC: polyvinyl chloride.

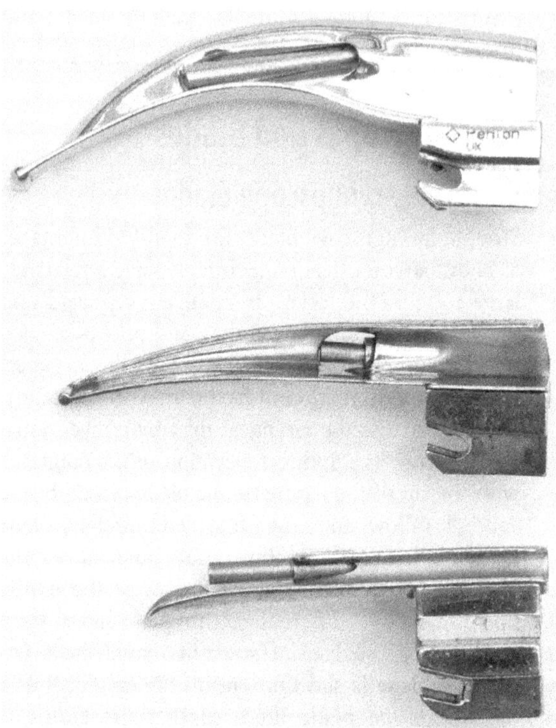

(a) Macintosh

(b) Robertshaw

(c) Miller

**Figure 11.4** Selection of laryngoscope blades used in paediatric anaesthesia.

There are several different straight blade laryngoscopes available (see Figure 11.4). The type selected is often based on personal preference. The Robertshaw and Seward blades have an open cross-section profile that allows for easier intraoral manipulation of the TT. The Miller laryngoscope blade is C-shaped in cross-section, which reduces the ease of such manipulation but the extended curve at the tip of the blade facilitates anterior lifting of the epiglottis.

### Curved Laryngoscope Blade (Macintosh Blade)

These are used from about the age of six months. The conventional technique for laryngoscopy should be employed. There are five sizes available: small infant size 0, infant size 1, child size 2, adult size 3 and large adult size 4. Polio blades and short-handled laryngoscopes may be useful.

## Specialised LARYNGOSCOPES

### The McCoy Blade

This is a standard Macintosh blade with a hinged tip that is useful for elevating the epiglottis if it is obstructing the view of the laryngeal inlet.

## Videolaryngoscopy

This traditionally describes the transmission of the view from the tip of the blade via a fibreoptic endoscope to a video display. Newer videolaryngoscopes use an image-sensing microchip camera with LED light source at the distal end; optical data are then transmitted electronically to a display system. This eliminates the fragility of fibreoptic bundles and provides a wider, clearer field of vision. Videolaryngoscopes are available in sizes suitable for all ages and are useful teaching aids when learning the techniques of paediatric intubation. Some such as the Glidescope® and D blade of CMAC® provide an angulated view of the larynx and may be useful in difficult intubation.

A combination of videolaryngoscope and flexible bougie or fibrescope (with TT railroaded) may be used for particularly challenging airway anatomy (see Chapter 22 regarding difficult airway in children).

Other videolaryngoscopes such as McGrath® and AirTraq® are portable and disposable or allow convenient disinfection after use.

## Aids to Intubation

Bougies and stylets are available in paediatric sizes. The smaller-sized bougies are rigid and often difficult to manipulate, and care must be taken to avoid trauma to the distal airway. A well-described technique in infants is a 'two-person' technique, where the first operator obtains the best possible laryngeal view during laryngoscopy using external pressure to the larynx, and a second anaesthetist passes the bougie. Stylets are useful for the introduction of flexible tubes. Care must be taken not to allow the hard tip of the stylet to protrude beyond the end of the TT to avoid trauma to the airway.

## Magill's Forceps

These are shaped anatomically to allow an object in the oropharynx to be gripped whilst staying away from the field of view. It is most commonly used to direct TT into the glottis, position the throat pack and assist in the retrieval of objects from the oropharynx. Adult as well as paediatric sizes should be available.

## Atomiser Devices

Nasal atomisers (MAD Nasal™) are used for trans-nasal administration of drugs like vasoconstrictors, local anaesthetics and premedication (dexmedetomidine). Laryngo-tracheal spray of local anaesthetic is used to anaesthetise the mucosa for diagnostic and therapeutic airway procedures. Devices with malleable stylet (MADgic®) are available in paediatric and adult sizes for this purpose.

## Airway Exchange Catheters

Airway exchange catheters, for example those manufactured by Cook®, are useful when employing fibreoptic techniques to manage a difficult airway. Their hollow central channel allows insufflation of oxygen and monitoring of end-tidal carbon dioxide ($ETCO_2$). The smallest size available is an 8 Fr catheter, which can be used to exchange a size 3 TT (see Table 11.5).

**Table 11.5** Airway exchange catheters

| Catheter gauge (French) | Catheter internal diameter (mm) | For replacing a TT with internal diameter (mm) |
|---|---|---|
| 8 | 1.6 | ≥ 3.0 |
| 111 | 2.3 | ≥ 4.0 |
| 4 | 3.0 | ≥ 5.0 |

## Suction Catheters

Suction catheters are available in a range of sizes. The following formula describes the relationship between the size of suction catheter and TT:

Suction catheter (French size) = 2 × internal diameter (in mm) of TT

Closed system suction catheters allow repeated suctioning without disconnections, thereby maintaining positive end expiratory pressure (PEEP), reducing wastage and preventing aerosolisation associated with disconnections.

# Breathing Systems

The ideal paediatric breathing system should have minimal functional or apparatus dead space, be either valveless or fitted with very low resistance valves and be constructed in such a way as to minimise gas turbulence and subsequent flow resistance.

Mapleson classified breathing systems into five types (A to E) according to their efficiency in eliminating carbon dioxide during spontaneous ventilation. Mapleson D, E and F systems are the most commonly used in paediatric practice as they most closely meet the criteria for an ideal paediatric system. However, the use of the circle system as the sole circuit for all age groups is increasingly common practice.

## The Jackson Rees Modification of the Ayre's T-Piece

The Mapleson E system is the Ayre's T-piece. This is a valveless breathing system used for children up to 25–30 kg. It consists of a T-shaped tubing with three opening ports: one port receives fresh gas from the anaesthetic machine; the second port leads to the patient's mask, LMA or TT; and the third port leads to reservoir tubing (see Figure 11.5). Mapleson F describes the Jackson Rees modification of system E by the addition of the open-ended reservoir bag to the end of the reservoir tubing.

The system requires a fresh gas flow (FGF) of 2.5–3 times the minute volume to prevent rebreathing with a minimum FGF flow of 4 l $min^{-1}$. The open-ended bag has a number of functions: it acts as a visual monitor during spontaneous ventilation, it can be used to provide CPAP during spontaneous ventilation and it can be used to

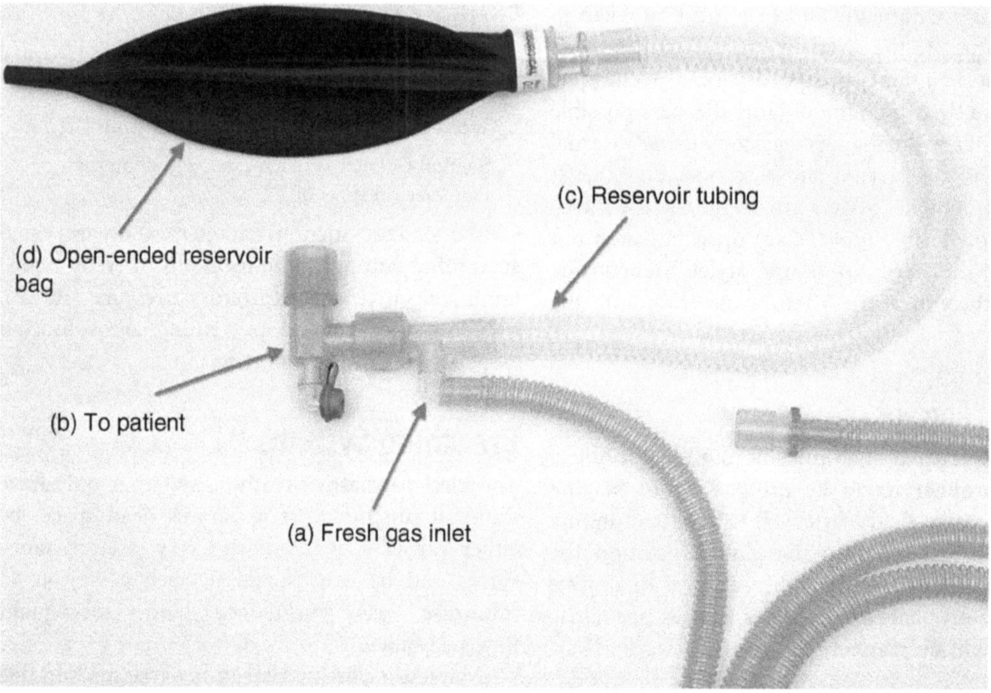


**Figure 11.5** The Ayre's T-piece with the Jackson Rees modification.

provide controlled ventilation, although experience is required to master the technique. The T-piece is not ideal for use in resuscitation for this reason.

## The Bain System

This is the coaxial version of the Mapleson D system. It may be used during induction of anaesthesia in children over 25–30 kg (although most practitioners now use the circle system for this purpose). The fresh gas flow to prevent rebreathing during spontaneous ventilation is 1.5–2 times the minute volume. Thus, a flow rate of 100–200 ml $kg^{-1}min^{-1}$ is required. During controlled ventilation, a fresh gas flow rate of 70–100 ml $kg^{-1}$ $min^{-1}$ is required.

## The Circle System

In this breathing system, soda lime is used to absorb the patient's exhaled carbon dioxide. The paediatric circle consists of lightweight 15 mm diameter tubing and a small 500 ml reservoir bag; 1 L bags are available for bigger children and adult tubing and reservoir bags (2 L) should be used in patients over 50 kg. The circle system/low-flow anaesthesia allows for improved preservation of heat and moisture, greater economy with less volatile agent used and reduced environmental pollution compared with the non-absorber systems. It is important to be vigilant if an uncuffed tube with a significant leak is used and very low-flow rates are employed.

Self-inflating resuscitating bags should be immediately available in adult, paediatric and infant sizes along with reservoir bags and supplemental oxygen connectors.

# Humidification

Humidification of inspired gases is important to prevent damage from dry gases and to minimise heat loss via the respiratory tract. The heat moisture exchanger (HME) is available in a range of sizes (volumes 7.8–100 ml) and is inserted at the point of connection of the airway device to the breathing circuit. The HME conserves approximately 50% of the water normally lost via the respiratory tract and prevents corresponding heat loss. This is of particular importance in neonates and small infants, who lose heat more rapidly than older children and adults because their ratio of minute volume to body surface area is higher. In addition, the HME protects against the inhalation of infective or hazardous particles and prevents cross-contamination between patients if re-usable breathing circuits are used. The HME is most efficient with smaller tidal volumes and higher respiratory rates and so is well suited to paediatric practice.

## Ventilators

The majority of children can be ventilated using modern adult circle ventilators provided:

- The ventilator can deliver high respiratory rates using pressure or volume-controlled ventilation.
- It allows adjustment of the I:E ratio.
- Lightweight 15 mm paediatric tubing is used.

Pressure-controlled ventilation is the preferred mode of ventilation in children as it can be adjusted more easily to compensate for leaks in the breathing circuit and minimises the risk of barotrauma.

Ventilation for term and preterm neonates can be challenging on conventional anaesthesia ventilators due to the requirement of accurate, small volume breaths delivered at a high rate with minimal dead-space/wasted ventilation. There are proprietary ventilators available for this niche requirement.

## Jet Ventilation

Low-frequency jet ventilation (LFJV) is a useful modality for laryngo-bronchoscopy (usually through a wide, short tube attached to the endoscope) and in 'can't intubate, can't ventilate' (CICV) situations (through a cricothyroidotomy cannula). Sanders injector or Manujet III are widely used hand-triggered devices. Particular attention should be paid to prevent disconnections, allow adequate time for exhalation and avoid barotrauma.

## CPAP and BiPAP machines

Children with obstructive airways, respiratory pathology or neuromuscular diseases may be supported with home ventilation and/or oxygen supplementation. These ventilators vary widely in their features, settings and emergency usage. Detailed discussion of these devices is beyond the scope of this text; however, anaesthetists should ensure they gain adequate understanding of their functioning, as children are likely to need this support whilst recovering from surgery and anaesthesia.

## High-Flow Nasal Oxygen Therapy (HFNOT)

Various devices are commercially available (e.g. OptiFlow™, Airvo™, Vapotherm, AquaVENT®, HI-Flow Star, AcuCare™, etc.) and are increasingly used to provide respiratory support in ward and ICU settings. These are open system devices that deliver heated (33–43°C), humidified (95–100%) oxygen at titratable $FiO_2$ and constant high flows (40–60 L/min). This combination allows improved oxygenation and patient compliance whilst reducing moisture loss and anatomical dead space. Attachments are available to adapt usage to tracheostomy tubes as well as nebulisers. Devices use different mechanisms to generate high flows (oxygen-air blender/entrainment system/built-in flow generator) and consequently differ in their operational characteristics. These devices have been used in various clinical settings:

- Supporting respiration in respiratory compromise when invasive ventilation is not indicated
- As an apnoeic oxygenation device during intubation or airway procedures
- Postoperative respiratory support to bridge transition to spontaneous ventilation

All the contraindications for non-invasive ventilation also apply to HFNOT, along with conditions like epistaxis or facial injury.

## Equipment for Vascular Access

### Intravenous Access

A range of sizes of cannula should be available. A 22-gauge cannula will suffice for the administration of drugs and fluid in most young children and infants. A 24-gauge, or even 26-gauge cannula, may be more appropriate in premature infants or those with difficult venous access. Larger-gauge cannulae are indicated for cases where significant blood loss is anticipated.

Specialised equipment is available for central venous access in children; catheters vary in length and size. A 4 Fr catheter is suitable for infants under 5 kg, 7 Fr for adolescents and 5 Fr catheters for all other ages. Ultrasound guidance should be used with a strict aseptic technique for the placement of central venous catheters in children, commonly via the internal jugular route or via the femoral vein.

Finding and cannulating paediatric veins can be challenging. This can be aided by 'vein finder' devices using principles of infrared light projection, transillumination or high-frequency ultrasound scanning.

## Intraosseous Access

Intraosseous (IO) access provides rapid, safe and effective vascular access in situations when intravenous access is difficult, for example during resuscitation. Various purpose made needles are available in 18G (0–6 months), 16G and 14G sizes. They possess a trocar that prevents bone from plugging the lumen of the needle. Traditional intraosseous needles (Cook®-type) are placed manually, the site, force required and depth of insertion being determined by the operator. Since 2006, a second type of device has been used in adult and paediatric practice. The EZ- IO® (Vidacare) has a battery-powered drill handle that powers needle insertion. Three different needle lengths are available, suitable for patients from 3 kg upwards.

Any drug or solution that can be given intravenously can be given by the IO route. Manual injection rather than passive infusion of fluid is required because of increased resistance. The resistance felt during injection is similar to that encountered during injection via an epidural catheter.

There is insufficient evidence to support use of IO samples for blood testing, and it should be reserved for when no other option is available. Results should be interpreted with caution and in the context of the clinical situation. Testing is invariably not calibrated for IO samples (samples may also be haemolysed or inadequate) and particulate matter can damage automated analysers.

## Equipment for Fluid Administration

It is important that intraoperative administration of fluids is carefully controlled and documented. Intravenous giving sets should incorporate a burette in smaller patients in order that accurately measured aliquots of fluid can be administered. A standard burette dispenses fluid at 20 drops per ml, and a microdrop burette dispenses fluid at 60 drops per ml. Blood and blood products should be infused using a system with an integral 170–200 mm filter.

Fluid warmers should be used in cases where large volumes of fluid or blood transfusion are anticipated. Many of the systems used in adult practice are not appropriate for use in the paediatric setting owing to cooling along the length of the IV tubing and relatively slow infusion rates in children. This problem is overcome by the use of counter-current warming systems (e.g. Hotline®) where warm water circulates around the entire length of the delivery line up to the point of administration to the patient.

## Drug Administration

Drug doses in paediatric practice are based on patient weight. Often only very small volumes of standard formulations of drug are required. Smaller-sized ampoules or paediatric formulations are available for some drugs, which help to reduce waste. It is important that a range of syringes from 1 ml upwards is available in order that dosing is accurate. Equipment to measure accurate weight and height must be available for all ages from preterm neonate to a teenager.

While using total intravenous anaesthesia (TIVA), appropriate paediatric-specific models should be loaded and used in syringe pumps.

## Equipment for Regional Anaesthesia

Epidural kits containing 19/20G Touhy needles are available with catheters ranging from 21G to 24G. These have 0.5 cm markings and are available in 50 or 80 mm length. Catheters can be multi-orifice or open-ended single orifice.

## Temperature Maintenance

Infants and small children are at particular risk of developing hypothermia owing to their large body surface area to volume ratio. It is important to avoid hypothermia as it increases postoperative oxygen consumption, affects recovery from anaesthetic drugs, impairs coagulation, may depress ventilation and can result in arrhythmias.

The ambient temperature in the operating theatre may be raised, which will help reduce heat loss due to radiation. However, the theatre should not be heated to such an extent as to compromise infection control policies and staff comfort. The ideal theatre temperature is between 19°C and 21°

C, and it should not exceed 23°C. Blankets, sheets, gauze pads and fluids are often warmed in a warming cabinet to prevent rapid cooling of an infant or small child.

Care should be taken during induction of anaesthesia to avoid unnecessary exposure of the child. It is important to remember to keep infants' heads covered. Intraoperatively, forced-air warming devices are most widely used. In smaller patients, most benefit is derived if the device is placed under the patient. Humidification of anaesthetic gases and fluid warmers should be used routinely, as discussed in the 'Humification' section. Clear plastic drapes are highly effective at reducing heat loss and prevent pooling of liquids which evaporate and further cool the patient. In conditions where forced-air warming is not feasible (transport, MRI suite, etc.), disposable transport warming mattresses can provide effective underbody warming (TransWarmer®); activation of the gel starts an exothermic reaction which provides warming for up to two hours without the need for a power source.

## Monitoring Equipment

Most monitors have been developed for adult practice and adapted for use in children. Essential monitoring is mandatory in all anaesthetised patients, but monitors are not a substitute for the presence of a vigilant anaesthetist, who should combine the information provided by the monitors with their own observations in order to direct the management of the patient. Essential monitoring for anaesthesia includes:

- Oximetry
- ECG
- Non-invasive blood pressure
- Capnography
- Airway pressure

### Pulse Oximetry

This provides a non-invasive measurement of peripheral saturation of arterial blood ($SpO_2$). It enables the detection of incipient and unsuspected arterial hypoxaemia, allowing early intervention before tissue damage occurs.

The 'peg-like' probes used in adult practice are suitable for use in children over 10 kg. A more reliable device for use in younger children is a wraparound probe in an adhesive strip. The strip can be attached to a digit, palm of a hand or sole of a foot, the site depending on the size of the patient. The sensors should be protected from interference from outside light sources. Motion artefact can also be a significant problem in the awake patient.

The presence of foetal haemoglobin or hyperbilirubinaemia in young infants has no clinical effect on the detection of hypoxaemia by the pulse oximeter. In patients with cyanotic congenital heart disease, the oximeter tends to overestimate readings at lower saturations. It should be remembered that in neonates with duct-dependent systemic circulation, the saturation measured may be appreciably different depending on the site of the probe; shunting of deoxygenated blood through a patent ductus arteriosus will result in lower saturations in the left hand and lower body.

### Electrocardiography

The electrocardiogram (ECG) provides a monitor of heart rate and rhythm and can indicate myocardial ischaemia. Neonates and young children display right-ventricular dominance on their ECG. This gradually declines with age; the QRS axis becomes similar to that of an adult by the age of five years. Neonatal and paediatric electrodes are available for babies and small infants.

Infants and young children are at risk of bradycardia during anaesthesia and surgery. Continuous ECG monitoring allows prompt intervention. Infants and young children desaturate rapidly and develop a bradycardia in response to hypoxia. Many practitioners advocate leaving both the pulse oximeter and ECG in place during emergence from anaesthesia; if technical problems or artefacts are encountered with the saturation probe and its accuracy is questioned, a slowing of heart rate will alert the practitioner to a 'patient' rather than 'equipment' problem.

### Capnography

Gases with molecules that contain at least two dissimilar atoms absorb radiation in the infrared region of the spectrum. This property forms the basis of capnography and the measurement of expired carbon dioxide concentration throughout the respiratory cycle. Capnography is an invaluable aid to detect oesophageal intubation, disconnection of the breathing circuit, rebreathing and hypoventilation and is a useful monitor to indicate low cardiac output.

The capnograph sampling chamber can be either positioned within the patient's gas stream (mainstream sampling) or connected to the distal end of the breathing system via a sampling tube (side-stream sampling). The latter is the most common arrangement in theatres. However, both systems have their drawbacks. With side-stream analysis, the $ETCO_2$ may be underestimated when the tidal volumes are very small (standard rate of sampling 150–200 ml $min^{-1}$). Mainstream (or inline) analysis is more accurate, but the sample cell is heavy and bulky and risks kinking the TT. Mainstream analysers are widely used in ICU and for monitoring during the transfer of intubated patients. The measurement of $ETCO_2$ levels in children may also be inaccurate if respiration is rapid or shallow, if there is a leak around the TT or when there is a large volume of apparatus dead space. In patients with cyanotic congenital heart disease, the $ETCO_2$ readings will be lower than arterial $PaCO_2$, sometimes by 2 kPa.

## Transcutaneous Carbon Dioxide Measurement

Arterial $CO_2$ tension can also be estimated from the continuous measurement of transcutaneous $CO_2$ ($TcCO_2$). This is a useful tool in the PICU but is of limited use in anaesthesia as calibration of the apparatus takes 10 minutes for each patient, and it requires good and constant skin perfusion. It may be useful in situations where $ETCO_2$ measurement is inaccurate, for instance during laparoscopic surgery in neonates. The position of the heated sensor (43–44°C) must be changed every three to four hours to avoid thermal injury.

### Non-invasive Blood Pressure Measurement

An appropriately sized blood pressure cuff is one that occupies two-thirds of the upper arm. A width of 4 cm is recommended in full-term neonates. If the cuff is too small, it overestimates blood pressure; if it is too large, readings are falsely low.

### Invasive Blood Pressure Measurement

An arterial line provides direct measurement of blood pressure and allows for intermittent blood sampling. The radial or the femoral arteries are the most common sites that are cannulated. The axillary artery can be used as an alternative, but the brachial route should be avoided as it has poor collateral vessels. A 22-gauge cannula is suitable for most infants and small children, a 24-gauge cannula should be used in neonates and preterm babies if the radial site is accessed. A cannula in the femoral artery can compromise blood flow to the leg, especially in infants of less than 3 kg, and placement of a cannula in this site should have a strong indication in these patients. Likewise, blood flow to the leg should be monitored when combined femoral venous and arterial access is used in older infants. Ultrasound is a useful tool for locating and confirming patency of arteries and with practice can be used to guide cannula insertion in peripheral sites even in very small babies. It is imperative that an arterial cannula does not possess an injection port and is clearly labelled. The transducer systems are the same as those used in adult practice and incorporate a column of bubble-free (heparinised) saline at a pressure of 300 mmHg. Care should be taken with the volume of fluid administered by the arterial flush system, and for this reason, an infusion pump delivering 1 ml $hour^{-1}$ is commonly used in the ICU setting.

## Monitoring Cardiac Output in Children

Monitoring cardiac output (CO) is technically challenging in children, and most paediatric anaesthetists monitor surrogates of flow such as pressure (arterial, central venous), capillary refill or markers of tissue oxygen delivery (base excess, lactate, central venous oxygen saturation). Technology is improving, though, and several techniques used in adults can now be applied to infants and children to provide accurate measurements of cardiac output:

- Thermal dilution – catheters limited to children >5 kg
- Lithium dilution (LiDCO)
- Transoesophageal, transthoracic echocardiography
- Transoesophageal doppler – probes limited to children >3 kg
- Pulse contour analysis (PiCCO)
- Venous oximetry
- Near-infrared spectroscopy (NIRS)

## Transoesophageal Doppler

Transoesophageal Doppler is used to measure the flow velocity in the descending aorta to estimate cardiac output. Aortic diameter may be measured directly or may be derived from an inbuilt nomogram by entering age, height and weight. Placement in the oesophagus is operator dependent, and CO values show reasonable correlation with those obtained by thermal dilution. Probes suitable for children >3 kg are now available.

## Pulse Contour Analysis

CO may be derived from arterial waveform analysis, and there are a number of different techniques available that measure real-time CO. Most depend on complex mathematical and physiological calculations, and few studies have validated these in children. These techniques may be useful during stable conditions, but monitors require recalibration and may have limited accuracy when vascular tone changes or with rapidly changing haemodynamics during surgery.

## Near-Infrared Spectroscopy

NIRS is a non-invasive optical method for continuous measurement of tissue oxygenation and has been used as a measure of cerebral and somatic perfusion in adults and children, particularly during cardiac surgery and intensive care. It relies on the principle that haemoglobin absorbs infrared light close to the visual spectrum, and that the absorption of light depends on the oxygenation status of haemoglobin, as most other biological tissues do not absorb light of this wavelength. Whereas pulse oximetry requires a pulsatile flow and provides a measure of arterial saturation, tissue oximetry does not require a pulsatile flow, and the value is mainly determined by venous oxygen saturation, haemoglobin and blood flow. Provided oxygen extraction and haemoglobin remain constant, the NIRS value becomes a surrogate measure of flow. The precise design of the equipment and the algorithms used to determine tissue oxygenation vary between manufacturers. Probes, including infant probes, are specifically designed for different tissue areas (cerebral, abdominal, renal, muscle) and will give inaccurate results if not used according to the manufacturer's instructions. The sensitivity and specificity of NIRS-derived measurements of low perfusion compared with invasive measurements of cardiac output are improved by monitoring at multiple sites. The technology is improving, but absolute values vary between manufacturers, and the upper and lower NIRS values are not clearly defined. The probes are expensive, and controversy remains about the value of NIRS in improving outcomes. However, NIRS does appear to have a role in monitoring trends in tissue perfusion, particularly as an early warning of low cardiac output or to detect catastrophic events, for instance during aortic cannulation in cardiac surgery.

## Depth of Anaesthesia Monitors

Traditionally, clinical signs (breathing pattern, pupillary size and reactivity, eye movement) and physiological response to surgical stimulation have been used to assess depth of anaesthesia. Several monitors have been developed by different manufacturers to assess depth of anaesthesia based on analysis of the EEG using information derived from adult EEG data. The Bispectral Index (BIS) has been studied extensively, but other monitors include the Narcotrend™, Cerebral State Monitor™, AEP/2 and M-entropy monitor. These monitors help to avoid awareness in high-risk patients and also, by avoiding unnecessarily deep anaesthesia, may improve recovery from anaesthesia. These monitors are affected by the use of neuromuscular blocking agents, some specific anaesthetic agents used (BIS is unaffected by nitrous oxide and high-dose opioids) and there may be paradoxical changes during sevoflurane anaesthesia (increased EEG activity associated with deep sevoflurane anaesthesia results in higher BIS values). The EEG changes during a child's development, and since they have been developed using adult data, depth of anaesthesia monitors may not be reliable in infants and younger children.

## Temperature Monitoring

Temperature monitoring is essential to detect both hypothermia and inadvertent hyperthermia in children undergoing general anaesthesia. Temperature is usually monitored in the nasopharynx, oesophagus or rectum or at a peripheral site. Oesophageal temperatures should be recorded in the lower third of the oesophagus to avoid falsely low readings caused by a leak around the tracheal tube. Rectal probes can cause perforation in neonates and should not be used in neutropenic patients.

## Urine Output

This should be monitored in all cases of major surgery or when significant blood loss is anticipated. Silastic catheters are used. The smaller catheters have a stylet, which should be removed prior to insertion to avoid creating a false passage. The smallest balloon catheter available is 6 Fr; this has a 1.5 ml balloon which is appropriate for most term neonates onwards. If a balloon catheter cannot be passed, then a 6 Fr feeding tube should be used (this is stiffer and smaller than the 6 Fr Foley as it does not have the extra thickness at the balloon). The balloon should always be inflated with water, not saline (and only after urine has been identified), as saline may crystallise, which can then block the channel and prevent balloon deflation. The same catheters are used for girls and boys. In male infants, the preputial orifice overlies the glandular meatus and thus the prepuce does not need to be fully retracted during catheter insertion. Once inserted, the catheter should be connected to a urometer that can collect and measure small volumes of urine.

## Point-of-Care Ultrasound

Ultrasonography (USG) is a useful bedside tool, assisting vascular access, regional anaesthesia, echocardiography, lung ultrasound and newer applications, including determination of gastric residual volume/contents, delineating tracheal anatomy and TT cuff localisation. The hockey-stick probe (7–10 MHz) has the smallest footprint and is most versatile, though a range of probes should be available for different applications. Bedside use of USG may become more commonplace with availability of portable and handheld units which interact via app-based interfaces on various devices. Apart from smaller structures, paediatric patients may have greater anatomical variations and mobile vasculature. Interventions with ultrasound require a motionless field, and general anaesthesia is often required to achieve the best conditions. Frequent practice and an understanding of USG principles and drawbacks, including reverberation artefacts, mistaking the shaft of the needle for the tip and acoustic shadowing, are vital to benefit from the use of USG.

## Anaesthetic Record and Configuration of Monitors

A clear record of all drugs and the doses administered should be part of the information recorded on the anaesthetic chart. The chart should also record the method of induction, airway management, monitoring equipment used and patient position in addition to documenting the physiological parameters measured throughout the procedure. Any problems encountered should be clearly documented as they may act as an alert for future anaesthetists. Electronic patient recordkeeping systems are being incorporated into many hospitals. These include anaesthetic charts for preassesment and intra- and postoperative care documentation. Staff should receive adequate training to use these systems. Where autopopulated data are incorrect, annotations may need to be made to improve accuracy. Various systems can be configured to allow secure communication with patients through apps and video conferencing, thereby making remote preassessments more routine. This may partly be aided by the evolution of medical grade remote monitors and wearable devices.

The presence of monitoring is not a substitute for an anaesthetist. Age-appropriate alarm limits should be set for each physiological variable to increase vigilance. The information provided by the monitors must be integrated with the anaesthetist's own observations so that appropriate interventions are made. It is worth noting that not all monitoring devices have established clinical testing standards for paediatric patients, and data may be extrapolated from adult counterparts.

## Distraction Technologies

Various distraction methods are available to help manage procedural anxiety and reduce stress in children. Toys, audio-visual stimulation and storytelling are often useful for infants and toddlers. Tablets, mobile phones, music players and gaming devices and virtual reality systems are available for older children. Pictures, videos and virtual reality simulations have been used preoperatively to familiarise children with specific hospital environments to help reduce anxiety.

### Key Points

- It is imperative that the correct equipment and monitoring are available to provide safe anaesthesia for children.
- Supraglottic airway size selection is based on patient weight; tracheal tube size selection is based on patient age.
- Most children can be ventilated using modern adult circle ventilators, as long as the appropriate settings are selected.

- Temperature monitoring and heat conservation techniques are important as infants and small children are at particular risk of developing hypothermia.
- Increasingly sophisticated monitors have been developed that are suitable for use in children, but no monitor is a substitute for the presence and vigilance of the anaesthetist.

## Further Reading

Association of Anaesthetists. Recommendations for standards of monitoring during anaesthesia and recovery 2021. 2021. Available at: https://anaesthetists.org/Portals/0/PDFs/Guidelines%20PDFs/Recommendations%20for%20standards%20of%20monitoring%20during%20anaesthesia%20and%20recovery%202021.pdf?ver=2021-05-26-141701-007. Accessed 14 March 2024.

Grasso C, Marchesini V, Disma N. Applications and limitations of neuro-monitoring in paediatric anaesthesia and intravenous anaesthesia: a narrative review. *Journal of Clinical Medicine* 2021; 10:2639.

Humphreys, S, Schibler, A, von Ungern-Sternberg, BS. Carbon dioxide monitoring in children: a narrative review of physiology, value, and pitfalls in clinical practice. *Paediatric Anaesthesia* 2021; 31:839–45.

Mittnacht AC. Near infrared spectroscopy in children at high risk of low perfusion. *Current Opinion in Anaesthesiology* 2010; 23:342–7.

Nishimura M. High-flow nasal cannula oxygen therapy devices. *Respiratory Care* 2019; 64:735–42.

Skowno JJ. Hemodynamic monitoring in children with heart disease: overview of newer technologies. *Paediatric Anaesthesia* 2019; 29:467–74.

Tobias JD. Pediatric airway anatomy may not be what we thought: implications for clinical practice and the use of cuffed endotracheal tubes. *Paediatric Anaesthesia* 2015; 25:9–19.

Chapter 12

# Vascular Access in Children

David Chisolm and Gema Munoz-Mozas

## Introduction

A substantial proportion of children will require vascular access at some time during their lives. This may be for resuscitation within minutes of being born, for intravenous antibiotics as an infant or perhaps to administer repeat courses of chemotherapy for treatment of leukaemia. This chapter will outline the routes available for vascular access, the factors influencing the choice of catheters and devices used and their associated complications. Choosing the most appropriate site and type of vascular access must be specific to each child and to their treatment requirements (see Table 12.1). The publication of 'The Michigan Appropriateness Guide for Intravenous Catheters in Pediatrics: miniMAGIC' in 2020 (see 'Further Reading') was a significant moment in paediatric vascular access. Evidence suggests that implementation of the adult version (MAGIC) published in 2015 has led to a significant reduction in inappropriate use, patient harm and costs associated with vascular access devices. It is hoped that miniMAGIC will have the same effect in children and encourage research into areas where evidence is limited.

The correct care of vascular access devices during and following insertion is extremely important and will have a major impact on functioning of the catheter as well as reducing potentially life-threatening complications. The use of care bundles incorporating evidence-based measures greatly reduces both infective and non-infective complications.

## Peripheral Intravenous Catheters and Midline Catheters

Short-term peripheral intravenous access is widely used in children of all ages. Short peripherally inserted intravenous catheters (PIVC) can be used for drug delivery, fluid infusion and blood sampling.

**Table 12.1** Types of vascular catheters

| Catheter type | Entry site | Duration of use |
|---|---|---|
| Peripherally inserted venous catheter (PIVC) | Veins on hands, feet and forearms. Scalp veins in infants. | 72–96 hours |
| Midline catheter | Basilic or cephalic veins at the antecubital fossa. Tip of catheter stops short of axillary vein. | Up to 28 days |
| Peripherally inserted central venous catheter (PICC) | Basilic or cephalic veins at the antecubital fossa. Long saphenous vein in infants. Tip of catheter in central vein. | Weeks to months |
| Umbilical catheter | Umbilical vein used within 1 week of birth. | Up to 14 days |
| Non-tunnelled central venous catheter | Percutaneous insertion into internal jugular, subclavian or femoral veins. | Days to weeks |
| Tunnelled central venous catheter | Subcutaneous tunnel with cuffed catheter into central vein. | Months to years |
| Totally implantable device | Port positioned on chest wall, abdomen or forearm with subcutaneous tunnelled access to central vein. | Months to years |
| Intraosseous cannula | Proximal anterior tibia. Distal end of femur. Medial malleolus | Up to 24 hours |

Total parenteral nutrition (TPN) of sufficiently low osmolarity and non-vesicant chemotherapy can also be given via this route. PIVCs are usually sited into small veins on the hands, forearms, feet and scalp in infants. Catheters inserted over joints tend to cause more discomfort and are more prone to phlebitis, thrombosis and dislodgement. Larger veins at the antecubital fossa should be preserved if a subsequent midline catheter or a peripherally inserted central catheter (PICC) is anticipated. In neonates, the long saphenous veins at the ankle or knee may also be required for PICC insertion at a later date.

## Peripheral Intravenous Catheters (PIVC)

Traditionally, peripheral catheters were used for only 72–96 hours, but insertion duration alone is not grounds for removing a functioning catheter if there is no evidence of phlebitis and it is still clinically required. PIVCs are short (2.5–7 cm) catheter over needle devices available in a wide variety of diameters (14–26G) and materials (Teflon™ and polyurethane). The choice of catheter size depends on the diameter of the intended vein and also the flow requirements. In general, small catheters cause less phlebitis, both chemical and mechanical, are more comfortable and last longer. Children requiring peripheral venous access require skilled management involving age-appropriate behavioural techniques and suitable analgesia. Poorly managed pain during cannulation causes distress at the time, more pain during future episodes and long-term phobic behaviour. Topical anaesthesia, using a eutectic mixture of local anaesthetics (EMLA™, topical tetracaine 4% gel (Ametop®) or lidocaine 4% cream (LMX 4®), is effective if given sufficient time to work, although the removal of the occlusive plastic dressings can cause significant distress. EMLA™ should not be used in preterm neonates or any other children at risk of methaemoglobinaemia. Needleless injection systems of ionised lidocaine (J-tip) are available that have the advantage of almost instant analgesia and compare favourably with EMLA. Ethyl chloride spray is effective, but its flammability precludes its use in environments with electrical equipment. Nitrous oxide (Entonox) has also been used successfully for pain control during cannulation. In difficult cases, the use of real-time ultrasound or a near-infrared or LED light device has been shown to improve success rates and decrease insertion times.

## Midline Catheters

These are longer, soft, peripheral catheters made of polyurethane or silicone, usually 3 or 4 French gauge (Fr) in diameter. They are inserted into the cephalic or basilic veins at or just above the antecubital fossa through a specific micro-introducer kit, which has a sheath that is peeled apart to leave the catheter in the vein. The midline catheter is cut to the correct length and should be positioned to stop short of the axillary vein. Midline catheters cause less chemical phlebitis than peripheral catheters and hence may be used for up to four weeks. The same restriction on the osmolarity of the infusate applies.

### *Complications*

The commonest complication of PIVCs is phlebitis. This presents as redness, swelling, induration and pain around the insertion site of the catheter and necessitates removal. Phlebitis is an inflammatory reaction that is not primarily an infective process, although secondary infection may occur. The incidence of catheter-related blood infection (CRBI) from peripheral catheters is about 0.2–0.5 per 1,000 catheter days. Midline catheters have a lower infection rate of around 0.1–0.2 per 1,000 catheter days. Subcutaneous extravasation of infusate is another common complication with PIVCs. This is a particular problem in neonates, where the incidence may be as high as 90%. Serious tissue damage with subsequent scarring may occur, especially with TPN and calcium-containing infusates. Rapid identification of the extravasation and treatment with injection of hyaluronidase (500–1,000 units) and 0.9% saline irrigation can prevent tissue loss. All hospitals should have a readily accessible protocol for the acute management and follow-up of extravasation injuries. Significant venous thrombosis is rare with PIVCs. Catheter fracture and air embolism are also rare but potentially serious complications.

## Peripherally Inserted Central Catheters (PICC)

PICCs are small diameter catheters (1.2–5 Fr) made of silicone or polyurethane. The larger catheters may have two or three lumens to allow separation of incompatible infusates. PICCs allow access to the central circulation without exposing the patient to some of the serious insertion complications of direct approaches to the central veins. The dilution of the infusate by the larger volume of blood in the central veins makes them suitable for the administration of TPN and hypertonic solutions. They are also useful in the presence of coagulopathies and low platelet count, as bleeding at the insertion site is rarely a serious problem and usually responds to direct pressure. Local infection and venous thrombosis proximal to the insertion site are contraindications to PICC insertion.

PICCs are most commonly inserted percutaneously into the cephalic, basilic or brachial veins in the arm. The long saphenous vein at the ankle or knee or the superficial temporal vein can be used in neonates and infants. Lower limb insertion sites in neonates have been shown to prolong catheter function and decrease overall complications when used for TPN. Real-time ultrasound is useful and allows the basilic and brachial veins to be accessed above the antecubital fossa. The insertion kits are similar to that of midline catheters, incorporating a split sheath introducer or splitable needle for the smallest catheters. The vein can be accessed by direct cannulation or by fine needle access and the use of a Seldinger wire micro-introducer set. Most PICCs are cut to length prior to insertion using surface landmarks for the final tip position. Groshong$^{TM}$ PICCs have a special valve near their tip that allows fluid to be injected or aspirated but is closed when not in use and hence must be cut to length at the hub end.

The tip of the PICC ideally is positioned in the lower third of the superior vena cava (SVC) from upper limb veins or in the proximal inferior vena cava (IVC) from the long saphenous vein. The use of surface landmarks with blind insertion results in a satisfactory tip position in only about 15% of cases. With fluoroscopic guidance, this can be increased to 90%. If fluoroscopy is not used, a post-insertion chest radiograph must be performed to verify tip position. Newer electrocardiogram (ECG) tip position confirmation systems can be used to navigate and track the tip of catheters to the low SVC. These are very accurate, but their current license in children requires a post-insertion chest radiograph. If the tip is in the right atrium, it must be withdrawn to avoid atrial perforation and cardiac tamponade, which has a mortality rate of over 80%. This is a particular concern in neonates having TPN or hypertonic glucose infusions and was the subject of a warning from the UK Department of Health in 2001. The PICC tip can be advanced significantly by adduction of the arm, and this may precipitate serious cardiac dysrhythmias. A non-central tip position markedly increases the risk of vessel thrombosis. The reported incidence of thrombosis associated with PICCs varies widely, from around 4% if clinical signs are used to up to 25% with surveillance venography. The cephalic venous system is reported to have a much higher thrombosis rate than the basilic system, probably owing to its tortuous course. Thrombus formation at the tip of the PICC can cause blockage requiring removal. This is a particular problem in neonates due to the small diameter of the catheters used. A continuous infusion of heparin at 0.5 IU $kg^{-1}$ $h^{-1}$ significantly reduces catheter occlusion. Another common problem is when the catheter flushes well, but blood withdrawal is not possible; this is known as a partial withdrawal occlusion (PWO). In these cases, the instillation of thrombolytics such as urokinase may restore function and avoid premature catheter removal.

The incidence of CRBI for outpatient PICCs is around 1.0 per 1,000 catheter days. For inpatient PICCs, the rate of infection is much higher at about 2.1 per 1,000 catheter days. Other serious complications of PICCs include catheter fracture with associated catheter or air embolism. Catheter rupture is associated with the flushing of small catheters with syringes smaller than 10 ml, as these can generate extremely high pressures. There are now PICCs available made of material with sufficient strength to be used for contrast injection for computed tomography (CT) scans. These CT-compatible PICCs remove the need for additional venous access for scans, as they are more resistant to fracture.

## Umbilical Vein Access

Central venous access in the newborn can be gained via the umbilical vein immediately after birth and for the first few days of life. The umbilical vein is a single, large, thin-walled vessel compared with the smaller paired muscular umbilical arteries. It gives off several large intrahepatic branches before converging with the left portal vein and continuing as the ductus venosus. This joins the IVC with the hepatic vein. An understanding of the anatomy of the umbilical vein is crucial for avoiding some of the more serious complications associated with the use of an umbilical vein catheter (UVC).

When a UVC is used for immediate resuscitation of a neonate at birth the position of the tip cannot be verified radiologically before use, and this is the only indication for a low catheter. With the umbilicus cut to 1–2 cm the tip must not be advanced beyond 3–5 cm below the skin to avoid intrahepatic placement. UVC tips positioned within the liver have been associated with liver abscess, liver necrosis and hepatic vein thrombosis leading to portal hypertension. UVCs in the portal venous system have been implicated in causing colonic perforation and necrotising enterocolitis. UVCs should not be inserted in the presence of omphalitis, an omphalocele or peritonitis.

For elective catheter placement the ideal tip position is just above the diaphragm in the IVC below the right atrium. There are graphs and formulae available to estimate catheter length based on umbilical to shoulder distance and weight. On a chest radiograph, the catheter should be visible just to the right of the vertebral column at the level of T9–10 vertebrae above the diaphragm. Malpositioned catheters can cause cardiac perforation, cardiac arrhythmias, thrombotic endocarditis and pulmonary infarction. Great care must be taken to avoid air embolism when inserting and using UVCs because of the negative pressure in the thorax during inspiration. Haemorrhage from the umbilical stump can be a problem at insertion. This is best controlled by a circular ligature around the umbilical stump, which is subsequently released to avoid necrosis.

There are both single- and double-lumen UVCs available between 3.5 and 5 Fr in size. Double lumen catheters decrease the need for additional venous access and are not associated with a significant increase in complications. Catheters with side holes should be avoided unless being used specifically for exchange transfusion as they have a higher incidence of thrombotic complications. Correctly sited high UVCs can be used for blood sampling, drug and fluid administration, TPN and hyperosmolar infusates. They can also be used for measuring central venous pressure (CVP).

Infection of UVCs occurs in up to 15% of patients and is related to prematurity, insertion duration and catheter handling. Prophylactic antibiotics do not seem to have a role in preventing infection. As well as a cause of general sepsis, infected UVCs can also cause widespread infective emboli. Transfer of infective emboli between the venous circulation and the systemic circulation can occur through a patent foramen ovale. UVCs should be removed as soon they are no longer required and should not be left in place for more than 14 days.

## Short-Term Central Venous Access

Secure access to the central venous system is often required during major surgery and during admissions to intensive care. This is usually provided by short- term non-tunnelled central venous catheters (CVC) made of a relatively stiff material such as polyurethane with a wide choice in diameter (3–8.5 Fr), length and number of lumens (one to five). The choice of catheter type and insertion site is determined by balancing the clinical need against the risk of insertion complications. Multiple lumen catheters are useful for drug infusions, especially if inotropic support is required. They also facilitate the measurement of CVP and venous blood sampling. Larger-diameter catheters should be used if rapid fluid administration is required as the flow is proportional to the fourth power of the radius. The length of the catheter is dependent on the size of the child and the insertion site. The tip of these short-term catheters must be in either the IVC or the SVC. Because of the risk of cardiac perforation, the tip must not lie within the heart. For short-term haemodialysis and haemodiafiltration, there are special large bore double lumen catheters that are designed for high flow rates without causing haemolysis.

Access to the central venous circulation is associated with an increased risk of bleeding both during catheter insertion and at the time of removal. The platelet count should be known prior to insertion and a clotting screen performed if there is a risk of coagulopathy. Traditionally a platelet count of greater than $50 \times 10^9\ l^{-1}$ has been used as a safe level, but there are studies of CVC insertions with platelet counts as low as $20 \times 10^9\ l^{-1}$ without any significant increase in haemorrhagic complications.

The most common insertion sites for short-term CVCs are:

- The femoral vein
- The internal jugular vein
- The external jugular vein
- The subclavian vein

For multi-lumen catheters, the Seldinger technique is utilised. Most catheter insertion kits have a J-tip Seldinger wire. In neonates and infants, the radius of the J-tip may be greater than the diameter of the vein, impeding advancement of the wire; often the other end of the wire is a soft straight tip, which may be easier to insert.

It is recommended that all short-term central catheters are connected to a pressure transducer to exclude arterial placement. This should be done prior to dilation of the vein if there is any suspicion of arterial puncture. Blood gas analysis is not helpful to differentiate between arterial and venous placement, especially if the child is hypoxic or supplementary oxygen is being administered. Full asepsis should be used during insertion.

## Femoral Vein

This is the most common site for short-term central venous access in children. The femoral approach has the major advantage of consistent anatomy with the vein found medial to the femoral artery and accessed below the inguinal ligament. There is no risk of pneumothorax in contrast to insertion sites in the neck. The major insertion complication is arterial puncture, which occurs in up to 10% of insertions using surface landmarks and femoral arterial pulsation as guidance. The use of ultrasound significantly reduces arterial puncture rates and decreases the number of insertion attempts. Bleeding from attempts at femoral venous access is usually easily controlled by digital pressure, but there are reports of substantial retroperitoneal bleeding causing cardiovascular collapse. The femoral vein is the preferred site for short-term haemodialysis catheters owing to the straight course of the femoral vein to the IVC. It is also the best route for CVC insertion during emergency resuscitation, as cardiopulmonary massage does not have to be interrupted during placement.

## Internal Jugular Vein

This is the next most common site to be used for short-term CVCs. It requires a higher level of technical expertise and practice compared with the femoral route. The anatomy of the internal jugular vein is more variable than that of the femoral vein. The relationship of the vein to the common carotid artery changes with age:

- In most infants, the vein either partially or completely overlies the artery at the level of the cricoid cartilage; rotating the head away from the midline increases the incidence of overlap.
- In older children and adults, there is substantial variation in position of the vein.
- In up to 5% of adults, the internal jugular vein lies medial to the common carotid artery, contrary to traditional teaching.

The use of the common carotid artery as a landmark for CVC insertion is therefore potentially flawed in many patients, and arterial puncture rates are between 5% and 15%. The dome of the lung lies posterior to the vein in the neck, and this approach is associated with pneumothorax rates of around 0.5–1%. The use of ultrasound significantly reduces arterial puncture, improves success rates and decreases insertion duration. Ideally, ultrasound should be used for visualisation during insertion rather than only for pre-insertion orientation. In the United Kingdom, National Institute for Health and Care Excellence (NICE) has recommended that ultrasound be used for every elective CVC insertion into the internal jugular vein in both adults and children. The size of the internal jugular vein can be increased by a head-down position, Valsalva manoeuvre or hepatic compression. The right internal jugular vein has a much straighter course to the SVC than the left side and is the preferred route. The left internal jugular vein should be avoided in children with a persistent left SVC as this usually drains to the coronary sinus.

## External Jugular Vein

This is more superficial than the internal jugular vein, although it is extremely variable in size and position. It can be used for short-term CVCs. Advancing a Seldinger wire down the vein through the clavi-pectoral fascia into a central vein can be problematic, and hence it is not often used for this purpose. The risk of pneumothorax is small but not negligible with this approach.

## Subclavian Vein

This is the continuation of the axillary vein from the upper limb. It becomes the subclavian vein at the outer border of the first rib and then arches up over the rib in front of the lung, anterior to and slightly below the subclavian artery. It joins the internal jugular vein to form the brachiocephalic vein and then combines with the opposite brachiocephalic vein to form the SVC. The clavicle overlies the subclavian vein for a substantial part of its extrathoracic course. From this description of the anatomy, it can be seen that the vein is a deep structure in close proximity both to the lung and subclavian artery. It cannot be visualised easily with ultrasound due to the overlying clavicle. Accessing the subclavian vein percutaneously requires a high degree of skill and expertise, and it is the approach associated with the highest failure rate. Of note:

- Damage to the vein or artery is not easily amenable to external pressure, and catastrophic bleeding can occur, especially if the blood collects in the pleural cavity.
- Pneumothorax rates are between 0.5% and 2% for this approach. The space between the clavicle and first rib is narrow in infants and small children and restricts the size of the catheter used.
- It can be difficult to dilate the tract to the vein, and pinching of the catheter can occur, causing pain, catheter malfunction and catheter damage.
- Because of the angle of entry of the subclavian vein into the thoracic cavity, the Seldinger wire is required to negotiate a 90° corner to enter the SVC. This can result in wire misplacement in around 10% of insertions with final catheter tip position in the opposite subclavian vein or either of the internal jugular veins. A chest radiograph should always be performed to verify catheter tip position.

Short-term non-tunnelled CVCs are extremely useful in critically ill children but are associated with many complications (see Table 12.2). The most common delayed complications are CRBI and venous thrombosis. Bloodstream infection rates are 3.4–11.3 per 1,000 catheter days, depending on the pre-existing patient risk factors. Children with burns and neonates less than 1,000 g are at the highest risk of CRBI. In children, there is not a great difference between infection rates at different insertion sites as opposed to adults, where the femoral route has a much higher infection rate. Thrombosis of the vein or around the catheter can occur in 2–35% of patients. In children with diabetic ketoacidosis, the use of the femoral vein for CVCs has been associated with a thrombosis incidence of around 50%, so this route should probably be avoided in these patients if possible. The recorded incidence is much higher if active surveillance is undertaken rather than relying on clinical signs. The presence of a catheter in a small vein may cause venous congestion of the distal venous system. This is particularly noticeable in neonates and infants with femoral catheters.

**Table 12.2** Complications of percutaneous central venous catheter insertion

| Immediate (usually within 24 hours) | Long term |
|---|---|
| Pneumothorax | Local infection at insertion site |
| Haemothorax | Bloodstream infection |
| Haemopneumothorax | Venous thrombosis and occlusion |
| Hydrothorax secondary to fluid | Arterio-venous fistula infusion |
| Chylothorax secondary to thoracic duct damage | Arterial false aneurysm formation |
| Arterial puncture with local haemorrhage | |
| Arterial endoluminal damage with flap occlusion | |
| Arterial thrombosis | |
| Arterial embolism | |
| Damage to great veins with massive haemorrhage | |
| Local haemorrhage at insertion site | |
| Cardiac perforation with tamponade | |
| Pericardial effusion | |
| Cardiac arrhythmias | |
| Pneumomediastinum | |
| Air embolism | |
| Catheter embolism | |
| Wire embolism | |

## Long-Term Central Venous Access

Some children will require central venous access for a period longer than a month. Consideration should be given early in their treatment to the insertion of a long-term central venous access device to avoid the trauma, both physical and emotional, of multiple short-term catheters. Cytotoxic chemotherapy, prolonged antibiotic therapy and parenteral nutrition are the most common indications in children. The devices used for long-term access are divided into skin-tunnelled catheters (STC) and implantable injection ports.

These catheters are usually made of soft silicone but can be made of polyurethane. Polyurethane catheters are stiffer, hence can have a larger lumen with the same external diameter allowing higher flow rates. They do not soften as much as silicone catheters in the blood at body temperature and thus are associated with a higher incidence of thrombosis, although this is less so with third-generation polyurethane catheters. The catheters may be open-ended or have a valve system such as the Groshong™ two-way valve.

## Long-Term Skin-Tunnelled Catheters

These have a Dacron™ cuff that is situated in the subcutaneous tunnel 3–4 cm from the exit site. Subcutaneous tissue grows in and around the cuff over a period of a few weeks. This secures the catheter in place, so no other external fixation is required. It also acts as a barrier to infective agents ascending the tunnel to cause bloodstream infections. The catheters may be single lumen, such as the small Broviac™ catheters (2.7 or 4.2 Fr) or larger double or triple lumen Hickman/Leonard™ style catheters (7–12 Fr).

## Implantable Ports

These are made of plastic or titanium so that they are MRI compatible (see Figure 12.1). The port is usually placed in a pocket fashioned on the chest wall and secured to the fascia with non-absorbable sutures to avoid rotation in the pocket. Less commonly, the port can be sited on the forearm or the upper abdomen. The port is attached to a tunnelled subcutaneous catheter (6–10 Fr) and is accessed percutaneously with a special Huber-type needle. This has a non-cutting atraumatic tip with a side hole to avoid damaging the diaphragm of the port. Ports are available as either high or low profile to aid palpability with varying thickness of subcutaneous tissue. Double-lumen ports are available, but they are rarely used in children. The implantable port system has the advantage of being a sealed system once the percutaneous needle is removed. They are associated with less local and systemic infection, and the child can swim and bathe freely when the port is not accessed.

Skin-tunnelled catheters are better for more intensive treatments, such as bone marrow transplantation, when multiple lumens are required. They are also preferred in needle-phobic children, as accessing an implantable port is not completely painless even with local anaesthetic creams. In children less than one year of age and in those with very little subcutaneous fat, there is a higher incidence of skin erosion over the port site; skin-tunnelled catheters may be more suitable in these cases.

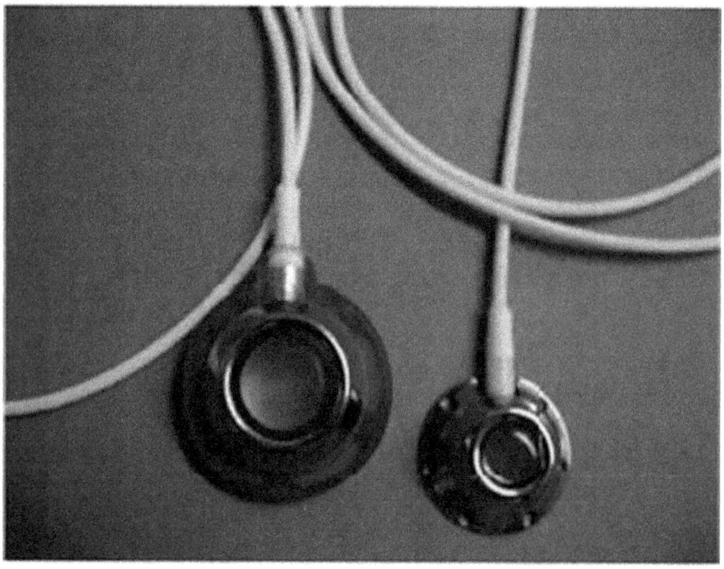

**Figure 12.1** Portacath for long-term vascular access.

## Insertion

Long-term catheters can be inserted either by open surgery or by a percutaneous technique and will require fluoroscopic support. Most children will require general anaesthesia for a port or tunnelled catheter insertion, although some older children will tolerate a percutaneous insertion with sedation and local anaesthesia. Open surgery can be used for accessing the internal and external jugular veins as well as the femoral vein. The subclavian vein is not suitable for open access. For the internal jugular and femoral veins, the catheter is inserted through a venotomy under direct vision with the vessel controlled between two vascular slings. The external jugular vein can be divided and tied off with the soft catheter threaded down the proximal segment.

For percutaneous insertion, access to the vein is identical to that for short-term catheters with the use of a Seldinger wire and ultrasound when using the internal jugular or femoral vein. The subclavian vein can also be accessed with the percutaneous technique, but due to the narrow space between the clavicle and first rib, the child usually needs to be above 20 kg for catheters of 7 Fr and larger. Whichever percutaneous insertion site is chosen, the position of the Seldinger wire should be confirmed with fluoroscopy prior to dilation. The catheter is then tunnelled up from the exit site for Hickman/Broviac lines or from the subcutaneous port site to a position next to the Seldinger wire. An integral vein dilator and peel-away sheath are inserted over the Seldinger wire, with great care being taken not to push the stiff dilator in too far or beyond the end of the wire. Serious damage to the mediastinum or heart with fatal consequences can occur if this system is misused. The wire and dilator are removed to leave the sheath in the vein. The soft catheter is inserted via the sheath, which is then peeled away, leaving the catheter in the vein. It is possible for large quantities of blood or air to flow rapidly through the peel-away sheath if the lumen is not well controlled.

The ideal position for the catheter tip of soft, long-term catheters is still controversial. There have been rare reports of cardiac perforation in neonates having TPN infusions with the tip positioned within the right atrium. In larger children, this is much less of a concern, and the catheters tend to function better if the tip is placed in the upper-right atrium. The catheter can be cut to length using the intermammary line as the surface landmark for the right atrium. A better technique for use with the Seldinger wire is to position the tip of the wire in the desired position, confirmed by fluoroscopy. The amount of wire on the exterior is then measured and deducted from the known length of the wire (usually 50 cm) to give the exact length for the catheter to be cut. This technique cannot be used for Groshong™ tip catheters, which are tunnelled backwards from the insertion site to the exit site or port. Fluoroscopy should always be used to confirm the final position of the catheter tip. It is not necessary to routinely perform a chest radiograph after insertion if fluoroscopy has been used, as this exposes the child to unnecessary radiation. A chest radiograph should be performed if there are any cardiorespiratory symptoms or signs postoperatively.

The insertion complications for long-term catheters are similar to those outlined for short-term catheters (see Table 12.2), with the addition of vascular damage and haemorrhage that can occur with any open surgery. The major long-term complications are CRBI, venous thrombosis and catheter malfunction. The incidence of CRBI for long-term venous catheters is around 1.5–3 per 1,000 catheter days for Hickman-type catheters and around 0.1–1 per 1,000 catheter days for implanted ports. There is no evidence that the use of prophylactic antibiotics at the time of insertion decreases the risk of infection.

The intravascular portion of a long-term catheter is rapidly covered in a fibrin sheath that can occlude the catheter tip. This can cause infusate to track back along the catheter and cause subcutaneous extravasation despite the catheter being intact. This can be confirmed by injection of X-ray contrast solution with fluoroscopy. Fibrin sheath or thrombus formation at the catheter tip or in the catheter lumen can sometimes be dissolved by fibrinolytic therapy. This involves the instillation of urokinase 5,000 IU $ml^{-1}$ or alteplase 1 mg $ml^{-1}$ into the dead space of the blocked lumen using a negative pressure technique. A three-way tap is connected to the catheter, and an empty 10 ml syringe used to generate a negative pressure within the lumen. The tap is then opened to the syringe containing the fibrinolytic agent, which is aspirated into the lumen by negative pressure and left in place for two to four hours or overnight. The catheter must then be carefully aspirated to remove any clots or remaining fibrinolytic agent prior to being flushed with saline or heparinised saline, depending on hospital policy. This procedure can be repeated if necessary, but if it is not successful the catheter should be removed. Massive thrombus formation can occur at the catheter tip, within the central veins or in the right atrium. This may present as pulmonary emboli, vena cava obstruction or cardiac insufficiency. The diagnosis is confirmed by ultrasound or echocardiogram. It can usually be treated effectively with systemic anti-coagulation and catheter removal, but occasionally cardiac surgery for open removal is required.

## Care Bundles for Venous Catheters

CRBI is a major source of morbidity and mortality in hospitalised patients, with a substantial social and economic cost. Additional hospital expenses in the United Kingdom related to a patient acquiring a CRBI have been estimated at over £15,000. Bloodstream infections account for around 6% of all hospital infections, with an estimated 42.3% of these being related to central venous catheters. Confirmation of CRBI requires the same organism to be isolated from peripheral blood culture as well as from the device in a patient with clinical signs of bacteraemia. Colonisation of venous catheters is present when an organism can be isolated from the internal lumen or the subcutaneous external surface of the catheter in the absence of clinical signs of bacteraemia. The micro-organisms that colonise venous catheters are responsible for most CRBI, with contamination occurring at the time of insertion or by migration along the catheter track. Contamination can also occur by the transfer of micro-organisms during handling of the catheter hubs. Catheter colonisation and infection by haematogenous spread from distant sites is thought to be rare. A 2006 UK prevalence study showed that coagulase-negative staphylococci were the most commonly isolated organism from all types of intravenous catheters (35%). Staphylococcus aureus was the second most common (25%), with methicillin-resistant organisms (MRSA) accounting for 40–45% of these infections. Candida species and enterococci are also common infective agents causing CRBI.

An evidence base compiled over the past few years resulted in the publication in 2014 of updated guidelines 'EPIC3: National Evidence-Based Guidelines for Preventing Healthcare-Associated Infections in NHS Hospitals in England'. These guidelines have been used to produce care bundles for both central venous catheters and peripheral intravenous cannulae ('NHS Improvement 2017 and Department of Health 2007, High Impact Interventions'; see Appendices 1 and 2). The concept of a care bundle is that it brings together all the scientifically based interventions that, when used together, improve clinical outcome. The care bundles are divided into insertion actions and ongoing care actions and are designed to be used in their entirety; assessment of compliance requires all elements to be completed for each patient. For these to be successful, there must be a proactive education programme for all staff involved in the care of intravenous catheters.

Concern has been raised that the use of care bundles has led to earlier removal of CVCs and increased use of peripheral venous cannulae on ICUs when patients still require venous access. This may be associated with an increased risk of phlebitis and subsequent CRBI. It is very important that peripheral cannulae are inspected daily and assessed for phlebitis using a visual infusion phlebitis (VIP) score as part of the ongoing care action. A VIP scoring system is invaluable in recording the daily state of peripheral cannula insertion sites (see Appendix 3).

## Intraosseous Access

Obtaining vascular access in emergency paediatric resuscitation can be extremely difficult due to collapsed small veins, which may be impossible to visualise because of overlying fat. This is frequently the case in infants with septic shock and trauma. The tracheal route offers an alternative emergency route for drug administration but requires the child to have a tracheal tube in situ. The absorption of drugs administered via the tracheal route is variable, and the amount of fluid permitted by this route is limited. The highly vascularised intraosseous (IO) space functions as a non-collapsible vein into which nearly all resuscitation drugs and unrestricted volumes of fluids can be infused.

The insertion of an IO cannula is painful, and if the child is not unconscious then local anaesthesia should be used. The best anatomical insertion site is the anteromedial aspect of the proximal tibia

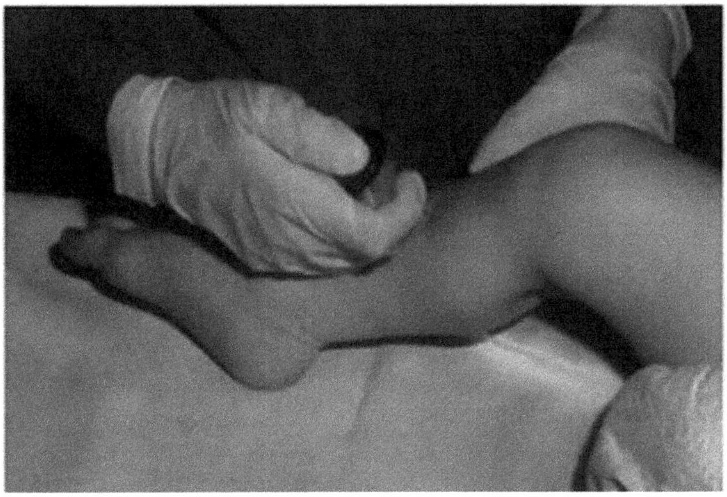

**Figure 12.2** Intraosseous needle insertion on the antero-medial aspect of the proximal tibia.

2–3 cm below the tibial tuberosity (see Figure 12.2). The tip of the needle should be directed away from the growth plate. Other insertion sites are the distal end of the femur 3 cm above the lateral condyle and the medial malleolus at the ankle. The sternum is not recommended in children. Contraindications to IO access are a proximal fracture or severe soft tissue injury; in these cases, the contralateral side should be used. A history of osteogenesis imperfecta or osteoporosis is associated with a higher risk of bone fracture.

There are commercially available IO cannulae of variable size (14–18G) and design; some have a cutting bevel designed for a rotating insertion technique. Bone marrow aspirate needles can be used as an alternative. In neonates and small infants, spinal needles have been successfully used but they tend to bend easily with the harder bones of older children. Any cannula used should have a central stylet to avoid plugging of the lumen with bone particles. Whatever the device or site chosen, a twisting technique is employed with sustained pressure until a sudden give is felt as the tip of the needle enters the medulla after passing through the harder cortex. Mechanical devices such as the EZ-IO® are available for use in children. Blood aspirated from the needle can be used for glucose and electrolyte estimation, cross-match and culture. Full blood count will reflect the marrow cell population rather than peripheral blood.

Infusion of fluids into the IO space requires higher pressure than normally used in intravenous infusions. Boluses of fluid can be given by syringe or the use of a pressurised system. All current resuscitation drugs and antibiotics can be given safely by the IO route. The IO route is extremely safe when used in short-term resuscitation, with complications in less than 1% of patients. Compartment syndrome requiring fasciotomy has been reported as well as injury to the growth plate, bone fracture and local haematoma formation. Osteomyelitis is a rare complication. Local extravasation is rarely serious unless vasoconstrictors or thiopentone are involved, when necrosis of the overlying skin may occur. Formal venous access should be established as soon as feasible to allow the IO access to be removed.

### Key Points

- Vascular access is an essential element of paediatric medical practice, but it is associated with a high complication rate.
- The choice of vascular access must be specific to each patient to balance the risks against the clinical requirements.
- The insertion complications of vascular access are potentially life-threatening, hence operators must be adequately trained and supervised for these procedures.
- There should be local protocols and care bundles for every type of vascular access.
- There should be an effective audit process in place to monitor complications from vascular access.

## Further Reading

Chopra V, Flanders SA, Saint S, et al. The Michigan appropriateness guide for intravenous catheters (MAGIC): results from a multispecialty panel using the RAND/UCLA appropriateness method. *Annals of Internal Medicine* 2015; 163 (suppl 6):S1–40.

Harding S. Procedures and iatrogenic disorders. In: Rennie JM, ed. *Roberton's Textbook of Neonatology*, 5th ed. Elsevier. 2012.

Loveday HP, Wilson JA, Pratt RJ, et al. EPIC3: national evidence-based guidelines for preventing healthcare-associated infections in NHS hospitals in England. *Journal of Hospital Infection* 2014; 86: Suppl 1:S1–70.

Munoz-Mozas G, Overland H and Hyde H. Vascular access devices. In Lister S, Hofland J and Grafton H eds. *The Royal Marsden Hospital Manual of Clinical Nursing Procedures*, 10th ed. Wiley Blackwell. 2020.

National Institute for Health and Care Excellence (NICE). 2017. Care Processes to Prevent Infection In: *Saving Lives: High Impact Interventions,* 4th ed. Available at: www.nice.org.uk.

Ullman AJ, Bernstein SJ, Brown E, et al. The Michigan appropriateness guide for intravenous catheters in pediatrics: miniMAGIC. *Pediatrics.* 2020; 145(Suppl 3): S269–84.

# Appendix 1 Central Venous Catheter Care Bundle

Modified from: Department of Health 2007 and NHS Improvement 2017. High Impact Intervention No. 1. Central venous catheter care bundle. http://data.parliament.uk/DepositedPapers/Files/DEP2008-0037/DEP2008-0037.pdf.

CR-BSI: catheter- related blood stream infection.

## Insertion Actions

### Catheter Type

- Use a single lumen catheter unless indicated otherwise.
- Consider an anti-microbial impregnated catheter if the catheter is to be used for one to three weeks and risk of CR-BSI is high.

### Insertion Site

- Subclavian or internal jugular.

### Skin Preparation

- Preferably use 2% chlorhexidine gluconate in 70% isopropyl alcohol. Allow to dry.
- If the patient is sensitive to chlorhexidine, use povidone-iodine.

### Personal Protective Equipment

- Gloves are single-use items and should be removed and discarded immediately after the care activity.
- Eye/face protection is indicated if there is a risk of splashing with blood or body fluids.

### Hand Hygiene

- Decontaminate hands before and after each patient contact.
- Use correct hand hygiene procedures.

### Aseptic Technique

- Gown, gloves and drapes should be used for the insertion of invasive devices.

### Dressing

- Use a sterile, transparent, semi-permeable dressing to allow observation of the insertion site.

### Safe Disposal of Sharps

- A sharps container should be available at point of use and should not be overfilled; do not disassemble the needle and syringe; do not pass sharps from hand to hand.

### Documentation

- Date of insertion should be recorded in the notes and on dressing if possible.

## Ongoing Care Actions

### Hand Hygiene

- Decontaminate hands before and after each patient contact.
- Use correct hand hygiene procedure.

### Catheter Site Inspection

- Observe the site for signs of infection, at least daily.

### Dressing

- Ensure transparent dressing is intact, dry and adherent.

### Catheter Access

- Use aseptic technique and swab ports or hub with 2% chlorhexidine gluconate in 70% isopropyl alcohol prior to accessing the line for administering fluids or injections.

### Administration Set Replacement

- Replace set immediately following administration of blood and blood products.
- Replace administration set after 24 hours following administration of TPN (up to 72 hours if there is no lipid).
- Replace all other sets within 96 hours.

### No Routine Catheter Replacement

# Appendix 2 Peripheral Intravenous Cannula Care Bundle

Modified from Department of Health 2007 and NHS Improvement 2017. High Impact Intervention No. 2. Peripheral intravenous cannula care bundle. http://data.parliament.uk/DepositedPapers/Files/DEP2008-0037/DEP2008-0037.pdf.

## Insertion Actions

### Hand Hygiene

- Decontaminate hands before and after each patient contact and before applying examination gloves.
- Use correct hand hygiene procedure.

### Personal Protective Equipment

- Wear examination gloves if there is a risk of exposure to body fluids.
- Gloves are single-use items and should be removed and discarded immediately after the care activity.
- Gowns, aprons, eye/face protection are indicated if there is a risk of splashing with blood or body fluids.

### Skin Preparation

- Use 2% chlorhexidine gluconate in 70% isopropyl alcohol. Allow drying.
- If patient is sensitive to chlorhexidine, use povidone-iodine.

### Dressing

- Use a sterile, semi-permeable, transparent dressing to allow observation of insertion site.

### Documentation

- Date of insertion should be recorded in notes and on dressing when possible.

## Ongoing Care Actions

### Hand Hygiene

- Decontaminate hands before and after each patient contact.
- Use correct hand hygiene procedure.

### Continuing Clinical Indication

- Check that all intravenous cannulae and associated devices are still indicated.
- If there is no indication, then the intravenous cannula should be removed.

### Site Inspection

- Observe the site for signs of infection, at least daily.

### Dressing

- An intact, dry, adherent transparent dressing should be present.

### Cannula Access

- Use 2% chlorhexidine gluconate in 70% isopropyl alcohol and allow it to dry prior to accessing the cannula for administering fluid or injections.

### Administration Set Replacement

- Replace the set immediately after administration of blood or blood products.
- Replace all other fluid sets after 96 hours.

### No Routine Cannula Replacement

- No need for routine replacement provided that the cannula is still clinically indicated and there are no signs of infection.

# Appendix 3 Visual Infusion Phlebitis (VIP) Score

From: Jackson A. Infection control; a battle in vein infusion phlebitis. *Nursing Times* 1994; 4:68–71.

| Appearance | Score | Comment | Action |
|---|---|---|---|
| IV site appears healthy | 0 | No signs of phlebitis | Observe |
| One of the following evident: slight pain or redness near IV site | 1 | Possible first signs of phlebitis | Observe |
| Two of the following evident: pain near IV site, erythema, swelling | 2 | Early stage of phlebitis | Resite cannula |
| All of the following evident: pain along cannula, erythema, induration | 3 | Moderate phlebitis – consider treatment | Resite cannula |
| All of the following evident, and extensive: pain along cannula, erythema, induration, palpable venous cord | 4 | Advanced phlebitis or start of thrombophlebitis | Resite cannula, consider treatment |
| All of the following are evident, and extensive: pain along cannula, erythema, induration, palpable venous cord, pyrexia | 5 | Advanced stage of thrombophlebitis | Initiate treatment, resite cannula |

Chapter

# 13 Perioperative Fluid Management in Children

Elena Fernandez

## Introduction

Intravenous fluids are given to children when the enteral route is not sufficient or is not an option, such as during surgery and anaesthesia. In the past, a lack of appreciation of the physiology of intravenous fluid management, particularly in the unwell child, has led to reports of serious morbidity and mortality, mainly due to acute hyponatraemia. Recent evidence has shown that giving children isotonic crystalloid fluids with a sodium concentration similar to plasma reduces the risk of hyponatraemia without increasing adverse effects. This has led to a change in intravenous fluid guidelines to now recommend that only isotonic fluids are used, with regular monitoring of fluid balance and electrolytes. This chapter considers the rationale for current recommendations for intravenous fluids in children, and fluid management and blood transfusion in the perioperative period and other special circumstances. The treatment of hyponatraemia is also considered.

## The Holliday and Segar Formula and the Choice of Fluid in Intravenous Fluid Management

In the 1950s, paediatricians were looking for a simple formula that could be used at the bedside to calculate fluid and electrolyte requirements in children rather than using calculations based on body surface area. Holliday and Segar linked water requirements and expenditure of calories to body weight, and electrolyte requirements to the concentration of sodium and potassium in human and cow's milk. They devised a simple formula for daily maintenance fluid requirements, which has been adapted to an hourly calculation (the '4-2-1 formula') (Table 13.1). The Holiday and Segar formula is still used as a guide to calculations for the volume of maintenance fluids required by children today.

The tonicity of intravenous (IV) fluids is mainly affected by the concentration of sodium and potassium. 'Hypotonic' crystalloids such as 0.45% sodium chloride with 2.5% or 5% glucose have lower sodium concentration than plasma. 'Isotonic' fluid contains sodium and potassium concentrations similar to plasma with a sodium concentration in the range 131–154 mmol $l^{-1}$. Examples include Hartmann's, Ringer's lactate, 0.9% saline and Plasmalyte (Table 13.2). Glucose in IV fluid does not contribute to tonicity because it is rapidly metabolised after entering the bloodstream.

Holiday and Segar suggested that hypotonic crystalloids should be used for intravenous maintenance in children, as there were concerns that excessive sodium intake in isotonic fluids would lead to hypernatraemia (if considering this as being equivalent to dietary sodium intake). However, following worldwide reports of hospital acquired hyponatraemia in children receiving hypotonic intravenous fluids, and high-quality randomised clinical trials, it has been recognised that the routine use of hypotonic fluids in children is not appropriate, particularly in the presence of raised antidiuretic hormone (ADH), such as in the postoperative period or in sick, hospitalised children. It has also been recognised that the '4-2-1 formula' may overestimate fluid requirements in certain situations. The updated UK National Institute for Health and Care Excellence (NICE) guidelines recommend isotonic crystalloids containing sodium in the range

**Table 13.1** The '4-2-1 formula' for calculating hourly fluid requirements in children

| Weight | Hourly fluid requirement (ml $h^{-1}$) |
|---|---|
| First 10 kg | 4 ml $kg^{-1}$ |
| 10–20 kg | 40 ml + 2 ml $kg^{-1}$ for each kg > 10 kg |
| >20 kg | 60 ml + 1 ml $kg^{-1}$ for each kg > 20 kg (max 100 ml $h^{-1}$) |

**Table 13.2** Composition of intravenous fluids

| Solution | Sodium (mmol/L) | Potassium (mmol/L) | Chloride (mmol/L) | Glucose (g/L) | Buffer | Tonicity (after glucose metabolism) |
|---|---|---|---|---|---|---|
| 5% glucose | 0 | 0 | 0 | **50** | – | **Hypotonic** |
| 10% glucose | 0 | 0 | 0 | **100** | – | **Hypotonic** |
| 0.18% sodium chloride with 4% glucose | 31 | 0 | 30 | **40** | – | **Hypotonic** |
| 0.45% sodium chloride with 2.5% glucose | 77 | 0 | 77 | **25** | – | **Hypotonic** |
| 0.45% sodium chloride with 5% glucose | 77 | 0 | 77 | **50** | – | **Hypotonic** |
| Lactated Ringer's | 130 | 4 | 109 | **0** | Lactate | **Isotonic** |
| Hartmann's | 131 | 5 | 111 | **0** | Lactate | **Isotonic** |
| Plasmalyte 148 | 140 | 5 | 98 | **0** | Acetate gluconate | **Isotonic** |
| Plasmalyte 148 with 5% glucose | 140 | 5 | 98 | **55** | Acetate gluconate | **Isotonic** |
| Sterofundin® ISO | 145 | 4 | 127 | **0** | Acetate malate | **Isotonic** |
| 0.9% sodium chloride with 5% glucose | 150 | 0 | 154 | **50** | – | **Isotonic** |
| Sodium chloride 0.9% | 154 | 0 | 154 | **0** | – | **Isotonic** |
| 4.5% albumin | 100–160 | 0 | 0 | **0** | – | **Isotonic** |
| Succinylated gelatin (gelofusine) | 154 | 0 | 120 | **0** | – | **Isotonic** |

131–154 mmol $l^{-1}$ as first choice for routine IV maintenance in children.

## Choice of Isotonic Crystalloid

There are a number of isotonic crystalloids with a sodium concentration of 131–154 mmol $l^{-1}$ used in clinical practice (Table 13.2). Normal saline (0.9% saline) is widely available and inexpensive. It contains 154 mmol $l^{-1}$ of sodium and chloride. 'Balanced' isotonic solutions have been formulated to more closely mimic the electrolyte composition and pH of normal plasma. They have lower concentrations of sodium and chloride; additional cations such as calcium, potassium or magnesium; and anions such as lactate, acetate or gluconate that are metabolised to bicarbonate to exert an additional buffering effect. The most common balanced isotonic solutions currently in use are Hartmann's, Ringer's Lactate and Plasmalyte 148.

Large volumes of 0.9% saline may lead to hyperchloraemia and subsequent metabolic acidosis. In vitro and animal studies have shown several adverse effects of hyperchloraemia on renal physiology, inflammation and haemolysis. In clinical use 0.9% saline may be associated with worse biochemical outcomes and higher incidence of acute kidney injury when compared to balanced isotonic solutions, although a difference in mortality has not been demonstrated.

In children with dehydration and hypovolaemia, the use of a balanced isotonic solution is thought to produce more physiological volume replacement and a faster improvement of metabolic acidosis than 0.9% saline. The Resuscitation Council UK 2021 Paediatric Advanced Life Support Guidelines recommend the use of balanced isotonic crystalloids as the first choice of fluid in volume resuscitation, with 0.9% saline as an acceptable alternative.

## The Need for Glucose in Intravenous Fluids

Restriction of glucose intake during fasting may lead to breakdown of fats in the liver to provide ketones as an alternative energy supply. Some children are at special risk of hypoglycaemia (see Table 13.3). Under normal circumstances, children under six years require glucose of at least 50 mg $ml^{-1}$ in maintenance fluids to prevent lipolysis. It is recommended that balanced isotonic crystalloids such as Hartmann's and Plasmalyte 148 (or 0.9% saline) with 5% glucose should be used as standard for maintenance therapy in children under six years to prevent hyponatraemia, maintain normoglycaemia and prevent ketosis. Children at special risk of hypoglycaemia should receive a balanced isotonic solution containing 5–10% glucose with regular glucose monitoring.

During surgery, most children are able maintain their blood glucose as a result of the stress response, and routine inclusion of 5% glucose in intravenous fluids has been shown to result in hyperglycaemia.

**Table 13.3** Children at risk of hypoglycaemia

| Children at risk of hypoglycaemia |
|---|
| Neonates in the first 48 hours of life |
| Infants undergoing prolonged/major surgery |
| Prolonged fasting |
| Children with sepsis |
| Children receiving parenteral nutrition |
| Children receiving glucose infusions |
| Low body weight (<3rd centile) |
| Extensive regional anaesthesia |
| Children with metabolic syndromes |

The 2011 European consensus statement for intraoperative fluid therapy in children recommended that intraoperative maintenance fluids in children should consist of balanced isotonic crystalloid with a lower concentration of glucose (1–2.5%) in order to both prevent hypoglycaemia and lipolysis and to avoid potential hyperglycaemia. However, solutions with 1–2.5% glucose are not yet commercially available in many countries.

Currently, for short minor procedures, children at low risk of hypoglycaemia usually receive glucose-free balanced isotonic crystalloids. For major or longer procedures in younger children especially, a second infusion of isotonic crystalloid with glucose should be considered for maintenance requirements, taking care to only give glucose-free isotonic solutions as boluses to replace intraoperative fluid losses. Blood glucose should be monitored.

## Colloids

Synthetic colloids include starches, dextrans, albumin and gelatins. They contain macromolecules from either plant or animal sources suspended in an electrolyte solution. Such colloids are used for volume expansion and fluid resuscitation. It was traditionally believed that colloids remain in the intravascular space longer than crystalloids due to their larger molecules which could not pass through the endothelium. However, emerging evidence considering new models of endothelial permeability in the presence of a damaged endothelial glycocalyx have demonstrated that crystalloids and colloids have similar volume-expanding and interstitial oedema-forming properties in critically ill patients.

Colloids are more expensive than crystalloids, and synthetic colloids carry a risk of anaphylaxis and have a dose-dependent effect on coagulation. Starches are associated with itching, the long-term side effects of which are not known. Albumin is the most commonly used non-synthetic colloid in children. It is often used in neonates, sepsis and in cardiac surgery, but there is no evidence for its use in children with traumatic brain injury, burns or in the postoperative period.

A 2018 Cochrane systematic review comparing colloids versus crystalloids for fluid resuscitation in critically ill people (including children) concluded that the choice of fluid probably makes no difference to mortality and that starches probably

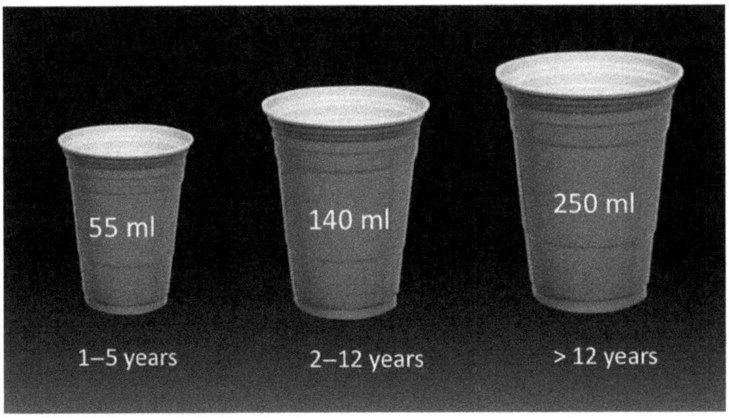


**Figure 13.1** Volumes of clear fluids based on age that children can be offered on arrival to hospital to ensure they drink up to one hour before elective surgery.

slightly increase the need for blood transfusion and renal replacement therapy. Synthetic colloids in children have now largely fallen out of use due to lack of evidence of benefit.

## Fluid Management in the Perioperative Period

Ideally, children should be allowed to control their own fluid balance by taking oral fluids for as long as possible before surgery and recommencing oral intake as soon as possible following surgery. When intravenous fluids are required, they should be prescribed with the same care as any drug.

## Preoperative Fasting and Clear Fluids

Children are fasted before surgery to minimise the risk of aspiration. Preoperative fasting in children has traditionally followed the rule of six hours nil by mouth for solids and formula milk, four hours for breast milk and two hours for clear fluids. However, in practice, children tend to be fasted for much longer than necessary, particularly those presenting to hospital on the day of surgery. Prolonged fasting has detrimental behavioural, metabolic and haemodynamic effects in children; it can make cannulation more difficult, and could potentially affect outcomes such as wound healing.

Recent evidence shows that after ingestion of 3–5 ml $kg^{-1}$ of clear fluid, residual gastric volume assessed by serial magnetic resonance or ultrasound imaging is back to baseline within one hour. A large prospective study involving over 10,000 children from birth to 16 years showed that liberal clear fluid intake preoperatively did not increase the risk of aspiration or related serious complications. In 2018, several European paediatric anaesthesia societies published a consensus statement affirming that, in the absence of increased risk of aspiration, it is safe for all children to be encouraged to have clear fluids up to one hour before elective surgery. One practical approach to save time for day-case units is to offer children a clear sugary drink when they arrive in hospital, with the volume based on the age of the child rather than the weight (Figure 13.1).

Current European Society of Anaesthesiology guidance on preoperative fasting in children recommends a six-hour nil by mouth time for solids and formula milk, three hours for breast milk and one hour for clear fluids. This guidance is practised in the fasting policy at this author's institution.

## Intraoperative Fluid Management

Intravenous fluids may be required during surgery for replacement of deficits/resuscitation, routine maintenance and to replace ongoing losses. Balanced isotonic solutions should be given, with blood given when necessary. Most children do not need glucose in their IV fluids during surgery (as indicated previously in the section 'The Need for Glucose in Intravenous Fluids').

The 'third space' for body fluids was traditionally used to describe a hypothetical transcellular space where fluid was sequestered intraoperatively. Third space losses were replaced at a variable rate depending on the magnitude of the surgical procedure, with high volumes of fluid sometimes being given. This concept has now been questioned, with tracer studies in adults showing that fluid is either in the intravascular, extracellular or intracellular space. There is also evidence that evaporative insensible losses during surgery are lower than previously thought. More restrictive intraoperative fluid regimens are now used, which have been associated with better outcomes.

**Minor surgery:** For healthy children who are undergoing minor procedures and will resume oral intake soon after surgery, 10–20 ml $kg^{-1}$ kg IV bolus during the procedure is acceptable and will reduce the need to drink immediately postoperatively and the risk of postoperative nausea and vomiting.

**Major surgery:** For children undergoing major surgery an initial fluid bolus of 10–20 ml $kg^{-1}$ is given, with subsequent fluid boluses of 10–20 ml $kg^{-1}$ balanced isotonic crystalloid or blood determined by clinical assessment (heart rate, capillary refill, blood pressure, core–peripheral temperature difference, base excess, urine output and haematocrit) and estimation of fluid losses (observation of the surgical field, weighing of swabs). Urine output may decrease due to raised ADH as part of the stress response and is an unreliable sign of volume status. It is important to avoid excessive volume loading as this will cause fluid retention and generalised oedema after surgery. Cardiac output monitoring should be considered for major surgery involving large volume losses, or for children with limited cardiac or renal reserve. A variety of cardiac output monitors have been validated for use in children (e.g., oesophageal Doppler, Lidco®). Monitors used to assess end organ perfusion such as near-infrared spectroscopy (NIRS) or central venous oxygen saturation monitoring (target $S_{CV}O_2$ >70%) may also be useful.

## Emergency Surgery

Children presenting for emergency surgery may be significantly dehydrated or hypovolaemic and require careful clinical assessment and replacement of fluid deficits before surgery. A similar approach of giving an isotonic crystalloid bolus of 10–20 ml $kg^{-1}$ may be used, with careful monitoring of electrolytes and haemoglobin and assessment of response before further fluid boluses are administered.

**Neurosurgery:** Neurosurgical patients are susceptible to a variety of conditions that affect sodium balance and in which fluid management requires special consideration, including diabetes insipidus, cerebral salt wasting and syndrome of inappropriate ADH (see Table 13.4).

## Postoperative Fluid Management

Children should resume oral intake of fluids as soon as possible in the postoperative period. Isotonic crystalloids containing glucose are recommended for postoperative maintenance if children are unable to resume full oral intake. The volume is calculated using the '4-2-1 formula' as a guide, restricted to 50–80% of full maintenance in children at risk of significant ADH secretion (e.g. those recovering from major surgery or who are critically unwell). Ongoing enteral losses should be replaced with 0.9% saline with added potassium ml for ml. Other losses (such as 'water' loss from sweating or inappropriate urinary losses with variable sodium and potassium content) should be considered on a case-by-case basis. Use of body surface area to calculate fluid requirements should be considered if the child is obese (over the 91st centile).

Hypovolaemia is treated with a bolus of 20 ml $kg^{-1}$ glucose-free isotonic crystalloid (e.g. Hartmann's, 0.9% saline) over less than 10 minutes, or blood products if required. Fluid balance, electrolytes and glucose should be monitored every 24 hours (or more frequently if abnormal) in all children receiving IV fluids, with daily weight if possible. Hypernatraemia during maintenance therapy is most likely due to inadequate volume and dehydration (see below). Fluids should be liberalised, and a hypotonic solution considered. Plasma sodium should be corrected slowly with frequent assessments of electrolytes. Correction should not exceed 12 mmol $l^{-1}$ in a 24-hour period.

## Enhanced Recovery after Surgery (ERAS)

The concept of enhanced recovery after surgery (ERAS) is that multiple small, evidence-based interventions combined in the perioperative period improve patient outcomes, reduce length of stay and increase patient satisfaction. The success of adult ERAS protocols has led to the development of paediatric ERAS pathways. Perioperative fluid management is a major component of ERAS and includes reducing fasting times for clear fluids, preoperative fluid and carbohydrate loading and judicious use of intravenous fluids during surgery, all of which are supported by existing good practice. Evidence of improved outcomes is starting to emerge from ERAS programmes in children.

**Table 13.4** Disorders of sodium and water balance

| | Diabetes insipidus | SIADH | Salt wasting |
|---|---|---|---|
| Description | Low ADH due to e.g.<br>- Craniopharyngioma<br>- Head injury<br>- Hypoxic brain injury | High ADH after e.g.<br>- Neurosurgery<br>- Head injury<br>- Meningitis | Natriuretic peptides release after e.g.<br>- Neurosurgery<br>- Head injury<br>- Meningitis |
| Plasma sodium | ↑ | ↓ | ↓ |
| Urine sodium | ↑ / normal | ↑ / normal | ↑↑ |
| Plasma osmolality | ↑ | ↓ | ↓ |
| Plasma glucose | Normal | Normal | Normal |
| Urine glucose | No | No | No |
| Urine output | ↑↑<br>Dilute polyuria | ↓<br>Concentrated oliguria | ↑↑<br>Concentrated polyuria |
| Urine SG | ↓ | ↑ | ↑ / normal |
| Fluid volume | Depleted | Overloaded | Depleted |
| Management | Fluids +/– DDAVP | Fluid restriction<br>3% saline if seizures/coma | Replace sodium & water with a bolus of isotonic fluid |

*Notes:* SIADH: Syndrome of inappropriate secretion of antidiuretic hormone; SG: specific gravity; DDAVP: desmopressin.

## Intravenous Fluid Management in the Newborn

Fluid requirements in the newborn period merit special consideration. Compared to older children, newborn infants have a greater percentage of total body water, with an expanded extracellular fluid compartment. During the first 24–96 hours of life, ADH levels are high, and urine output is low. This represents an appropriate evolutionary response to a period of low fluid intake whilst lactation is established. After the first few days of life, pressure changes in the heart results in increased secretion of atrial natriuretic peptide, stimulating a brisk diuresis of sodium and water and a period of postnatal weight loss.

Renal function is immature, and neonates cannot excrete a large water or sodium load. Conversely, neonates do not tolerate dehydration well as urine can only be concentrated to half its adult capacity. Excessive sodium intake in the first few days of life may result in hypernatraemia. Premature neonates have limited capacity for sodium re-absorption in the kidneys, so they may require sodium supplements in the first weeks of life to avoid hyponatraemia.

The premature or sick neonate is particularly vulnerable to hypoglycaemia due to low glycogen stores, reduced liver gluconeogenesis and limited glucose re-absorption causing glycosuria. Hypoglycaemia is defined as a blood glucose level <2.6 mmol $l^{-1}$ in a neonate and can lead to profound neurodevelopmental impairment. Neonates require frequent measurements of blood glucose and should receive routine maintenance containing 10% glucose in isotonic crystalloid if required (see the section 'Maintenance Fluids in Neonates' for the first few days of life). Acute hypoglycaemia should be treated with 2 ml $kg^{-1}$ of 10% glucose.

## Replacement of Fluid Deficit/ Resuscitation in Neonates

A bolus of 10–20 ml $kg^{-1}$ of glucose-free isotonic crystalloid should be given over less than 10 minutes. Reassess and repeat if necessary. The 2020 International Consensus for Neonatal Resuscitation recommends early volume replacement with isotonic crystalloid or red cells for newborn infants with blood loss who are not responding to resuscitation.

## Maintenance Fluids in Neonates

In the first few days of life, maintenance fluids should contain 10% glucose with minimal or no added sodium to ensure basal requirements are

**Table 13.5** Maintenance fluids rates in term neonates (based on NICE guidance NG29); commonly given as 10% glucose with sodium and potassium added from day 1

| Age | Total fluid required (ml $kg^{-1}day^{-1}$) |
|---|---|
| Day 0–1 | 60 ml $kg^{-1}day^{-1}$ |
| Day 2 | 70–80 ml $kg^{-1}day^{-1}$ |
| Day 3 | 80–100 ml $kg^{-1}day^{-1}$ |
| Day 4 | 100–120 ml $kg^{-1}day^{-1}$ |
| Day 5 | 120–150 ml $kg^{-1}day^{-1}$ |

met and to avoid hypoglycaemia (see Table 13.5). Sodium and potassium are usually added from day 1 after the postnatal diuresis, but this should be reviewed on an individual basis. Intravenous fluids are normally started at 60 ml $kg^{-1}$ $day^{-1}$ on the first day of life unless the baby is critically unwell, in which case 40 ml $kg^{-1}$ $day^{-1}$ should be considered. Fluid volumes should be reviewed daily and can be increased until full enteral requirements have been met, and unless there are any contraindications this should be up to a maximum of 150 ml $kg^{-1}$ $day^{-1}$. Enteral losses should be replaced with 0.9% saline with added potassium.

## Perioperative Fluids in Neonates

Neonates receiving intermittent feeds do not need IV fluids routinely preoperatively, but IV fluids should be given if fasting is prolonged. Intraoperatively, an infusion of 10% glucose in isotonic crystalloid at 50–100% of maintenance rate should be considered, with regular glucose monitoring. The use of infusion pumps is recommended to prevent inadvertent boluses of glucose. A balanced isotonic crystalloid solution without glucose (or blood/blood products) should be used as boluses of 10–20 ml $kg^{-1}$ to replace losses during surgery. Large volumes of fluid should be avoided as this may cause fluid retention and generalised oedema after surgery.

## Fluid Management in Special Situations

### Dehydration

Dehydration occurs when fluid is lost from all fluid compartments, often over a prolonged period of time, most commonly due to gastrointestinal causes. The mainstay of treatment is fluid replacement, ideally via the oral route if possible. The most accurate assessment of the degree of dehydration is based on the difference between the previous (last two weeks) and current body weight:

Water deficit (ml) = [Previous weight (kg) – current weight (kg)] × 1,000

If a previous weight is not available:

Water deficit (ml) = weight (kg) × % dehydration × 10

Signs and symptoms of dehydration and shock in children are shown in Table 13.6. Individual signs are unreliable; the higher the number and the greater the severity of signs, especially in the presence of red flags, indicate a greater degree of dehydration. Hypotension is a late sign in dehydration.

- For children with mild or moderate dehydration, enteral (oral or nasogastric) rehydration is preferable.
- Children with severe dehydration or shock may require a bolus of 20 ml $kg^{-1}$ glucose-free isotonic crystalloid (i.e. Hartmann's, 0.9% sodium chloride). Further boluses may be given if signs of shock persist. After initial treatment of shock, the remaining deficit is replaced slowly over 24–48 hours. Replace half the calculated requirement (not including losses) over 24 hours and then reassess and consider replacing the rest in the following 24 hours.

### Pyloric Stenosis

If long-standing, pyloric stenosis results in a characteristic pattern of dehydration with hypochloraemic hypokalemic metabolic alkalosis. There may not be any electrolyte changes if diagnosed early (first few weeks of life). The plasma sodium may be normal, high or low. If the baby is shocked, they should receive a bolus of 20 ml $kg^{-1}$ isotonic crystalloid. Mild dehydration may be corrected with intravenous fluid given over 6–12 hours, but severe dehydration should be corrected over 36–72 hours. The fluid deficit should be estimated (a record of body weight may be available) and given in addition to maintenance. The choice of fluid depends on plasma sodium and should be given as isotonic crystalloid with 5% glucose in the first instance. Potassium should be added once the baby is passing urine, and fluid balance and electrolytes must be monitored. Ongoing metabolic alkalosis is associated with postoperative apnoeas, so surgery should only be undertaken when the metabolic alkalosis is

**Table 13.6** Signs and symptoms of dehydration and shock in children

| Degree of dehydration | Mild (not clinically detectable) | Moderate clinical dehydration | Hypovolaemic shock |
|---|---|---|---|
| Weight loss | 5% | 10% | 15% |
| Volume deficit | 50 ml $kg^{-1}$ | 100 ml $kg^{-1}$ | 150 ml $kg^{-1}$ |
| Clinical state | Appears well | Unwell or deteriorating* | Shocked |
| Mental state | Alert and responsive | Altered: irritable, lethargic* | Decreased consciousness |
| Heart rate | Normal | Tachycardia* | Tachycardia |
| Breathing pattern | Normal | Tachypnoea* | Tachypnoea |
| Eyes | Normal | Sunken* | Deeply sunken |
| Skin turgor | Normal | Reduced* | Doughy |
| Peripheral pulses | Normal | Normal | Weak |
| Capillary refill time | <2 s | 2–4 s | >4 s |
| Anterior fontanelle | Normal | Normal | Sunken |
| Tears | Present | Decreased | Absent |
| Mucous membranes | Moist | Dry | Parched |
| Blood pressure | Normal | Normal | Hypotension (decompensated shock) |
| Urine output | Normal | Decreased | Oliguric/anuric |
| Skin colour | Normal | Normal | Pale or mottled skin |
| Extremities | Warm | Warm | Cold |

* These signs of dehydration are 'red flags' to help to identify children at increased risk of progression to shock. (Based on the NICE guidance NG29.)

corrected (bicarbonate <26 mmol $l^{-1}$ and chloride >90 mmol $l^{-1}$).

## Diabetic Ketoacidosis

Dehydration due to the osmotic diuresis in diabetic ketoacidosis (DKA) has developed over a period of many weeks and must not be corrected rapidly. Water moves from the intracellular to the extracellular fluid compartment as part of the physiological adaptation, and rapid rehydration, especially when plasma sodium is allowed to fall, will result in cerebral oedema, the leading cause of death in children with DKA. Shock is rare, but if it occurs, a fluid bolus will be required, but should be limited to 7.5–10 ml $kg^{-1}$. The fluid deficit should be replaced over a minimum of 48 hours with isotonic fluid only. The blood sugar should be reduced slowly using an infusion of insulin with glucose introduced as it falls. Children with severe DKA should be monitored closely in an intensive care unit.

## Hyponatraemia

Hyponatremia is defined as a plasma sodium concentration <135 mmol $l^{-1}$. Hyponatraemia produces osmotic movement of free water across the cell membranes from the extracellular to the intracellular compartments and cell swelling. Symptomatic cerebral oedema develops relatively rapidly in children with hyponatraemia. The brain is relatively large compared to the skull, and cellular physiology is immature, so there is limited ability to adapt to excess free water. A low index of suspicion and lack of timely treatment may have contributed to poor outcomes in children in the past.

### Symptoms of Acute Hyponatraemic Encephalopathy in Children

- Headache
- Nausea and vomiting
- Confusion and disorientation

- Irritability
- Lethargy
- Reduced consciousness
- Convulsions
- Coma
- Apnoea

### Antidiuretic Hormone

Plasma sodium concentration depends on the balance between sodium and water content. In a healthy child, plasma osmolality is around 300 mOsmol $l^{-1}$ and water intake (determined by thirst) is matched by water loss (insensible losses and urinary losses determined by the action of ADH). ADH is released in response to a rise in plasma osmolality and activates water retention in the kidneys. ADH is also released in response to a variety of 'non-osmotic' stimuli that are common in hospitalised children such as:

- Postoperative pain, stress and nausea
- Drugs: opioids, non-steroidal anti-inflammatory drugs (NSAIDs), carbamazepine, vincristine
- Respiratory disorders: pneumonia, bronchiolitis, intermittent positive pressure ventilation (IPPV)
- Neurological disorders: tumours, trauma, meningitis, haemorrhage
- Endocrine and metabolic disorders

The non-osmotic release of ADH overrides osmotic control; if hypotonic IV fluids are administered to patients in the presence of non-osmotic release of ADH, concentrated urine will be excreted, and the extra free water load will be retained. Major surgery is frequently associated with increased ADH secretion and water retention. Hypotonic fluids and inappropriately high volumes of fluids should be avoided (Table 13.7).

The management of hyponatremia depends on the sodium concentration and the severity of the symptoms and is based on NICE guidance NG29.

**Table 13.7** Factors contributing to hyponatraemia in children

| Factors contributing to hyponatraemia in children |
|---|
| • Hypotonic IV fluids |
| • High volume of IV fluids |
| • Non-osmotic ADH secretion |
| • Non-specific symptoms of hyponatraemia |
| • Higher risk of cerebral oedema due to: |
| o Higher brain-to-skull ratio |
| o Lower levels of Na/K ATPase |
| o 10% less CSF |
| • Failure to monitor electrolytes and fluid balance |
| • Failure to act appropriately to abnormal results |
| • Lack of training and education in IV fluid therapy in children |

*Notes:* IV: intravenous; ADH: antidiuretic hormone; Na: sodium; K: potassium; CSF: cerebrospinal fluid

## Management of Asymptomatic Hyponatraemia

- If a child has been prescribed a hypotonic fluid, change to an isotonic fluid.
- Restrict IV fluids to 50–80% of routine maintenance in children who are hypervolaemic or at risk of hypervolaemia (for example, if there is a risk of increased ADH secretion).

## Management of Acute Symptomatic Hyponatraemic Encephalopathy

- Seek immediate expert advice (for instance, from the paediatric intensive care team).
- Give a bolus of 2 ml $kg^{-1}$ 2.7% saline (hypertonic saline) over 10–15 minutes (maximum 100 ml).
- Give a further bolus of 2 ml $kg^{-1}$ 2.7% saline over the next 10–15 minutes (maximum 100 ml) if symptoms are still present after the initial bolus.
- If symptoms are still present after the second bolus, check the plasma sodium level and consider a third bolus of 2 ml $kg^{-1}$ 2.7% saline over 10–15 minutes (maximum 100 ml).
- Measure the plasma sodium concentration at least hourly.
- As symptoms resolve, decrease the frequency of plasma sodium measurements based on the response to treatment.
- Do not manage acute hyponatraemic encephalopathy using fluid restriction alone.
- After the acute symptoms of hyponatraemia have resolved, ensure that the rate of increase

of plasma sodium does not exceed 12 mmol $l^{-1}$ in a 24-hour period. Faster correction may result in osmotic demyelination syndrome (quadriplegia and locked-in state).

- One ml $kg^{-1}$ of 2.7% sodium chloride will normally raise the serum sodium by 1 mmol $l^{-1}$.
- The sodium correction required can be calculated using the formula:

$$\text{mmol of sodium required} = (130 - \text{current serum sodium}) \times 0.6 \times \text{weight (kg)}.$$

## Prevention of Hyponatraemia

- Use isotonic maintenance fluids.
- Give 50–80% restriction of maintenance fluids in children at risk of ADH secretion.
- Monitor fluid balance and electrolytes at least every 24 hours whilst the child is receiving IV fluids.

**Table 13.8** Transfusion triggers in children

| | Haemoglobin g $l^{-1}$ |
|---|---|
| First 24h of life | 120 |
| Neonates in intensive care | 100–120 |
| Neonates not requiring oxygen | 75–85 |
| Acutely ill child | 70 |
| Cyanotic congenital heart disease | 100–120 |

**Table 13.9** Estimated blood volume (EBV) at different ages

| Age | EBV ml $kg^{-1}$ |
|---|---|
| Preterm neonate | 90–100 |
| Term neonate | 80–90 |
| Infant and children | 70–80 |
| Adult | 70 |

## Transfusion of Blood and Blood Components

Children may need a blood transfusion to replace blood loss during surgery, following trauma or to treat certain blood disorders. Compared to adults, blood transfusion is associated with a higher rate of adverse events in children, especially in the first year of life.

Transfusion should be minimised in all patients if possible, in line with NHS Blood and Transplant 'Better Blood Transfusion' initiatives. Strategies include optimising cardiovascular or respiratory disease, correction of preoperative anaemia (iron therapy, erythropoietin), nutritional advice, stopping NSAIDs prior to surgery, a perioperative plan for children who are anticoagulated, meticulous surgical technique, acute normovolaemic haemodilution and cell salvage. Treating iron deficiency anaemia with supplemental oral iron can increase haemoglobin by 10 g $l^{-1}$ per week.

Haemoglobin concentration of 70 g $l^{-1}$ should be used as a threshold for transfusion in stable patients without a major comorbidity or active bleeding. Healthy children can usually compensate for acute anaemia better than adults because they have normal cardiorespiratory physiology and effective oxygen delivery. A haemoglobin concentration of 70 g $l^{-1}$ is well tolerated outside the immediate neonatal period. A higher trigger for transfusion is used in neonates or children with cyanotic heart disease. The decision to transfuse should not be based solely on the haemoglobin level; it should also take into account the clinical situation, coexisting pathology, likelihood of continued bleeding, patient age and physiological parameters. Suggested triggers for transfusion in different circumstances are shown in Table 13.8.

In the surgical setting, it is useful to estimate the maximum allowable blood loss (MABL) as a guide to when blood is likely to be needed:

$$\text{MABL} = \frac{\text{initial haemoglobin} - \text{final haemoglobin}}{\text{initial haemoglobin}} \times \text{EBV}$$

The estimated blood volume (EBV) is calculated using the body weight and age (Table 13.9).

Transfusion volumes for children should be calculated carefully and prescribed in millilitres, not component units, to minimise dosing errors and reduce the risk of circulatory overload. In the absence of ongoing losses, 4 ml $kg^{-1}$ of packed red cells will raise the haemoglobin level by approximately 10 g $l^{-1}$.

If arterial or central venous access is available, regular haemoglobin estimation ensures that the smallest volume of blood necessary is transfused. However, in smaller infants, donor exposure can

**Table 13.10** Blood component therapy in children

| Component | Volume |
|---|---|
| Packed red blood cells | 4 ml $kg^{-1}$ raises haemoglobin by 10 g $l^{-1}$ |
| Platelets | 10–15 ml $kg^{-1}$ |
| Fresh frozen plasma | 15–20 ml $kg^{-1}$ |
| Cryoprecipitate | 5–10 ml $kg^{-1}$ |

be minimised by using as much blood as possible from one unit, although the posttransfusion haemoglobin should not exceed 200 g $l^{-1.}$ Recommended transfusion volumes of blood components are shown in Table 13.10.

Blood products should be warmed to 37°C to prevent hypothermia, as this may worsen coagulopathy or cardiac arrhythmias. Large-volume transfusion in neonates and small infants and rapid transfusions into a central catheter in older children may cause metabolic derangements, in particular hyperkalaemia and hypocalcaemia.

Cell salvage for neonates and children with large-volume blood loss is technically feasible and should be used to reduce allogeneic transfusion. Contraindications include sickle cell disease and other conditions characterised by red cell fragility. As in adults, careful risk assessment is essential in malignancy and abdominal injury when the salvaged blood may contain a high concentration of malignant cells or bacteria.

## Blood Components and Specifications

Blood components provided for the foetal, neonatal and infant age group in the United Kingdom have additional safety features and are suitable for all recipients under one year of age:

- All blood components (except granulocytes) in the United Kingdom are leucodepleted to reduce transfusion reactions and reduce the risk of variant Creutzfeldt–Jacob disease (vCJD). Fresh frozen plasma (FFP) and cryoprecipitate are currently sourced in the United Kingdom as the risk of vCJD has reduced.
- Cytomegalovirus (CMV) negative red cells and platelets should be provided for neonates.
- Irradiated blood is required in children with known or suspected T-cell immunodeficiency, such as DiGeorge syndrome, or those at risk of transfusion-associated graft-versus-host disease.

## Consent for Transfusion

Consent for blood transfusion should be obtained to include a description of risks, benefits and alternatives to blood transfusion.

A clear management plan and a full and timely discussion with the family are crucial where children or their parents refuse to consent to transfusion (e.g. Jehovah's Witnesses). The principles of 'patient blood management' should be used to optimise preoperative haemoglobin levels, minimise blood sampling, correct any coagulopathy and minimise blood loss to reduce the chance of a blood transfusion being required for all patients, and a 'best interest' approach for the child taken (see Chapter 4). Blood and blood components can be given in an emergency to save a child's life, despite parental refusal or refusal of the child. However, a plan needs to be agreed in advance of elective surgery that may require blood transfusion such as cardiac surgery or cardiopulmonary bypass; this may require court approval for surgery and any related transfusions in the case of parental refusal. It is not acceptable to wait until it is an emergency and then to use that as a reason for giving the blood without consent. Individual cases involving parental refusal should always be discussed with the Trust/Health Board legal department to obtain clarity prior to surgery. The Jehovah's Witness Hospital Liaison Committee can be a useful source of advice where relevant.

## Blood Transfusion in Neonates

Normal haemoglobin values are significantly higher at birth (160–200 g $l^{-1}$) and decrease gradually over the first few months of life to reach their lowest values (90–110 g $l^{-1}$) at around two to three months of age ('physiological anaemia'). At birth, the prevalent haemoglobin is foetal haemoglobin, which has a higher affinity for oxygen than adult haemoglobin, essential for oxygen uptake from the placenta in utero, but which results in decreased extraction of oxygen by the tissues after birth. Delayed cord clamping of at least one minute is recommended for the term and preterm neonate not requiring resuscitation and has been shown to result in a significantly increased haemoglobin after birth and decreased iron deficiency at two to six months of age. Fetal haemoglobin falls rapidly during the first few months of life with only trace amounts present at six months. Transfusion thresholds in neonates vary according to the cardiorespiratory status and postnatal age of the infant (Table 13.11). Neonatal transfusions are usually given as small volume 'top-up' transfusions to maintain the haemoglobin above a particular threshold or in the presence of surrogate markers of anaemia, such as poor growth, lethargy or increased episodes of apnoea. In preterm infants, low haemoglobin levels are a risk factor for post-operative apnoea. Potential benefits of transfusion in this group include improved tissue oxygenation and a lower cardiac output to maintain the same level of oxygenation.

Normal neonates have different age-related values for common coagulation screening tests compared to older children and adults. At birth, vitamin K-dependent clotting factors are 40–50% of adult levels and are lowest in preterm infants. The prothrombin time (PT), thrombin time (TT) and activated partial thromboplastin time (APTT) may be longer, although overall haemostatic function may be normal. Vitamin K is recommended for every newborn infant. Disseminated intravascular coagulation (DIC) is common in sick neonates, and haemorrhagic disease of the newborn due to vitamin K deficiency can cause major bleeding in babies who have not received appropriate vitamin K prophylaxis at birth. Major vitamin K deficiency bleeding requires urgent treatment. Four factor prothrombin complex concentrate (PCC) is preferable to FFP. Platelets are present in normal numbers at birth and reach adult reactivity at two weeks of age. For neonates where there are no bleeding concerns, platelet transfusion should not be administered if platelet count is $\geq 25 \times 10^9\ l^{-1}$.

## Major Haemorrhage

Major haemorrhage may be defined as the loss of either a single circulating blood volume (approximately 80 ml kg$^{-1}$) in 24 hours, 40 ml kg$^{-1}$ in three hours or 2–3 ml kg$^{-1}$ min$^{-1}$. In practice, the usual triggers for activation of major haemorrhage protocols are rapid blood loss with shock or with no likelihood of control or anticipated/actual administration of 40 ml kg$^{-1}$ of blood.

Major haemorrhage related to trauma is uncommon in children (see Chapter 39). In paediatric surgery, massive blood loss mostly occurs in craniofacial, neurosurgery, tumour resection, spinal, liver and cardiac surgery.

## Key Principles for the Management of Major Haemorrhage in Children

- Early recognition and activation of the major haemorrhage protocol (including the necessary clinical and transfusion teams)
- Active resuscitation to restore circulating volume
- Control of bleeding
- Rapid provision of Group O Rhesus negative or group-specific red cells
- Anticipation and treatment of coagulopathy and thrombocytopenia with early use of FFP and consideration of platelets and cryoprecipitate in ongoing bleeding
- Prevention/correction of the metabolic consequences of massive blood transfusion (hypothermia, hypocalcaemia, acidosis and hyperkalaemia)

Current major haemorrhage protocols, based on adult trauma research, recommend the early use of FFP and platelets prior to the results of coagulation tests where bleeding is ongoing. Table 13.12

**Table 13.11** Suggested transfusion thresholds for surgery in neonates (based on the 2016 Guidelines from the British Committee for Standards in Haematology)

| | Haemoglobin g l$^{-1}$ | | |
|---|---|---|---|
| **Postnatal age** | **Ventilated** | **Receiving oxygen/NIPPV** | **Not receiving oxygen** |
| First 24 hours | <120 | <120 | <100 |
| ≤Week 1 | <120 | <100 | <100 |
| Week 2 | <100 | <95 | <75–85 |
| ≥Week 3 | <100 | <85 | <75–85 |

*Note:* NIPPV: Non-invasive positive pressure ventilation.

shows suggested aliquots of blood and blood components to treat major haemorrhage in children. These aliquots should be repeated in recommended ratios as necessary until bleeding is controlled. Ratios should be modified accordingly once laboratory parameters are available. The therapeutic aims should be:

- Hb >80 g $l^{-1}$
- Fibrinogen >1·5 g $l^{-1}$
- PT ratio <1·5
- Platelet count >75 × 1,09 $l^{-1}$

Early use of tranexamic acid has been shown to reduce mortality in adult trauma, and this beneficial effect may also apply in children. It should be considered in all neonates and children undergoing surgery where there is risk of significant bleeding. An initial dose of 15 mg $kg^{-1}$ (maximum 1 g) intravenously over 10 minutes should be given as soon as possible, followed by 2 mg $kg^{-1}h^{-1}$ for at least eight hours or until bleeding stops.

Careful monitoring for adequacy of resuscitation and for circulatory overload is essential. Unintended over-transfusion of red cells is common in small infants. Volume replacement should be guided by clinical endpoints and laboratory or point-of-care testing. All large-volume transfusions should be given via a blood warmer to avoid hypothermia, and the core temperature should be monitored.

Potential electrolyte disturbances from massive blood transfusion include:

**Table 13.12** Blood, clotting factors and tranexamic acid dosing in major haemorrhage

| Component | Volume |
|---|---|
| Emergency transfusion (1:1 ratio) | |
| PRBC* | 20 ml $kg^{-1}$ |
| FFP | 20 ml $kg^{-1}$ |
| For ongoing bleeding: | |
| Continue PRBC: FFP 1:1 | |
| Platelets | 15 ml $kg^{-1}$ |
| Cryoprecipitate | 10 ml $kg^{-1}$ |
| Fibrinogen concentrate | 70 mg $kg^{-1}$ |
| Prothrombin concentrate | 25–50 IU $kg^{-1}$ |
| Factor VII | 90 mcg $kg^{-1}$ |
| Tranexamic acid | Loading dose 15 mg $kg^{-1}$<br>Infusion 2 mg $kg^{-1}$ $h^{-1}$ |

*Notes:* * Use emergency O D-negative blood until group-compatible blood is available; PRBC: packed red blood cells.

- **Hyperkalaemia**
  There is a risk of hyperkalaemia due to high extracellular potassium in old stored or irradiated blood following large-volume transfusions, particularly if infused rapidly. It is recommended that red cells for large-volume neonatal and infant transfusions be used before the end of day 5 following donation (and within 24 hours of irradiation) in order to reduce this risk.
  Rapid transfusion via a central line may represent a particular risk of cardiac arrest. Emergency treatment of hyperkalaemia with 10% calcium gluconate (0.5 ml $kg^{-1}$), nebulised salbutamol, glucose-insulin infusion or bicarbonate for metabolic acidosis may be required.
- **Hypocalcaemia**
  Low-ionised calcium (<1 mmol $l^{-1}$) is due to citrate overload from large blood transfusion and can result in myocardial dysfunction.
  It should be corrected with calcium chloride 5–10 mg $kg^{-1}$ by slow intravenous infusion via a central line.
- **Hypomagnesaemia**
  This is also due to citrate toxicity and may result in ventricular arrhythmias.
  Hypomagnesaemia is treated with intravenous magnesium 25–50 mg $kg^{-1}$ (maximum 2 g).

## Key Points

- It's safe and recommended to allow children to drink clear fluids up to one hour before elective surgery.
- Isotonic crystalloids with a sodium concentration similar to plasma reduce the risk of hyponatraemia without increasing adverse effects and are the first choice for fluid replacement and maintenance in children.
- Intraoperative fluid management in children should be individualised and aim for normovolaemia.
- ADH secretion in postoperative or unwell children causes water retention and increases their risk of hyponatraemia. The calculated rate for postoperative maintenance fluids should be reduced to 50–80% for at risk patients.
- Children receiving IV fluids should have electrolytes and fluid balance measured daily.

- Most children do not require glucose-containing fluids intraoperatively unless they are at risk of hypoglycaemia (for instance neonates).
- If the child has signs of severe dehydration (presence of red flags) or shock, 10–20 ml $kg^{-1}$ of a glucose-free isotonic crystalloid should be given immediately. Further boluses may be given if signs of shock persist.
- Acute symptomatic hyponatraemia should be treated with hypertonic saline in a high-dependency unit.
- Strategies to reduce blood transfusion include treatment of preoperative iron deficiency, use of appropriate transfusion thresholds, cell salvage and administration of tranexamic acid.

## Further Reading


Arumainathan R, Stendall R, Visram, A. Management of fluids in neonatal surgery. *BJA Education* 2018; 18(7):199–203.

Blain S, Paterson N. Paediatric massive transfusion. *BJA Education* 2016; 16 (8):269–75.

Faraoni D, Meier J, New H et al. Patient blood management for neonates and children undergoing cardiac surgery: 2019 NATA guidelines. *Journal of Cardiothoracic and Vascular Anesthesia* 2019; 33:3249–63.

Feld LG, Neuspiel DR, Foster BA et al. Clinical practice guideline: maintenance intravenous fluids in children. American Academy of Pediatrics. *Pediatrics* 2018; 142(6):e20183083.

Lewis SR, Pritchard MW, Evans DJW et al. Colloids or crystalloids for fluid resuscitation in critically ill people. *Cochrane Systematic Review* 2018, 3 August; 8(8):CD000567. Available at: www.cochranelibrary.com/cdsr/doi/10.1002/14651858.CD000567.pub7/full. Accessed 10 March 2024.

McNab S, Duke T, South M et al. 140 mmol/L of sodium versus 77 mmol/L of sodium in maintenance intravenous fluid therapy for children in hospital (PIMS): a randomised controlled double-blind trial. *Lancet* 2015; 28;385(9974):1190–7.

McNab S, Ware RS, Neville KA et al. Isotonic versus hypotonic solutions for maintenance intravenous fluid administration in children. *Cochrane Systematic Review* 2014, 18 December;(12): CD009457. Available at: www.cochranelibrary.com/cdsr/doi/10.1002/14651858.CD009457.pub2/full. Accessed 10 March 2024.

National Institute for Health and Care Excellence. Intravenous fluid therapy in children and young people in hospital. NICE Guideline 29 2015. Updated 2020. Available at: www.nice.org.uk/guidance/ng29. Accessed 10 March 2024.

New HV, Berryman J, Bolton-Maggs PHB et al on behalf of the British Committee for Standards in Haematology. Guidelines on transfusion for fetuses, neonates and older children. *British Journal of Haematology* 2016; 175: 784–828.

Sümpelmann R, Becke K, Crean P et al. European consensus statement for intraoperative fluid therapy in children. *European Journal of Anaesthesiology* 2011; 28(9):637–9.

Thomas, M, Morrison, C, Newton, R et al. Consensus statement on clear fluids fasting for elective pediatric general anesthesia. *Pediatric Anesthesia* 2018; 28:411–14.

Chapter 14

# Total Intravenous Anaesthesia in Children

Vaithianadan Mani, Alistair Baxter and Jon McCormack

## Introduction

Anaesthesia in children has traditionally been achieved using volatile agents. Total intravenous anaesthesia (TIVA) has recently gained popularity in children due to:

- Availability of newer anaesthetic and analgesic drugs with favourable pharmacokinetic (PK) and pharmacodynamics (PD) properties
- Better understanding of the pharmacokinetics of these drugs in children, resulting in the availability of newer PK and PK-PD models to achieve the desired clinical effect
- Widely available and user-friendly infusion devices with these pharmacokinetic models suitable for use in children

In addition, there are specific advantages of TIVA over volatile agents, which include:

- Reduced emergence delirium
- Reduced incidence of airway complications
- Reduced incidence of postoperative nausea and vomiting
- Reduced pollution
- Minimal interference with neurophysiological monitoring under anaesthesia
- Reliable delivery of anaesthesia in children undergoing airway procedures using bronchoscopes/suspension laryngoscopes

TIVA can be used for all procedures but is particularly useful for:

- Children undergoing microlaryngoscopy, bronchoscopy and other airway procedures
- Frequent and brief radiological or painful procedures where rapid recovery is needed (e.g. MRI, CT scans, endoscopy, paediatric oncology procedures and radiotherapy)
- During neurosurgical procedures to assist with control of intra-cranial pressure and for cerebral protection and smooth emergence from anaesthesia
- During transfer of anaesthetised children including transfer for remote site procedures (e.g. scans)
- Children at very high risk of postoperative nausea and vomiting

TIVA is absolutely indicated now for the following:

- Any neurosurgical procedure where evoked potential monitoring is required
- Spinal instrumentation surgery where evoked potential monitoring is used
- Children at risk of malignant hyperthermia
- Children at risk of rhabdomyolysis due to volatile agent exposure (e.g. Duchenne muscular dystrophy)

The most used drugs for TIVA include propofol, remifentanil and dexmedetomidine. Drugs such as alfentanil, ketamine and midazolam are occasionally used. These can be given by simple manual infusion schemes or by a target-controlled infusion (TCI) method, currently only available for propofol in children.

## Basic Science of TIVA and TCI

We will briefly describe the important concepts needed to understand TIVA and TCI.

### Pharmacokinetics (PK)

Sometimes described as 'what the body does to the drug', PK is more accurately defined as the movement of a drug within the body, including its elimination. A PK model can be used to predict the plasma or effect-site concentration profile of a drug after a bolus dose or an infusion. The behaviour of most drugs used for TIVA can be described

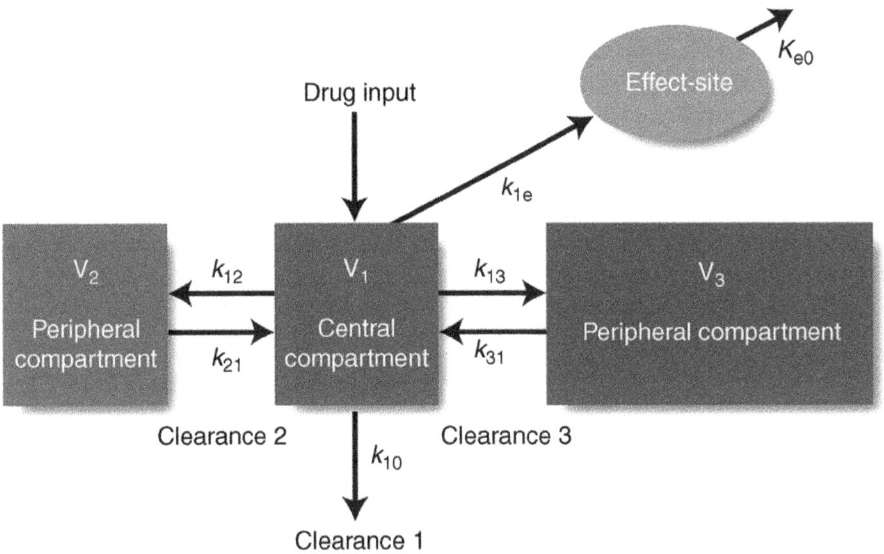


**Figure 14.1** Three-compartment pharmacokinetic model (see text for details).

by models using either two or three theoretical compartments. Each model is described by:

- The compartments and their volumes
- The rate of transfer between compartments
- The rate of drug elimination

The drug is delivered and eliminated from a central compartment (V1) and distributes to and redistributes from two peripheral compartments (V2 and V3, Figure 14.1). V2 (the 'fast' compartment) represents well-perfused organs and tissues, whilst V3 (the 'slow' compartment) represents the less perfused tissue, mainly fat. A drug that is highly lipid soluble or highly protein bound will have a large volume of distribution. It should be noted that V1 includes blood volume but may be far larger than blood volume for these drugs. The rate of transfer between compartments and elimination can be described using rate constants. By convention, *k*10 means rate constant for elimination, whereas *k*12, *k*21, *k*13 and *k*31 are used to denote the rate constants for drug transfer between V1 and V2, V2 and V1, V1 and V3 and V3 and V1 respectively.

Elimination by metabolism in the liver and excretion via the kidneys is assessed by the clearance (Cl), which is the volume of blood from which the drug is eliminated per unit time. The time required for the blood concentration of a drug to decrease by 50% is its elimination half-life ($_{1/2}$). The context-sensitive half-time (CSHT) is another helpful concept. When a drug is administered by infusion, it distributes from the central compartment to all the peripheral compartments. Once the infusion is stopped, the drug must distribute back from the peripheral compartment into the central compartment before it is eliminated. The half-time of the decrease in drug concentration is therefore related to the *duration* of the infusion for most drugs (except remifentanil). For an individual drug in an individual patient, CSHTs can be determined by graphing the elimination half-lives against the duration of the infusion. This CSHT graph will eventually become parallel to the time ($x$) axis. At that time, the infusion has become context *in*sensitive. This pattern is observed for nearly all intravenous anaesthetics. The exception is remifentanil, for which the half-time becomes context insensitive almost immediately after starting the infusion because its elimination is rapid and complete. Alfentanil's CSHT becomes constant after approximately 90 minutes' infusion.

Prolongation of the elimination of a drug reflects either an increase in the volume of distribution or a reduction in clearance, or both, and is evident in neonates and infants (due to both increased volume of distribution and reduced clearance) and patients with liver or renal dysfunction (reduced clearance). Propofol has a larger volume of distribution and higher clearance in children than in adults. In neonates, the variety of enzymatic phenotypes responsible for glucuronidation further complicates the picture by leading to variations in the speed of metabolism and subsequent elimination of the drugs. This is especially noticeable in the metabolism of propofol, which rather than following the glucuronidation pathway of older children and adults, will be hydroxylated slowing drug clearance and elimination. This concept is further complicated by the speed at which these enzyme systems begin to mature and explains the covariates of propofol elimination and the impact of postconceptual age versus postnatal age.

## Concept of Effect-Site

The clinical effect of a drug depends on the concentration at the effect-site. After intravenous administration, there is usually a delay in clinical effect as the drug must reach the effect-site from V1. The rate of equilibration between plasma and effect-site depends on several factors. These include the factors that influence the rate of delivery of the drug to the effect-site, such as cardiac output and cerebral blood flow, and the pharmacological properties of the drug, such as those that determine the rate of transfer across the blood–brain barrier (lipid solubility and degree of ionisation).

The time course of plasma/effect-site equilibration can be mathematically described by a rate constant typically referred to as *k*e0. This term should strictly be used to describe the rate of removal of drug from the effect-site, but the effect-site is usually regarded as a volumeless additional compartment, and so there is no need for separate rate constants describing movement into and out of the effect-site compartment.

## Pharmacokinetic-Pharmacodynamic (PK-PD) Modelling

Pharmacodynamics can be thought of as 'what the drug does to the body', or its biological effect. It is not possible to directly measure the concentration of the drug at the effect-site in vivo, but the time course of the changes in the effect-site concentration can be estimated from measures of clinical effect (PD effect) such as evoked EEG parameters and bispectral index (BIS). When the blood concentration in a group of subjects is known, then PD measurements can be used to estimate the *k*e0 for that drug. This is the basis of PK-PD modelling. The $_{1/2}$ *k*e0 (which is 0.693/*k*e0) is sometimes used to express this rate constant. As *k*e0 increases, $t_{1/2}$ *k*e0 decreases, and equilibration between blood and effect-site is quicker. Recently, age-related *k*e0 values have been derived for children. Neonates, critically ill children or those with major organ failure need significantly smaller doses of intravenous anaesthetic agents, and particular care is needed in children receiving vasodilator medication and in those with some types of congenital heart disease, as hypotension is a significant risk.

## Target-Controlled Infusion (TCI)

TCI is administered using a microprocessor-controlled infusion pump incorporating a PK-PD model. The user enters the patient parameters and chooses the appropriate paediatric TCI model. The pump then calculates the bolus dose and infusion rate needed to achieve a user-defined plasma or effect-site drug concentration.

## Plasma Target TCI

When plasma target TCI is used, one selects the desired PK model and inputs the selected drug, its concentration and the patient's age and weight. The microprocessor then calculates the bolus required to fill the central compartment rapidly. Once the target plasma concentration is reached, the system stops the rapid bolus and commences a stepwise-reducing infusion rate to replace drug that is lost by elimination and intercompartmental transfer (Figure 14.2). To increase depth of anaesthesia, a bolus is given and the infusion rate recalculated to maintain a higher target blood concentration. To reduce depth of anaesthesia, the system stops the infusion until the calculated new lower target concentration is reached. The rate at which the plasma concentration falls depends on the rate of elimination and the intercompartmental drug concentration gradients.

## Effect-Site-Targeted TCI

When plasma TCI is used, there is a delay before the effect-site and plasma concentrations equilibrate. With effect-site targeting, the TCI system calculates the plasma concentration to bring about the user-defined effect-site concentration as rapidly as possible (Figure 14.3)

This results in a relatively larger loading bolus dose with a higher peak plasma concentration. Whilst healthy children may be able to tolerate

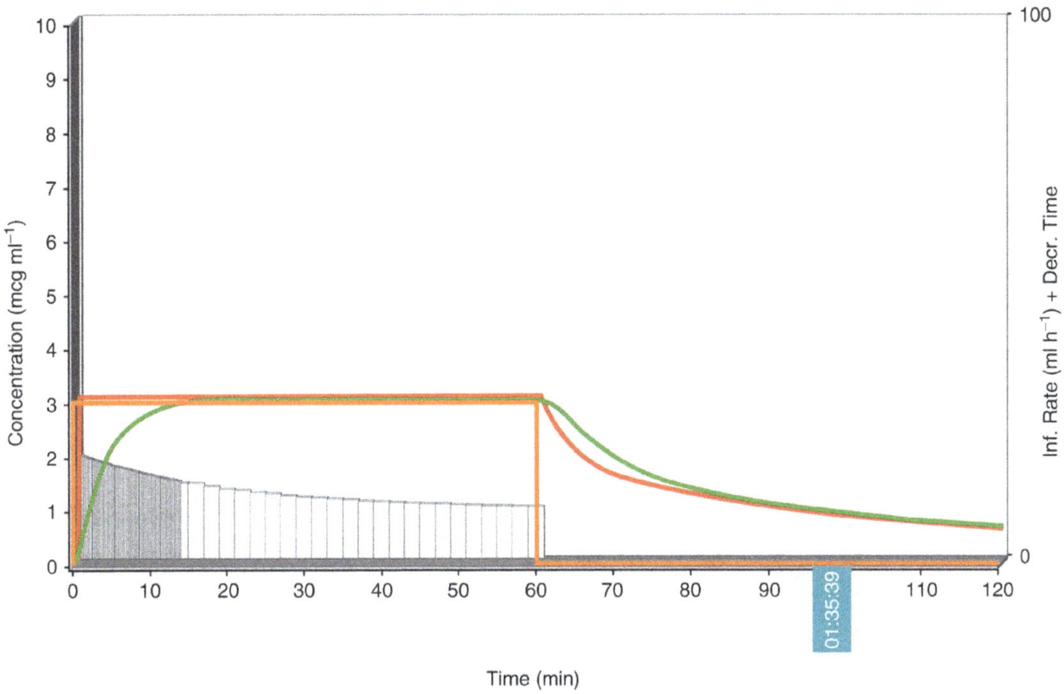


**Figure 14.2** Blood-targeted infusion of propofol in a child using the Paedfusor PK model. This diagram represents a 60-minute infusion of propofol where the blood-target concentration (the orange line) has been set at 3 mcg ml$^{-1}$, and then the infusion is switched off (blood target 0). The red line represents the predicted blood concentration, whilst the green line represents the effect-site concentration, which correlates with depth of sedation or anaesthesia. The effect-site concentration lags behind the blood concentration, and it takes around 10 minutes to reach an effect-site concentration equal to the target. The context-sensitive half-time is represented by the time it takes for the blood concentration to drop from 2 mcg ml$^{-1}$ to 1.5 mcg ml$^{-1}$, which is in this case after 60 minutes of infusion approximately 20 minutes. Inf = infusion.

this higher peak blood concentration, it may cause cardiovascular instability with hypotension and bradycardia in those who are ill.

The commercially available plasma target models for propofol are Paedfusor and Kataria. Paedfusor uses age and weight as covariates; it can be used between 5–61 kg and 1–16 years of age. Kataria can be used from 3 to 16 years of age and works with a minimum weight of 15 kg.

The newer Eleveld TCI model for a wide patient age group is now commercially available. This second-generation model was developed by combining the PK-PD data of different studies from diverse populations, including neonates, children, adults and the elderly. This model incorporates the variables of weight, age, post-menstrual age (PMA), height, sex and BMI. The predictive performance, which was measured across children, adults, elderly and high-BMI individuals, performed within acceptable limits. The PD target in this model is Ce50 (corresponding with a predicted BIS of 47), which is an age-specific effect-site concentration corresponding with 50% of maximal effect for the induction of anaesthesia. It can be seen in Figure 14.4 that with increasing age, the Ce50 required is less. This model can also be used in obese children, where it calculates the propofol infusion rates using allometric scales, with maximum body weight to be 40% above the ideal body weight for patient age, height and sex.

# Drugs Used for TIVA

## Propofol

### Manual Propofol Infusion

The simple '10–8–6' scheme devised by Roberts for propofol infusion in adults is very effective in maintaining a propofol blood concentration of 3 mcg ml$^{-1}$, which in most adults produces a state of anaesthesia. This scheme involves a loading dose of around 1 mg kg$^{-1}$ of propofol followed by an infusion of 10 mg kg$^{-1}$ hr$^{-1}$ for 10 minutes, then 8 mg kg$^{-1}$ hr$^{-1}$ for 10 minutes and 6 mg kg$^{-1}$ hr$^{-1}$ thereafter. When this regimen is used in

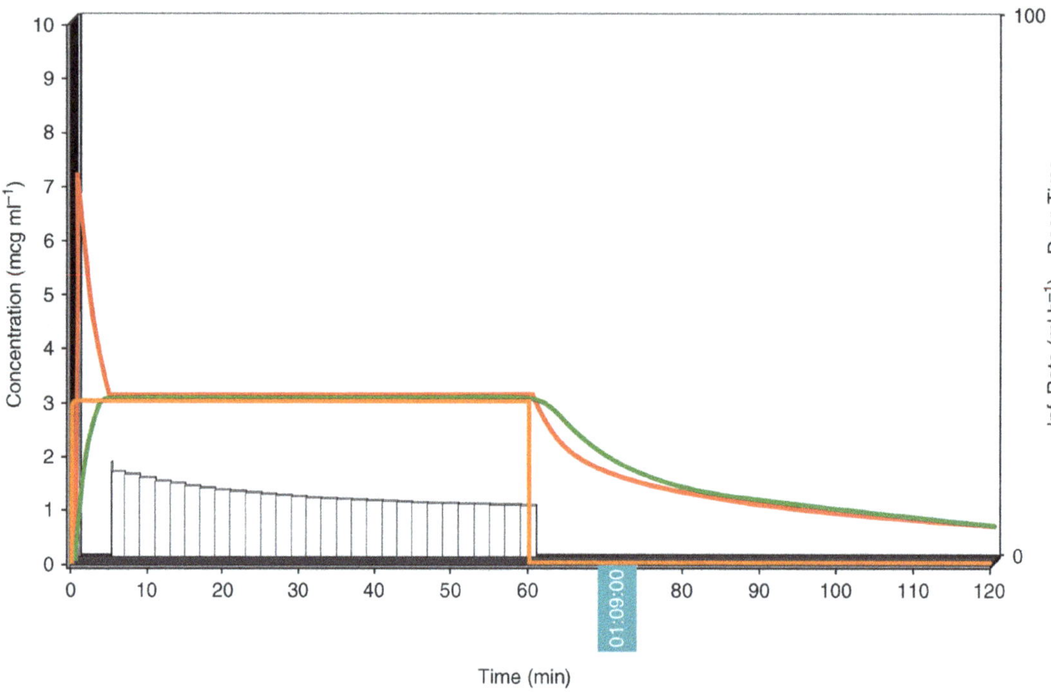


**Figure 14.3** Effect-site targeted infusion of propofol in a child using the Paedfusor PK model. This diagram represents a 60-minute infusion of propofol where the effect-site target concentration (the orange line) has been set at 3 mcg $ml^{-1}$, and then the infusion is switched off (blood target 0). As in Figure 14.2, the red line represents the predicted blood concentration, whilst the green line represents the effect-site concentration, which correlates with depth of sedation or anaesthesia. Although the effect-site concentration still lags behind the blood concentration, it takes only around three minutes to reach an effect-site concentration equal to the target. This is because a larger bolus is given to increase the blood concentration quickly to a higher peak, which drives the propofol along a concentration gradient into the effect-site much more quickly. Thus induction of anaesthesia will be quicker but at the expense of potential adverse effects related to the higher peak blood concentration, such as hypotension and bradycardia.

children, however, a subtherapeutic blood concentration of propofol is achieved. This low concentration is because of the larger V1 and increased clearance of propofol in children.

Using the Paedfusor data, it has been found that to achieve a plasma concentration of 3 mcg $ml^{-1}$, the dosing of propofol infusion in children must be approximately twice that in adults (a '19–15–12' regimen). Recent studies have shown that the target concentrations to produce anaesthesia in children above one year old are slightly higher than in adults (Figure 14.4).

The other simple manual infusion scheme to obtain a propofol blood concentration of 3 mcg $ml^{-1}$ was devised by McFarlan and validated by Engelhardt, using the Kataria dataset in children aged one to six years. In the McFarlan model, anaesthesia is induced with a bolus dose of 2.5 mg $kg^{-1}$ and then maintained with a propofol infusion regimen (commenced within one minute of the propofol bolus) of: 15 mg $kg^{-1}$ $hr^{-1}$ for the first 15 minutes, 13 mg $kg^{-1}$ $hr^{-1}$ for the next 15 minutes, 11 mg $kg^{-1}$ $hr^{-1}$ from 30 to 60 minutes, 10 mg $kg^{-1}$ $hr^{-1}$ from 1 to 2 hours and 9 mg $kg^{-1}$ $hr^{-1}$ from 2 to 4 hours. This results in a near steady-state blood concentration of 3 mcg $ml^{-1}$.

For children under three years, Steur et al. suggested a dosing regimen which has been used in neonates (see Table 14.1).

## Propofol TCI

Currently the Paedfusor and Kataria models are the most popular for achieving plasma-targeted propofol TCI. Effect-site targeting is now possible in paediatrics using the Eleveld model as discussed earlier in this chapter.

## Depth of Anaesthesia Monitoring

The popular modalities available for monitoring depth of anaesthesia (DOA) are BIS and entropy. These were used in only 1% of the paediatric anaesthesia cases reported in NAP5 in 2015. Both the

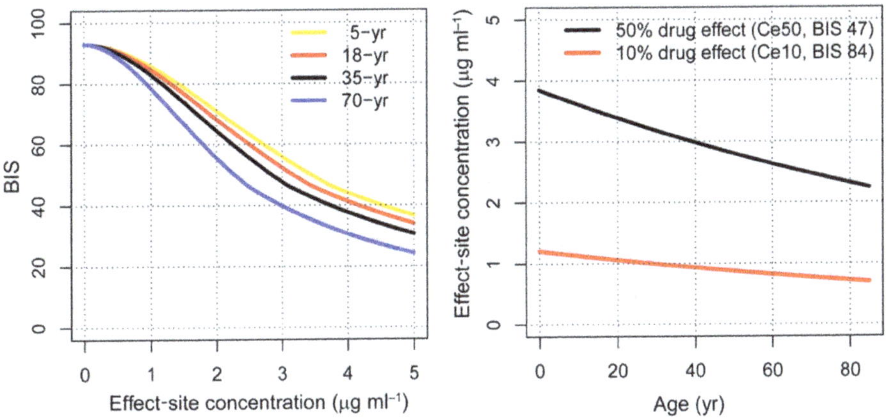


**Figure 14.4** The relationship between target concentration and age for the Eleveld PK-PD model showing the expected drug effect and suppression of BIS values.

**Table 14.1** The Steur regimen for propofol TIVA in children under three years, which has been used in neonates (all doses in mg $kg^{-1}$ $hr^{-1}$)

| Time (mins) | 0–3 months | 3–6 months | 6–12 months | 1–3 years |
|---|---|---|---|---|
| 0–10 | 25 | 20 | 15 | 12 |
| 10–20 | 20 | 15 | 10 | 9 |
| 20–30 | 15 | 10 | 10 | 9 |
| 30–40 | 10 | 10 | 10 | 9 |
| 40–50 | 5 | 5 | 5 | 9 |
| 50–60 | 5 | 5 | 5 | 9 |
| 60–120 | 5 | 5 | 5 | 9 |
| 120–240 | 2.5 | 2.5 | 2.5 | 6 |

Bispectral Index™ monitor (BIS monitor, Covidien, Ireland) and Narcotrend™ (Monitor Technik, Germany) have shown a close relationship to effect-site target concentration and can serve as a measure of anaesthetic drug effect in children older than one year. Clinical signs are currently required for depth of anaesthesia assessment in infants and neonates, as processed electroencephalograms (EEGs) are unreliable. BIS has only been validated in children above three years of age and therefore should only be used to titrate propofol dosing in this cohort. DOA monitoring is especially useful when TIVA is used with neuromuscular blockade. The National Institute for Health and Care Excellence (NICE) recommends using DOA to reduce awareness, even in cases where it has not been validated. Awareness has been reported when using TIVA. These case reports suggest that awareness possibly happens at the time of transition from inhalational induction to TIVA, when a maintenance infusion of propofol is started without administering a bolus first.

## Propofol-Related Infusion Syndrome (PRIS)

TIVA with propofol is a safe anaesthetic technique, but it is important to be aware of PRIS when infusing propofol in children. This was originally reported following its use for sedation in paediatric intensive care and is defined as the occurrence of bradycardia associated with lipaemia, fatty liver enlargement, metabolic acidosis with a negative base excess of more than 10 mmol $l^{-1}$, rhabdomyolysis or myoglobinuria.

Risk factors for developing PRIS are:

- Respiratory tract infection
- A dosage of propofol > 5 mg $kg^{-1}$ $hr^{-1}$ for > 48 hours
- Severe head injury
- Concomitant use of corticosteroids with increased catecholamine and glucocorticoid serum levels
- Low carbohydrate levels

The pathophysiology seen in PRIS is due to an increase in malonyl carnitine, which inhibits carnitine palmitoyl transferase 1 (CPT1), leading to a failure of long-chain fatty acid transport mechanisms via impairment of co-enzyme Q. This results in the accumulation of free fatty acids in mitochondria and cytolysis of cardiac and skeletal muscle. Caution is required in children with disorders of fat or carbohydrate metabolism, but it must be remembered that PRIS is rare in children undergoing anaesthesia. If children with these disorders present for anaesthesia in which propofol is absolutely indicated, then this can be mitigated by infusing a constant source of carbohydrate (dextrose infusion).

Treatment for PRIS is to stop propofol and institute the necessary supportive measures dependent on the clinical features present. These may include cardiac pacing, inotropic support, carbohydrate substitution and haemofiltration. Extracorporeal membrane oxygenation (ECMO) support may be required.

## Propofol and Lipid-Sparing Techniques

Adjuncts may be used to reduce propofol requirement. Opioids, particularly remifentanil, have been studied extensively and found to reduce the dose of propofol needed to produce unconsciousness when used in TCI. In one study, a plasma remifentanil concentration of 4 ng ml$^{-1}$ was found to reduce the propofol target concentration for loss of response to verbal command from 2.9 mcg ml$^{-1}$ to 2.2 mcg ml$^{-1}$.

Mixtures of propofol with short-acting opioids have also been used for many years to achieve a maximum effect with minimum doses, utilising their synergistic effects on sedation. Propofol (10 mg ml$^{-1}$) mixed with alfentanil (20 mcg ml$^{-1}$) or propofol (10 mg ml$^{-1}$) with remifentanil (5 mcg ml$^{-1}$) have been used successfully to provide anaesthesia, with the latter shown to be non-inferior to volatile agents. The lower propofol dose improves haemodynamic stability. Alpha-2 agonists, such as clonidine and dexmedetomidine, also have a propofol-sparing effect, as does regional anaesthesia.

Propofol 1% is a solution of 10 mg ml$^{-1}$ propofol in an emulsion containing 0.1 g ml$^{-1}$ lipid. Propofol 2% solution contains 20 mg ml$^{-1}$ propofol but the same lipid content and is therefore preferred for longer-duration anaesthesia, as this halves the lipid load to the child. The disadvantage of propofol 2% is severe pain on injection. This can be reduced by techniques described later in this chapter.

## Opioids for TIVA

Short-acting opioids used for TIVA include remifentanil, alfentanil, sufentanil and fentanyl. Appropriate postoperative analgesia must be considered, especially when ultra-short-acting opioids such as remifentanil are used. Suggested doses for opioids when used for TIVA are summarised in Table 14.2. Recent evidence suggests that infants and younger children outside the neonatal period are more resistant to the effects of remifentanil, even when combined with propofol. This is possibly due to the clearance of remifentanil being highest in neonates, decreasing with age to reach adult rates in adolescence. Spontaneous breathing can be maintained at doses that are adequate to suppress somatic responses to painful procedures, but large interindividual variation of respiratory depressant effects mandates individualised dose titration. The drug dose is more linearly related to variation in the respiratory rhythm and respiratory rate than to minute volume or end-tidal carbon dioxide. Apnoeic episodes are less likely when respiratory depressant drugs are administered slowly.

The maximum dose of remifentanil tolerated by children breathing spontaneously under anaesthesia varies widely (between 0.05 and 0.3 mcg kg$^{-1}$ min$^{-1}$). A dose of 0.05 mcg kg$^{-1}$ min$^{-1}$ will allow spontaneous breathing in more than 90% of children; a dose of 0.3 mcg kg$^{-1}$ min$^{-1}$ will produce apnoea in 90% of children. Younger children, especially those <3 years old, maintain spontaneous breathing at higher doses of remifentanil, up to 0.35 mcg kg$^{-1}$ min$^{-1}$; this is in contrast to the lower dose ranges tolerated in adults. The dose required to produce significant respiratory depression in children of the same age and weight is highly variable, despite the predictable plasma half-life of remifentanil. This variation may be due to an intrinsic difference in receptor sensitivity.

## Dexmedetomidine

Dexmedetomidine is a highly selective alpha-2 agonist with sedative, anxiolytic and analgesic properties. It does not produce respiratory depression and provides stable haemodynamics when given as a continuous infusion, except in children who are hypovolaemic or have heart block (Table 14.2).

## Ketamine

Ketamine can produce dissociative sedation and analgesia when given as an intravenous loading

**Table 14.2** Commonly used doses for TIVA in children

| Drug | Loading dose | Maintenance infusion | Notes |
|---|---|---|---|
| Propofol (Roberts) | 1 mg kg$^{-1}$ | 13 mg kg$^{-1}$ h$^{-1}$ for 10 min, then 11 mg kg$^{-1}$ h$^{-1}$ for 10 min, then 9 mg kg$^{-1}$ h$^{-1}$ thereafter | Concurrently with alfentanil infusion |
| Propofol (McFarlan) | 2.5 mg kg$^{-1}$ | 15 mg kg$^{-1}$ h$^{-1}$ for the first 15 min, 13 mg kg$^{-1}$ h$^{-1}$ for the next 15 min, 11 mg kg$^{-1}$ h$^{-1}$ from 30 to 60 min, 10 mg kg$^{-1}$ h$^{-1}$ from 1 to 2 hours, 9 mg kg$^{-1}$ h$^{-1}$ from 2 to 4 hours | Achieves blood concentration of around 3 mcg ml$^{-1}$ |
| Alfentanil | 10–50 mcg kg$^{-1}$ | 1–5 mcg kg$^{-1}$ min$^{-1}$ | Results in blood concentration of 50–200 ng ml$^{-1}$ |
| Remifentanil | 0.5 mcg kg$^{-1}$ min$^{-1}$ for 3 minutes | 0.25 mcg kg$^{-1}$ min$^{-1}$ | Produces blood concentrations of 6–9 ng ml$^{-1}$ |
| Remifentanil | 0.5–1.0 mcg kg$^{-1}$ over 1 minute | 0.1–0.5 mcg kg$^{-1}$ min$^{-1}$ | Produces blood concentrations of 5–10 ng ml$^{-1}$ |
| Sufentanil | 0.1–0.5 mcg kg$^{-1}$ | 0.005–0.01 mcg kg$^{-1}$ min$^{-1}$ | Results in blood concentration of 0.2 ng ml$^{-1}$ |
| Sufentanil | 1–5 mcg kg$^{-1}$ | 0.01–0.05 mcg kg$^{-1}$ min$^{-1}$ | Results in blood concentration of 0.6–3.0 ng ml$^{-1}$ |
| Fentanyl | 1–10 mcg kg$^{-1}$ | 0.1–0.2 mcg kg$^{-1}$ min$^{-1}$ | |
| Ketamine | 2 mg kg$^{-1}$ | 11 mg kg$^{-1}$ h$^{-1}$ for first 20 min, then 7 mg kg$^{-1}$ h$^{-1}$ for next 20 min, 5 mg kg$^{-1}$ h$^{-1}$ for the next 20 min, 4 mg kg$^{-1}$ h$^{-1}$ for the next hour, then at 3.5 mg kg$^{-1}$ h$^{-1}$ | Produces blood concentration of 3 mg l$^{-1}$ |
| Ketamine (anaesthetic dose when administered with $N_2O$ or midazolam) | 2 mg kg$^{-1}$ | 7 mg kg$^{-1}$ h$^{-1}$ for first 20 min, then 5 mg kg$^{-1}$ h$^{-1}$ for next 20 min, 4 mg kg$^{-1}$ h$^{-1}$ for the next 20 min, 3 mg kg$^{-1}$ h$^{-1}$ from then on | Produces blood concentration of 2–2.2 mg l$^{-1}$ |
| Midazolam | 0.05–0.1 mg kg$^{-1}$ | 0.1–0.3 mg kg$^{-1}$ h$^{-1}$ | |
| Dexmedetomidine (sedation for non-invasive procedures) | 0.5–1 mcg kg$^{-1}$ over 10 min | 0.5–1 mcg kg$^{-1}$ h$^{-1}$ | |
| Dexmedetomidine (sedation for invasive procedures) | 1–2 mcg kg$^{-1}$ over 10 min | 1–2 mcg kg$^{-1}$ h$^{-1}$ | |

dose of 1 mg kg$^{-1}$ and a maintenance infusion of 0.1 mg kg$^{-1}$ h$^{-1}$, with additional boluses of 1–2 mg kg$^{-1}$ and increases in maintenance rate to 0.2 mg kg$^{-1}$ h$^{-1}$ if required. To achieve anaesthetic target blood concentrations, a higher loading dose and infusion rates are needed (see Table 14.2).

TCI PK models for ketamine are described for adults; there are no PK models for children. In their simulator study using PK parameters from published studies, Dallimore suggested an infusion regimen aiming to attain a plasma concentration of 3 mg l$^{-1}$. They suggested that a lower rate of infusion could be employed when ketamine is used alongside nitrous oxide and/or midazolam. The large clearance and hence short context-sensitive half-time for infusions under two hours of racemic ketamine in children make it a good choice as a sedative or anaesthetic agent for shorter procedures. In a study on sedation in the emergency department using racemic ketamine, Dallimore found that smaller bolus doses and repeated top-ups resulted in faster recovery. In children aged 12, 6 and 2 years, the study suggested that a dosing regimen of 0.275, 0.3 and 0.35 mg $kg^{-1}$ respectively, followed by an infusion of 2.75, 3 and 3.5 mg $kg^{-1}$ $h^{-1}$ for 15 minutes, gives stable sedation with rapid recovery (20 minutes to being awake).

**Table 14.3** Morse regimen for manual infusion scheme for propofol

| Duration (min) | Dosing in neonates | Dosing in 1–2 year olds |
|---|---|---|
| Loading dose | 2 mg $kg^{-1}$ | 2.5 mg $kg^{-1}$ |
| 0–15 | 9 mg/kg/hr | 13 mg/kg/hr |
| 15–30 | 7 mg/kg/hr | 12 mg/kg/hr |
| 30–60 | 6 mg/kg/hr | 11 mg/kg/hr |
| 60–120 | 5 mg $kg^{-1}$ $hr^{-1}$ | 10 mg $kg^{-1}$ $hr^{-1}$ |

# Special Circumstances

## Neonates

There is concern about the use of TIVA in neonates, due to immaturity of the enzymes responsible for glucuronidation leading to slower drug clearance. This is further complicated by the speed at which these enzyme systems begin to mature and explains the variability of propofol elimination in neonates with respect to postmenstrual age as compared to postnatal age. This implies that preterm neonates and neonates in the first week of postnatal life are at an increased risk of propofol accumulation during either intermittent bolus or continuous administration. Adverse effects to propofol, such as hypotension, are also more common in neonates. These can lead to delayed recovery after anesthesia.

The Eleveld model could be used for TCI in neonates and infants even though it has not been validated in a neonatal population. Commercial TCI pumps for neonates and infants younger than one year are not yet available.

There are two manual infusion regimens which can be used in cases when there is an indication for TIVA: the Steur regimen is shown in Table 14.1 and the Morse regimen in Table 14.3.

Morse and colleagues used pooled clinical data to determine a manual infusion regimen to achieve steady plasma concentrations in neonates and infants. Their work highlights the difficulties experienced by all anaesthetists in dealing with such diverse populations, and the use of these techniques is only recommended for experienced users of TIVA in neonates. Propofol and remifentanil infusions are useful in this patient group for examinations of the airway, and remifentanil can be used for intubation without muscle relaxant.

### Adolescents and Children Large for Their Age

Children vary significantly with regards to height and weight for a given age; this is particularly so around puberty, when children may be significantly larger than predicted by their age model. There is therefore a risk that these children are underdosed using paediatric TCI models. Whilst some clinicians advocate using paediatric TCI models in adolescents and entering higher target values to compensate for the underdosing, we believe it may be better in bigger adolescents to use an adult TCI model and input actual patient weight, but with age entered as 16 years (which is the lowest that Schneider/Marsh models allow). Alternatively, the newly validated Eleveld model can be used, as this has been proposed to have high precision across these cohorts.

### Obese Children

Obesity creates difficulties in estimating drug doses. None of the current paediatric TCI models can be reliably used in obese children; however, the Eleveld model has been reported to deliver TCI with some precision in these patients. Regardless of what model is used, we suggest using BIS or entropy to titrate the propofol target in these children where interindividual variability may be high.

# Practical Aspects

## Equipment

Most departments have access to programmable TCI pumps. These must be programmed with appropriate paediatric infusion models, and the practitioner must be familiar with their setup. It is best practice to use luer lock syringes for TIVA to avoid disconnection at the syringe end and potential underdosing. Some pumps are programmed to accept a variety of sizes and manufacturers of syringes, others are not. It is essential to know which syringes work with your pump when using TIVA techniques.

IV access is obviously required for TIVA. Local anaesthetic creams and distraction techniques have made this more tolerable for awake children, but this may not be possible in all cases, and a cannula may need to be placed under inhalational anaesthesia for some children. If this is the case, a bolus dose of propofol is required before starting the manual infusion, or plasma levels of propofol will not reach adequate anaesthetic levels soon enough. When using TCI after gas induction, it may be better to start with a slightly lower target, such as 3 mcg $ml^{-1}$ and then to titrate further according to BIS, entropy or clinical markers. Return of consciousness after prolonged anaesthesia with propofol and remifentanil is determined primarily by the context-sensitive half-time of propofol. Context-sensitive half-time is longer in children than adults because children have proportionally greater propofol accumulation in peripheral tissues due to their higher dose requirements.

The output from TIVA infusion lines should be placed as close as possible to the venous cannula (rather than on IV extensions) with one-way non-return valves to prevent backflow up intravenous fluid lines. It is important to have access to the IV cannula. The infusion site is not always easily accessible in small children where limbs may be covered by surgical drapes and inadvertent dislodgement, obstruction or extravasation may occur. If central venous access is available, then it should be used where possible as it provides a dedicated port for TIVA and reduces the risks posed by peripheral IV access malfunction. When using a PICC line for TIVA, it is common for the pump's high-pressure alarm to sound due to the small radius and long tubing. It also is important to consider the dead space of the tubing used and the syringe size and type, as they can have an impact on the initial clinical response time. The dead space of all TIVA lines needs to be primed with the anaesthetic agents, including small extension sets, CVCs, PICCs and IV giving sets. The bolus dose programmed by the TCI pump will not compensate for the dead space, and so underdosing and miscalculation of plasma and effect site concentrations may occur if this is neglected.

We suggest opioids are diluted to an appropriate concentration (around 1–2 mcg $kg^{-1}$ $ml^{-1}$ for remifentanil) so that when a change of target or infusion rate is made, an adequate volume is delivered to ensure a quicker drug effect.

## Target Concentrations

All anaesthetists are familiar with the use of expired anaesthetic gas concentration as an estimate of effect-site concentration when providing inhalational anaesthesia. This differs from TIVA users, who instead use predicted plasma concentration targets (and effect-site concentrations if using the Marsh adult TCI model or the Eleveld universal model) as programmed into and displayed by the TCI pump.

The plasma concentration will take time to equilibrate with the effect-site concentration, approximately four minutes, as a rule of thumb. The use of adjuvant drugs such as opioids must be taken into account, especially if the patient has received neuromuscular blocking drugs, and depth of anaesthesia monitoring is strongly recommended to avoid accidental awareness. If the patient is not paralysed, movement in response to stimulation gives a good indication of inadequacy of anaesthesia or analgesia, which can be adjusted accordingly.

The authors' practice is to use a mixture of propofol 1% and remifentanil 5 mcg $ml^{-1}$ in the same syringe using the Paedfusor TCI program; a target of 3 mcg $ml^{-1}$ is suitable for less stimulating procedures (e.g. endoscopy or MRI), whilst 4 mcg $ml^{-1}$ is suitable for surgery requiring anaesthesia with spontaneous ventilation and a supraglottic airway device (SAD). If intubation without muscle relaxants is required (mastoid surgery), then a concentration target of 6 mcg $ml^{-1}$ is usually adequate.

It must be remembered that these are only guides; experience with TCI TIVA is essential, and as with all anaesthetic agents there is individual variation of pharmacodynamics and pharmacokinetics requiring titration to effect.

### Disadvantages of TIVA

- Injection pain with propofol, minimised by using:
  - Lidocaine 1 mg $kg^{-1}$
  - An appropriate dose of opioids before starting TIVA

  - Using a large bore vein
  - Using propofol 1% instead of 2% propofol for induction and then switching to 2% propofol for maintenance
- Potential for disconnection from cannula
- Drug extravasation due to high pressures from the infusion pump
- Need for infusion pumps capable of delivering TIVA/TCI
- Need for training and knowledge to use TIVA/TCI
- Risk of awareness, minimised by:
  - Avoiding muscle relaxants if possible
  - Using depth of anaesthesia monitoring
- Lipid load

### Key Points

- TIVA is becoming more popular in paediatric anaesthesia, and TCI pumps with appropriate open-source paediatric software are now available.
- TCI propofol is possible for those at least one year of age.
- Blood-targeted propofol infusions may be replaced by effect-site targeted infusions as age-appropriate software is introduced.
- Techniques should be used to limit the propofol and lipid dose, and 2% propofol solutions are recommended.
- Injection pain can and should be minimised using a range of techniques.

## Further Reading

Absalom A, Struys M. *An Overview of TCI and TIVA*. Academic Press. 2005.

Anderson BJ, Holford NHG. What is the best size predictor for dose in the obese child? *Pediatric Anesthesia* 2017; 27: 1176–84.

Elevel DJ et al. Pharmacokinetic-pharmacodynamic model for propofol for broad application in anaesthesia and sedation. *British Journal of Anaesthesia* 2018; 120(5):942–59.

Jeleazcov C, Ihmsen H, Schmidt J et al. Pharmacodynamic modelling of the bispectral index response to propofol-based anaesthesia during general surgery in children. *British Journal of Anaesthetics* 2008; 100(4):509–16.

Kam PC, Cardone D. Propofol infusion syndrome. *Anaesthesia* 2007; 62(7):690–701.

Lerman J, Johr M. Inhalational anesthesia vs total intravenous anesthesia (TIVA) for pediatric anesthesia. *Paediatric Anaesthesia* 2009; 19(5): 521–34.

Mani V, Morton NS. Overview of total intravenous anesthesia in children. *Paediatric Anaesthesia* 2009; 20(3):211–22.

Munoz HR, Cortinez LI, Ibacache ME, Leon PJ. Effect site concentrations of propofol producing hypnosis in children and adults: comparison using the Bispectral Index. *Acta Anaesthesiologica Scandinavica* 2006; 50(7):882–7.

Tirel O, Wodey E, Harris R, Bansard JY, Ecoffey C, Senhadji L. Variation of Bispectral Index under TIVA with propofol in a paediatric population. *British Journal of Anaesthesia* 2008; 100(1):82–7.

Chapter 15

# Regional Anaesthesia in Children

Naveen Raj and Steve Roberts

## Introduction

Regional anaesthesia is an important aspect of paediatric anaesthesia and should be considered for all suitable cases. The benefits of excellent analgesia need to be balanced against the potential risks; where possible, the most appropriate and peripheral technique should be used. Peripheral nerve blocks (PNB) should only be performed by those with the correct training, equipment and assistance. It is essential that the signs and management of local anaesthesia toxicity are understood by those performing and assisting with PNB.

In the United Kingdom, the bulk of paediatric PNBs are performed under general anaesthesia (GA). In the rare circumstance where blocks are performed awake (e.g. minor surgery on older, cooperative children), age-appropriate preoperative information, a quiet theatre environment and reassurance are essential to minimise the child's and their carers' anxiety.

Ultrasound (US) imaging is the gold standard for the majority of blocks and as such will in general be the only description outlined in this chapter.

The nerve blocks to be discussed are listed in Table 15.1.

**Table 15.1** Common regional blocks

| | |
|---|---|
| Head and neck | Superficial cervical plexus<br>Auriculotemporal |
| Upper limb blocks | Interscalene<br>Supraclavicular<br>Axilla<br>Forearm<br>Ring block |
| Truncal blocks | Thoracic paravertebral<br>Erector spinae plane<br>Serratus anterior plane |
| Abdominal blocks | Rectus sheath<br>Quadratus lumborum<br>Penile |
| Lower limb blocks | Lateral femoral cutaneous nerve<br>Femoral<br>Adductor canal<br>Fascia iliaca<br>Lumbar plexus<br>Sciatic – proximal and distal<br>Ankle<br>Metatarsal and ring blocks |
| Central blocks | Caudal – single shot |

## General Points

For all blocks, a thorough history and examination are mandatory to identify any contraindications to regional anaesthesia (see Table 15.2) along with appropriate preparation of the child and care:

- *History:* allergies, previous regional/general anaesthesia, comorbidities, current medications.
- *Planned procedure*: to determine the most suitable block, and whether a catheter technique would be beneficial for continued pain relief in the postoperative period e.g. to facilitate physiotherapy.

**Table 15.2** General contraindications to regional anaesthesia

| Absolute contraindications | Relative contraindications |
|---|---|
| Lesions (infective) at the site of injection | Neuromuscular disorders |
| History of allergy to LA | Systemic infection (catheter techniques) |
| Lack of consent | Bleeding disorders (US can avoid inadvertent damage to blood vessels) |

- *Examination:* of the operative site and potential puncture site, to exclude local infection.
- *Weight:* to calculate maximum dose of local anaesthetic (LA).
- *Consent:* to explain potential advantages, side effects, complications and alternative methods of pain relief if the block fails. General complications include failure, nerve damage, LA toxicity, haematoma, infection and anaphylaxis.
- *Preoperatively:* where a GA can be avoided, the patient can be prepared by a play specialist if necessary and age-suitable distraction provided. Before coming to theatre, topical anaesthesia can be applied to the proposed puncture site. In these circumstances, parental presence can be reassuring. Administration of paracetamol and an NSAID to supplement the block should be considered.
- *Anaesthetic room:* a trained assistant should be present, along with accessibility to resuscitation equipment and drugs, including 20% Intralipid. Prior to performing the block, the airway and IV access should be secured and full monitoring instituted. Inadvertent wrong-sided nerve blocks are uncommon but do occur; a systematic check confirming the surgical site marking and consent form should be performed immediately before needle insertion ('stop before you block' process).
- *Equipment:* an insulated short-bevelled needle with extension tubing, gauze swabs, antiseptic solution, sterile gloves, sterile drapes, syringe, LA, a peripheral nerve stimulator (PNS) (for mixed nerves) and a US machine (with high-frequency probe, sterile gel and probe cover).
- *Procedure:* for those children not having a GA, the skin should be infiltrated with lidocaine first; the administration of Entonox can smooth proceedings.
- *Asepsis:* single-shot techniques require a basic sterile technique, but those involving catheters should have a full aseptic technique.

## Technique

- As regional needles are quite blunt, it is useful to nick the skin first with a hypodermic needle. This ensures that the fascial planes are appreciated as the short-bevelled needle is advanced.
- If a PNS is used, an initial current of 2 mA is set; as the needle is advanced and the relevant motor response elicited, the current is decreased to 0.5 mA.
- After initial aspiration, 1 ml of LA is injected, abolishing the motor response. The injection is made slowly with intermittent aspiration to exclude intravascular placement.
- Usually a long-acting LA is appropriate, providing analgesia for 6–12 hours. If prolonged analgesia is required, the insertion of a catheter should be considered.
- To minimise the risk of dislodgement, the catheter should be tunnelled 3–4 cm subcutaneously. The use of a drop of Indermil® tissue glue over the puncture site limits the leak; this prevents the LA escaping and causing the dressing to lift off and the catheter to fall out.
- If planning a postoperative infusion, start it intraoperatively as this may highlight any occlusion issues.

## Postoperative

In the recovery area, a failed block can be difficult to differentiate from emergence delirium; if in doubt, pain should be assumed and treated promptly with either 0.25–0.5 mg kg$^{-1}$ of ketamine or 0.5 mcg kg$^{-1}$ of fentanyl. This achieves quick control and the need for morphine can then be considered. Carers and patients should be advised to protect the anaesthetised area; this should include warning of decreased sensation (especially temperature) and motor weakness. Upper limbs should be kept in a sling. Where lower limb blockade is used, ensure means of ambulation and discharge are in place.

## Local Anaesthetics

Levobupivacaine is our LA of choice owing to its longer duration of action, and low cardio/neurotoxicity. As the blocks usually accompany a GA, concentrations of 0.125–0.25% are adequate; low concentrations are essential if there is a risk of compartment syndrome. Ropivacaine is preferred in some centres as it may cause less profound motor block. Lidocaine is indicated for infiltration before performing a block in awake children (see Table 15.3).

Neonates and infants are at greater risk of LA toxicity because of lower protein binding and the

**Table 15.3** Local anaesthetics

| Local anaesthetic dose.LA | Single-shot block (mg $kg^{-1}$) | PNB catheter infusions (mg $kg^{-1}$ $h^{-1}$) | Maximum dose per 4 hours (mg $kg^{-1}$) |
|---|---|---|---|
| L-bupivacaine | 2.5* | 0.125–0.4 | 2.0 |
| Ropivacaine | 3 | 0.4 | 1.6 |
| Lidocaine | 4 | NA | NA |

*Note:* * halve dose in neonates.

immature blood–brain barrier and liver. Consideration should be given to halving LA doses in these patients and limiting LA infusions to 48 hours.

For non-minor surgery, the duration of analgesia can be extended by administration of dexamethasone IV and an alpha-2 adrenergic agonist IV. Clonidine 1–2 mcg $kg^{-1}$ may be added to caudals.

**Table 15.4** Signs of local anaesthesia toxicity

| |
|---|
| Restlessness or agitation, followed by slurred speech or loss of consciousness |
| Muscle twitching, which may progress to seizures |
| Respiratory depression |
| Bradycardia, heart block, hypotension |
| Ventricular tachyarrhythmias, progressing to cardiac arrest |

## Local Anaesthetic Toxicity

Prevention is preferable:

- Never exceed the maximum dose of LA (see Table 15.3).
- Always aspirate before injection.
- Use US to observe the injection (note that this is not infallible).
- Maintain a high level of suspicion.

Systemic toxicity results in depression of both the central nervous and cardiovascular systems with recognisable symptoms and signs, increasing in severity from somnolence through to convulsion and cardiac arrhythmia (see Table 15.4). However, as most children receive regional anaesthesia under GA, the earlier warning signs may be masked, and thus the first manifestation of a problem may be cardiovascular collapse.

In the event of toxicity, management should follow an established protocol such as that in Figure 15.1. Arrhythmias may be refractory, and resuscitation may be very prolonged.

## Specific Blocks

### Head and Neck Blocks

#### Superficial Cervical Plexus Block

##### Anatomy

The superficial cervical plexus (SCP) is formed by the anterior rami of cervical nerves C1–4, emerging at the midpoint of the posterior border of the sternocleidomastoid muscle (SCM) at the level of thyroid cartilage. The four terminal branches of this plexus provide innervation to the skin and superficial structures over the anterolateral part of the neck and the area immediately underneath the clavicle:

- Greater auricular: auricle of the ear
- Lesser occipital: superior posterior neck and scalp behind the auricle
- Transverse cervical: anterolateral aspect of the neck from the sternum to the mandible
- Supraclavicular: cape of the neck and shoulder to the level of the second intercostal space

##### Indications

For surgical procedures in the front of the neck, including excision of thyroglossal/branchial cyst, tracheostomy, thyroidectomy, carotid and vascular surgery, lymph node biopsy, tympanic and mastoid procedure, pinnaplasty, clavicular fracture and posterior neurosurgical incisions.

##### Technique

The aim of the SCP block is to inject LA behind the midpoint of the posterior border of the SCM between the muscle and the prevertebral fascia.

Posterior in-plane (IP) approach: place the patient in a position similar for insertion of a

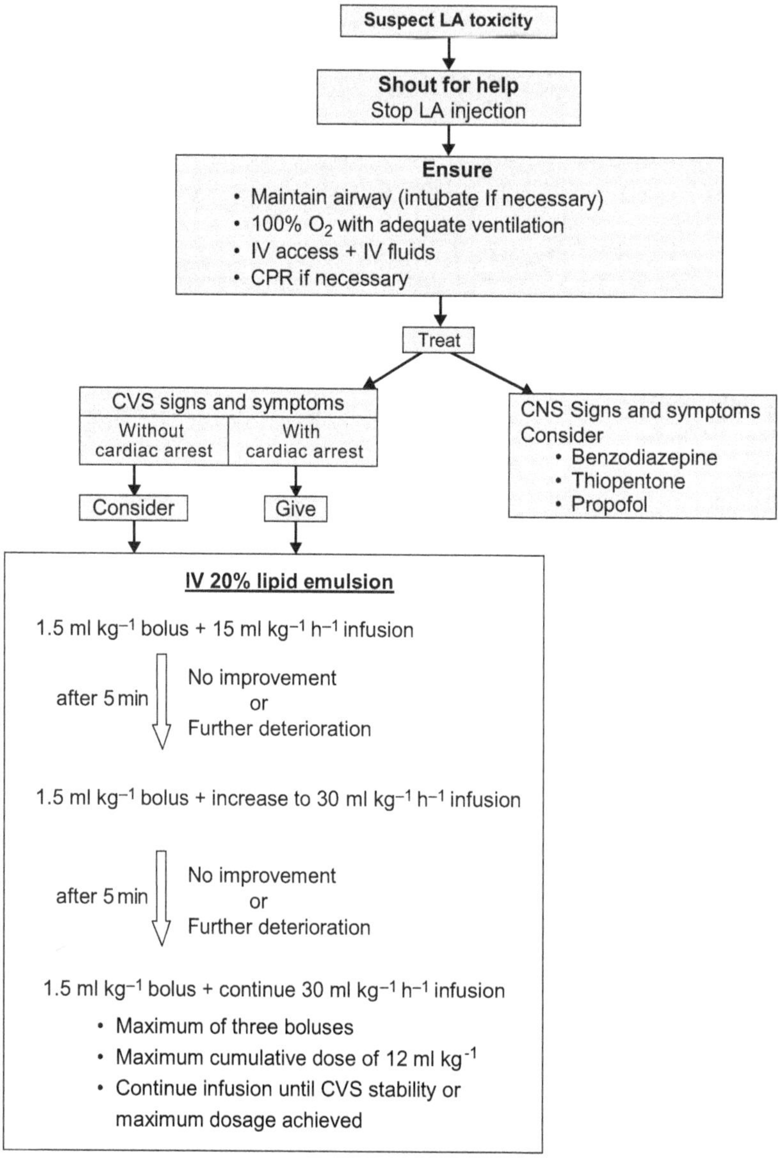


**Figure 15.1** Management of LA toxicity.

central venous pressure (CVP) line in the neck with the face turned slightly away from the block site. A linear transducer probe of appropriate length is placed transversely over the front of the neck to identify the thyroid cartilage (the midpoint of a line from the sternoclavicular joint to the mastoid process) and moved laterally to visualise the tapering edge of the sternocleidomastoid muscle in the middle of the screen. The needle is inserted IP from the posterolateral edge of the probe position aiming for the tapered tip of SCM, to traverse a short distance along the posterior border of SCM directed towards the carotid artery. Needle position is confirmed with SCM being hydrodissected away from the prevertebral fascia before completion of injection as the needle is withdrawn towards the tapering tip, with a maximum of 5 ml of LA.

### Specific Complications

Deeper injection without visualisation of the needle tip may lead to inadvertent vascular puncture or blockade of deeper neural structures, e.g. phrenic nerve, deep cervical plexus, brachial plexus and the recurrent laryngeal nerve.

#### Auriculotemporal Nerve Block

The SCP can be combined with an auriculotemporal nerve block for surgery on the ear and mastoid. This nerve supplies the superior two-thirds of the anterior surface of the ear, the external auditory canal and the temporal region of the forehead. It is blocked by subcutaneous infiltration of LA in front of the tragus behind the superficial temporal artery.

## Upper Limb Blocks

### Brachial Plexus Anatomy

The anterior primary rami of C5 to T1 form the brachial plexus. They emerge from the intervertebral foramina between the scalenus anterior and medius muscles enclosed within a fascial sheath. The roots come together to form trunks:

- C5 and C6 unite to form the superior trunk.
- C7 forms the middle trunk.
- C8 and T1 roots unite to form the lower trunk.

From the interscalene groove, the trunks pass over the first rib superoposterior to the subclavian artery. At the lateral border of the first rib, the trunks divide into anterior and posterior divisions. The anterior divisions of the upper and middle trunks join to become the *lateral cord*, the anterior division of the lower trunk continues as the *medial cord*. The posterior divisions of the three trunks join to form the *posterior cord*. The cords are named according to their position in relation to the axillary artery; they divide into the nerves that supply the arm.

- Lateral cord: becomes the *lateral root of median nerve and musculocutaneous nerve.*
- Medial cord: becomes the *medial root of median nerve, ulnar nerve and medial cutaneous nerves of arm and forearm.*
- Posterior cord: becomes the *axillary and radial nerves.*

#### Interscalene Block

##### Indications

Shoulder surgery and the upper medial aspect of the arm.

##### Technique

LA is injected into the interscalene groove between the scalenus anterior and scalenus medius muscles at the level of C6 (cricoid cartilage level) to block the nerve roots, resulting in analgesia over most of the shoulder region and the medial aspect of the arm, but with no block to the ulnar aspect of the arm, forearm or the hand.

The patient is placed supine with the head turned slightly to the opposite side of the block. A linear US probe is positioned transversely over the middle of the neck and slid laterally past the carotid artery and internal jugular vein following the SCM, until the tapered tip of the SCM is seen in the middle of the screen. The two scalenus muscles should be identified just underneath the tip of the SCM and the probe tilted or rotated slightly to appreciate the C5–7 nerve roots of the brachial plexus as hypoechoic circles stacked one above other vertically in the interscalene groove (Figure 15.2). If it is difficult to identify in this area, then the probe can be slid into the base of the neck as described for the supraclavicular block; once the plexus is identified, it can be easily traced back to the level of C6 vertebrae.

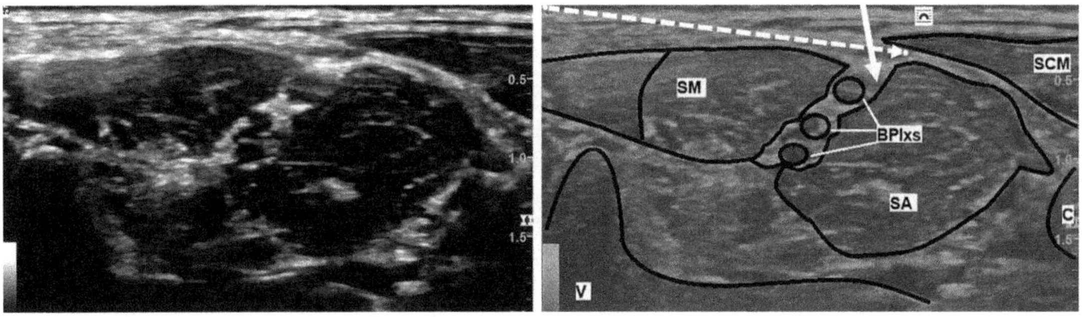


**Figure 15.2** Ultrasound appearance of the brachial plexus in the interscalene region (BPlxs); scalenus medius (SM), scalenus anterior (SA), sternocleidomastoid(SCM), vertebra (V) and carotid artery (C).

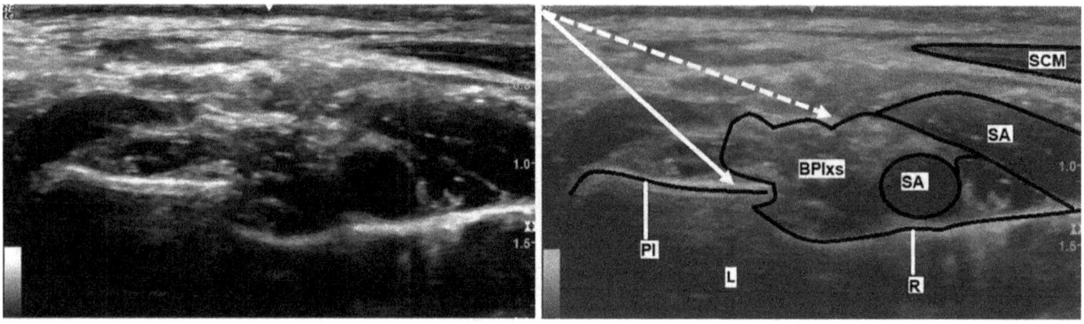


**Figure 15.3** Ultrasound appearance of the brachial plexus in the supraclavicular region (BPlxs); subclavian artery (SA), pleura (Pl), lung (L), rib (R) and sternocleidomastoid muscle (SCM).

The needle can be inserted out of plane directed to one side of the most superficial nerve root in the interscalene groove and then advanced deep along the side of the hypoechoic circles with hydrodissection until all of the nerve roots are covered with sufficient LA. The needle is then withdrawn and the procedure repeated on the other side of the nerve roots ensuring they are covered with LA on both sides.

An IP approach from the lateral edge of the probe with the needle advanced through the scalenus medius to reach the nerve roots in the interscalene groove is feasible. Risk of damage to long thoracic and dorsal scapular nerves exists with the latter approach, since these nerves pass through the scalenus medius muscle.

#### Specific Complications

Inadvertent neuraxial block by intrathecal injection may occur. Phrenic nerve block with resultant ipsilateral diaphragmatic palsy is common and should be taken into account if the patient has poor baseline respiratory reserve. Less common are ipsilateral Horner syndrome due to block of cervical sympathetic ganglion, and hoarseness due to involvement of the recurrent laryngeal nerve.

### Supraclavicular Block

The brachial plexus at this point is close to the subclavian artery and pleura. For this reason, a block at this level should only be performed by experienced practitioners, and arguably only with ultrasound. Classically it is said that this approach can miss the lower nerve roots. However, with US poor LA distribution can be observed and corrected. Specific relative contraindications include previous neck surgery and contralateral pneumothorax.

When performed with US, the whole upper limb can be anaesthetised, with the exception of the shoulder.

#### Technique

The patient lies supine with a roll between the shoulders and the head turned to the opposite side to the intended surgery; this allows adequate room for needle manipulation. The US machine and equipment are positioned ergonomically.

A linear probe of appropriate size footprint is placed parallel to the clavicle. The three main structures to identify are the pleura, the subclavian and dorsal scapular arteries. The brachial plexus is seen as a group of hypoechoic (black) bubbles posterior and slightly superficial to the subclavian artery (Figure 15.3). The dorsal scapular artery often passes through the brachial plexus, so it should always be identified using colour Doppler. The needle is inserted using an IP technique, travelling in a posterolateral to anteromedial direction. The tip of the needle is aimed between the bubbles where the subclavian artery and pleura come together. LA injection is observed and appropriate needle manipulation made to ensure uniform spread.

#### Specific Complications

Pneumothorax, phrenic and recurrent laryngeal nerve blockade, and Horner syndrome.

### Axillary Block

The three main branches of the brachial plexus lie close to the axillary artery. In the supine child the three main branches are commonly positioned with the median and musculocutaneous nerves superior, the ulnar nerve inferior and the radial nerve posterior to the artery. Note that the musculocutaneous and axillary nerves leave the

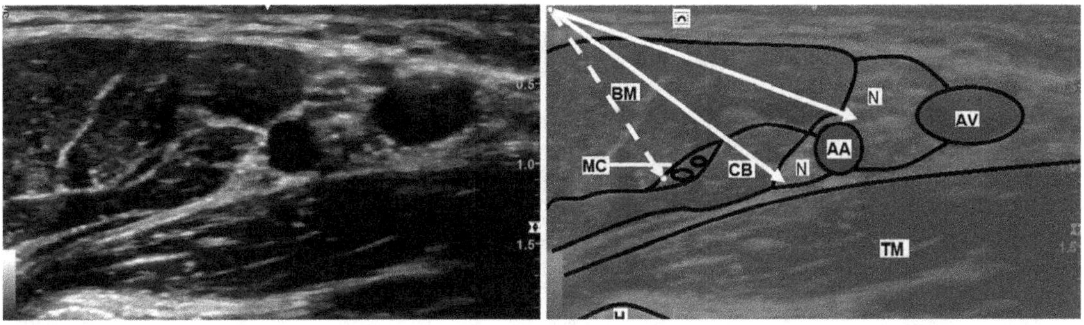


**Figure 15.4** Ultrasound appearances of the brachial plexus in the axillary region showing axillary artery (AA), axillary vein (AV), biceps muscle (BM), musculocutaneous nerve (MC), coracobrachialis muscle (CB), triceps muscle (TM), humerus (H) and radial, median and ulnar nerves (N).

'sheath' at the level of the coracoid process, hence the absence of block in these nerves in up to 50% of blocks.

#### Indications

This block is appropriate for hand and forearm surgery.

#### Technique

The patient is positioned with the arm abducted and flexed to 90° at the elbow. With a linear probe held transversely across the upper arm at the level of insertion of the pectoralis major muscle, an IP needling technique can be used to block the four main nerves individually (Figure 15.4). The musculocutaneous nerve is easily identified and blocked as it passes between the biceps and coracobrachialis muscles, ensuring coverage of the lateral forearm. The musculocutaneous nerve is oval in appearance, changing to a triangular shape distally. As the arrangement of the nerves in the axilla is very variable, the most reliable way of identifying them is to follow their path distally with the US. The median nerve passes along with the artery to the elbow, the ulnar nerve becomes more superficial and moves away from the artery and the radial nerve can be seen to drop down towards the humeral groove with gentle to-and-fro movement of the probe. If it is not possible to visualise the nerves, then injection around the axillary artery with care after piercing the sheath can be performed to aid nerve block. The deepest nerve structures are blocked first in case an air artefact subsequently obscures the view. Each nerve can be blocked with as little as 1–2 ml.

### Forearm

The three nerves can be blocked individually anywhere along their path within the forearm.

#### Indication

Hand surgery, or as rescue blocks for failed upper limb blocks.

#### Technique

Either an out-of-plane (OOP) or IP needling technique is suitable.

The *median nerve* is most easily blocked mid-forearm, where it sits between the deep and superficial flexor muscles. The probe is placed in a transverse plane mid-forearm (Figure 15.5). At this point, there is little vasculature to hit and few tendons to confuse with the nerve.

The *ulnar nerve* is best blocked in the proximal third of the forearm as the associated artery does not join the nerve till farther down. By placing the probe at the midpoint of the ulnar aspect of the forearm, the ulnar nerve can be imaged lying on the deep aspect of flexor carpi ulnaris muscle (Figure 15.6). The ulnar artery is adjacent, and the LA is injected where the nerve is separate from the artery.

The *radial nerve* is blocked preferably just above the elbow joint with the transducer probe placed transversely across the lateral epicondyle of the humerus. The nerve is seen as a triangular hyperechoic structure which can be traced up proximally into the posterior spiral groove of the humerus. Alternatively, the probe is placed transversely over the groove between the tendons of biceps brachii and brachioradialis. The division of the radial nerve into superficial and deep branches can be imaged at this point; an

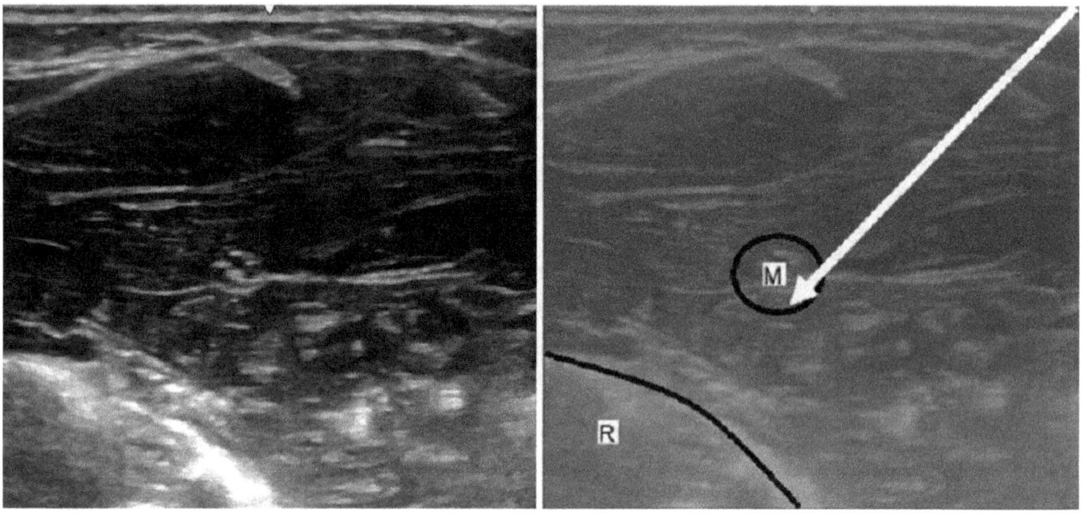


**Figure 15.5** Ultrasound appearance of the median nerve (M) and radius bone (R) at mid-forearm.

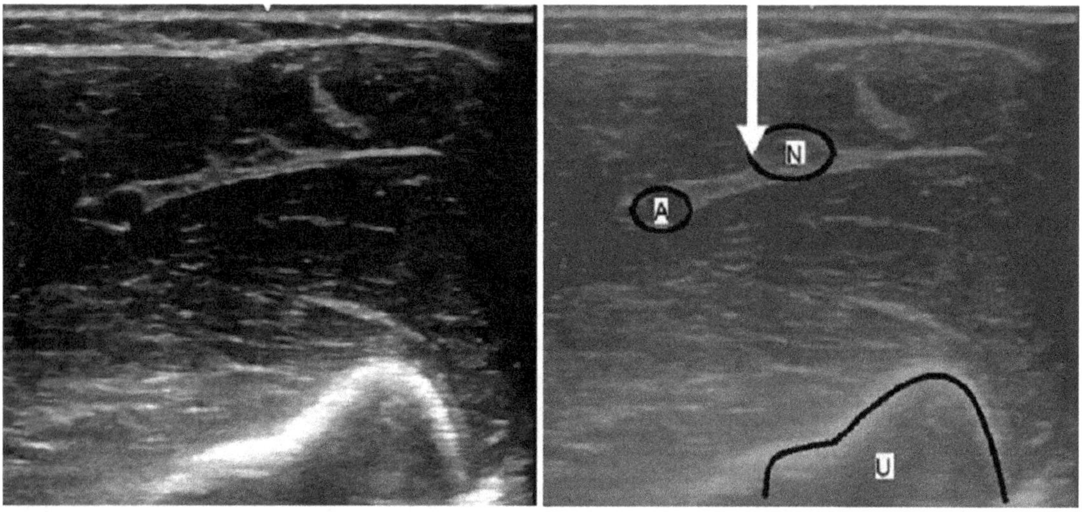


**Figure 15.6** Ultrasound appearance of the ulnar nerve (N), ulnar artery (A) and ulnar bone (U) at mid-forearm.

accompanying artery is present and must be avoided (Figure 15.7).

## Ring Block

This simple block is used for operations on the fingers, such as nail bed repair. The digital nerves are branches of the median and ulna nerves ventrally and the ulna and radial nerves dorsally. Each digit is supplied by four nerves in the 2, 5, 7 and 10 o'clock positions in relation to the phalanx.

The needle is inserted medially and laterally to the extensor tendon. The needle is passed subcutaneously down both the medial and lateral aspects of the phalanx.

The needle is inserted as far as the volar skin before being slowly withdrawn as LA is injected.

In the awake patient, this is a painful block to perform, therefore topical anaesthesia should be placed around the base of the finger. *Vasoconstrictors must not be used.*

## Truncal Blocks

### Anatomy

The upper thoracic nerves (mainly T2–6) provide the innervation of the skin and musculature over the chest wall. The thoracic spinal nerves divide into dorsal and ventral branches on exiting the intervertebral foramen. The dorsal branch divides into a medial and lateral branch to supply the skin over the back, from the midline to the border of the latissimus dorsi muscle. The ventral intercostal nerve passes underneath the inferior border of the corresponding rib with the intercostal vessels, initially between the pleura and posterior intercostal membrane and then between the internal and innermost intercostal muscles. They give a lateral branch at the angle of the rib (mid-axillary line) and terminate at the edge of the sternum as the anterior cutaneous branches. The lateral cutaneous branch (except T2) divides into anterior and posterior branches supplying the skin over the anterolateral chest wall. The intercostobrachial nerve is the undivided lateral branch of T2, which in addition runs through the axilla and innervates portions of the axilla, tail of the breast, lateral chest wall and upper-medial side of the arm.

### Thoracic Paravertebral Block

The aim is to inject LA into the wedge-shaped paravertebral space found either side of the vertebral column. The base is formed by the posterolateral part of the vertebral body, the disc and the intervertebral foramina with its contents, the anterolateral boundary by the parietal pleura and the posterior wall by the superior-costotransverse ligament (Figure 15.8). The LA spreads to at least two vertebral levels above and below, the intercostal space laterally and potentially to the epidural space medially and the contralateral paravertebral space.

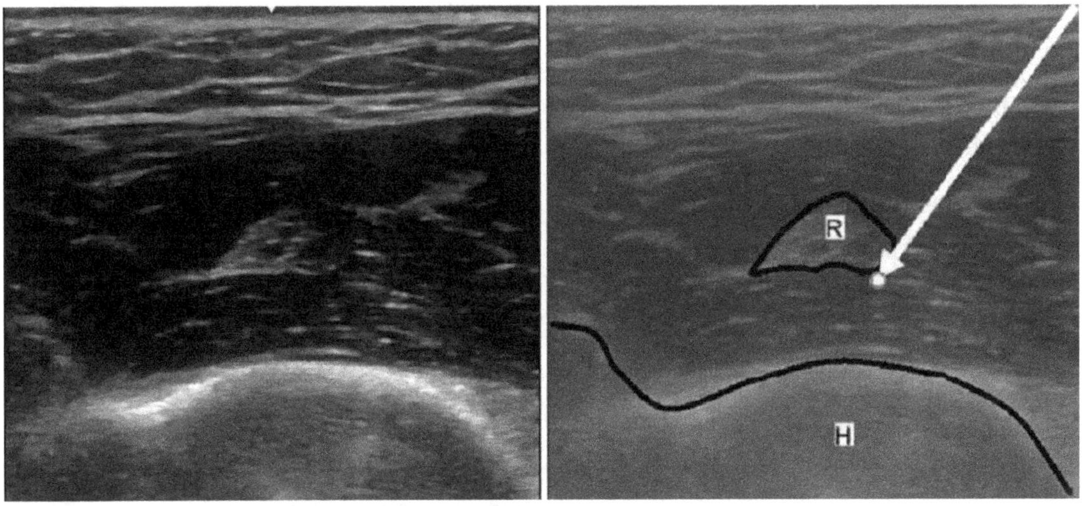


**Figure 15.7** Ultrasound appearance of the radial nerve (R) and humerus (H) at the elbow.

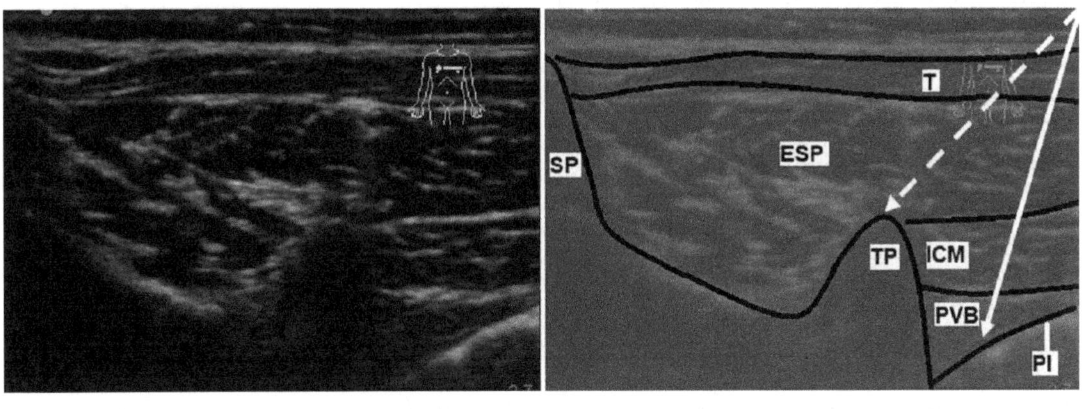


**Figure 15.8** Ultrasound appearance of the paravertebral region; spinous process (SP), transverse process (TP), pleura (Pl), trapezius (T), erector spinae (ESP), intercostal muscle (ICM) and paravertebral space (PVB).

Empyema and tumour occupying the space are contraindications. It may not be possible to find the space easily in children with kyphoscoliosis or be successful in children with a history of previous thoracotomy.

#### Indications

Thoracic and abdominal procedures, utilising unilateral or bilateral injections as appropriate. A catheter can be placed by the anesthetist or by the surgeon under direct vision during a thoracotomy.

#### Technique

The anaesthetised child is placed in the lateral decubitus position with the knees bent up and the side to be blocked uppermost. A linear probe is placed at an appropriate level in the midline (T4–5 for sternotomy, T6–7 for thoracotomy and T9–10 for abdominal procedures) to view the hypoechoic peak formed by the spinous process of the vertebrae and traced laterally to see the shiny lamina of the vertebral body and a more shallow second peak of the transverse process (TP) deep to the muscles of the back. Lateral to this the intercostal muscles are seen with a very hyperechoic pleura, and a characteristic lung shadow below disappearing medially underneath the shadow of the TP. The paravertebral space is the triangular space with the TP as the base, the pleura anteriorly and the lower border of intercostal muscle (internal intercostals membrane) posteriorly. A needle can be inserted IP from the lateral edge of the probe into the space, and the position confirmed by observing anterior displacement of the pleura on injection. Once the pleura is displaced, the needle is advanced just under the shadow of the TP and the rest of the LA injected. A volume of 0.3–0.5 ml $kg^{-1}$ per side to a maximum of 20 ml is recommended. It can also be performed with the probe placed in the paramedian plane with the vertebral level of interest at the middle of the probe, and the needle inserted IP in a craniocaudal direction into the paravertebral space; position is again confirmed with anterior displacement of the pleura before the rest of the LA is injected.

#### Specific Complications

Pneumothorax, contralateral paravertebral spread, epidural spread and dural tap.

### Erector Spinae Plane Block (ESPB)

ESPB is an interfascial plane block where LA is injected between the erector spinae muscle and the TP of the vertebrae; it is proposed as an alternative to paravertebral block. There is no clear consensus on its mechanism of action, but it is thought to be by diffusion into the paravertebral space. A low incidence of adverse events is reported with this block.

#### Anatomy

The erector spinae (ES) group of muscles are the intermediate layer of the intrinsic muscles of the back originating from the posterior part of the iliac crest and sacrum. They ascend between the spinous process medially and the angle of the rib laterally to insert into the base of the skull, the mastoid process, spinous process of upper thoracic vertebrae, TP of cervical and thoracic vertebrae and ribs.

#### Indications

Thoracic and lumbar ESPB have been used for various surgical procedures, including cardiothoracic, breast, fractured ribs, spinal, abdominal, gynaecological and hip surgery.

#### Technique

Similar to the paravertebral block, the transducer probe is placed in either transverse or paramedian position lateral to the relevant spinous process. Once placed, the anatomy is similar to the paravertebral block, with the focus on the TP laterally and the erector spinae muscle superficial to it. A needle is inserted IP aimed at the superficial surface of the TP (see Figure 15.8) and the position confirmed by visualising the hydrodissection of the ES muscle from the TP by the LA.

### Serratus Anterior Plane Block (SAPB)

This blocks the lateral cutaneous branches of the intercostal nerves which pass through the serratus anterior muscle (SAM) to reach the subcutaneous area, in addition to the thoracodorsal and long thoracic nerves.

#### Indications

It is an alternative to epidural and paravertebral blocks for breast surgery, thoracotomy and thoracoscopic procedures.

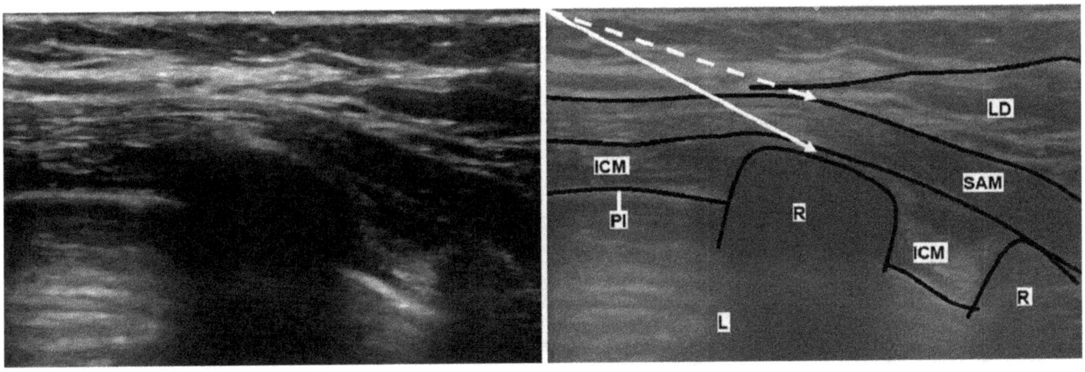


**Figure 15.9** Ultrasound appearance of the serratus anterior plane block, showing serratus anterior muscle (SAM), latissimus dorsi (LD), intercostal muscle (ICM), rib (R), pleura (Pl) and lung (L).

#### Technique

The patient is positioned supine with the ipsilateral arm abducted. A linear transducer probe is placed in a transverse plane at the fifth intercostal space in the mid-axillary line. The SAM is identified above the rib shadows. Deep to the SAM, the intercostal muscles and pleura can be identified. Superficial to the SAM, the lateral part of the latissimus dorsi muscle should be seen, confirming correct probe position. The needle is placed IP directed to the plane between the SAM and the surface of the rib (Figure 15.9) and the position confirmed with separation of the SAM from the rib. An injection superficial to the SAM can be performed, but a deep injection avoids blocking the long thoracic nerve and hence winging of the scapula.

## Abdominal Blocks

#### Anatomy

The ventral rami of the lower thoracic nerves (T7–12) and first lumbar nerve provide segmental innervation to the skin and muscle of the anterior and lateral abdomen. The intercostal nerves pass between the digitations of the diaphragm and the transverse abdominis muscles (TAM) to run anteriorly in the fascial plane between the TAM and internal oblique muscles (IOM). Lateral cutaneous branches arise at the mid-axillary line to pierce the oblique muscles and divide into anterior and posterior branches to supply the anterolateral (to the margin of the rectus sheath) and posterior (latissimus dorsi region) parts of the abdomen. The nerves terminate as anterior cutaneous branches supplying the anterior abdominal wall from midline to the border of rectus muscle after entering the lateral aspect of the rectus sheath via the posterior laminae of the internal oblique muscle and traversing the rectus muscle. The 12th thoracic nerve (subcostal) gives a branch to the first lumbar nerve forming part of the lumbar plexus. Its lateral branch does not divide into an anterior and posterior branch but, after piercing the oblique muscles, descends over the iliac crest to supply the skin of the anterior part of the gluteal region. The iliohypogastric and ilioinguinal nerves emerge from the lateral border of the psoas muscle and pass anteriorly over the quadratus lumborum (QL) to pierce the TAM at the level of the iliac crest. The iliohypogastric divides into a lateral cutaneous branch, which pierces the IOM and external oblique muscle (EOM) to supply skin over the gluteal region, and an anterior cutaneous branch, which passes between TAM and IOM to then pierce the EOM aponeurosis to supply skin over the hypogastric region. The Ilioinguinal nerve, after passing into the TAP, pierces the IO to supply the skin over the inguinal region, upper and medial thigh and some parts of the genital region. The skin over the back of the abdomen is supplied by the dorsal branches of these nerves.

### Rectus Sheath Block

The rectus sheath is formed from the aponeuroses of the TAM and has an anterior and posterior wall. The sheath encloses the rectus muscle and fuses in the midline to form the linea alba. The rectus muscle is adherent to the anterior sheath at the level of the xiphisternum, the umbilicus and midway between these two points. The anterior cutaneous branches of the lower five thoracic nerves can be blocked.

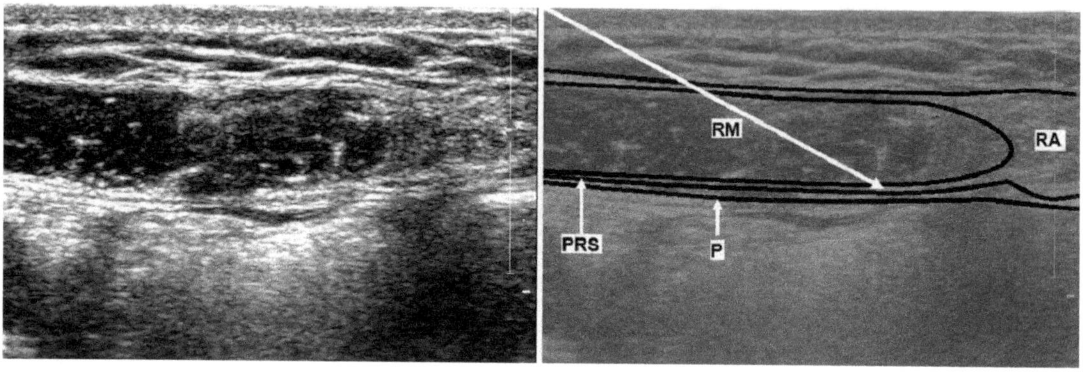


**Figure 15.10** Ultrasound appearance of the rectus muscle (RM), posterior rectus sheath (PRS), peritoneum (P) and linea alba of the rectus abdominis (RA).

#### Indications

Pyloromyotomy, umbilical hernia, epigastric hernia repair, umbilical laparoscopic port site, and midline mini-laparotomy incisions.

#### Technique

A high-frequency linear probe is placed transversely just above the umbilicus. The linea alba is identified and the probe moved laterally to appreciate the rectus muscle enclosed in its sheath, which appears as a hyperechoic line above and below the muscle (Figure 15.10). The peritoneum, with the bowel underneath, can be seen deep to the posterior sheath. The inferior epigastric vessels can be identified with Doppler. As the probe is moved laterally, the lateral abdominal muscles are imaged. A 22 g regional block needle is inserted IP and advanced through the anterior sheath and the rectus muscle to reach the plane between the muscle and posterior sheath. After aspiration, 0.5 ml LA is injected to ensure the muscle splits from the posterior sheath. The rest of the LA is then injected (0.1–0.3 ml $kg^{-1}$ per side). Placing the probe longitudinally allows assessment of spread. The procedure is then repeated on the opposite side.

#### Specific Complications

Peritoneal puncture and organ damage.

### Quadratus Lumborum Block

LA can be injected at either posterior, lateral or anterior injections points underneath the thoracolumbar fascia (TLF) around the quadratus lumborum muscle (QLM) resulting in varying degrees of block in the T5–L4 distribution (consistent block T12–L2 since iliohypogastric, ilioinguinal and subcostal nerves lie on the anterior aspect of QLM within the endothoracic fascia). The TLF is formed by the aponeurosis and fascia enveloping the back muscles and is described as having either two or three layers. It blends with the endothoracic fascia and diaphragm above and with the fascia iliaca below, aiding the spread of LA to lower thoracic and lumbar nerves. Visceral analgesia may result from spread of LA via the splanchnic nerves to the coeliac ganglion and sympathetic nerves, or from blockade of the adrenergic pain and mechanoreceptors present in the TLF.

#### Indication

Described for procedures in the abdomen and pelvis, as well as for hip and femur surgery. Paediatric trials demonstrate non-inferiority compared with caudal analgesia.

#### Technique

The patient is placed supine with a roll under the hip to elevate it and create a lateral tilt to the torso to aid probe position and needling. The probe is initially placed transversely resting on the iliac crest, and the anterior abdominal muscles (EOM, IOM, TAM) are visualised. The probe is then slid posteriorly to see the tapered end of the TAM, with the QLM seen in a deeper and lower position. The probe is adjusted to better visualise QLM, including its anterior borders, keeping the tapered end of the TAM in view (Figure 15.11). A needle is then inserted IP in an anteroposterior direction to inject LA and visualise hydrodissection, in one of the following locations.

- Lateral – the needle is positioned immediately underneath the fascia covering the lateral border of QL close to the tapered end of the

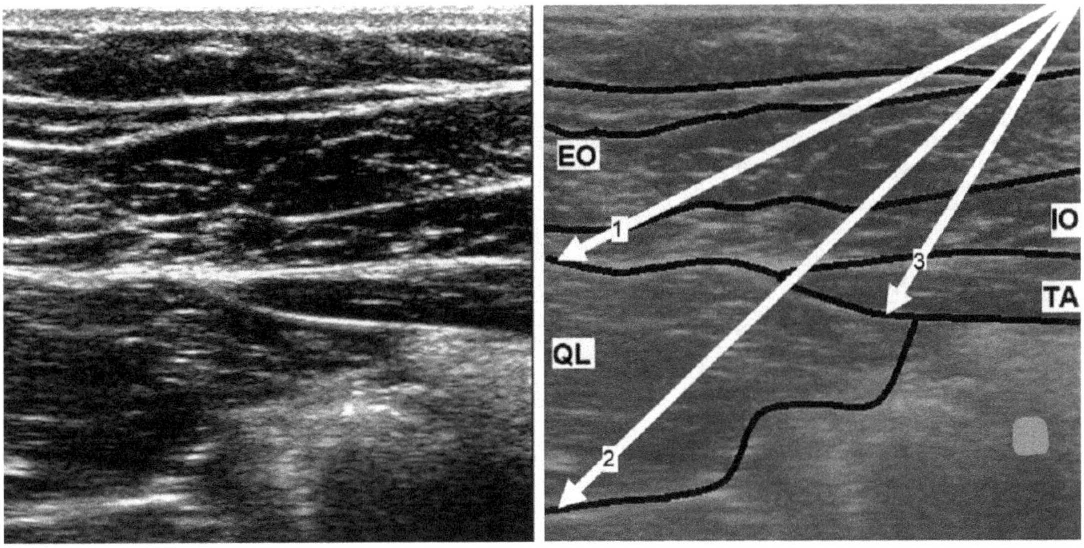


**Figure 15.11** Ultrasound appearance of the quadratus lumborum (QL), external oblique (EO), internal oblique (IO) and transversus abdominis (TA).

TAM to allow spread along the TAM plane and subcutaneous area.

- Posterior – the needle is directed more posteriorly, towards the erector spinatus muscle, to a position between the TLF and posterior border of QL muscle to allow spread along the TLF midtransverse area.
- Anterior – the needle is passed through the QL muscle to reach anteriorly between the anterior border of QL and anterior TLF or fascia transversalis, close to psoas muscle, to block lumbar nerve roots and branches in addition to a paravertebral spread through the endothoracic fascia.

A lateral position and curvilinear probe may be required when there is an increased depth to access the QLM. A paramedian IP approach in the semi-prone position is also described for this block. Catheters can be placed after hydrodissection.

#### Specific Complications

Lumbar vessels may travel close to or in the QLM, and colour doppler inspection is important before proceeding with the block. Lower extremity weakness has been reported.

### Penile Block

The aim is to block the dorsal nerves of the penis, which are branches of the pudendal nerve (S2–4) in the subpubic space.

This block is primarily used for circumcisions, although it may be used for distal hypospadias repair after discussion with the surgeon. It is useful when a caudal block is contraindicated. It requires injection into the subpubic space; this space is divided into left and right by the suspensory ligament. It is within this space that the dorsal penile nerves pass. It should be remembered that the vessels travel in the midline, and midline injection should be avoided. The penis is gently pulled caudally so that the skin is taut; the short-bevelled needle is then carefully placed under the skin in the midline aiming for the inferior aspect of the pubic symphysis. Once through the skin the needle is redirected deeper to the pubis, from the perpendicular so that it points laterally (10°) and slightly cephalad; it is then advanced until a 'pop' is felt as it passes through the Scarpa's fascia. The depth of the fascia is independent of age and weight (generally 8–30 mm). After aspiration, 1 ml + 0.1 ml $kg^{-1}$ of LA is injected (preferably the highest concentration available); the process is then repeated for the contralateral side. Following this, a hypodermic needle is inserted subcutaneously into the ventral aspect of the base of the penis, and LA is injected whilst withdrawing the needle to form of a partial ring block bilaterally. *Vasoconstrictors should not be used.*

A US technique has been described, which is generally easier in older children. A linear transducer is placed transversely at the base of the penis (apply gentle traction). The midline dorsal vein with the dorsal arteries on either side above deep Buck's fascia over the corpus callosum is identified. The needle is inserted from either side of the probe using an IP technique and directed towards the dorsal artery, and LA is then injected just lateral to these arteries.

## Lower Limb Blocks

The nerve supply to the lower limb is derived from the lumbosacral plexus.

### Lateral Femoral Cutaneous Nerve

This is a purely sensory nerve arising from the dorsal divisions of L2 and L3. The nerve emerges from the lateral border of the psoas muscle and then runs down and lateral across the iliac fossa before passing beneath the inguinal ligament just medial to the anterior superior iliac spine (ASIS). It divides into an anterior branch supplying the anterolateral thigh and a posterior branch supplying the lateral area from the greater trochanter to the mid-thigh region.

#### Indications

Slipped upper femoral epiphysis (used in conjunction with a femoral block).

#### Technique

A linear probe is placed just inferior to the ASIS in a transverse plane. The space between sartorius and tensor fascia lata is identified; within this fascial plane, a small elliptical nerve may be identified (Figure 15.12). An IP needling technique is used to deliver 0.1–0.3 ml $kg^{-1}$ of LA.

### Femoral Nerve Block

The femoral nerve is the largest branch of the lumbar plexus arising from the dorsal divisions of the second to fourth lumbar nerves. It emerges from the lower border of psoas and passes underneath the inguinal ligament into the femoral triangle. At the level of the inguinal ligament, it lies deep to fascia lata and iliaca in a groove between the iliacus and the psoas muscle; it is separated from the femoral vessels, which lie in a separate fascial compartment medial to the nerve. It supplies the anterior compartment of the thigh.

#### Indications

Femoral fracture or osteotomy. Patella reconstruction.

#### Technique

A linear multi-frequency transducer is placed on the inguinal crease. The femoral vein and artery are identified. The nerve is found lateral to the femoral artery in a triangular hyperechoic area (Figure 15.13). The needle is inserted OOP/IP (from lateral to medial). Often more than two 'pops' are felt as the needle pierces the fascias; ensure that the LA is deposited under the fascia iliaca and not in the iliacus muscle deep to the nerve. The increased contrast between the LA and nerve allows the latter to be imaged better. The nerve should be surrounded with LA.

### Adductor Canal Block

The aim of this block is to minimise loss of motor function. As such, the nerves usually involved are the saphenous nerve and the nerve to vastus medialis.

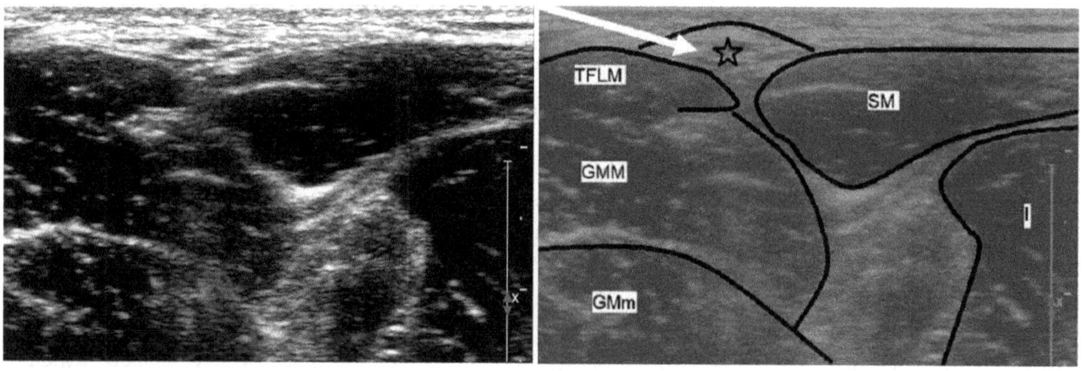


**Figure 15.12** Ultrasound appearance of the lateral cutaneous nerve of the thigh ( ), tensor fascia lata muscle (TFLM), gluteus maximus (GMM), gluteus medius (GMm), sartorius (SM) and iliacus (I).

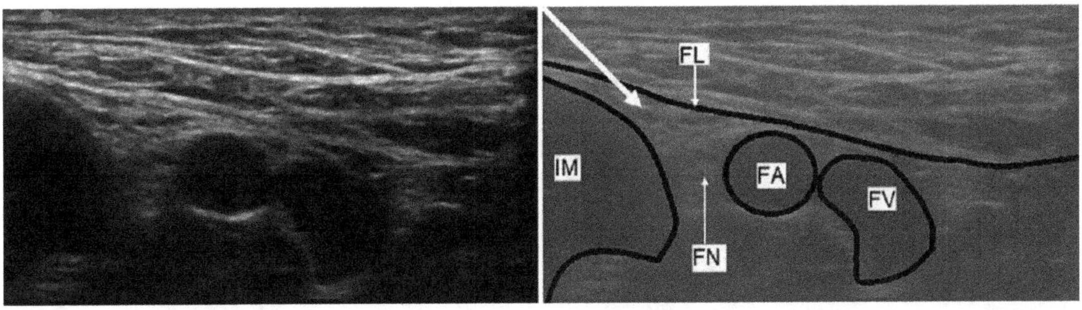


**Figure 15.13** Ultrasound appearance of the femoral canal, showing the fascia lata (FL), iliacus muscle (IM), femoral nerve (FN), femoral artery (FA) and femoral vein (FV).

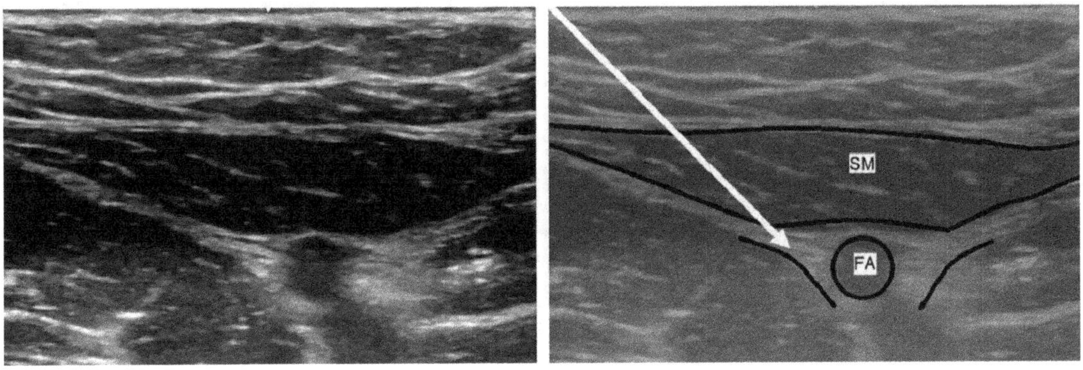


**Figure 15.14** Ultrasound appearance of the adductor canal, showing sartorius muscle (SM) and the femoral artery (FA).

#### Indications

Knee surgery, such as ACL reconstruction.

#### Technique

The leg is positioned slightly externally rotated. A linear transducer is placed transversely over the junction of the middle and distal third of the thigh. The femoral vein and artery are identified lying beneath the sartorius muscle. The nerves are found anterolateral to the femoral artery (Figure 15.14). The needle is inserted IP and LA injected to surround the structures.

### Fascia Iliaca Block

This block is used for above-knee surgery as it blocks the femoral (100%), lateral femoral cutaneous (90%) and obturator (75%) nerves with a single injection. It is more successful than the '3-in-1' block. The nerves lie in a compartment which is bound superficially by the fascia iliaca (investing the iliacus muscle), superiorly by the iliac crest and posteriorly by the psoas muscle.

#### Technique

A linear probe is placed in a longitudinal plane just medial to the ASIS. The iliacus muscle is identified and the probe moved cephalad, following the muscle as it passes over the pelvic brim. The needle is inserted IP from caudad to cephalad so the tip is positioned beneath the fascia iliaca. The LA is injected and the fascia lifted off the muscle; the needle can then be carefully advanced farther and the fascial plane dissected open farther. A large volume of LA (0.5 ml $kg^{-1}$, maximum 20 mls) is needed to get the required spread (Figure 15.15).

### Sciatic Nerve Blocks

The sciatic nerve has tibial and common peroneal components. It enters the gluteal region from the pelvis through the greater sciatic foramen and runs down between the ischial tuberosity and the greater trochanter of the femur. It usually divides at the apex of the popliteal fossa, though this can occur anywhere along the course of the nerve. As it exits the gluteal region, it is usually accompanied by the posterior cutaneous nerve of the thigh on its medial side.

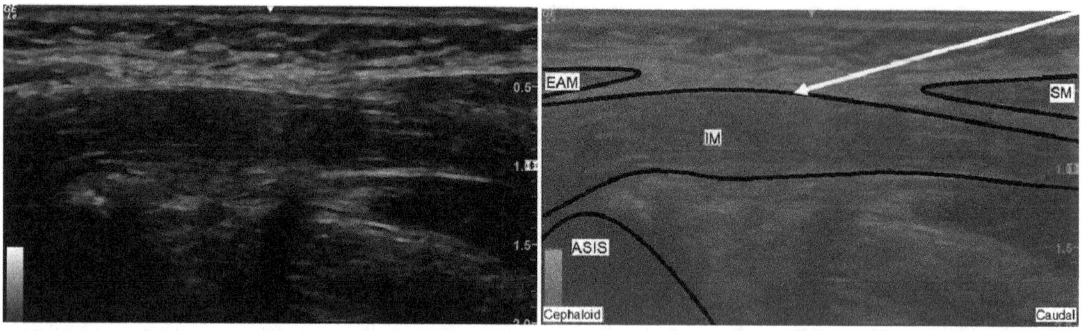


**Figure 15.15** Ultrasound appearance of the fascia iliaca overlying the iliacus muscle (IM), the external abdominal oblique muscle (EAM), sartorius muscle (SM) and the anterior superior iliac spine (ASIS).

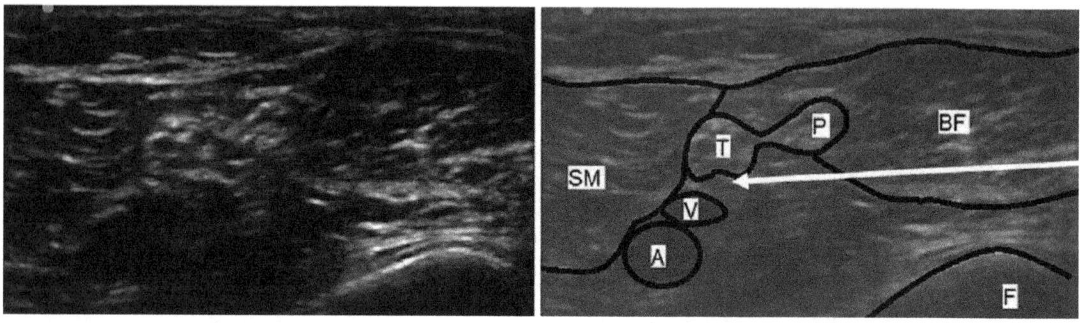


**Figure 15.16** Ultrasound appearance of the popliteal fossa showing semimembranosus muscle (SM), biceps femoris (BF), tibial (T) and popliteal (P) nerves, popliteal artery (A) and vein (V) and the femur (F).

The nerve supplies the skin on the posterior thigh, the hamstrings, the biceps femoris muscles and most of the leg below the knee joint except for the area supplied by the saphenous nerve.

## Popliteal Block

### Indications

When used with a saphenous or femoral nerve block, a popliteal block can be used for any operation below the knee, such as club foot surgery.

### Technique

The child is placed in the lateral position with the leg to be blocked on the top and straight. The linear probe is placed slightly superior on the popliteal crease. The popliteal vessels are identified. The tibial branch of the sciatic nerve is usually found slightly superior and lateral to the popliteal vein. Once identified, continue scanning proximally along the nerve to find the common peroneal nerve, which appears to join the tibial to form the sciatic nerve. Measure the depth to the nerve at this point, as this is probably the best site for injection (Figure 15.16). A 22G regional block needle is inserted in-plane into the lateral side of the thigh at the depth previously measured. The needle is advanced deep to the nerve until a subtle give is felt and half the LA is injected. The injection normally improves visualisation of the nerve. The needle is then withdrawn and directed superficially to the nerve where the rest of the LA is injected.

If it is difficult to identify the nerve above the popliteal crease, tilting the probe caudad or cephalad may help. Also, dorsiflexion and plantar flexion of the foot will produce the 'seesaw sign', where the tibial and peroneal components slide against one another and help with their identification. In cerebral palsy patients, nerve identification may be challenging owing to muscle fibrosis obscuring the nerve. The branching of the sciatic can occur more proximally, so scanning the nerve through its entire course is advised.

## Infragluteal Block

### Indications

Hamstring release.

### Technique

The sciatic nerve is targeted in the groove where it lies between the ischial tuberosity and the greater trochanter of the femur. With the child lying supine, the leg is held straight. In patients under 50 kg, a linear probe will suffice; thereafter, a curvilinear probe may serve better. The probe is placed transversely just below the subgluteal crease; substantial pressure needs to be applied. The main difficulty with this block is the lack of vascular markers to indicate where the nerve may be found. Firstly, identify the femur, then observe the fascial planes as they come together to a point level with the anterior surface of the femur (Figure 15.17). The sciatic nerve is found at this juncture of fascial planes; due to its anisotropy, the probe will need to be angled to improve visualisation. Where the nerve is still not visible, reposition the probe longitudinally and scan from lateral to medial; as the nerve is passed over, a thick hyperechoic band will be seen. Stop at this point and rotate the probe transversely to see the nerve. Note the nerve depth and insert the needle IP from lateral to medial so that it comes in parallel to the probe at the nerve depth. LA (maximum 0.5 mg $kg^{-1}$) must be injected around the nerve.

## Ankle Block

The foot is supplied by the terminal branches of the femoral and sciatic nerves. The tibial branch of the sciatic nerve divides into a posterior tibial and sural nerve in the leg.

The posterior tibial nerve lies on the medial side of the Achilles tendon, posterior to the posterior tibial artery, and supplies the heel, the skin of the sole of the foot and the deep structures of the foot. It is blocked at the level of the medial malleolus. The probe is placed in a transverse plane over the medial aspect of the ankle, just posterior to the malleolus. As it is the only motor nerve to the foot, a nerve stimulator can be used. The nerve is identified deep to the tibial artery and veins. An OOP approach is simplest.

The sural nerve receives a branch from the common peroneal nerve and passes lateral to the Achilles tendon behind the lateral malleolus to supply the lateral border of foot up to the tip of the little toe. Place a linear probe in a transverse plane over this area; the nerve travels with the short saphenous vein in a fascial channel superficially between tendons. An IP or OOP approach is used.

The deep peroneal nerve passes beneath the external retinaculum midway between the lateral and medial malleolus to lie lateral to the dorsalis pedis artery. The linear probe is placed over the dorsum of the foot and the dorsalis pedis artery identified; as the probe is moved proximally over the talus, the artery comes into contact with the bone. It is at this point the nerve can be seen to travel from lateral to medial over the artery. The deep peroneal nerve is blocked at mid-foot immediately lateral to the dorsalis pedis artery. The saphenous nerve, which is the terminal branch of the femoral nerve, runs downwards in front of the saphenous vein anterior to the medial malleolus and supplies the medial border up to the base of the great toe. The ultrasound probe is placed transversely over the vein and LA injected around the vein using an IP approach.

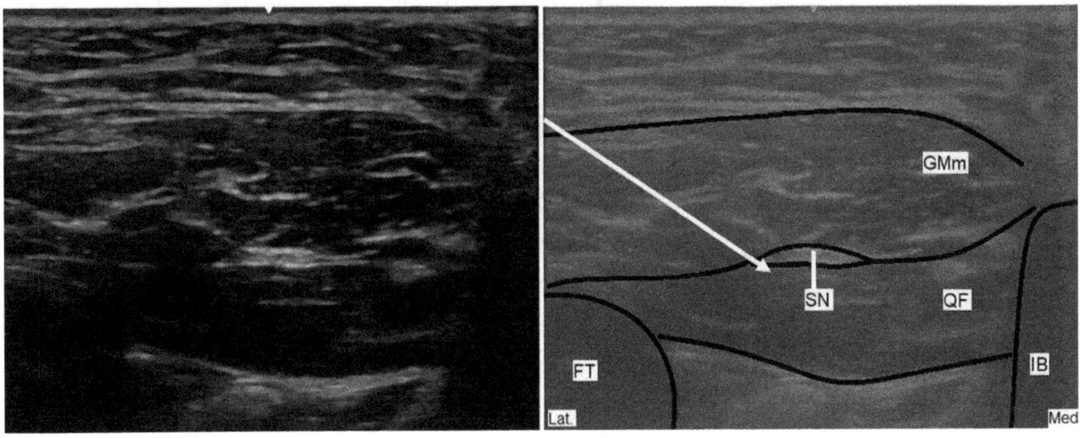


**Figure 15.17** Ultrasound appearance of the sciatic nerve (SN) as it passes between the gluteus maximus muscle (GMm) and quadratus femoris (QF); the ischium bone (IB) and greater trochanter of the femur (FT) lie medially and laterally respectively.

The superficial peroneal nerve pierces the deep fascia in the lower part of the leg and runs in the superficial fascia over the dorsum of the foot. It supplies skin over most of the dorsum of the foot, except the cleft between the first and second toes, which is supplied by the deep peroneal nerve, and the medial and lateral borders of the foot. The US probe is placed over the lateral aspect of the lower leg in a transverse plane. Identify the anterior corner of the fibula and the fascial plane between the anterior and lateral peroneal compartments. As the probe is moved distally, the nerve can be seen to travel superficially to lie just beneath the skin.

## Caudal Block

The sacrum is made up of five cartilaginous vertebrae that eventually ossify and fuse in adulthood. The posterior arch of the fifth and occasionally the fourth vertebra fails to fuse: this is the sacral hiatus. This area is covered by the sacrococcygeal membrane. At birth, the dural sac is low, at the S3/S4 vertebral level; by three years of age, it has ascended to the S2 vertebral level.

### Indication

For surgery on the lower abdomen, pelvis and lower limbs.

Contraindications are as for any central block. Specific contraindications are the presence of cutaneous stigmata of spinal dysraphism, such as sacral pit and anorectal malformations. In these circumstances, the spine should be cleared by US and/or MRI prior to caudal.

### Technique

The child is positioned in the lateral position with the knees drawn up towards the chest. The sacral hiatus is palpated in the midline; it forms the apex of a triangle formed by it and the two posterior superior iliac crests. For neonates, a 24G cannula is used, 22G thereafter. For the occasional older child where a caudal is appropriate, a 20G cannula is used. The US probe is placed in a transverse position at the bottom of the sacrum to identify the two hyperechoic sacral cornua (the 'frog eye' sign) with two transverse hyperechoic bands in between: the superficial sacrococcygeal membrane and the deeper (brighter) dorsal surface of the sacrum (Figure 15.18). The probe is then turned 90° to a longitudinal midline view of the sacral hiatus, the coccyx and the sacrococcygeal membrane. Scanning cephalad will allow the level of the dural sac to be identified. The cauda equina and the filum terminale can be appreciated in children under two years of age. A tethered cord is suspected where there is:

- An absence of cord pulsatility
- An excessively anterior placement of the cord within the vertebral column
- An abnormally low level of dural sac termination, or
- A thickened filum terminale

In these circumstances, the risks and benefits should be carefully considered before proceeding. The cannula is inserted IP from the coccygeal edge of the probe to pierce the sacrococcygeal ligament; it is

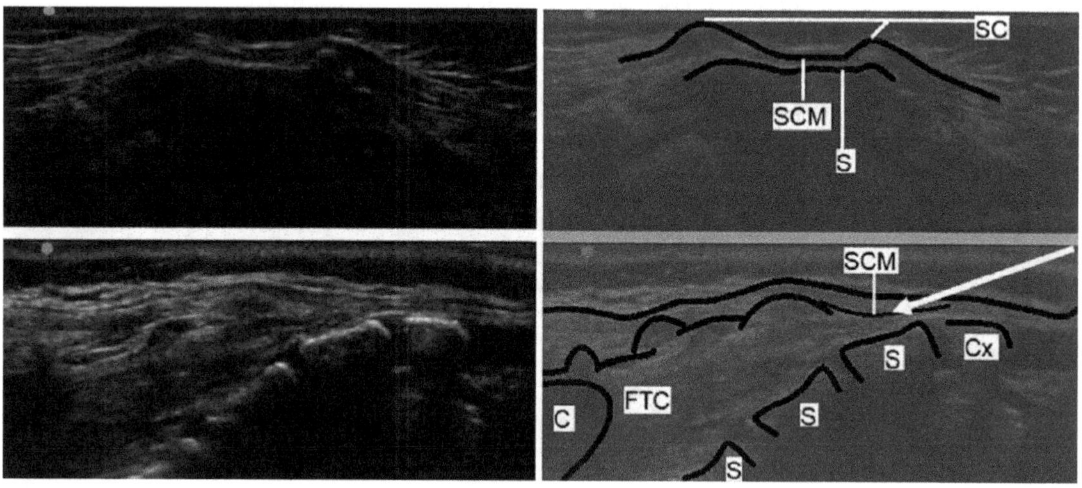


**Figure 15.18** Ultrasound appearance of the caudal space, showing the sacral cornua (SC), sacrococcygeal membrane (SCM), sacrum (S), conus medullaris (C), filum terminale (FTC) and coccyx (Cx).

advanced a short distance with care not to puncture the dural sac. Needle position is confirmed initially with a 0.2 ml bolus of saline; correct placement is indicated by the anterior displacement of the posterior dura. LA can then be injected and its spread monitored by sliding the probe cephalad (this often requires a paravertebral probe angulation). Generally, 0.5 ml $kg^{-1}$ is used to cover the sacral roots, and 1 ml $kg^{-1}$ for high lumbar roots. Consider adding clonidine 1–2 mcg $kg^{-1}$ to the LA.

#### Specific Complications

Dural tap, total spinal blockade, intravascular/intraosseous injection and perforation of the rectum.

**Key Points**

- Regional anaesthesia is an important component of paediatric anaesthesia and should be considered for all suitable cases.
- Neonates and infants are at greater risk of LA toxicity, owing to their lower protein binding and the immature blood–brain barrier.
- Cardiac arrhythmias and circulatory collapse may be refractory to treatment, and resuscitation should be prolonged.

## Further Reading


Brown DL. *Atlas of Regional Anesthesia*, 2nd ed. Saunders. 1999. Available at: www.nysora.com/ regional_anesthesia/sub-specialties/pediatric_anesthesia/index.1.html.

Hadzic A. *Textbook of Regional Anesthesia and Acute Pain Management*. McGraw-Hill Professional. 2006.

Harmon D, Frizelle H, Sandhu N, Colreavy F, Griffin M. *Peri-operative Diagnostic and Interventional Ultrasound*. Elsevier. 2007.

Jones, MR, Novitch, MB, Sen, S. et al. Upper extremity regional anesthesia techniques: a comprehensive review for clinical anesthesiologists. *Best Practices & Research Clinical Anaesthesiology* 2020 March; 34 (1):e13–e29.

Kamarkar, MK. Ultrasound guided Paravertebral block. *Techniques in Regional Anesthesia and Pain Management* 2009; 13:142–9.

Mian A, Chaudhry I, Huang R, Rizk E, Tubbs S, Loukas M. Brachial plexus anesthesia: a review of the relevant anatomy, complications, and anatomical variations. *Clinical Anatomy* 2014 March; 27 (2):210–21.

Saadawi M, Layera S, Aliste J, Bravo D, Leurcharusmee P, Tran DQ. Erector spinae plane block: a narrative review with systematic analysis of the evidence pertaining to clinical indications and alternative truncal blocks. *Journal of Clinical Anesthesia* 2021 February; 68:110063.

Tran DQ, Bravo D, Leurcharusmee P, Neal JM. Transversus abdominis plane block: a narrative review. *Anesthesiology* 2019 November; 131(5): 1166–90.

Urits I, Ostling PS, Novitch MB et al. Truncal regional nerve blocks in clinical anesthesia practice. *Best Practices & Research Clinical Anaesthesiology* 2019 December; 33(4):559–71.

Wiegele M, Marhofer P, Lönnqvist P-A. Caudal epidural blocks in paediatric patients: a review and practical considerations. *British Journal of Anaesthesia* 2019 April; 122(4): 509–17.

Woodworth GE, Ivie RMJ, Nelson SM, Walker CM, Maniker RB. Perioperative breast analgesia: a qualitative review of anatomy and regional techniques. *Regional Anesthesia & Pain Medicine* 2017 September/ October; 42(5):609–31.

Xie C, Ran G, Chen D, Lu Y. A narrative review of ultrasound-guided serratus anterior plane block. *Annals of Palliative Medicine* 2021 January; 10(1):700–6.

Chapter 16

# Sedation for Procedures in Children*

Grant Stuart

## Introduction

Children often need support to cooperate with medical professionals for clinical procedures. This may be due to their age, developmental immaturity, illnesses or anxiety. In most circumstances, it is not acceptable to forcibly restrain a child. Clinicians have therefore developed a variety of non-pharmacological and pharmacological techniques (including sedation and general anaesthesia) to help facilitate procedural comfort for children (Table 16.1).

Recent years have seen an increase in the demand for paediatric sedation, particularly for painless imaging procedures such as MRI, which has become the standard of care for investigation, diagnosis, staging, surgical planning and post-operative monitoring or surveillance of many medical conditions. Sedation can also be a useful tool in clinical situations when general anaesthesia is a high-risk option. This increasing demand, the availability of newer drugs and sedation techniques and the reality that sedation is being practised by an array of health care professionals (anaesthetists, intensivists, nurse specialists, dentists, emergency physicians, gastroenterologists) for increasingly complex patients in varied locations have necessitated recent international guideline changes and consensus statements on this topic. It is vital for paediatric anaesthetists to have a comprehensive understanding of sedation techniques and to take the lead in maintaining and advancing the standards of safety and education of health care teams providing sedation for children.

* Many thanks to Dr Mike R. J. Sury, who wrote the first edition of this book chapter, much of the content of which has been used in this version.

## Background Knowledge

### Definitions

Sedation is a spectrum between being fully awake and cooperative and being fully anaesthetised. Current definitions of the depth of sedation (Table 16.2) attempt to identify where on this spectrum a patient's level of sedation might fall. Identifying the depth of sedation based on these definitions is not always easy, as stimulating a child undergoing procedural sedation might be counterintuitive. Ideally a minimal sedation drug technique should have a margin of safety wide enough to make loss of consciousness unlikely. It remains possible, though, for a patient's depth of sedation to vary between moderate and deep during a sedation episode depending on factors, including patient comorbidities, the drugs and doses given, and the presence of stimuli around them.

### Special Considerations for Moderate Sedation

In moderate sedation, the child should be easily rousable and be able to show some degree of cooperation. Failure can be common. Moderate sedation requires patience and skill, and the time invested is worthwhile when the failure rate is low. If a child will not cooperate, the dose of sedative can be increased or an additional sedative administered, but this risks deep sedation. In general, it is not possible to be certain what dose of sedation can cause deep sedation. Nitrous oxide alone is the exception – 50% nitrous oxide does not cause an unrousable state in otherwise normal children. Sedation may therefore be unpredictable, varying between conscious and deep depending on the sedative dose administered, drug combinations used and degree of stimulation. Techniques combining an opioid

**Table 16.1** Management options for procedural anxiety in children

| Non-pharmacological techniques | Pharmacological options for sedation |
|---|---|
| Prehospital information and preparation<br>• Child friendly information leaflets, books or videos<br>• Hospital tours (e.g. MRI suite)<br>• Engagement with clinical psychologists<br>• Cognitive behavioral therapy | Simple oral sedatives<br>• Chloral hydrate<br>• Melatonin<br>• Trimeprazine, chlorphenamine and other sedating antihistamines |
| Communication aids<br>• Information about child's needs, routines and communication strategies<br>• Makaton and symbol charts | Nitrous oxide (in oxygen) |
| Play therapy and preparation<br>• Interaction with child life specialists<br>• 'Medical games' that mimic the procedure<br>• Immersive reality play (MRI machine becomes the child's rocket ship) | Benzodiazepines<br>• Midazolam<br>• Diazepam<br>• Temazepam |
| Involvement of parents/carers<br>• Parental presence and role for sedation period | Ketamine |
| Distraction techniques<br>• Toys, videos, video games, phones/tablets, virtual reality<br>• Immersive games<br>• Blowing bubbles<br>• Clowns and magic | Alpha 2 adrenergic agonists<br>• Clonidine<br>• Dexmedetomidine |
| Environmental adjustment<br>• Sleep promoting behaviors<br>• Adopt the child's normal nighttime routine (toys/stories)<br>• Reduce sensory input<br>• Soft lighting<br>• Minimise ambient noise and avoid unnecessary staff<br>• Soft music therapy<br>• Hypnosis | Opioids<br>• Morphine<br>• Fentanyl<br>• Sufentanil |
| Relaxation techniques<br>• Breathing and relaxation exercises<br>• Hypnosis<br>• Acupuncture | Barbiturates<br>• Pentobarbitol |
| Engagement with sedation technique<br>• Allow child to engage with or help with aspects of the procedure | Anaesthetic agents<br>• Sevoflurane<br>• Propofol |

and benzodiazepine are notorious for causing delayed respiratory depression after the pain of a procedure has subsided.

## Special Considerations for Deep Sedation

Potent drugs, such as propofol and sevoflurane, can be used to achieve moderate to deep sedation, and these advanced techniques can be used by anaesthetists in hospital practice. For anaesthetists, the boundary between sedation and anaesthesia need not be clear. If the facilities and personnel can deliver anaesthesia, the sedation level achieved is not important provided the child is safe, comfortable and recovers quickly. This can be achieved using short-acting potent drugs. These specialist

**Table 16.2** The American Society of Anesthesiologists (ASA) levels of sedation and some historical terms

| | Conscious state | Respiratory depression |
|---|---|---|
| Minimal sedation | • Remains awake, calmed by sedative<br>• Normal response to verbal commands<br>• Cognitive function and coordination may be impaired | • None |
| Moderate sedation | • Sleepy<br>• Responds purposefully to verbal commands or light tactile stimulation<br>• Reflex withdrawal from a painful stimulus is not a purposeful response | • Detected<br>• Intervention rarely necessary |
| Deep sedation | • Asleep<br>• Cannot be easily roused<br>• Responds purposefully to repeated or painful stimulation | • Common<br>• Intervention often necessary<br>• Cardiovascular function is usually maintained |
| Anaesthesia | • Asleep<br>• Unrousable | • Usual<br>• Routine airway intervention<br>• Cardiovascular depression common |

Some alternative and outdated terms to describe sedation

| | Conscious state | Respiratory and circulatory intervention |
|---|---|---|
| Conscious sedation | • Sleepy<br>• Opens mouth to verbal commands (see 'Dental Procedures') | • Rarely necessary with basic techniques<br>• To be expected with advanced techniques |
| Safe sleep | • Asleep<br>• Rousability not tested | • Rarely necessary |
| Ketamine sedation | • Eyes open<br>• Unresponsive<br>• Immobile | • 1% brief apnoea and/or laryngospasm |
| Minimal anaesthesia | • Asleep with short-acting drug/s<br>• Not easily roused or briefly unrousable<br>• Rapid recovery when drug delivery stops | • Routine airway intervention<br>• Cardiovascular depression common but intervention unnecessary |

techniques which cause a state that fluctuates between sedation and anaesthesia are valuable and are described in this chapter. They have been called minimal anaesthesia, and this may be a more appropriate term depending upon the circumstances.

# Patient Preparation

## Assessment

All children must have a full medical assessment and focused examination prior to sedation. Some medical conditions require caution and specialist advice should be sought before proceeding; these are described in Table 16.3.

It is important to evaluate a child's ability to cooperate. This may be influenced by age, anxiety, behavioural disorders or learning difficulties. It is also important to consider the nature of the procedure, how long it will take, how immobile they need to be, any pain or noise involved, the need for intravenous access and the need for airway protection.

Part of an assessment should consider if the child would benefit from psychological preparation. Do they know what to expect or what they will experience? What should they do during the procedure? How will they cope? Can their parents be around to provide reassurance and help during the procedure? The time invested in gaining a child's trust and cooperation is invaluable. The

**Table 16.3** Conditions requiring caution and specialist advice prior to sedation

| System | Details |
|---|---|
| General factors | • ASA III or greater<br>• Neonates and Infants less than 1 year old<br>• Severe anxiety<br>• Autistic spectrum disorder<br>• Developmental delay |
| Difficult airway or risk of airway obstruction | • Snoring or stridor<br>• Blocked nose<br>• Obstructive sleep apnoeas<br>• Small mandible<br>• Large tongue |
| Respiratory compromise | • $SpO_2$ less than 94% in air<br>• High respiratory rate<br>• Oxygen treatment<br>• Unable to cough or cry<br>• Apnoeic spells<br>• Recent respiratory tract infection (within 2 weeks) |
| High intracranial pressure | • Drowsiness<br>• Headache<br>• Vomiting |
| Epilepsy | • Major neurological or neuromuscular disease<br>• Previous adverse reaction to sedation<br>• Requiring resuscitation within the past month<br>• Cyanosis more frequent than once per day<br>• Convulsion less than 4 hours before sedation<br>• Failure to regain full consciousness and mobility after a recent convulsion |
| Risk of pulmonary aspiration of gastric contents | • Abdominal distension<br>• Appreciable volumes draining from nasogastric (NG) tube<br>• Vomiting<br>• Oesophageal disease<br>• Polyhandicap<br>• Unfasted |
| Severe metabolic, liver or renal disease | • Requiring IV fluids or dextrose<br>• Jaundice or abdominal distension<br>• Requiring peritoneal or haemodialysis |

assistance of child life specialists and play preparation are useful tools at this stage.

## Fasting

Fasting is rarely required for minimal sedation, nitrous oxide or moderate sedation techniques, and hungry and thirsty children are less likely to be cooperative. Nil by mouth status has not been shown to be a predictor of aspiration or major adverse events for paediatric sedation, and children having procedural sedation are often unintentionally fasted for longer than instructed.

A recent international multidisciplinary consensus statement on fasting before procedural sedation in adults and children has provided evidence-based guidelines. The patient's fasting recommendations are based on and stratified according to their individual risk factors and those of the proposed procedure and sedation technique (Figure 16.1).

## Consent

Parents, and if appropriate the child, should understand what the procedure involves, the

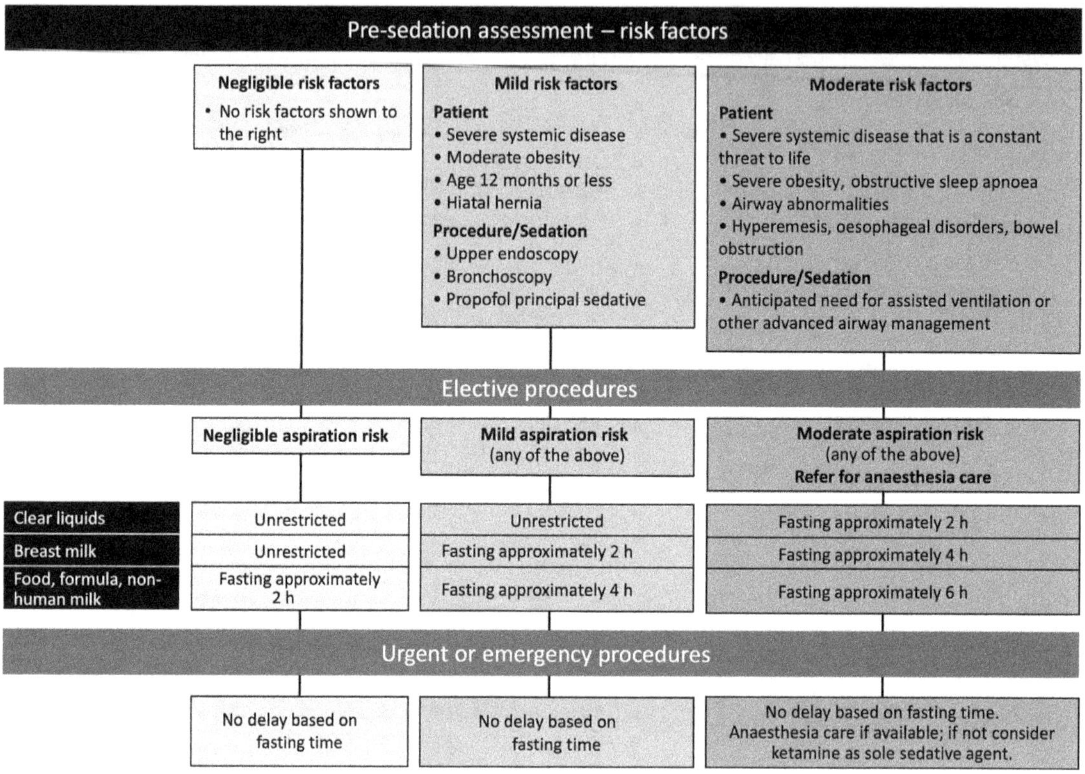


**Figure 16.1** Fasting for procedural sedation risk stratification algorithm.
*Source:* Used with permission from John Wiley & Sons Ltd from *Anaesthesia* 2020; 75:376.

proposed sedation technique, the risks and benefits involved and alternatives to sedation. Informed consent should be documented in writing.

## Safety in Sedation

It is essential that practitioners of sedation have a comprehensive knowledge of the pharmacology of the drugs that they use. They must understand and have practical experience of the medical assessment, monitoring, recovery care and complications of sedation and their immediate management. They must have life support skills training and be able to manage an airway. Where agents such as sevoflurane and propofol are used as sedatives, these clinicians must be appropriately trained to deliver anaesthetic agents.

Children must be monitored whilst undergoing sedation. For moderate sedation, monitoring should include a regular assessment of:

- Depth of sedation, pain, coping and distress
- Respiration
- Pulse oximetry
- Heart rate

For patients having deep sedation, high-risk patients (ASA III–IV), or when using drugs that have a narrow margin of safety, additional monitoring should include:

- Electrocardiogram (ECG)
- Capnography
- Blood pressure

Resuscitation equipment should be available including oxygen supply and delivery equipment, oro-/nasopharyngeal airways, face masks, supraglottic airway devices, self-inflating bags, tracheal tubes, laryngoscopes, suction apparatus, intravenous access equipment, blood gas analysis, emergency drugs and defibrillators.

Most complications related to sedation can be managed simply by opening the airway, giving supplemental oxygen and occasionally supporting breathing.

## Common Scenarios in Paediatric Sedation

Sedation should meet the needs of the procedure. Some require immobility, others require analgesia. Any chosen technique will also vary depending on the patient's requirements and the sedationist and their hospital's experience and preferences; individual case-by-case judgement is always required. Examples of sedation techniques for four common procedural scenarios are described in the following subsections. The procedures are:

- Painless imaging (e.g. magnetic resonance imaging [MRI])
- Painful procedures (e.g. suture of laceration, manipulation of a fracture)
- Gastrointestinal endoscopy (e.g. gastroscopy and colonoscopy)
- Dental procedures

## Painless Imaging

MRI and similar imaging techniques need the child to keep sufficiently still in a confined noisy space. There are four methods to achieve this:

- The 'feed and wrap' technique. Infants less than three months old may naturally sleep deeply after a feed, and this technique can be attempted if the scan is not urgent. Feed the infant 30 minutes before the scan and wrap them up warmly. If this fails, sedation or anaesthesia must be delayed for at least six hours (four hours after breast milk).
- Awake imaging. Some younger children and most older children will lie still without the need for sedation or anaesthesia. It is possible to select children who can be calmed by behavioral techniques, and play specialists are remarkably successful. If the scan is not urgent, this allows time for the child to get used to what is expected of them. It may take several sessions, and the principle of encouragement and reward helps. If this is not possible or practical, the child will require pharmacological interventions.
- Procedural sedation.
- General anaesthesia.

Within a busy radiology department, there will need to be an efficient selection process to identify the best strategy. Remember that intravenous contrast agents may be necessary, and so it is important to establish the need for intravenous access and how best to site it in advance.

## Moderate Sedation versus Deep Sedation (Minimal Anaesthesia)

If an anaesthesia service is available, the depth of sedation is not important, as deeper sedation can be safely delivered, and it is rather the success and complication rates that dictate the technique. Potent short-acting drugs such as propofol or sevoflurane are familiar to anaesthetists, and, unless contraindicated, there is no need to use low doses of either to sedate the child. In most cases, anaesthetic doses are recommended to achieve sleep and immobility. Where these doses are not advisable, then sedation doses could be considered. An example might be in a child with cardiomyopathy (low-dose propofol is useful) or an infant with poor venous access (sevoflurane delivered by nasal cannulae could be considered) – but these situations are rare.

## Deep Sedation (Minimal Anaesthesia) Techniques

Propofol infusion (bolus dose 2–3 mg $kg^{-1}$ followed by 10 mg $kg^{-1}$ $h^{-1}$ IV) has the advantage of a high success rate and rapid pleasant recovery; the disadvantage is the need for IV access. An artificial airway is unnecessary for the majority of children who have normal airway anatomy. If an airway device is used, the dose of propofol may need to be higher in order to tolerate it. Remote monitoring of breathing using capnography is essential (use nasal speculae).

Occasionally propofol does not immobilise the child, and the addition of ketamine, an opioid or midazolam, is necessary; use low doses to maintain spontaneous breathing.

Sevoflurane inhalational anaesthesia has obvious advantages in those with needle phobia or difficult venous access. Once anaesthesia is induced, it can be converted to a propofol technique if necessary. Propofol has the advantage over sevoflurane of being associated with less post-procedural emergence delirium.

## Moderate Sedation Techniques

If non-anaesthetists provide a service, the depth of sedation is important, and the technique should ideally be limited to moderate sedation. Frequently testing the level of sedation with stimulation is counterproductive when scanning though.

Vigilance is therefore always required, as the true level of sedation might be unclear.

The following sedation methods can be considered:

- Chloral hydrate. Use 100 mg kg$^{-1}$ PO (maximum dose 1 g). Limited to children less than 15 kg. Sleep begins within 10 minutes in most cases and lasts for up to 60 minutes. Vomiting is common. Intravenous cannulation and top-up with midazolam is necessary in 5–10% of children. Expect a failure rate of 5%.
- Midazolam. Intravenous doses should be titrated to effect. Start with 25–50 mcg kg$^{-1}$ and increase in small steps (maximum of 6 mg, 7.5 mg and 10 mg for children aged <6 years, 6–12 years and 12–18 years respectively).

## Dexmedetomidine Sedation Techniques

The use and popularity of this highly specific alpha-2 adrenergic agonist for sedation has grown in the past decade, although it is not yet incorporated into national guidance in the United Kingdom and its use for paediatric sedation remains off-label. Dexmedetomidine's sedative action simulates natural non-rapid eye movement sleep whilst maintaining respiratory function, making it a very safe and desirable drug for procedural sedation, especially for painless imaging. The effects of dexmedetomidine include haemodynamic changes. There is a biphasic blood pressure response (initial increase in blood pressure, followed by a decrease from baseline) and reduction of heart rate or bradycardia. These cardiovascular effects are rarely clinically significant and if associated with other concerning changes in vital signs can be attenuated by stopping the drug and administering 10 ml kg$^{-1}$ of a balanced salt solution. Bradycardias are rarely associated with a reduction in blood pressure; anticholinergic treatment is not recommended and is associated with a significant hypertensive response.

It is particularly important when using dexmedetomidine that attention is taken to provide a 'sleep-promoting' environment, including soft lighting, minimising ambient noises and reducing stimulation of the patient; treat these children as you would a normal sleeping child, as they are very rousable. If roused, the child should settle down with calm reassurance, although additional boluses are sometimes needed. Suggested sedation strategies with dexmedetomidine include:

- Undiluted atomised intranasal dexmedetomidine 4 mcg kg$^{-1}$ to a maximum of 200 mcg. The dose may need to be limited by what is a reasonable volume to give via the intranasal route. This technique is useful for children having short scans who do not require intravenous access. A dose of 0.2 mcg kg$^{-1}$ of buccal midazolam may be needed if the dexmedetomidine alone fails to achieve the desired level of sedation. This combination has been found to be reliable and safe.
- For longer scans and when intravenous access is required for contrast agents, an intravenous loading dose of 3 mcg kg$^{-1}$ dexmedetomidine over 10 minutes followed by a 2mcg kg$^{-1}$ hr$^{-1}$ maintenance infusion can be given. These children usually fall asleep around five minutes into the loading dose and can be taken into the scanner after the loading dose has been completed. Occasionally a second loading dose is necessary if the desired level of sedation is not achieved. The recovery period for dexmedetomidine can vary between one and two hours, as these children remain rousable but very sleepy. Allow an initial 30-minute rest and recovery period following completion of the scan, then encourage active engagement and stimulation of the child, including play, eating and drinking.

## Painful Procedures

Some painful procedures in emergency departments and in hospital wards can be managed using moderate sedation. Manipulation of a fracture and suturing of a wound are common examples. Local anaesthetic should be used whenever possible. In addition, the following may be required:

Minimal sedation is appropriate in cooperative children and can be achieved with:

- Nitrous oxide. In a maximum concentration of 50% in oxygen, it should be 'self-administered' by the patient.
- Oral midazolam (0.5 mg kg$^{-1}$) is an effective anxiolytic, acting within 30 minutes. The buccal route is also useful.

When these are not effective, two techniques can be considered:

- Ketamine causes a unique 'dissociative' sedation. Children are immobile, calm and unreactive to pain, yet their eyes may remain open. Airway and breathing reflexes are usually maintained. Ketamine is not considered to be conscious sedation, yet appreciable airway and respiratory effects are uncommon at recommended doses. It can be administered by the intravenous or intramuscular routes. Expect a low incidence of laryngospasm caused by airway secretions. Recovery is usually within 90 minutes.

  - IV: 2 mg $kg^{-1}$; give additional doses of 1 mg $kg^{-1}$ if necessary.
  - IM: 5–10 mg $kg^{-1}$.

- Intravenous midazolam with or without fentanyl is an effective conscious sedation technique but is less reliable than ketamine, and respiratory interventions are more likely. Titrate both drugs carefully.
  - A starting dose of midazolam is 25–50 mcg $kg^{-1}$.
  - A starting dose of fentanyl is 0.25–0.5 mcg $kg^{-1}$. The effect of fentanyl may outlast the pain of the procedure and may cause respiratory depression once the procedure is over.

When these techniques are unsuitable or ineffective, a specialist technique or anaesthesia should be used. A combination of propofol and an opioid such as fentanyl, alfentanil or remifentanil is effective and suitable for short procedures. Lumbar puncture and bone marrow aspirate procedures, common in oncology departments, can be achieved using short-acting anaesthesia with propofol (2–3 mg $kg^{-1}$) and remifentanil (1 mcg $kg^{-1}$). Apnoea almost always occurs with remifentanil, and a short period of assisted ventilation is necessary. Delivered via indwelling central venous catheters, this technique allows fast recovery, and children can eat and drink shortly afterwards. Postoperative analgesia other than local anaesthesia is not usually necessary.

## Dental Procedures

In the United Kingdom, conscious sedation for dentistry is divided into basic and advanced techniques. Basic conscious sedation requires the cooperation of the child and involves one of two techniques:

- Nitrous oxide is administered via a nasal mask in concentrations up to 70%. Usually only 30% is necessary. Higher concentrations cause dysphoria.
- Midazolam, titrated intravenously, is recommended for anxious adolescent children and young people. A starting dose is 25–50 mcg $kg^{-1}$ IV.

Both techniques are effective and safe. If they are not suitable or sufficient, either an advanced sedation technique or anaesthesia should be considered. The specialist techniques themselves involve the use of combinations of potent drugs, and there may be a risk of unintended deep sedation, depending on the drugs and their doses. Specialist techniques should only be used by specially trained teams and are only safe in fully equipped facilities.

## Endoscopy

Whilst many adults can swallow an endoscope or tolerate the discomfort of colonoscopy without sedation, children almost always require sedation or anaesthesia.

Endoscopy is possible under *moderate sedation* in older children using intravenous midazolam; an opioid is sometimes necessary. Both drugs should be titrated carefully. Two techniques are recommended:

- Upper gastrointestinal endoscopy. Intravenous midazolam, starting dose 25–50 mcg $kg^{-1}$ IV.
- Lower gastrointestinal endoscopy. Intravenous midazolam combined with fentanyl (or equivalent opioid), starting dose of fentanyl 0.25–0.5 mcg $kg^{-1}$ IV.

Propofol sedation or minimal anaesthesia without tracheal intubation is widely used for endoscopy for younger children or where *deeper sedation* is required. Older children can be positioned on their side and monitoring attached prior to drug administration. Nasal speculae are used to deliver oxygen and monitor capnography. Intubation is advised for children less than one year.

For gastroscopy:

- Use propofol to induce sedation/anaesthesia with 1–2 mg $kg^{-1}$ IV, or if using propofol TCI titrate up to effect aiming for a target concentration of 6 mcg.$ml^{-1}$.
- A dose of 0.5 mcg $kg^{-1}$ IV fentanyl is a useful adjunct if the child is breathing well and not having colonic manometry.
- Insert a mouth gag to protect the endoscope.
- The depth of anaesthesia can be tested by inserting a suction catheter into the pharynx.

- Give 1–2 mg $kg^{-1}$ IV increments of propofol or increase TCI concentration if there is too much movement.
- Some gag reflex should be preserved but not enough to make the procedure difficult, and this can be attenuated with a dose of 1 mg $kg^{-1}$ lidocaine IV.
- Insert the gastroscope.
- A soft suction catheter can be used to remove pharyngeal secretions and to help prevent laryngospasm.
- It may be necessary to perform a jaw thrust to maintain the airway.
- Inject further boluses of propofol as required (1 mg $kg^{-1}$ IV). A total dose of 3–4 mg $kg^{-1}$ IV is usually required for a 10-minute procedure.
- Duodenoscopy may cause retching.

Colonoscopy is uncomfortable but not usually painful, except when the colon is stretched, often during biopsy of the terminal ileum. For colonoscopy:

- Maintain anaesthesia with propofol 10 mg $kg^{-1}$ $h^{-1}$ IV infusion, or if using propofol TCI reduce the target concentration to 3 mcg $kg^{-1}$.
- Entering the terminal ileum is usually the most stimulating part of the procedure. Colonic distension is painful, and further boluses or analgesia may be necessary. Opioids affect colonic motility and should be avoided for colonic manometry.
- Propofol 8–9 mg $kg^{-1}$ IV is commonly required for colonoscopy of 45 minutes duration.

## Discharge Criteria after Sedation

After sedation, children should be recovered and monitored in a fully equipped recovery area until they have regained control of their airway and breathing reflexes, are haemodynamically stable and are easily roused. Written 'safety netting' advice with contact numbers is useful for families to take home. Before being discharged, children must meet the following criteria:

- Vital signs have returned to normal.
- They are awake or have returned to their baseline level of consciousness and are not at risk of further reduced level of consciousness (the ability to eat, socially interact, ambulate and pass urine are useful signs).
- Any nausea, vomiting, pain or other complications of the sedation or procedure have been adequately managed.

**Key Points**

- Sedation is one of many useful and effective tools to help children cope with medical procedures.
- Fasting protocols should be guided by the depth of sedation required, patient comorbidities and procedural requirements.
- Practitioners should be trained and ready to prevent or manage complications of potent sedative drugs.

## Further Reading


European Society for Paediatric Anaesthesiology. Safe pediatric procedural sedation and analgesia by anesthesiologists for elective procedures: A clinical practice statement from the European Society for Paediatric Anaesthesiology. *Pediatric Anesthesia* 2019; 29:583–90.

Green M, Leroy L, Roback MG et al. An international multidisciplinary consensus statement on fasting before procedural sedation in adults and children. *Anaesthesia* 2020; 75:374–85. Available at: https://associationofanaesthetists-publications.onlinelibrary.wiley.com/doi/epdf/10.1111/anae.14892. Accessed 25 April 2024.

Mahmoud M, Mason KP. Dexmedetomidine: review, update, and future considerations of paediatric perioperative and periprocedural applications and limitations. *British Journal of Anaesthesia* 2015; 171–82.

Mason, KP, Seth, N. Future of paediatric sedation: towards a unified goal of improving practice. *British Journal of Anaesthesia* 2019; 122(5):652–61. Available at: www.bjanaesthesia.org/action/showPdf?pii=S0007-0912%2819%2930066-2. Accessed 25 April 2025.

National Institute for Clinical Excellence (NICE). Sedation for diagnostic and therapeutic procedures in children and young people. 2010, updated February 2019. Available at: www.nice.org.uk/guidance/cg112/. Accessed 14 March 2024.

Chapter 17

# Perioperative Analgesia in Children

Glyn Williams and Helen Laycock

## Introduction

Pain following surgery continues to be a common experience in children, despite advances in acute pain management. The effective and safe management of pain in children of all ages requires significant knowledge of the biopsychosocial experience of pain and strategies available for its management. Numerous factors can influence the success of analgesic treatment:

- Developmental age has a profound effect on both the processing of nociceptive information and the response to analgesia.
- The pharmacology of all drugs is age and size dependent, requiring appropriate dosage adjustments.
- Communication with the very young or those with developmental delay can influence the ability to assess pain and monitor the response to treatment.

## Pain Perception

Nociceptive pathways are present from birth, and even the most premature infant is born with the capacity to detect and respond to painful stimulation. During foetal, neonatal and infant life, the nervous system is continually evolving. This allows structural and functional changes to occur continuously in response to the child's needs as it grows and develops. The pain pathways mirror these changes, with different components developing along differing time frames. The structural components required to perceive pain are present from early fetal life, although pathways involved in modifying pain perception are still developing during infancy. The expression of the many molecules and receptors involved in the pain pathways vary in their number, type and distribution between early life and adulthood. These structural and functional changes will affect both the immediate and short-term responses to pain and analgesic effect in infancy. Conversely, pain or analgesic treatment at this time may also predispose to persistent or long-term changes affecting the function of the somatosensory nervous system in later life.

## Perioperative Pain Management

Perioperative pain management can be considered in three parts: preoperative assessment, intraoperative management and postoperative care. Successful pain management is based on the formulation of a sensible analgesic plan for each individual. It is best to take a practical and pragmatic approach depending on the patient, the type of surgery and the resources available. The primary aims are to:

- Recognise pain in children
- Prevent pain where it is predictable
- Minimise moderate and severe pain safely in all children
- Bring pain rapidly under control
- Continue pain control after discharge from hospital
- Reduce the risk of children developing a persistent pain presentation

The two primary aims of preoperative pain assessment are:

- Planning the analgesic strategy for the child both during and after their procedure
- Identifying children with risk factors for developing increased postoperative pain and/or persistent pain post discharge

Risk factors for poor perioperative pain management in children are not well described; however, evidence suggests these include the presence of preoperative pain and/or analgesic use; previous difficulties with pain control following procedures; psychological risk factors such as pain catastrophising or anxiety (parent and/or child); and surgical factors, including anatomical location, duration, surgical approach and repeated surgery.

Preoperative assessment may also allow exploration of previously used pain management strategies and provide an opportunity to give general pain management education and information on postoperative pain strategies. This may help to alleviate anxiety. Early involvement of the hospital pain team can be useful for both those children with risk factors for challenging perioperative pain management and those at risk of developing chronic postsurgical pain (see the section 'Discharge Care and Chronic Postsurgical Pain').

## Analgesic Plan

An individual analgesic plan should be devised for each patient (Table 17.1). The plan will depend on a number of factors and should be discussed with the patient, parents and staff to confirm acceptability, consider preferences, answer questions and take into account previous experiences. It should allow treatment to be titrated to effect, include provision for the rapid control of breakthrough pain and enable the identification and treatment of side effects. In established paediatric centres with a high level of resources, a dedicated paediatric pain service is the standard of care. Where this is not available, significant improvements in pain management can be made by the establishment of clinical routines and protocols for the treatment and assessment of postoperative pain, alongside a network of interested medical and nursing staff to provide ongoing education.

**Table 17.1** Factors to consider in designing an analgesic plan

| | |
|---|---|
| The pain | Type, severity, location, onset, duration |
| The patient | Age, development, medical history, drug history and ongoing treatment, cognitive ability |
| The setting | Home, hospital, available staff and resources |
| The techniques/ drugs available | Pharmacology, resources, safety, routes of administration |

## Multimodal Pain Management

Pain management involves considering the neurobiology of pain pathways and basic pharmacology to design an approach that targets multiple areas along the pain pathways. Perioperative care needs to appreciate that pain is a biopsychosocial experience that not only involves biological pathways but is influenced by psychological and social factors related to both the child and caregivers. Consequently, a comprehensive pain management strategy needs to appreciate all the facets that make up a child's pain experience and utilise a variety of methods to achieve analgesia.

Although a significant focus should be on providing effective multimodal pharmacological strategies, the integration of other aspects such as rehabilitation, physical therapy and effective psychosocial interventions (including psychological strategies, play and distraction) are key to comprehensive management. The use of valid and appropriate pain assessment tools alongside evaluating the impact of pain on a child's general recovery and function is important to achieving timely hospital discharge, which needs to be accompanied by individualised plans for follow-up.

Multimodal or balanced pharmacological analgesia involves the simultaneous use of a number of analgesic interventions to achieve optimal pain management. Analgesics acting independently and synchronously on pain mechanisms at different points on the pain pathway are likely to be more effective than a single drug. Potentially, this also minimises the doses of drugs used, thereby reducing side effects and possibly accelerating recovery. Multimodal analgesia also allows for the use of non-pharmacological pain control strategies where possible.

Using a multimodal approach, effective pain management is achievable for most cases, and the technique can be adapted for day cases, major cases, the critically ill child or the very young. In current practice, most analgesic techniques in children are based on different combinations of four main classes of analgesics:

- Paracetamol
- Non-steroidal anti-inflammatory drugs (NSAIDs)
- Opioids
- Local anaesthetics

Other analgesic adjuncts can also be considered. Unless there is a contraindication to do so, a local/regional analgesic technique should be used in all cases (see also Chapter 15). For many minor and day-case procedures, this may allow opioids to be omitted, particularly if used in combination with paracetamol and NSAIDs.

## Routes of Administration

Analgesic drugs can be given by a variety of routes, and the choice of route can have a significant impact on the efficacy of pain management. The choice(s) must be acceptable to the patient, parents and staff. Where possible, prescriptions should allow for more than one choice of route.

The routes in common use are:

*Oral:* This is generally the preferred route but is not always achievable in the perioperative period due to the child being 'nil by mouth' for some of this time. Different formulations are available for most analgesics in terms of flavour and liquids or tablets to allow for the varied tastes of children.

*Rectal:* Although a useful and convenient alternative when the oral route is unavailable, rectal absorption of many drugs is slow, erratic and unreliable. Rectal administration can also be unpleasant or unacceptable to some patients, although its use under general anaesthesia is usually more palatable if discussed prior to surgery.

*Intravenous:* This allows for rapid onset and high efficacy and is therefore the preferred route intraoperatively, provided suitable formulations are available. Postoperative use will be dependent on the availability of trained staff, suitable resources and monitoring. Securing intravenous access is easily achieved under general anaesthetic but may prove problematic at other times.

*Subcutaneous:* This allows for continuous and intermittent infusion of low volumes of drugs. Subcutaneous access is easier to establish compared with intravenous access. Provided tissue perfusion is good, absorption seems to be predictable and rapid, but the pharmacokinetics of subcutaneous analgesics in children have not been well studied.

*Epidural:* This provides extensive and profound analgesia at the site of surgical insult with little systemic effect and the option of long-term infusion. It requires a skilled anaesthetist and trained staff with adequate resources and monitoring for subsequent management. Epidurals are inserted under general anaesthesia in the majority of children and have a good safety profile.

*Transdermal and Transmucosal:* Lipid-soluble drugs can be rapidly absorbed in small volumes from highly vascular sites. This allows a potentially rapid onset and high efficacy without the need for painful access. Intranasal diamorphine has been used with success in the emergency room and for painful procedures. Significant opioid-related side effects are still common. Transdermal absorption is slower, but newer technologies in delivery systems are improving this. Topical application of local anaesthetics is frequently used for minor painful procedures.

*Inhalation:* Nitrous oxide/oxygen (Entonox) inhalation has been used successfully for the management of brief painful procedures in children. Acceptability is often good, but trained staff with specialist equipment and a suitable environment are required.

## Analgesic Drugs and Techniques

Pain intensity and duration in the perioperative period are usually predictable, and planning analgesic requirements is relatively straightforward. Many combinations of drugs and techniques are possible. Potent analgesic combinations are usually required initially, with gradual reduction over time as healing occurs, and pain finally being managed by simple, readily available analgesics. Opioids, paracetamol and NSAIDs are usually administered regularly as part of a multimodal strategy. Local anaesthesia can be used in the form of a 'single-shot' technique at the time of surgery or as a postoperative infusion either centrally or peripherally. Other agents such as NMDA antagonists (ketamine), $\alpha_2$-adrenergic agonists (clonidine/dexmedetomidine), magnesium, intravenous lidocaine and gabapentinoids can be considered as additives to supplement the multimodal strategy.

Whatever analgesic medication combinations are decided upon, it is important to ensure that, at a minimum, simple analgesia is prescribed at regular intervals. Research suggests 'as-needed' prescriptions can lead to analgesia not being given or children receiving as little analgesia as possible.

Regular administration reduces peaks and troughs of plasma drug levels and ensures that the child receives the medication. Medications prescribed 'as-needed' should be for management of breakthrough pain, that is, intermittent and unpredictable pain.

## Paracetamol

Paracetamol is the most widely prescribed drug in paediatric hospitals and has become the mainstay base analgesic for almost all procedures. The analgesic potency is low, and it is effective against mild pain. In combination with NSAIDs and weak opioids, it has been shown to be effective for moderate pain and is opioid sparing when used in tandem with more potent opioids. Paracetamol has a mainly central mode of action, producing both analgesic and antipyretic effects. Its oral bioavailability is very good, being rapidly absorbed from the small bowel. Rectal absorption is slow and incomplete, except in neonates. Therefore, where possible, paracetamol should be given orally preoperatively or intravenously at the time of surgery. Intravenous paracetamol may have a higher analgesic potency than both the oral and rectal preparations, as uptake into the cerebrospinal fluid is greater and faster following intravenous administration than via the other routes. Paracetamol is very safe in children; however, data supporting its use in neonates are limited, and caution is required for those under 32 weeks' gestation, with use accompanied by monitoring of liver function.

## Non-steroidal Anti-inflammatory Drugs

NSAIDs act mainly in the periphery inhibiting prostaglandin synthesis and reducing inflammation, although central effects have been postulated involving the opioid, serotonin and nitric oxide pathways. They are highly efficacious in the treatment of mild to moderate pain in children. NSAIDs have a reported opioid-sparing effect of 30–40% when used in combination with opioids. They also reduce opioid-related adverse effects and facilitate more rapid weaning of opioid infusions. They are highly effective in combination with a local or regional nerve block, and combination with paracetamol produces better analgesia than either drug alone. There are limitations to their use in paediatric populations. In the United Kingdom, ibuprofen is now available in over-the-counter formulations for ages three months and above, and it is used in children above one month in the hospital setting. At present, diclofenac and other NSAIDs are not recommended for children less than six months of age. Care should be taken in patients who are asthmatic or have a known aspirin or NSAID allergy, and those with hypovolaemia, dehydration, renal impairment, coagulopathy or where there is a significant risk of haemorrhage. A careful history of previous NSAID use should be taken in every case. Different NSAIDs have different side-effect profiles, and the relative risks associated with each of the contraindications given will differ between drugs. In the United Kingdom, the Committee on the Safety of Medicines has classified ibuprofen and diclofenac as having the best side-effects profile. Both rectal and oral bioavailability are good, though for short cases they are best given orally preoperatively. The dose is higher than expected in children if scaled by body weight from adult doses; recommended dose ranges for children should be used. Other routes of administration are available, such as intravenous and topical, although their use in children so far has been limited.

COX-2 selective inhibitors such as parecoxib have improved side-effect profiles compared to NSAIDs in adults. There is limited safety data in children; however, they have been used safely in paediatric rheumatology populations. Parecoxib works through an active metabolite; clearance of the active metabolite is reduced in younger age groups, requiring dose reduction or increased dose interval in children under two years. If parecoxib is given intraoperatively, a 12-hour delay is required before subsequent NSAIDs are used.

## Opioids

Opioids remain the mainstay of analgesic treatment for the majority of all but minor surgical procedures. Whilst the tension between benefit and threat of opioid use and misuse is relevant to a paediatric population, this class of drugs remains the best and safest option to manage moderate to severe pain in children. Safe use therefore relies on health care professionals to ensure appropriate in-hospital safety systems and stewardship for rare instances where children are discharged with continued opioid medications.

The choice of opioid will depend on the patient's medical history, type of surgery, drug availability, any locally devised protocols and often individual anaesthetic preference. The pharmacology of these agents changes during early life, and these changes are not consistent between different drugs. Understanding the pharmacology of each particular opioid in neonates and infants is important to ensure both efficacy and safety. It has been shown that individuals with central nervous system disease or disability may be more sensitive to the side effects of opioids, such as respiratory depression, and doses and/or dose intervals may need to be adjusted.

Morphine remains the most commonly used opioid. Morphine clearance is decreased and the elimination half-life is increased in neonates compared with infants and older children. In neonates, the glucuronidation pathways, the main metabolic pathways for morphine, are still developing, slowing morphine metabolism and giving a relatively increased production of morphine-6-glucuronide, an active metabolite. These differences may to some extent account for the increased efficacy of morphine seen clinically in neonates.

Oxycodone is similar in structure to codeine, although the analgesic effect is via the parent molecule rather than its metabolites. It has been shown to be effective for treatment of moderate to severe pain in children.

Tramadol has a dual mode of action. It is an agonist at mu receptors but also works by enhancing descending inhibition via the serotonergic and noradrenergic systems. In children, it has been shown to be efficacious for mild to moderate pain with a good safety profile.

Historically, codeine was commonly prescribed as a weak opioid to children. It works via its active metabolite morphine. The cytochrome P-450 enzyme, CYP2D6, responsible for this conversion demonstrates genetic polymorphism, leading to marked variability in activity. Although this can lead to reduced activity and thus little or no morphine being produced from a dose of codeine, far more concerning is increased activity leading to morphine toxicity and overdose. Consequently, codeine is currently not recommended for use in children under 12 years old in the United Kingdom.

## Opioid Infusions

The requirements for opioid infusion analgesia include:

- Clear protocols for infusion rates and the detection and treatment of side effects
- Staff educated in the use of opioid infusion techniques
- Appropriate monitoring
- A safe nursing environment

If all these factors are in place, then opioid infusions can be effectively and safely used in even the most premature neonate.

*Continuous infusion:* Morphine at infusion rates of 10–40 mcg $kg^{-1}$ $h^{-1}$ will provide effective analgesia for most postoperative pain. Lower infusion rates (5–15 mcg $kg^{-1}$ $h^{-1}$) should be used in neonates. Fentanyl (0.5–2 mcg $kg^{-1}$ $h^{-1}$) and oxycodone (10–40 mcg $kg^{-1}$ $h^{-1}$) are useful alternatives to morphine. Infusion analgesia can be comparable with the more flexible nurse-controlled and patient-controlled analgesia (NCA and PCA) techniques, but changes in infusion rate alter plasma levels slowly in comparison with methods that include supplemental boluses.

*Nurse-controlled analgesia:* This increases the flexibility of a continuous infusion by combining a moderate background infusion with the ability to give two or three extra demand-led boluses per hour. Efficacy is improved by the use of reliable pain assessment.

*Patient-controlled analgesia:* In children, a small background infusion (4 mcg $kg^{-1}$ $h^{-1}$) has been shown to improve nighttime sleep patterns without increasing side effects. Aside from this, traditional adult PCA settings are used. With the right supervision and monitoring, PCA can be used in children as young as five years.

Opioid-related side effects such as nausea and vomiting, itching, sedation and respiratory depression can occur in a dose-dependent fashion. Sedation scoring and monitoring of the respiratory rate should be undertaken in all patients receiving parenteral opioids. Oxygen and opioid antagonist must be easily accessible in case of emergency, alongside antiemetics and antipruritics. The subcutaneous route is an alternative to intravenous administration, but it should not be used in hypovolaemic patients.

## $\alpha_2$-Adrenergic Agonists

Clonidine, an $\alpha_2$-adrenergic agonist, has a long history of safe use in children. It can be used as part of a multimodal strategy for perioperative pain by oral and intravenous routes (dose ranges 1–2 mcg $kg^{-1}$ every six to eight hours) or epidural routes. Clonidine is used as an adjunct to local anaesthetics. It is also used for premedication owing to its sedative properties. Dexmedetomidine, another drug in this class, has been shown to reduce postoperative pain, and despite associated cardiac issues such as variability in blood pressure and heart rate, has safety data from widespread use in paediatric intensive care. Although absorbed orally and intranasally, its main route of administration is via intravenous infusion, which limits its use for analgesia outside the critical care setting.

## Ketamine

Ketamine is an NMDA receptor antagonist. It has analgesic properties in its own right at lower doses than those used for anaesthesia. It prevents the induction of central sensitisation, wind-up and the development of opioid tolerance. Efficacy has been shown in children when combined with opioids or with local anaesthetics when used as part of a multimodal strategy. At low doses used for analgesia, the potential psychomimetic effects of ketamine are rare. It has also been used successfully for premedication.

## Intravenous Lidocaine

Intravenous lidocaine works by decreasing excitability in the dorsal horn and is thought to be anti-inflammatory, reducing nociceptor stimulation by inflammatory proteins. Data regarding its use in acute pain management continue to be equivocal in adults, and there are currently no trial data in children. Intravenous lidocaine should be regarded as a 'high-risk' medicine for use in selected patients only as part of a multimodal pain management strategy. It may be useful in procedures associated with significant postoperative pain. Dosing should be no more than a 1.5 mg $kg^{-1}$ IV bolus given over 10 minutes, with a possible further infusion of 1 mg $kg^{-1}$ $h^{-1}$ for no longer than eight hours. It should not be used concurrently with other local anaesthetic techniques. Current use is off-label, and close monitoring of patients is required to identify cardiovascular conduction abnormalities or local anaesthetic toxicity.

## Gabapentin and Pregabalin

Gabapentin and pregabalin work on ascending and descending pathways via voltage-gated calcium channels, influencing both nociceptive and affective components of pain. They rose to prominence when small trials in adults suggested gabapentin may be protective against developing chronic postsurgical pain. Use in patients at risk of developing acute neuropathic pain appears sensible, although evidence is scarce. Evidence regarding general use for acute postoperative pain in children is lacking. Gabapentin and pregabalin are associated with abuse and diversion. They have a significant side-effect profile, including weight gain, inability to concentrate, sleepiness and some evidence of increased suicidal ideation in adolescents, so they have a limited application in children.

## Magnesium

Magnesium is a non-competitive NMDA receptor antagonist that has anti-inflammatory effects. Although some evidence supports opioid-sparing effects and reduced pain scores in adults, evidence is lacking in paediatric practice.

## Local Anaesthetics

Nerve blockade is appropriate for nearly all surgical procedures and forms an important component of a balanced analgesic technique. It allows site-specific analgesia, demonstrates a lack of sedative and respiratory side effects and reduces systematic analgesic requirements. Many techniques of nerve blockade have been described in children of all ages, and they are generally simple, safe and effective (see Chapter 15).

Bupivacaine, ropivacaine and levobupivacaine remain the local anaesthetics of choice in paediatric practice. They all demonstrate efficacy and safety in children. Local anaesthetic agents have an increased half-life and decreased clearance and protein binding in neonates, requiring adjustment of dosing schedules to reduce the risk of systemic toxicity.

*Single-shot techniques:* Single-shot central blocks (epidural/caudal), regional or local blocks can be used to provide excellent intraoperative and early postoperative analgesia. They decrease the use of other analgesics and the incidence of side effects and potentially avoid the use of opioids. The analgesic plan, however, must allow for sufficient analgesia to be in use when the effect of the block wears off.

Caudal analgesia remains popular owing to its versatility and simplicity. Adjuncts are often added to extend the spread and duration of the block. Ketamine and clonidine have been shown to be effective adjuncts, with a low incidence of side effects at low doses. Concern has been expressed about both drugs in relation to their effects on the developing nervous system and potential side effects in neonates and infants, thus questioning their use by the neuraxial route in these age groups. Clonidine appears to be safe in older children, but ketamine has potential neurotoxic effects at any age and would not be advised for use by this route unless there was a specific reason. Caudal opioids are associated with an increased incidence of side effects and are now not commonly used.

*Infusion techniques:* Continuous local anaesthetic infusions can be used to extend the duration of nerve blockade for days into the postoperative period. Accumulation of local anaesthetic is a factor in children and potential toxicity can limit the duration and efficacy of an infusion. Local infection at the insertion site and catheter occlusion or dislodgement can also occur, especially in smaller children. Lumbar and thoracic epidural infusions are well established in children for severe acute pain. Efficacy and postoperative respiratory benefits have been demonstrated in children, but the relative benefits and risks in comparison with other techniques have not been well studied. Insertion is usually performed under general anaesthesia, and most practitioners use a continuous loss of resistance to saline technique. There is now increased use of ultrasound-guided insertion to improve success and safety of the technique. Shorter (5 cm) 18 G and 19 G Toughy needles are available for use in small children, with standard 8 cm 16 G and 18 G for older children. Catheter size varies according to needle size (23 G with 19 G needle and 21 G with 18 G needle). The 23 G catheter has been reported as having a high incidence of displacement. As with adults, at least 3 cm should be left in the epidural space to decrease the risk of the catheter falling out. Epidural infusions in children are prone to leaking but are often effective despite this. Opioids and clonidine have been used as adjuncts with the local anaesthetic to improve efficacy and limit local anaesthetic usage. Epidural clonidine is best avoided in neonates and infants, as discussed in the section '$\alpha_2$-Adrenergic Agonists'. Clear established protocols for the safe management of epidural infusions must be in place, along with trained staff, appropriate monitoring and a safe environment. Treatment protocols for side effects should also be used, and if opioids are added, urinary catheterisation is recommended. Continuous catheter-based infusion techniques in other anatomical locations, such as paravertebral and fascia iliaca compartment block, have been reported in children (see Chapter 15).

## Non-pharmacological Pain Management Strategies

Effective multimodal analgesia for acute pain should include not only pharmacological strategies but also consider rehabilitation, psychology, spirituality and integrative ('non-pharmacological') modalities. These all act synergistically to provide effective paediatric pain control leading to fewer side effects compared to a single analgesic or modality. It is recognised that each technique in isolation is unlikely to be adequate, but many of these strategies have low side-effect profiles, and their addition to overall pain management may be helpful. Over recent years, psychologists have become important members of the multidisciplinary acute pain team, acknowledging how preoperative anxiety, depression and fear of postoperative pain in both children and caregivers can impact on postoperative experiences. Early involvement and psychological interventions may be helpful, especially in patients with underlying chronic pain, previous difficult postoperative pain control and those undergoing complex or repeated surgery. Physical therapy and exercise are key to both acute and chronic paediatric pain management in all settings. Increased activity improves pain, speeds up return to normal function and positively impacts on mood. Other physical therapies including transcutaneous electrical nerve stimulation (TENS) and massage can be helpful. Breast feeding, kangaroo care and facilitated swaddling are useful additional strategies in infants. Finally, supporting a family's spirituality or life philosophy can be important in pain relief and overall care.

## Pain Assessment

Appropriate clinical assessment of pain improves both the safety and efficacy of pain management in children. It allows for the prompt administration of analgesia and is an effective method of monitoring treatment. Effective pain assessment involves regular clinical monitoring of the child by trained staff allied with the use of an appropriate pain-scoring tool. Tools for routine clinical use should be practical, valid for the clinical setting and age range of the patients and acceptable to staff, patients and carers. Current validated tools in children focus on pain intensity, although overall pain assessment should also include a child's function, including ability to drink, eat and mobilise; emotional response; and global satisfaction of pain management by both the child and caregivers.

Pain is subjective in nature, and self-reporting pain tools are generally regarded as the gold standard measure. This requires a degree of both cognitive and physical development. 'Child-friendly' adaptations of these scores – for example, a face type scale (Figure 17.1) – have been designed for younger patients and have been used down to ages as low as four years of age. Older children are often able to use numerical pain scales effectively. At younger ages, the scales may not be truly linear and are not directly interchangeable or numerically comparable with other scales.

In younger, especially non-verbal children, or those with cognitive or communication difficulties, other approaches are necessary and tools using behavioural and/or physiological measures have been developed, such as the face, legs, activity, consolability (FLACC) pain measurement tool (Table 17.2). It is important to remember that these behaviours are affected by a number of factors:

- Age of the child
- Other factors such as hunger, distress and anxiety
- Concurrent drug treatment
- Individual interpretation by health care workers using the tools

## Postoperative Nausea and Vomiting

Postoperative nausea and vomiting (PONV) are common in children. The causes are multifactorial with analgesia potentially involved, especially opioids. Pain can also be a contributory factor, and adequate analgesia has been shown to reduce the incidence of PONV. Other risk factors are increasing age (age greater than three years), a history of PONV or motion sickness, the duration and type of surgery and the use of volatile anaesthetics. The effect of nitrous oxide in increasing PONV has not been proven in children. A multimodal-type strategy may give better outcomes for treatment of PONV owing to the complexity of the pathogenesis of PONV. Ondansetron and dexamethasone are the most commonly used drugs perioperatively. Combination therapy has been shown to be superior to either drug alone.

## Discharge Care and Chronic Postsurgical Pain

Pain management is integral to discharge planning following surgery. This should include clear documentation of which medicines are to be continued and which are to be stopped, the time analgesia use is expected to continue for and whether it should be slowly tapered or simply stopped. Instructions for parents should be both verbal and written and include contact details should pain continue to be problematic after a predetermined time frame. Early follow-up by surgical teams should include children discharged using strong opioids or other analgesic adjuncts such as gabapentinoids, those who had a

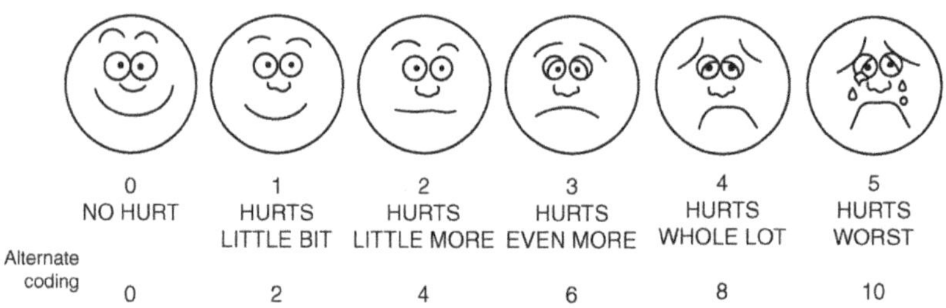


**Figure 17.1** Wong-Baker faces pain rating scale.
*Source:* Originally published in Whaley and Wong's *Nursing Care of Infants and Children*. © Elsevier Inc., 2023. Reproduced with permission.

**Table 17.2** FLACC behavioural scale

| | Scoring | | |
|---|---|---|---|
| **Categories** | **0** | **1** | **2** |
| **Face** | No particular expression or smile | Occasional grimace or frown, withdrawn, disinterested | Frequent to constant frown, clenched jaw, quivering chin |
| **Legs** | Normal position or relaxed | Uneasy, restless, tense | Kicking, or legs drawn up |
| **Activity** | Lying quietly, normal position, moves easily | Squirming, shifting back and forth, tense | Arched, rigid or jerking |
| **Cry** | No cry (awake or asleep) | Moans or whimpers, occasional complaint | Crying steadily, screams or sobs, frequent complaints |
| **Consolability** | Content, relaxed | Reassured by occasional touching, hugging, or being talked to, distractable | Difficult to console or comfort |

*Note:* Each of the five categories – (F) face; (L) legs; (A) activity; (C) cry; (C) consolability – is scored from 0–2, which results in a total score between zero and 10.

difficult or prolonged postoperative pain journey and children who are at risk of developing chronic pain conditions, including chronic post-surgical pain (CPSP) or complex regional pain syndrome.

CPSP is pain that develops or increases in intensity after a surgical procedure and persists beyond the healing process. The current definition stipulates its occurrence continuing at least three months after the initiating event, the pain being localised either in the surgical field or projected to the area of innervation of a nerve from this area and where other causes of the pain have been excluded. Prevalence depends on the surgery undertaken but may occur in up to one in five children. Risk factors have been extensively explored in adults but less so in children. Current evidence in paediatric populations suggests these include pre-existing anxiety, parental pain catastrophising, poorer pain coping efficacy and possibly pre-existing pain prior to surgery.

Ideally hospitals will have transitional pain clinics to review patients who develop chronic pain after surgery; however, when these are not available, there should be mechanisms in place to ensure rapid referral and review by an experienced chronic pain team.

### Key Points

- Nociceptive pathways are present from birth, and even the most premature infant has the capacity to detect and respond to painful stimulation.
- Developmental age has a profound effect on both the processing of nociceptive information and the response to analgesia.
- It is essential to understand the pharmacology of analgesic drugs in children of all ages.
- An analgesic plan is required in all cases and should be flexible, sufficient and safe.
- Adopting a multimodal approach to treatment provides optimal pain management.
- Regular pain assessment improves the safety and efficacy of pain management in children.
- Complex pain management requires the use of clear protocols and the detection and treatment of side effects. It also requires educated staff, appropriate monitoring and a safe nursing environment.

## Further Reading

Association of Paediatric Anaesthetists of Great Britain and Ireland. Good practice in postoperative and procedural pain management, 2nd edition. *Paediatric Anaesthesia*. 2012 July; 22 (Suppl 1):1–79.

Howard RF. Complex pain management. In: Bingham R, Lloyd-Thomas A, Sury M, eds. Hatch and Sumner's Textbook of Paediatric Anaesthesia, 3rd ed. Hodder Arnold. 2008; 407–23.

Lonnqvist P-A, Morton NS. Postoperative analgesia in infants and children. *British Journal of Anaesthesia*. 2005; 95:59–68.

Schug SA, Scott DA, Mott JF, Halliwell R, Palmer GM, Alcock M, APM:SE Working Group of the Australian and New Zealand College of Anaesthetists and Faculty of Pain Medicine. Acute Pain Management: Scientific Evidence, 5th ed., Section 10. ANZCA ans FPM. 2020.

Chapter

# 18 Neonatal Anaesthesia*

Joy Dawes

## Introduction

Some neonates may require specialist surgery during the first days or weeks of life. Many neonates presenting for repair of congenital abnormalities are born prematurely, which leads to additional challenges (discussed in Chapter 19). In this chapter, we consider common neonatal surgical conditions and their anaesthetic management.

## General Considerations

Conditions requiring major general surgery in the neonatal period are:

- Oesophageal atresia (OA), with or without tracheoesophageal fistula (TOF)
- Congenital diaphragmatic hernia (CDH)
- Intestinal atresias
- Meconium ileus
- Malrotation and volvulus
- Hirschsprung's disease
- Imperforate anus
- Exomphalos and gastroschisis
- Necrotising enterocolitis (NEC)

Anaesthetic techniques should be tailored to the relevant surgical condition, but most of the key management principles are similar and require an in-depth knowledge of the anatomical, physiological and pharmacological differences particular to this vulnerable group of patients (discussed in Chapters 1 and 2). The following differences are of specific importance with respect to anaesthesia for neonatal general surgery.

### Respiratory

- The intercostal muscles are poorly developed in neonates and contribute very little to the mechanics of respiration. Diaphragmatic breathing predominates and surgical conditions resulting in abdominal distension can significantly compromise ventilation.
- Oxygen consumption is twice that of the adult. Hypoxia develops very quickly if alveolar ventilation is compromised and may lead to profound bradycardia.
- All neonates are at risk of postoperative apnoea, and this is compounded by the presence of anaemia (Hb $<100$ g $l^{-1}$). Premature and ex-premature neonates are particularly susceptible; the incidence is decreased at 60 weeks postmenstrual age [PMA]).

### Cardiovascular

- Many neonates with congenital defects presenting for surgery also have congenital heart disease (CHD). For some lesions, such as TOF and exomphalos, CHD may be present in 50% of cases. Cardiac lesions are often diagnosed antenatally. The presence of cyanosis should raise the possibility of undiagnosed CHD, although many cardiac defects are acyanotic. Neonatal surgery should be undertaken in specialist centres with preoperative echocardiography as standard practice. Surgery is not usually postponed in the presence of a cardiac lesion, but the cardiac physiology must be fully appreciated in order to ensure optimal management in the perioperative period (see Chapter 33).
- Occasionally, a prostaglandin infusion will be required to maintain patency of the ductus arteriosus. In lesions associated with very poor pulmonary blood flow such as severe tetralogy of Fallot, it may be necessary to perform a systemic to pulmonary artery shunt prior to general surgery. Close communication with the cardiologists is important to ascertain which lesion takes surgical priority.

* Many thanks to Dr Mark Thomas, who wrote the first edition of this book chapter, much of the content of which has been used in this revision.

## Thermoregulation

- Neonates have limited capacity to regulate body temperature, have poor thermal insulation and lose heat readily. Normothermia can be maintained by increasing ambient temperature, using warmed fluids and active warming strategies.
- The response to hypoxaemia is temperature dependent in neonates; under normal conditions peripheral chemoreceptors stimulate hyperventilation, but under hypothermic conditions hypoxaemia may result in hypoventilation and apnoeas.

## Metabolic

- Neonates are at risk of hypoglycaemia in the first 48 hours of life, if they have low body weight (less than the third centile), if they have undergone prolonged surgery or if they have received extensive regional anaesthesia with a reduced stress response. Blood glucose should be monitored regularly, and glucose-containing fluids given to those at risk.

## Haematological

- The haemoglobin level in neonates may be as high as 200 g $l^{-1}$, but it is predominantly fetal haemoglobin (60–90%) which confers relatively poor tissue oxygen delivery. Blood transfusion may be restricted to maintain Hb $> 90$ g $l^{-1}$ in a term neonate with no oxygen requirement, and $> 110$ g $l^{-1}$ if the neonate is aged under 1 week old, is intubated or has an oxygen requirement.
- Vitamin-K dependent clotting factors levels are very low at birth. Vitamin K (1 mg IM) should be given prior to surgery if it has not already been given at birth.
- Blood should be cross-matched for most surgery in the neonatal period. Coagulation may be disordered in neonates with bowel necrosis, and blood products are frequently necessary.

## Neurological and Pain

- Nociceptive pathways develop within the first trimester and are particularly susceptible to maladaptive changes that may have long-term consequences for the neonate. Adequate analgesia must be provided.

# Conduct of Anaesthesia

## Preoperative Preparation

- **Fasting.** Breast-fed babies should be fasted for four hours prior to elective surgery, and babies receiving formula milk should be fasted for six hours. Clear fluids may be given up to one hour preoperatively.

## Intraoperative Management

- **Airway.** The majority of neonatal surgical procedures require tracheal intubation and ventilation, as neonates have limited respiratory reserve and are prone to airway obstruction.
- **Induction.** Patients with small bowel obstruction are at risk of aspiration at induction. A modified rapid sequence induction should be performed, with gentle ventilation and the use of a non-depolarising muscle relaxant such as atracurium. It is reasonable to ask the parents to leave the anaesthetic room prior to induction so that full attention can be paid to the neonate at this critical time.
- **Volatiles.** The minimum alveolar concentration (MAC) for all inhalational agents is slightly greater in neonates than in adults. The neonatal myocardium is particularly sensitive to the depressant and vagotonic effects of inhalational agents. Sevoflurane is commonly used for induction followed by either sevoflurane or isoflurane for maintenance.
- **Analgesia.** A balanced anaesthesia technique using fentanyl will enable a reduced concentration of volatiles to be given, with the caveat that high-dose opioids will increase the requirement for postoperative respiratory support.
- **Neurotoxicity.** There has been concern in recent years that volatile agents may have a detrimental effect on the developing brain. Some anaesthetists advocate the use of spinal anaesthesia for surgical procedures such as inguinal hernia repair to avoid the potential disadvantages of general anaesthesia, but the

surgery must be completed within one hour for this to be successful. The multicentre GAS trial investigating the effects of one hour of general anaesthesia with sevoflurane compared with awake regional anaesthesia for infants undergoing inguinal hernia repair showed no difference in neurodevelopmental outcome at five years. The rates of early postoperative apnoea were lower in the regional anaesthesia group.

- **Vascular access.** Ideally, two venous lines should be available and accessible during surgery (22G or 24G gauge). The anaesthetist should take care to preserve veins that may be used for long lines, particularly if use of parenteral nutrition is anticipated. For most major cases, an arterial line is extremely helpful, with distal arterial cannulation sites preferred. Complications associated with both arterial and venous access in neonates are common, and lines should be removed when they are no longer necessary.
- **Monitoring.** Standard monitoring should be applied and haematocrit, blood gases, lactate and blood glucose checked regularly.
- **Temperature regulation.** Maintaining normothermia is often a challenge during neonatal surgery. Fluid warmers and forced-air warming mattresses should be used and core temperature monitored.

## Postoperative Analgesia

- **Paracetamol.** Comprehensive data analysis has been undertaken for the use of intravenous (IV) paracetamol in neonates, with specific dosing regimens suggested according to PMA. Intravenous paracetamol preparations have a concentration of 10 mg ml$^{-1}$, and great care should be taken to prevent accidental overdose due to confusion between the dose in ml and dose in mcg of the drug. There are reassuringly few reports of hepatotoxicity after overdose, particularly when the antidote, N-acetylcysteine (NAC) is administered promptly. Paracetamol should be prescribed regularly, not 'as required'.
- **Ibuprofen.** Ibuprofen is not licenced for use in infants under three months of age.
- **Opioids.** Intravenous morphine delivered via nurse-controlled analgesia (NCA) is used commonly after major surgery. Morphine increases the risk of postoperative apnoea in unventilated neonates; oxygen saturation and apnoea monitoring in a high-dependency unit (HDU) environment is essential. It is our practice to use morphine boluses of 10 mcg kg$^{-1}$ with a 20 minute lockout and to avoid a background infusion. Oral morphine can be given at an effect-titrated dose of 0.05–0.1 mg kg$^{-1}$ every four to six hours in carefully monitored term neonates. Extreme caution should be taken when giving oral morphine to non-ventilated premature infants due to the increased risk of adverse respiratory events.
- **Regional.** Epidurals are effective in neonates and may avoid the requirement for postoperative ventilation. Neonates have lower levels of plasma-binding proteins (in particular, alpha-1 glycoprotein), and higher free-plasma levels of local analgesic are possible. Our preference is to use plain 0.125% levobupivacaine, up to 0.3 ml kg$^{-1}$ hr$^{-1}$. Local anaesthetic infiltration up to a maximum of 0.8 ml kg$^{-1}$ of 0.25% levobupivacaine and NCA can be used as an alternative to an epidural.

## Minimally Invasive Surgery (MIS)

Neonatal surgery is increasingly performed thoracoscopically or laparoscopically for procedures such as repair of TOF, congenital diaphragmatic hernia, duodenal atresia and malrotation. It is essential that the anaesthetist and surgeon work closely together to minimise complications during MIS. Anaesthetic considerations for MIS include:

- **Patient positioning and access.** The neonate may be positioned head up, head down or semi-prone and will be surrounded by equipment and monitors. There will be limited access to the tracheal tube (TT) and lines once the drapes are in place, so these must be checked and fixed securely prior to surgery.
- **Effects of pneumothorax/ pneumoperitoneum.** Specific complications from MIS in neonates include hypercarbia, desaturation, hypotension, metabolic acidosis and hypothermia and are seen more often during thoracoscopic procedures.
  - *Respiratory effects*: A cuffed or well-fitting uncuffed tracheal tube should be used to ensure that adequate tidal volumes are delivered during periods of reduced

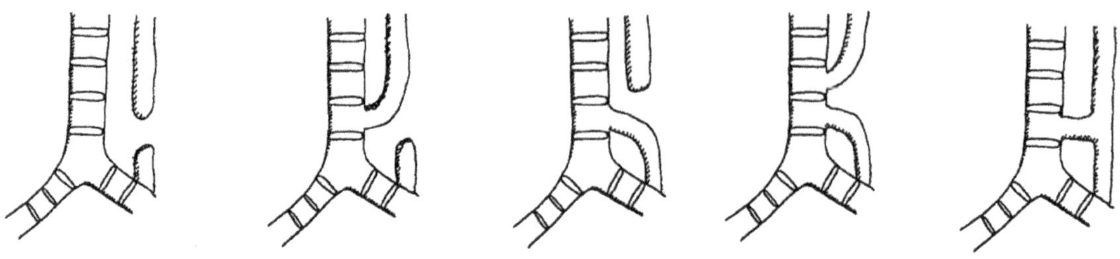

Type A Type B Type C Type D H Type (Type E)

**Figure 18.1** Gross's classification of oesophageal atresia and tracheal-oesophageal fistula.
*Source*: Gross RE. *The Surgery of Infancy and Childhood.* WB Saunders, 1954; figure by Thomas M.

respiratory compliance. The $CO_2$ insufflation pressure should be limited to 8 mm Hg. Systemic absorption of $CO_2$ can rapidly lead to high $PaCO_2$. Arterial blood sampling or transcutaneous $CO_2$ monitoring are invaluable for monitoring trends in these parameters. Minute ventilation will need to be increased to compensate for increased $PaCO_2$. It may be necessary to intermittently reduce the $CO_2$ insufflation to facilitate $CO_2$ clearance.
  - *Cardiovascular effects*: Increased intra-abdominal pressure leads to reduced venous return, which may be particularly significant in neonates with CHD; isolated cardiac arrests have occurred during laparoscopic procedures. It is advisable to augment the preload with 10 ml $kg^{-1}$ IV crystalloid before insufflation to preserve cardiovascular stability.
  - *Thermoregulation*: The $CO_2$ insufflation gas is cold and may result in a reduction in body temperature.
- **Prolonged surgery.** Operating time should be limited to less than 100 minutes to minimise the adverse cardiorespiratory sequelae from insufflation.

# Specific Neonatal Conditions

## Oesophageal Atresia and Tracheoesophageal Fistula

Tracheal-oesophageal fistula (TOF) is a common congenital anomaly of the respiratory tract with an incidence of approximately 1:4500 live births. Oesophageal atresia (OA) and TOF are classified according to the anatomical configuration (Figure 18.1). The most common is the combination of a proximal oesophageal pouch with a distal TOF (Type C), which represents more than 80–85% of cases. Antenatal ultrasound may identify polyhydramnios, although many cases are not detected prenatally. Infants with OA become symptomatic immediately after birth, with excessive secretions that cause drooling, choking, respiratory distress and the inability to feed. Diagnosis is made by the failure to pass a nasogastric (NG) tube and a chest X-ray (CXR) which shows the NG tube coiled in the proximal oesophageal pouch (Figure 18.2). Patients with H-type fistulae may present early if the defect is large, but smaller defects may not be diagnosed until infancy or early childhood.

Additional clinical features relate to the presence of the VACTERL association (vertebral, anorectal, cardiac, tracheal-oesophageal fistula, renal and limb defects) or CHARGE syndrome (coloboma, heart defects, choanal atresia, growth retardation, genital abnormalities and ear abnormalities). Congenital heart disease is seen in up to 40% of patients with TOF, most commonly ventricular septal defect (VSD) or tetralogy of Fallot. Echocardiography and renal ultrasonography should be performed in all infants in whom a TOF has been identified. The modified Spitz criteria can be used to identify risk factors for mortality, specifically birth weight <1.5 kg and the presence of major cardiac morbidity.

Neonates with TOF/OA require a Replogle suction catheter in the blind-ending oesophageal pouch preoperatively to help prevent pooling and overspill of secretions. This is a double-barrelled

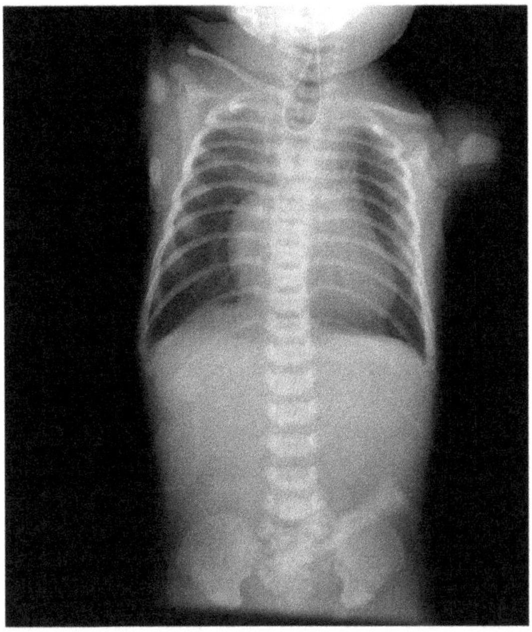

**Figure 18.2** A coiled nasogastric tube suggestive of oesophageal atresia in a neonate with Down syndrome.
*Source:* Thanks to Dr Frank Galliard, http://radiopaedia.org, reproduced with permission in the first edition.

oesophageal tube that is kept on continuous low-level suction. Inadvertent ventilation of the gastrointestinal tract may occur if the baby requires respiratory support preoperatively. This will result in bowel distension and further respiratory compromise. The requirement for preoperative ventilation is an indication for urgent surgery to close the fistula.

There is a role for microlaryngoscopy and bronchoscopy (MLB) prior to surgery to define the site and size of the fistula, exclude multiple fistulae and provide information to guide positioning of the TT. A recent multicentre audit in the United Kingdom showed that bronchoscopy was used in approximately 50% of cases. There is no standard of practice in anaesthesia or surgery in relation to the use of rigid or flexible bronchoscopy.

## Anaesthesia

If an MLB is being performed, a gentle gas induction with sevoflurane in 100% oxygen is used, followed by topicalisation of the vocal cords with 1% lignocaine (2–3 mg $kg^{-1}$) when sufficient depth of anaesthesia is reached. An uncuffed TT is used as a nasopharyngeal airway and is passed into the posterior pharyngeal space, with anaesthesia maintained with 100% oxygen and sevoflurane. In our practice, the ENT surgeon then performs rigid bronchoscopy whilst spontaneous ventilation is maintained. Once the fistula has been identified, the surgeon or anaesthetist can advance the TT through the vocal cords into an appropriate position with the bevel of the TT facing anteriorly. Some centres advocate the use of a Fogarty catheter to block a large fistula, but this is not the usual practice at our institution. Other strategies include endobronchial intubation with withdrawal of the tube until bilateral air entry is obtained, keeping the bevel of the TT facing anteriorly. The fistula is usually in the posterior wall of the trachea, close to the carina, and this technique ensures that the tube is as distal as possible and less likely to result in ventilation of the fistula. Very rarely, it may be necessary to selectively intubate the bronchus in order to provide adequate ventilation for the procedure.

A non-depolarising neuromuscular relaxant should be given and the lungs ventilated with gentle manual positive pressure ventilation. Neonates with a large fistula may have problems due to gastric distension. If gastric distension does occur, disconnect the TT and apply gentle pressure to decompress the stomach via the TT. Whilst tempting, emergency surgical decompression via a gastrostomy will not be useful in this situation, as the gastrostomy offers a route of low resistance via the fistula, which will be ventilated in preference to the lungs. This is a particular concern in premature neonates with reduced lung compliance. Gastrostomy may, rarely, be useful to avoid life-threatening gastric rupture.

## Surgery

Repair of the fistula can be performed using either an open or thoracoscopic technique. The main advantage of using a thoracoscopic approach is a reduction in the musculoskeletal sequelae. Suggested selection criteria include short-gap OA, birth weight $> 2$ kg, cardiorespiratory stability with no major cardiac or pulmonary malformation and no more than one major malformation (such as duodenal or anal atresia). Some centres electively use high-frequency oscillatory ventilation (HFOV) to reduce hypercapnia and respiratory acidosis during thoracoscopic repair. This requires expertise in delivering HFOV in the theatre environment and a total intravenous anaesthetic (TIVA) technique to facilitate surgery and is not the current practice in our institution.

For open repair, surgical access is through a right thoracotomy (unless there is a right-sided aortic arch) with the baby in the left lateral position and their right arm above their head. The right lung is retracted. Gentle ventilation should be used until the fistula can be ligated. At the time of ligation, it is advisable to gently ventilate by hand to establish that it is not the right main bronchus or tracheal that is about to be tied off. Close cooperation with the surgeon is important if the patient is having frequent desaturations; intermittent reinflation of the compressed lung may be necessary. After successful ligation of the fistula, a primary oesophageal anastomosis is usually performed if the oesophageal gap is small. A transanastomotic tube (TAT) is gently placed with assistance from the surgeon; it must not be removed postoperatively and must be clearly labelled. In long-gap oesophageal atresia, a feeding gastrostomy is sited at the time of fistula ligation, and oesophageal anastomosis is delayed for a few weeks. The blind end of the oesophageal pouch is brought out into the neck to form an oesophagostomy to facilitate drainage of oral secretions.

Most babies will remain intubated, ventilated and sedated for one to two days postoperatively. Neonates who have an oesophageal anastomosis under tension are electively paralysed and ventilated for two to five days. It is better to err on the side of caution rather than risk disruption of the freshly sutured trachea should reintubation be necessary in the days immediately after surgery.

Infants commonly display a characteristic barking 'TOF cough' after TOF repair. Some will develop tracheomalacia, which may require aortopexy if symptoms are severe. Oesophageal strictures also occur, necessitating repeated oesophageal dilatations for dysphagia.

## Congenital Diaphragmatic Hernia

Congenital diaphragmatic hernia (CDH) affects approximately 1:3,600 births and occurs when a defect in the diaphragm allows abdominal organs to protrude into the thoracic cavity. The exact aetiology is unclear, but the 'dual hit hypothesis' suggests that pulmonary hypoplasia is the primary disturbance, which then hinders the formation of the diaphragm. The resulting protrusion of abdominal contents into the chest further impairs lung development. Approximately 10% of patients have associated genetic or chromosomal abnormalities (trisomy 13, 18 and 21, Fryns syndrome, Cornelia de Lange syndrome, Beckwith–Weidemann syndrome or CHARGE syndrome) and a third of patients have one or more structural abnormality (cardiovascular abnormalities in 14% of patients). There are two types of CDH. Bochdalek hernias occur in 95% of cases, are posterolateral and almost always left-sided. Morgagni hernias are retro- or parasternal, usually smaller, predominantly right-sided and are associated with a better outcome.

Approximately 50% of cases of CDH are diagnosed antenatally. The absence of liver herniation is the most reliable predictor of survival. Cardiac defects have been shown to worsen outcome, and the presence of a small contralateral lung or a bilateral CDH are also poor prognostic signs. Some fetuses with a predicted poor outcome may benefit from the experimental intrauterine intervention of fetoscopic endoluminal tracheal occlusion (FETO). Its aim is to promote lung growth and consequently limit the developing pulmonary hypoplasia but is complicated by the risk of preterm delivery and concerns about tracheomegaly and tracheomalacia postnatally.

If not diagnosed antenatally, CDH usually presents with respiratory distress in the newborn, possibly in the presence of a scaphoid abdomen. A CXR characteristically shows bowel and sometimes other abdominal organs within the hemithorax, and the mediastinum may be displaced (see Figure 18.3). Resuscitation and medical stabilisation are required before definitive surgical repair. The majority of neonates will require tracheal intubation and ventilation immediately after delivery. The insertion of an NG tube may help to decompress the bowel and relieve pressure on the lungs. The pulmonary vasculature is usually underdeveloped, so pulmonary vascular resistance is high and pulmonary hypertension is common. Inhaled nitric oxide is often used, and IV sildenafil or prostacyclin may be required in severe refractory cases. Inotropes help to maintain organ perfusion and can decrease right to left shunting, thereby improving post ductal oxygen saturations. Neuromuscular blocking agents can improve synchronisation with respiratory support and optimise chest wall compliance when ventilation is challenging but should be avoided in the delivery room. Protective ventilation strategies should be

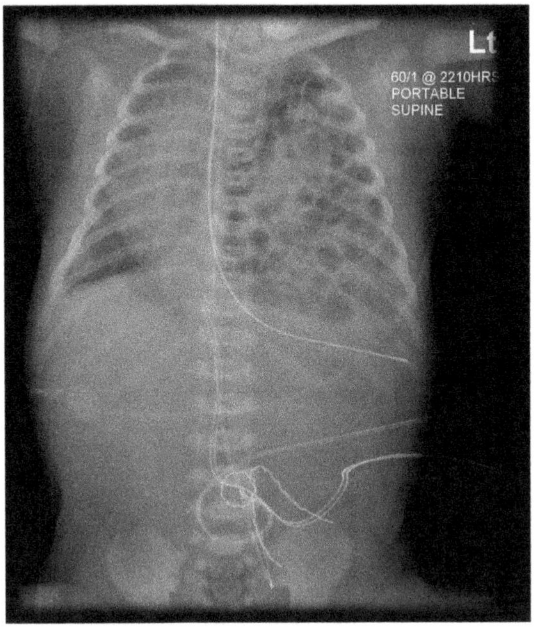


**Figure 18.3** Left-sided congenital diaphragmatic hernia: the bowel can be seen herniating into the left hemithorax with displacement of the cardiac silhouette to the right.
*Source:* With thanks to Dr Frank Galliard, http://radiopaedia.org, reproduced with permission in the first edition.

used to avoid further lung injury, aiming to limit peak inspiratory pressures to 25 $cmH_2O$ and allowing permissive hypercapnia. The VICI trial comparing HFOV to conventional mechanical ventilation found no significant difference in mortality when HFOV was used as an initial mode of ventilation. 'Gentle' mechanical ventilation is recommended as the initial ventilation strategy, with HFOV considered as rescue therapy if required. Extracorporeal membrane oxygenation (ECMO) may confer a survival advantage in the most severe cases of CDH, but its value in more moderate disease is less clear because of the high rates of ECMO-related complications.

The CDH EURO Consortium has published comprehensive consensus guidelines for postnatal management of infants with CDH. Elective surgical closure should be considered after clinical stabilisation once cardiorespiratory function is stable with clinical evidence that pulmonary hypertension is resolving. The CDH EURO consortium defines clinical stabilisation as normal blood pressure for gestational age, preductal $SpO_2$ 85–95% with $FiO_2$ <0.5, lactate <3 mmol $l^{-1}$ and normal urine output. Repair on ECMO is a viable treatment option in selected patients.

### Surgery

Primary closure of a large defect may not be possible, and a patch is frequently needed to close the diaphragm. Open surgery is necessary for large hernias, particularly in the presence of liver herniation, and for sicker patients requiring higher ventilatory or cardiovascular support. Occasionally it may not be possible to close the abdominal wall without compromise to respiratory or cardiovascular stability and the risk of abdominal compartment syndrome. In this situation, the viscera can be covered and the patient left with a laparostomy, with definitive closure at a later date. Thoracoscopic repair has many theoretical advantages but is associated with more severe hypercapnia and acidosis, decreased cerebral oxygen saturations and longer surgery, the significance of which is unclear. Careful patient selection and multidisciplinary input is important in determining the appropriate surgical approach.

### Anaesthesia

Periods of manual hyperventilation may be necessary to reduce hypercapnia during thoracoscopic repair, and conversion to an open procedure must be considered. Inhaled nitric oxide should always be available in theatre and started if a pulmonary hypertensive crisis is suspected. Simple interventions such as increasing $FiO_2$ and depth of anaesthesia, opioid administration and correction of acidosis are usually effective. Fluid overload should be avoided, as it may result in pulmonary congestion postoperatively. Inotropes may be required to optimise organ perfusion and manage intraoperative shunting. Pulmonary hypertension may persist in the postoperative period, potentially requiring further ECMO.

## Intestinal Atresias

Congenital intestinal stenosis or atresia can occur at any point along the gastrointestinal tract. The neonate presents with bowel obstruction and specific clinical features depending on the level of obstruction.

**Duodenal atresia** occurs in approximately 1:6,000 live births. It has a male preponderance, and up to 45% of babies are born prematurely. Half of the patients have associated anomalies, particularly trisomy 21, malrotation and cardiac defects. Neonates present with bilious or non-bilious vomiting depending on whether the obstruction is distal or proximal to the ampulla of Vater. Abdominal X-ray demonstrates the characteristic 'double bubble' with an absence of gas distally. The patient should be resuscitated and stabilised, with intravenous replacement of fluid losses in addition to maintenance fluids, and an NG tube passed. Ultimate management is surgical. A laparotomy and duodenostomy are the primary procedures performed via a supraumbilical transverse or umbilical incision. There may be complete atresia or an intraluminal web that will need excising. The minimally invasive approach is feasible and increasingly being used. If the baby is otherwise well and stable, the aim should be to extubate at the end of surgery.

**Jejunal/ileal atresia** is a common cause of neonatal intestinal obstruction occurring in 1:3,000 live births. There may be a family history, and multiple atresias are not uncommon. Chromosomal abnormalities are much less common compared to duodenal atresia; however, patients with ileal atresia may also have cystic fibrosis. The atresia is thought to be caused by an intrauterine 'vascular accident' with interruption of the blood supply to affected segments. Neonates present with signs of intestinal obstruction and may have significant respiratory compromise necessitating respiratory support. Medical management includes NG decompression, IV resuscitation and maintenance fluids. Good outcomes can be obtained with excision and primary anastomosis at laparotomy. A proximal stoma and mucous fistula are formed as a temporising measure if the patient is unstable or the distal bowel is significantly compromised, and bowel continuity is restored at a later date. Postoperative ventilation may be required after prolonged surgery with significant fluid shifts. The primary cause of morbidity and mortality is short bowel syndrome or intestinal failure requiring parenteral nutrition, with associated risks of sepsis and liver disease.

## Meconium Ileus

Meconium ileus is an intraluminal obstruction of the distal small bowel due to the presence of thick tenacious meconium. The majority are due to intestinal and pancreatic dysfunction secondary to cystic fibrosis. Once the obstruction has been treated, the infant should have genetic screening and a sweat test. Almost all such patients will require pancreatic enzyme replacement when feeds are introduced. The respiratory physicians should be involved early, although respiratory complications are uncommon in the neonatal period. Simple meconium ileus presents with distal intestinal obstruction. Abdominal X-ray demonstrates multiple dilated bowel loops with a 'soap bubble' appearance in the right-lower quadrant caused by mixing of air and meconium. Bowel perforation and meconium peritonitis may result in giant pseudocyst formation. Simple meconium ileus may be relieved with bowel washouts. Hypertonic enemas increase the risk of hypovolaemic shock due to sequestration of fluid in the gut. Surgery may be required if non-operative measures fail or in meconium ileus complicated by persistent bowel obstruction, perforation, atresia or volvulus. Surgical options include manual disimpaction via a proximal enterotomy or with the intraluminal injection of 4% N-acetylcysteine. Resection and anastomosis or stoma formation may be required for complicated cases.

## Malrotation/Volvulus

Malrotation is congenital failure of the normal rotation and fixation of the bowel, resulting in a shortened mesenteric base and a tendency of the small bowel to twist around it (volvulus). This causes obstruction of the blood supply and lymphatic drainage to the small bowel in addition to luminal bowel obstruction, which can lead to ischaemia with necrosis of the entire midgut. It occurs in 1:6,000 live births but may be discovered incidentally. These neonates usually present with bilious vomiting, abdominal distension and pain. Fluid may be sequestered within the obstructed bowel, which can result in significant hypovolaemia and shock. Such neonates require resuscitation with large volumes of IV fluid and inotropic support. Systemic compromise and blood in the stools are later signs of volvulus in which significant ischaemia has already occurred. The gold standard for diagnosis is an upper GI contrast study which demonstrates the 'bird's beak' or 'corkscrew' appearance of duodenal obstruction. Malrotation with midgut volvulus constitutes a true surgical emergency, as the consequences are potentially catastrophic with loss of the entire small bowel.

The classic surgical approach is Ladd's procedure with derotation of the volvulus via laparotomy.

Laparoscopy is increasingly being used, but the technique is still controversial, and early conversion to an open approach must occur if technical difficulties are encountered. The surgical options to address the ischaemic/necrotic bowel include excision of the necrotic segment, with or without anastomosis, or conservative management with a 'second look' laparotomy after 36–48 hours to determine whether perfusion has improved.

Anaesthetic considerations in the unstable neonate should focus on simultaneous resuscitation and expedited preparation and transfer to theatre. Coagulopathy is common in the presence of necrotic bowel, so blood and blood products must be available. The abdomen should be decompressed with an NG tube and respiratory support provided as needed. Invasive monitoring is very useful, and inotropic support may be required. Avoid deep inhalational anaesthesia in critically ill neonates. Derotation of the volvulus may lead to acute cardiovascular instability due to release of vasoactive compounds and lactic acid; intravenous calcium chloride and bicarbonate may be required to manage acidosis and hyperkalaemia. The infant who presents late with necrotic bowel may remain critically ill even after successful surgery and will require maximal support in NICU until perfusion is restored.

## Hirschsprung's Disease

Hirschsprung's disease is due to aganglionosis, usually of distal bowel, and results in functional bowel obstruction. It is a multigenic disorder that is caused by a dysfunction in signalling pathways which are critical in the development of the enteric nervous system. Varying lengths of bowel are affected; short-segment disease affects the rectosigmoid region (80%), and long-segment disease extends proximal to the rectosigmoid region. Serial bowel biopsies are taken at the time of surgery to establish the line of demarcation between abnormal and normally innervated bowel. The most common presentation in neonates is bilious vomiting with failure to pass meconium in the first 24 hours of life. Signs of enterocolitis (fever, abdominal distension and diarrhoea) may also be present. This is a potentially fatal complication that must be identified early and managed aggressively to reduce the risk of sepsis, intestinal necrosis and perforation. Treatment is with fluid resuscitation and broad-spectrum antibiotics. Abdominal X-ray may show dilated bowel loops with an absence of air in the rectum. In the neonatal period, a suction rectal biopsy provides a definitive diagnosis when it fails to demonstrate ganglion cells.

Initial management aims to relieve the functional bowel obstruction, either with warm saline washouts or a defunctioning stoma into ganglionic bowel. A stoma is indicated if the neonate is unwell or has developed enterocolitis and perforation and has a grossly dilated colon or suspected long-segment disease. Definitive surgery consists of resection of the aganglionic segment, either after initial stoma formation or ideally as a primary procedure. Several 'pull-through' techniques have been described, usually performed when the infant is approximately three months of age or around 5–6 kg in weight. The timing and exact procedure undertaken varies between institutions and according to the length of abnormal bowel. The Duhamel procedure, in which the native rectum remains unchanged and a side-to-side anastomosis is stapled to the ganglionic bowel, is often the preferred technique for long-segment disease. Each technique can be performed open or with laparoscopic assisted intra-abdominal dissection and biopsies or entirely laparoscopically. For the laparoscopic approach, the patient is positioned in a steep Trendelenburg position. Blood loss is usually minimal. Caudal or epidural regional anaesthesia provides excellent perioperative analgesia after this surgery. Extubation at the end of surgery is usual.

## Anorectal Anomalies

Anorectal anomalies occur in approximately 1:4,000 neonates and are diagnosed on clinical examination after birth. Imperforate anus with rectourethral fistula (males) or rectovesicular fistula (females) are the most common defects. Associated anomalies (genitourinary, spinosacral, cardiac, gastrointestinal and chromosomal) should be sought and further investigations (ECHO, abdominal X-ray, renal ultrasound) may be required. Initial management is supportive with IV fluids and gastric decompression with an NG tube. Surgical decompression and reconstruction are necessary. For 'low' anomalies, this involves a primary anoplasty with or without a diverting colostomy and a distal mucous fistula. For 'high' anomalies, a colostomy and a mucous fistula are formed, with later reconstructive surgery at one to two months of age. Several types of reconstructive surgery have been proposed, of which posterior sagittal anorectoplasty (PSARP) is the most common.

Stoma formation is considered relatively minor surgery in the neonatal period. Provided there are no significant sacral abnormalities, a caudal block provides excellent analgesia. Reconstructive surgery (PSARP) is usually performed in the prone position or as a combined abdominoperineal or laparoscopic-assisted procedure and may take several hours. Tracheal intubation is required, and IV access should ideally be placed in the upper limbs. Blood transfusion is rarely needed. The aim should be to extubate the baby at the end of surgery. Perioperative analgesia can be achieved with an epidural infusion or morphine NCA.

## Cloacal Malformation

Cloacal anomaly is uncommon, occurring in 1:50,000 live births. It is seen exclusively in girls when the rectum, urethra and vagina fail to develop separately and instead drain via a single common channel onto the perineum. There is a high incidence of associated anomalies, so ECHO, renal and spinal ultrasounds are required. Initial management is supportive, with IV fluids, antibiotics, an NG tube to decompress the bowel and a urinary catheter to drain the urinary tract. When the baby is stable, a protective proximal transverse colostomy is performed to allow for adequate length for subsequent reconstruction. Endoscopy of the common channel is also undertaken to assess the internal anatomy and determine the length of the common channel. Definitive reconstruction (cloacal repair) to create three separate channels usually occurs at around two to three months of age.

## Abdominal Wall Defects

### Gastroschisis

Gastroschisis occurs in approximately 1:5,000 live births, is usually diagnosed on antenatal ultrasound and presents with herniation of bowel through a defect in the abdominal wall (usually right-sided), lateral to the umbilicus (Figure 18.4). The thickened bowel wall is covered in fibrin 'peel' due to exposure to amniotic fluid in utero. Gastroschisis is associated with prematurity, but the presence of other congenital abnormalities is unusual. The herniated bowel should be wrapped in cling film to minimise the large evaporative water and protein losses from the exposed bowel wall and to avoid damage to the bowel prior to surgery. Significant volumes of IV fluid may be required perioperatively.

### Exomphalos

Exomphalos is rare, occurring in 1:10,000 live births. It is a midline periumbilical abdominal wall defect of variable size, covered by a membranous sac consisting of amnion (outer layer) and peritoneum (inner layer), with Wharton's jelly in between, and containing abdominal contents (Figure 18.5). The membraneous sac reduces evaporative losses and allows semi-urgent repair, unless

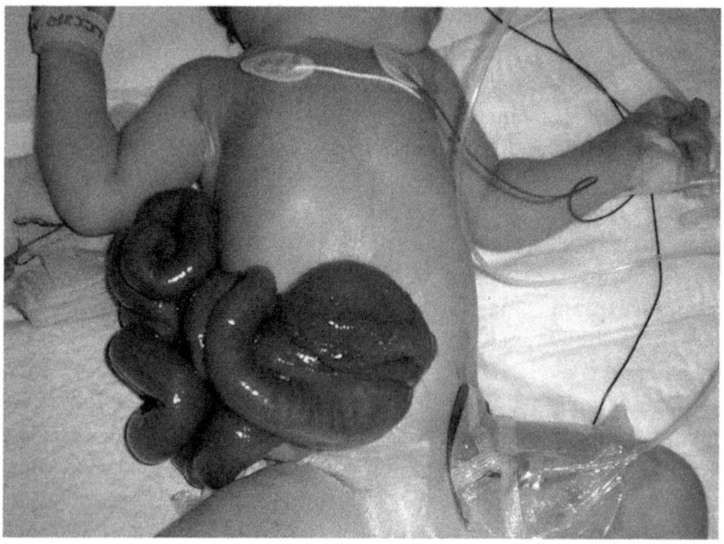

**Figure 18.4** A neonate with gastroschisis.

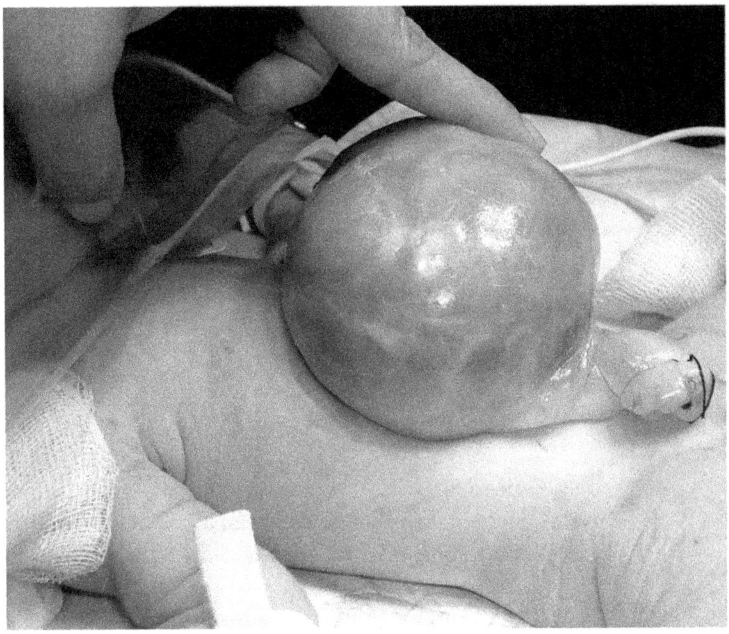

**Figure 18.5** A neonate with exomphalos major.

the sac has ruptured. The defect may involve only minor herniation of the bowel (exomphalos minor) or may be large (> 4 cm diameter) and contain a herniated liver (exomphalos major). Giant exomphalos describes defects > 6 cm diameter. Associated congenital anomalies are common (> 50% of children) and include chromosomal abnormalities (trisomies 13, 18 and 21) and structural abnormalities, such as other midline defects and major cardiac defects. Beckwith–Wiedemann syndrome, an abnormality of chromosome 11 associated with gigantism, macroglossia, pancreatic islet cell hyperplasia with hyperinsulinism, organomegaly and hemihypertrophy, occurs in around 15% of cases. Exomphalos major is associated with pulmonary hypoplasia.

### Surgery and Anaesthesia

The perioperative management for both of these abdominal wall defects is broadly similar. Initial management is supportive, with IV fluids, broad-spectrum antibiotics and an NG tube to decompress the stomach. Either a gas induction (avoiding nitrous oxide) or a gentle IV induction, followed by full muscle relaxation and ventilation, should be employed.

In exomphalos minor, the surgeon will attempt to reduce the herniated contents and close the defect in a single operation. In exomphalos major and gastroschisis, surgical closure in one stage may result in diaphragmatic dysfunction and compartment syndrome. Consequently, the bowel is placed in a temporary silo (prolene mesh sac), which is sutured to the abdominal wall. The anaesthetist and surgeon must work closely together to decide which option is the most preferable as determined by changes in lung compliance and gas exchange. Full muscle relaxation is essential at this stage. Some centres measure abdominal compartment pressure, for example with intravesical or intragastric pressure monitoring, to aid decision-making.

In the immediate postoperative period, these neonates should remain intubated and ventilated, particularly if primary closure has been performed. An opioid infusion for analgesia is usual. Many surgeons will request muscle relaxation for the first 24 hours after surgery. The silo is suspended above the baby to allow the bowel to be reduced under gravity, and a series of silo 'tucks' are performed on NICU over subsequent days (see Figure 18.6), facilitating early extubation. The baby then returns to theatre three to five days later for formal abdominal wall closure. Gut motility is commonly impaired after reduction of gastroschisis, and parenteral nutrition is commonly required.

## Necrotising Enterocolitis

Necrotising enterocolitis (NEC) is predominantly a disease of prematurity and is covered in Chapter 19.

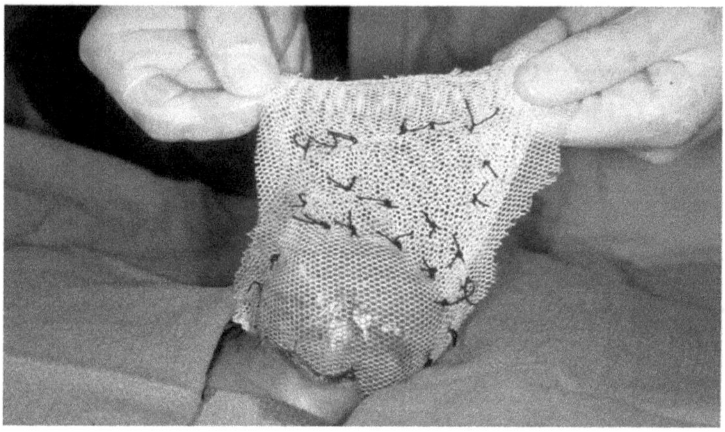

**Figure 18.6** Management of gastroschisis with silo and sequential tucks.

## Sacrococcygeal Teratoma

Sacrococcygeal teratoma (SCT) occurs in 1-2:40,000 live births. It is the most common neonatal tumour and is more frequently seen in females. Structurally, SCTs are classified as cystic (15%), solid (majority) or mixed. Perinatal mortality is around 30% and is more likely in rapidly growing vascular teratomas that act as arteriovenous malformations. These malformations lead to hydrops, high-output cardiac failure, preterm birth, and death. Caesarean section is indicated for large tumours to avoid rupture. At delivery, 90% of SCTs are benign, but 75% are malignant by one year of age if not resected. At birth, 90% are external midline sacral masses. Investigations should be performed to define the borders of the mass within the pelvis. Complications relate to vascularity, size and position of the teratomas.

### Anaesthesia

Excision of SCT is high-risk surgery as it can haemorrhage acutely and dramatically. The perioperative risks relate to major haemorrhage from the highly vascular tumour in neonates who may be preterm and have pulmonary hypertension, high-output cardiac failure, coagulopathy and renal and hepatic impairment.

Once the airway is secured, arterial and central venous access is established, and the bladder is catheterised. The neonate is then turned prone, so vascular lines must be adequate and secure, as access to the baby will be limited. It is essential to plan for major blood loss, with cross-matched blood and blood products readily available. Intraoperative cardiac arrest has been reported from hyperkalaemia and hypocalcaemia secondary to massive blood transfusion. Hyperkalaemia has also been associated with surgical manipulation of a necrotic tumour. Blood must be transfused slowly, ideally via a peripheral cannula (not via a central line), particularly if the blood is not fresh; ideally fresh blood should be available. At the end of surgery, the neonate should be transferred to NICU in the prone position.

### Surgery

The coccyx should be removed with the tumour for a complete excision. If the tumour has a small intrapelvic component, it should be resectable in the prone position. An abdominal approach may be indicated for larger intrapelvic tumours or in cases where early vascular control is required.

**Key Points**

- Neonates have specific physiological and pharmacological requirements.
- Congenital abnormalities requiring general surgery are often associated with cardiac and other anomalies.
- Neonatal anaesthesia is high risk and should be undertaken in specialist centres.
- Postoperative apnoea is common following neonatal surgery; many of these patients will require postoperative ventilatory support.
- Multimodal analgesia should be used for pain management.
- Vascular access can be challenging in neonates. Lines should be removed when they are no longer required.

## Further Reading


Ahmad N, Dobby N, Walker E et al. A multicenter audit of the use of bronchoscopy during open and thoracoscopic repair of esophageal atresia with tracheoesophageal fistula. *Pediatric Anesthesia* 2019; 29:640–7.

Arumainathan R, Stendall C, Visram A. Management of fluids in neonatal surgery. *BJA Education* 2018; 18:199–203.

Brindle ME, McDiarmid C, Short K et al. Consensus guidelines for perioperative care in neonatal intestinal surgery: enhanced recovery after surgery (ERAS®) recommendations. *World Journal of Surgery* 2020; 44:2482–92.

Cross K, Smith J Walker I. Thoracoabdominal and general surgery. In: Lerman J, ed. *Neonatal Anesthesia*. Springer, 2015; 225–71.

Gleich SJ, Wong AV, Handlogten KS, Thum DE, Nemergut, ME. Major short-term complications of arterial cannulation for monitoring in children. *Anesthesiology* 2021; 134:26–34.

Hartley C, Moultrie F, Hoskin, A et al. Analgesic efficacy and safety of morphine in the Procedural Pain in Premature Infants (POPPI) study: randomised placebo-controlled trial. *Lancet* 2018; 392:2595–605.

McCann ME, De Graaff JC, Dorris L et al. Neurodevelopmental outcome at 5 years of age after general anaesthesia or awake-regional anaesthesia in infancy (GAS): an international, multicentre, randomised, controlled equivalence trial. *Lancet* 2019; 393:664–77.

Quinney M, Wellesley H. Anaesthetic management of patients with a congenital diaphragmatic hernia. *BJA Education* 2018; 18(4):95–101.

Veyckemans F, Anderson BJ, Wolf AR, Allegaert K. Intravenous paracetamol dosage in the neonate and small infant. *British Journal of Anaesthesia* 2014; 112:380–1.

Walker SM. Neonatal pain. *Paediatric Anaesthia* 2014; 24:39–48.

Chapter 19

# The Premature and Ex-Premature Infant*

Joy Dawes

## Introduction

The impact of prematurity can be lifelong, and although the risk of acute complications decreases throughout infancy and early childhood, long-term morbidity remains high. Low gestational age at birth is an independent risk factor for increased mortality from respiratory, cardiovascular, endocrine and congenital disorders in childhood and early adulthood. This chapter will describe the clinical manifestations unique to the premature and ex-premature infant and specific considerations for anaesthetic management in this particularly vulnerable group.

## Definitions

Definitions from the American Association of Pediatrics (AAP) are as follows:

- Gestational age: time from the first day of the last normal menstrual period to the day of delivery.
- Conceptional age: time between conception and day of delivery.
- Chronological age: time elapsed since birth.
- Postmenstrual age (PMA): gestational age + chronological age. Used to describe age during the perinatal hospital stay. For example, a baby born at 28 weeks who is now four weeks of age has a PMA of 32 weeks.
- Corrected age: chronological age reduced by the number of weeks born before 40 weeks of gestation. Used to describe the age of children who were born preterm up to the age of three years. For example, a baby born at 28 weeks who has a chronological age of 6 months has a corrected age of (26 weeks – (40–28 weeks) = 14 weeks.

* Many thanks to Dr Isabeau Walker, who wrote the first edition of this book chapter, much of the content of which has been used in this revision.

**Table 19.1** Terminology used for classification of preterm neonates

| Terminology based on gestational age | |
|---|---|
| Full term neonate | 37–42 weeks' gestation and age <1 month |
| Premature neonate | <37 weeks' gestation |
| Extreme preterm neonate | <28 weeks' gestation |
| Terminology based on weight | |
| Low birth weight (LBW) | <2,500 g |
| Very low birth weight (VLBW) | <1,500 g |
| Extremely low birth weight (ELBW) | <1,000 g |

The terminology used to describe neonates and preterms is based on either gestational age or weight (Table 19.1).

## Risk Factors for Premature Delivery

Risk factors for premature delivery include maternal factors, complications of pregnancy and fetal factors:

### Maternal Factors

- Maternal age <17 or >35 years of age
- Lower socioeconomic status
- BMI <19 kg $m^{-2}$ or pre-pregnancy weight <50 kg
- Previous preterm birth
- Prior cervical surgery or uterine anomalies

### Pregnancy Factors

- Multiple gestation
- Vaginal bleeding
- Oligo- or polyhydramnios

- Chorioamnionitis
- Maternal medical conditions: hypertension, diabetes, thyroid disease, asthma
- Maternal abdominal surgery during pregnancy
- Adverse behaviours: smoking, heavy alcohol consumption, cocaine, heroin

**Fetal Factors**

- Chromosome anomaly, structural abnormality, intrauterine growth restriction (IUGR)

## Clinical Consequences of Premature Delivery

Preterm birth is relatively common, occurring in 5–18% of births worldwide. The clinical consequences of prematurity depend on the gestational age at birth and any underlying abnormalities that may have resulted in premature delivery. All bodily systems may be affected as important aspects of development are not yet complete.

## Thermoregulatory Instability

Rapid heat loss can occur in preterm neonates because of their large body surface area to body weight ratio and limited heat production through brown fat metabolism. Heat loss is by increased thermal conductance, increased evaporation through non-keratinised skin, convection and radiation. Hypothermia is associated with intraventricular haemorrhage (IVH), pulmonary insufficiency and coagulopathy and may contribute to metabolic disorders such as hypoglycaemia or acidosis.

## Respiratory Abnormalities

- Respiratory distress syndrome (RDS) occurs in 60% of infants born at <30 weeks of age and is caused by immaturity of the lungs and surfactant deficiency. It presents with increased work of breathing, cyanosis and 'grunting'. The chest X-ray (CXR) shows widespread atelectasis with a granular appearance and widespread air bronchograms. Histologically, the lungs contain hyaline membranes, hence the previous terminology of hyaline membrane disease. RDS may be complicated by air leak (pneumothorax, pneumomediastinum, pulmonary interstitial emphysema) and is the precursor to bronchopulmonary dysplasia. Antenatal corticosteroids are given to mothers in preterm labour to induce surfactant production, which is associated with improved outcomes from RDS. Additionally, exogenous surfactant is administered prophylactically to infants <28 weeks gestation within hours of birth or as rescue in RDS. The strategy for ventilation in premature infants is to minimise ventilator induced lung injury. High-frequency oscillatory ventilation (HFOV) is used to reduce barotrauma and oxygen requirements. Inhaled nitric oxide (iNO) may be used as rescue therapy but may increase IVH and does not appear to improve long-term outcomes.
- Bronchopulmonary dysplasia (BPD), also known as chronic lung disease (CLD), is a late respiratory complication that occurs in 15–50% of VLBW infants. It is defined as oxygen dependency at 36 weeks PMA. Early CXR changes include a ground glass appearance, later progressing to patchy atelectasis, cystic changes, hyperexpansion and areas of emphysema. Long-term intubation and positive pressure ventilation are avoided if possible, as they are more likely to be associated with barotrauma, oxygen toxicity and the development of BPD. Postnatal steroids have been found to have adverse effects on development of the brain in premature infants and are no longer recommended to facilitate weaning from prolonged ventilation. BPD is associated with long-term morbidity that continues into later life. Infants may remain oxygen dependent for many months, although it is unusual to require oxygen after two years of age.
- Apnoea of prematurity occurs in approximately 25% of premature infants and 90% of ELBW infants. It is defined as a pause in breathing of more than 20 seconds or a pause associated with bradycardia and/or desaturation. Apnoeas may be:
  - Central: due to brainstem or peripheral chemoreceptor immaturity.
  - Obstructive: due to reduced airway tone, asynchrony of diaphragmatic or upper airway activity, excessive neck flexion or structural abnormalities.
  - Mixed: central and obstructive. This is the most common type.

Premature infants respond to hypoxia by a brief increase in ventilation followed by apnoea

and have a blunted response to hypercapnia. Apnoea may have a number of triggers, including hypoxia, sepsis, intracranial haemorrhage, metabolic abnormalities, hypo/hyperthermia, upper airway obstruction, heart failure, anaemia, vasovagal reflexes and drugs (including prostaglandins and anaesthetic agents). Central control of ventilation matures with age, and normal responses to hypercapnia and hypoxia (increased ventilation) are seen by three weeks of age in term infants.
- Pulmonary haemorrhage occurs most commonly in ELBW infants and is associated with increased mortality.

## Cardiovascular Abnormalities

- Patent ductus arteriosus (PDA). The ductus arteriosus is one of the fetal shunts and usually closes in response to increased oxygen tension and a fall in circulating prostaglandins by 48 hours in the majority of babies. Patent ductus arteriosus is common in preterm neonates, occurring in approximately 30% of VLBW infants due to low oxygen tension, continuing high prostaglandin levels, acidosis or expansion of the circulating volume. The PDA shunts blood from left to right, resulting in increased flow through the pulmonary circulation, decreased perfusion of the systemic circulation and a low diastolic pressure. PDA typically becomes symptomatic when pulmonary vascular resistance (PVR) falls at 5–10 days. Clinical manifestations include increased work of breathing and ventilatory requirements, bounding pulses, a continuous murmur with cardiomegaly and increased vascular markings seen on CXR. Diagnosis is confirmed by echocardiography. The physiologic consequences of the PDA depend upon the size of the shunt and the response of the heart and lungs to the shunt. Significant shunting may present with apnoea, respiratory distress or heart failure. Treatment for symptomatic PDA includes fluid restriction, diuretics and 'medical closure' with indomethacin, ibuprofen or paracetamol. Surgical closure is indicated if medical management fails or NSAIDs are contraindicated.

## Central Nervous System Abnormalities

- Germinal matrix haemorrhage and intraventricular haemorrhage (GMH-IVH) usually occurs within the first few days of life due to germinal matrix fragility and disturbances of cerebral blood flow. The risk is inversely proportional to gestational age, as cerebral autoregulation has not yet developed and it is an important cause of brain injury in premature infants. Risk factors for IVH include hypotension, fluctuating blood pressure, hypoxia and hypocapnia. GMH-IVH is classified into four grades:
  - Grade I: germinal matrix haemorrhage
  - Grade II: IVH without ventricular enlargement
  - Grade III: IVH with ventricular enlargement
  - Periventricular haemorrhagic infarction (PVHI, previously Grade IV): IVH with extension into the periventricular white matter

  Patients with severe GMH-IVH (grades III and PVHI) have poorer neurodevelopmental outcomes. Management is supportive and focused on reducing further brain injury through preservation of cerebral perfusion and oxygenation; providing appropriate fluid, metabolic and nutritional support; and treating seizures.

  Post haemorrhagic ventricular dilatation (PHVD), the most common complication, occurs in approximately 25% of infants with GMH-IVH. Management involves early identification with regular cranial ultrasounds and intervention based on evidence of progressive dilatation. Neurosurgical intervention consists of temporising procedures such as serial lumbar punctures, ventricular access devices, ventricular reservoirs or subgaleal shunts. Subgaleal shunts reduce the need for daily CSF aspiration and prolong the time period before permanent shunt placement.
- Periventricular leukomalacia (PVL) describes histological changes in periventricular white matter seen in premature infants. It is associated with hypoxic-ischaemic injury, infection, impaired cerebral autoregulation,

cerebral 'steal' due to a large PDA and severe hypocapnia. Bilateral occipital cystic PVL is a very strong predictor of cerebral palsy, particularly spastic diplegia.

- Retinopathy of prematurity (ROP) is a developmental proliferative vascular disorder that occurs in the retina of preterm infants with incomplete retinal vascularisation. It is predominantly seen in LBW infants <32 weeks' gestation and is a common cause of potentially preventable childhood blindness worldwide. Risk factors for ROP are not completely understood; hyperoxia in the newborn period seems to increase the risk, with increased oxygen free radical activity believed to be an underlying mechanism. However, supplemental oxygen alone is not sufficient or required to cause ROP, and no 'safe' threshold for oxygen has been determined.

  ROP is classified into stages 1–5 according to four features: zone, stage, extent and presence or absence of 'plus' disease (vascular congestion and dilatation). Good neonatal care and ophthalmic screening and treatment can largely prevent ROP. However, 6% of premature babies have advanced disease (grades 3–5) and require intervention. Treatment consists of retinal ablative therapy (laser photocoagulation or cryotherapy) or intravitreal injection of an anti-vascular endothelial growth factor (VEGF) agent. In the later stages, other treatment options include scleral buckle or vitrectomy.

## Gastrointestinal Abnormalities

- Necrotising enterocolitis (NEC) is a disease of prematurity and is associated with a high mortality. The risk of death increases with decreasing gestational age. It is associated with ischaemia or hypoxic injury to gut mucosa causing inflammation and transmural necrosis, affecting any part of the intestine but typically the terminal ileum, caecum or ascending colon. The severity of disease may be described using the modified Bell staging criteria (stages 1–3). NEC is associated with early feeding with formula milk and colonisation with pathogenic bacteria. It typically presents with abdominal distension, bloody stool and bilious aspirates during the second or third week of life when full feeds are commenced. Signs of sepsis may predominate and progress to apnoea with shock and disseminated intravascular coagulation. Abdominal X-ray shows thickened dilated bowel loops with intramural gas. Free gas indicates gut perforation and a poor outcome. There may be thrombocytopenia, coagulopathy, raised inflammatory markers and metabolic acidosis.

  Medical management includes fluid resuscitation with or without inotropes, correction of deranged clotting and platelets, parenteral nutrition (PN) and antibiotics. Fifty per cent of neonates with NEC require surgery due to perforation or failure of medical management. Surgical options include resection of necrotic bowel and formation of proximal stoma and distal mucous fistula, gut resection with primary anastomosis or proximal defunctioning jejunostomy and 'second look' at 24 hours if critically ill. Prognosis of NEC has improved with earlier recognition and treatment, with survival rates of approximately 70–80% in affected infants. Long-term complications include short bowel syndrome, intestinal strictures, poor growth and impaired neurodevelopmental outcome. However, approximately half of survivors have no significant sequelae.

## Metabolic Abnormalities

- Hypoglycaemia. Hepatic glycogen stores develop in the last few weeks of gestation, and therefore premature infants are prone to hypoglycaemia (blood glucose <2.6 mmol $l^{-1}$) if exogenous glucose is not delivered. Maintenance fluids with 10% dextrose are usually required with added sodium after 24 hours. Hyperglycaemia can also have adverse consequences, including osmotic diuresis, IVH and ROP.

## Haematological and Coagulation Abnormalities

- Anaemia of prematurity (AOP). The haematocrit falls soon after birth in newborn infants, predominantly due to impaired production of erythropoietin. The decline occurs earlier and is more pronounced in preterm infants and is referred to as AOP. Premature infants have a lower haemoglobin concentration (130–150 g $l^{-1}$) compared to term infants (180–200 g $l^{-1}$). They are at particular risk of impaired oxygen delivery due to the increased likelihood of concomitant respiratory disease, higher concentrations of haemoglobin F (70–80%) and the need to avoid hyperoxia, which increases the risk of BPD and ROP.

- Coagulation abnormalities. The activity of vitamin K–dependent clotting factors in preterm infants is approximately 30% that of adult levels, and plasma concentrations are significantly lower at birth. Neonatal coagulation reference ranges for healthy preterm and term neonates should be used. Prophylactic transfusion of fresh frozen plasma (FFP) to correct abnormalities is not usually required unless bleeding is encountered. All neonates are given a dose of vitamin K after birth to prevent vitamin K–deficient bleeding (previously known as haemorrhagic disease of the newborn).

## Infection

- Sepsis is a major cause of morbidity and mortality in premature infants and is associated with increased likelihood of poor neurodevelopmental outcome and growth impairment. It may present with non-specific signs, including hypothermia, hyperthermia, tachycardia, bradycardia, apnoea, increased oxygen requirements, metabolic acidosis or feeding problems. A decrease in platelet count of >30% is frequently seen, for which the differential diagnosis is IVH or NEC. Early onset infection is usually acquired from the mother, such as Group B streptococci and *Escherichia coli*. Nosocomial infections, such as *Staphylococcus aureus*, Klebsiella or Pseudomonas, often present after the first week of life. Late onset infection may be due to *Candida albicans* or Gram-negative organisms, particularly in association with indwelling catheters.

## Outcomes

Advances in neonatal intensive care have extended the survival of preterm infants such that around 50% of babies born at 24 weeks and around 90% of those born at 27 weeks survive; however, the levels of morbidity are high. Outcomes are better in female infants, singleton pregnancies and when antenatal steroids have been given. ELBW neonates are more susceptible to complications. First year survival for babies with a birth weight of <500 g is approximately 15%, 500–749 g is 50% and >750 g is 85%.

## Conduct of Anaesthesia in the Premature Infant

### Preoperative Assessment and Preparation

Anaesthesia and surgery in the premature neonate are high risk. Evidence-based guidelines on how best to anaesthetise this patient group are lacking. Close collaboration with the neonatologists and careful attention to detail is required. Consent should be discussed with the parents in accordance with GMC guidance and questions answered fully.

Operative location: For the ELBW and LBW infants, it is advantageous for surgery to take place on NICU. This reduces the need for transfer and handling, minimising heat loss; enables ventilation to continue on the neonatal ventilator; and provides ready availability of the neonatal team. If these vulnerable infants must be taken to theatre, the utmost care should be taken not to displace intravenous lines or the tracheal tube (TT) during transport and positioning.

Temperature control: Provide under-warming with either a 3M Bair Hugger® or TransWarmer®, warm the theatre environment to 25°C, minimise heat loss (use a heat moisture exchanger and cover the head), warm IV fluids and use clear surgical drapes (lightweight, to improve visualisation of baby and TT during surgery). Take care when removing drapes to preserve fragile skin.

Monitoring: Check that monitoring is reliable as access to the baby will be limited once surgery is under way. Two oxygen saturation probes should be placed: one preductal on the right hand and the other postductal. End-tidal $CO_2$ monitoring is mandatory; however, this may significantly under-read. Transcutaneous $CO_2$ monitoring provides a very useful trend, particularly where changes in lung compliance are anticipated. Ensure that an appropriately sized blood pressure (BP) cuff is used. Measure core temperature either nasally or rectally. Near-infrared spectroscopy (NIRS) may provide another useful 'trend monitor'; however, it is not properly validated in neonates <2.5 kg, and specific thresholds for intervention are not known.

Vascular access: Invasive monitoring is extremely useful in the septic baby requiring inotropes or when cardiovascular instability is anticipated. The ability to take blood samples intraoperatively is the gold standard but is not always possible. Due consideration must be given when inserting arterial lines in premature infants due to the risk of thrombosis and distal ischaemia. Anaesthetists should aim to preserve peripheral veins, as neonatal long lines are likely to be required for PN. Extension lines with three-way taps should be placed on all cannulae and should be bubble-free.

## Intraoperative Management

Airway: Premature neonates will often be intubated and ventilated already. An oral uncuffed TT of 2.5–3 mm internal diameter is usual. If intubation is required, checklists are helpful to ensure that all staff are fully prepared. Once the TT is secure, check the position meticulously as minor changes in head position may result in endobronchial intubation or accidental extubation. Recheck the position every time the baby is moved. Use equipment with as little dead space as possible.

Ventilation: Ventilation may be provided via a neonatal ventilator or HFOV on NICU, or an anaesthetic machine in theatre. Ventilatory strategies should aim to avoid hyperventilation, $SpO_2$ > 95%, high peak inspiratory pressures and barotrauma. Permissive hypercapnia is acceptable. The baby may need to be hand ventilated via an Ayres T piece if compliance is variable. An air/oxygen mix should be used and hyperoxia avoided.

The optimal $SpO_2$ for preterm infants who receive supplemental oxygen therapy has not been fully established. However, based on the available evidence, the most prudent target range is between 90–95%. This range minimises both the low and high extreme oxygenation levels that have been associated with adverse outcomes and mortality.

Circulation: It is important to avoid haemodynamic instability and conditions that impair cerebral autoregulation, such as hypotension and fluctuations in BP. Hypotension due to hypovolaemia (e.g. acute blood loss) should be treated with volume expansion, taking care to avoid excessive volume loading. Fluid shifts up to 60–80 ml $kg^{-1}$ may be significant in laparotomy for NEC but will vary according to the type of surgery. Isotonic fluids should be used (0.9% saline, Hartmann's or Ringer's lactate) given as boluses of 10 ml $kg^{-1}$ and titrated to BP, heart rate, capillary refill time and base excess. However, in many cases, volume expansion alone is insufficient to maintain adequate BP levels, and inotropic therapy is required.

Blood should be transfused to maintain a Hct of 35–45% in newborn infants, replacing calcium as necessary. Babies with NEC may require blood, platelets, FFP and cryoprecipitate during surgery. The World Society of Surgery suggests a target Hb of 110 g $l^{-1}$ for neonates with an oxygen requirement or those that are ventilated.

Blood glucose should be monitored regularly and glucose-containing maintenance fluids continued during surgery. This fluid should not be used for bolus administration. Usual rates for preterms are 100 ml $kg^{-1}day^{-1}$ or 4–5 ml $kg^{-1}hr^{-1}$.

Anaesthesia and analgesia: Volatile anaesthesia can be provided if surgery is being undertaken in theatre. If operating in NICU, continuation of morphine infusions with additional fentanyl boluses is usual. Intraoperative remifentanil may be a useful alternative. Some anaesthetists will also give boluses of ketamine, with the rationale that surgical stress and unmanaged pain is likely to have more deleterious effects than any concerns about neurotoxicity. Multimodal analgesia is favoured. Paracetamol should be dosed according to gestational age with special care taken to avoid accidental overdose. Regional anaesthesia is particularly useful if extubation is planned at the end of surgery. A morphine nurse-controlled analgesia (NCA) can be set up with NICU settings (smaller boluses, no background if <5 kg).

Neurotoxicity: The effect of anaesthetic drugs such as midazolam, isoflurane and ketamine on the developing brain have been investigated in the last decade. These agents were found to cause widespread apoptosis with persistent memory and learning impairment in animal models. The existence of an association between general anaesthesia at a young age and subsequent neurodevelopmental deficits has not been fully elucidated; however, the GAS study has shown no association at five years follow-up. The relevance to clinical practice in other settings remains unclear, but only essential surgery should be performed in early life.

## Postoperative Management

A thorough handover to NICU is mandatory, with all members of the multidisciplinary team present. Extremely premature neonates will usually remain intubated and ventilated until a time when they can safely be weaned from invasive ventilation.

# Conduct of Anaesthesia in the Ex-Premature Infant

## Preoperative Assessment

Clinical features of ex-premature infants include:

- Ongoing oxygen requirements, CLD with reduced lung compliance, asthma, tracheomalacia, susceptibility to respiratory infection
- Acquired subglottic stenosis (SGS) as a consequence of prolonged intubation in infancy
- Residual shunts or pulmonary hypertension
- Gastro-oesophageal reflux disease
- Neurodevelopmental delay and/or seizures
- Impaired renal concentrating ability
- Chronic anaemia
- Failure to thrive

## Intraoperative Management

- Anticipate difficulty with vascular access.
- A smaller TT size may be required if SGS is present.
- Ventilation may be difficult with cases of CLD, particularly in laparoscopic surgery.
- The infant may have increased sensitivity to opioids.
- Use regional blocks where possible. Spinal anaesthesia for inguinal hernia repair may be suitable in experienced hands and can reduce postoperative apnoeas, provided supplemental sedation is avoided.

## Postoperative Management

- Ex-premature infants are susceptible to postoperative apnoeas up to 60 weeks PMA and may require nasal continuous positive airway pressure (CPAP) or ventilation after surgery. Local protocols regarding postoperative destination, apnoea monitoring and overnight stay should be in place.

### Key Points

- The impact of premature birth is lifelong, affects multiple organ systems and is associated with reduced life expectancy.
- Modern neonatal intensive care has improved survival of extremely premature and low birth weight babies, although problems associated with CLD, poor growth and developmental delay are common.
- Premature babies commonly present for surgery in association with PDA, NEC or ROP.
- Surgery is high risk, and close collaboration with the neonatal team is required to ensure the baby is in optimal condition for surgery.
- Ex-premature infants may have a wide range of disabilities and be susceptible to postoperative apnoeas. Poor venous access should be expected.

## Further Reading


Arumainathan R, Stendall C, Visram A. Management of fluids in neonatal surgery. *BJA Education* 2018; 18:199–203.

Brindle ME, McDiarmid C, Short K et al. Consensus guidelines for perioperative care in neonatal intestinal surgery: enhanced recovery after surgery (ERAS®) recommendations. *World Journal of Surgery* 2020; 44:2482–92.

Cummings JJ, Polin RA, Committee on Fetus and Newborn. Oxygen targeting in extremely low birthweight infants. *Pediatrics* 2016; 138: e20161576.

Jones LJ, Craven PD, Lakkundi A, Foster JP, Badawi N. Regional (spinal, epidural, caudal) versus general anaesthesia in preterm infants undergoing inguinal herniorrhaphy in early infancy (review). *Cochrane Database of Systematic Reviews* 2015; 6: CD003669.

Lonnqvist P. A different perspective: anaesthesia for extreme premature infants: is there an age limitation or how low should we go? *Current Opinion in Anesthesiology* 2018; 31: 308–12.

Mandy GT, Martin R, Kim MS. Short term complications of the premature infant. Available at: www.uptodate.com/contents/

overview-of-short-term-complications-in-preterm-infants. Accessed 18 March 2024.

McCann ME et al. Neurodevelopmental outcome at 5 years of age after general anaesthesia or awake-regional anaesthesia in infancy (GAS): an international, multicentre, randomised, controlled equivalence trial. *Lancet* 2019; 393: 664–77.

Pang LM, Sun LS, Crowley M. Anaesthesia for ex-premature infants and children. Available at: www.uptodate.com/contents/anesthesia-for-ex-premature-infants-and-children. Accessed 21 March 2024.

Chapter

# 20 Anaesthesia for General Surgery in Children

Alice Miskovic and Usman Ali

## Introduction

Children presenting for general paediatric surgery range in both age and complexity from neonates undergoing hernia repair, to older children undergoing appendicectomy or excision of extensive neuroblastoma. Many patients presenting with congenital defects will require surgery in the neonatal period. Specific issues related to anaesthesia for neonatal surgery are discussed in Chapter 18. In this chapter, we provide an overview of general surgery for infants and children after the neonatal period.

## Anaesthesia

For elective cases, breast-fed babies need only be fasted for three hours, whereas for babies receiving formula milk the usual six hours should apply. Clear fluids may be given up to one hour preoperatively. Clear fluids are defined as water, clear non-opaque fruit juice or squash/cordial, ready diluted drinks and non-fizzy sports drinks. Fluids must be non-thickened and non-carbonated. The maximum volume of clear fluids is 3 ml $kg^{-1}$.

Most general surgery in children is best managed by tracheal intubation and ventilation. Supraglottic airway devices can be used for shorter cases where aspiration risk is deemed low.

The minimum alveolar concentration (MAC) for all the volatile agents is slightly higher in neonates than adults, increasing with age to reach a maximum at one to six months of age before declining over the rest of life. It is common to use sevoflurane for induction and then either sevoflurane or isoflurane for maintenance. A balanced technique using fentanyl will enable a lower dose of volatile agents to be given, although high-dose opioid techniques may increase the likelihood of needing postoperative ventilation.

Some anaesthetists advocate the use of spinal anaesthesia for surgical procedures such as inguinal hernia repair to avoid any disadvantages posed by general anaesthesia; when used, surgery must be completed within one hour of the spinal. Ultrasound guided transverse abdominus plane (TAP), quadratus lumborum, rectus sheath and ilioinguinal blocks are being increasingly used as part of perioperative analgesia for general surgical procedures.

Venous capacitance is relatively low in neonates and infants, and arterial blood pressure will often fall in the face of a small drop in circulating volume. For major cases, an arterial line is indicated.

Finally, maintaining normothermia is a challenge for major general surgical cases. Forced air warmers or overhead heaters should be used during induction and siting of lines, and fluid warmers and forced-air warming mattresses should both be used intraoperatively.

## Postoperative Analgesia

After major surgery, analgesia may be achieved by intravenous nurse- or patient-controlled analgesia (NCA/PCA). Morphine increases the risk of postoperative apnoea. An additional background infusion may be added if required. Ibuprofen is not licensed for use below three months of age.

Epidurals work well even in very young children and may avoid a need for postoperative ventilation. Due to lower levels of plasma-binding proteins in younger children and neonates (in particular, alpha-1 glycoprotein), higher free plasma levels of local anaesthetic are possible. Our preference is to use plain 0.125% levobupivacaine, up to 0.4 ml $kg^{-1}$ $h^{-1}$.

## Laparoscopic Surgery

An increasing number of procedures are carried out laparoscopically, including Nissen fundoplication, inguinal hernia repair, appendicectomy, colectomy and pyloromyotomy, as well as primary neonatal surgical procedures.

Anaesthesia considerations for laparoscopic surgery are as follows:

*Increased intra-abdominal pressure.* A cuffed or snug-fitting tracheal tube should be used to facilitate ventilation in the face of possible reduced respiratory compliance.

*The insufflation gas.* This is almost always carbon dioxide; systemic absorption can rapidly lead to high arterial partial pressure of carbon dioxide, $P_aCO_2$. This should be monitored regularly, with either arterial sampling or using a transcutaneous $CO_2$ monitor. It may be necessary to deflate the abdomen periodically to enable $CO_2$ to be cleared, or sometimes to convert to an open procedure, particularly in small children with poor lung function such as those with congenital diaphragmatic hernia (CDH).

*Cardiovascular consequences.* Increased intra-abdominal pressure may reduce venous return and may also stimulate vagal reflexes because of peritoneal stretching. This may be relevant in neonates and children with congenital heart disease, such as those with a single ventricle circulation who are dependent on venous return for adequate pulmonary blood flow and cardiac output.

*Temperature.* The insufflation gas is cold. Body temperature needs to be monitored, and the child should be kept warm in the usual ways.

*Gas embolism.* This should be considered if there is a sudden drop in the end-tidal carbon dioxide level.

*Inadvertent gastric perforation.* Insertion of a nasogastric tube to deflate the stomach prior to insertion of the trocar will help reduce this risk. Nitrous oxide must not be used.

# Specific Conditions

## Pyloric Stenosis

Pyloric stenosis is due to hypertrophy of the pyloric sphincter and leads to gastric outlet obstruction. It occurs in approximately one in 500 live births. It classically presents with projectile vomiting in the immediate postneonatal period, but only rarely after the age of six months. These babies develop metabolic alkalosis with hypochloraemia as a result of losing hydrochloric acid from the gastric contents. Untreated, they can become severely dehydrated. Renal compensation includes excretion of bicarbonate ions along with sodium. As vomiting continues, renal compensation switches from sodium excretion to excretion of potassium and hydrogen, further worsening the initial alkalosis and causing hypokalaemia with possible hyponatraemia. This is a medical rather than surgical emergency.

- The child needs careful rehydration with 0.45% saline with 5% dextrose at 1.5 times the normal maintenance rate.
- If the baby is hyponatraemic, the deficit should be made up with 0.9% saline until the sodium is in the normal range.
- A bolus of 0.9% saline may be required if the baby is shocked.
- Additional potassium may be needed as guided by capillary or venous gas levels.
- These babies should only be considered for surgery when rehydrated and with a serum chloride level of greater than 100 mmol $l^{-1}$ and serum bicarbonate less than 28 mmol $l^{-1}$. The patient is at risk of postoperative apnoea if surgery is performed before the metabolic alkalosis is resolved.

An umbilical approach is usually taken, although the classic Ramstedt procedure or laparoscopic approach may also be used. The pylorus is incised down to the mucosa. The surgeon may ask for air to be introduced via a nasogastric tube to look for a leak in the mucosal layer. Fentanyl 1–2 mcg $kg^{-1}$ IV, local infiltration and paracetamol usually provide sufficient analgesia. Saturation and respiratory rate should be monitored postoperatively.

## Inguinal Hernia Repair

Inguinal hernias are common in children, occurring in approximately 3% of the paediatric population. This incidence rises to 30% in babies born prematurely. Repair of an obstructed hernia is undertaken as an emergency, and babies should be treated as if they have a full stomach. Effective analgesia for a unilateral repair undertaken as an open procedure is provided by a caudal block or unilateral ilioinguinal/iliohypogastric nerve block. Analgesia for bilateral repair may be provided by bilateral blocks or a caudal using 1.0 ml $kg^{-1}$ of 0.25% levobupivacaine.

## Acute Appendicitis

This is the most common indication for emergency surgery in children. The peak incidence is at 10–12 years of age with a 7% chance of developing the disease during a lifetime. A child younger than 6 years with symptoms for more than 48 hours is more likely to have perforated appendicitis. Urgent surgery is required since peritonitis and sepsis will ensue if left untreated.

- Preoperative rehydration is essential, and these children will often come to the anaesthetic room with intravenous fluid running.
- A modified or rapid sequence induction should be used.
- A nasogastric tube should be considered if one is not present on arrival to the anaesthetic room.
- The operation is commonly performed laparoscopically but can also be open.
- A reliable analgesic regimen consists of 1–2 mcg $kg^{-1}$ of fentanyl followed by a loading dose of 50–100 mcg $kg^{-1}$ of morphine and regular paracetamol with an NSAID.
- Postoperative NCA or PCA should be considered for open procedures.

Local analgesic infiltration or a TAP block may be used for perioperative analgesia, provided contamination of the wound is avoided.

## Intussusception

This usually occurs in children aged from six months to two years but can occur in the neonatal period. Typically, the bowel 'telescopes' in on itself, and the resultant wall oedema causes obstruction. Children usually present with abdominal pain and a palpable mass. They may have rectal bleeding because of mucosal sloughing; the so-called red currant jelly stool. They may require fluid resuscitation and occasionally blood transfusion. The internal herniation can be reduced with a combination of air and saline or contrast enema in the X-ray department in up to 75% of cases, but if this fails then surgical reduction is necessary. Ninety per cent have no identifiable lead point for the apex, but a Meckel diverticulum or polyp should always be sought at laparotomy or laparoscopy.

## Nissen Fundoplication

Gastro-oesophageal reflux disease (GORD) is common in children with neurodevelopmental problems, particularly cerebral palsy, congenital diaphragmatic hernia and tracheoesophageal fistula/oesophageal atresia, although reflux may also occur in healthy children. It may be associated with failure to thrive, oesophagitis, oesophageal stricture and chronic lung disease due to recurrent aspiration. Some infants may have life-threatening aspiration episodes. GORD should be confirmed, for instance by a 24-hour pH probe. If GORD is unresponsive to medical therapy, the child may require Nissen fundoplication. In this procedure, the fundus is wrapped around the lower oesophagus to reinforce the lower oesophageal sphincter. A laparoscopic approach is often preferred, although there is significant soft tissue dissection, and morphine NCA will be required postoperatively. Epidural analgesia is reserved for open cases, particularly for children with chronic lung disease.

## Anorectal Anomaly

Approximately one in 3,000 babies are born with anorectal anomaly; it can be low or high. A low anorectal anomaly is where the anus is closed over, in a slightly different position or narrower than usual. There may also be a fistula to the skin. In high anorectal anomaly, the bowel has a closed end and does not connect with the anus; it may connect with another part of the body, usually the bladder, urethra or vagina, through a fistula. Most children require a series of operations. The first operation is to create a loop stoma or end colostomy usually in the days after birth. The second is a posterior sagittal anorectoplasty (PSARP) operation to join the bowel to a newly created anus. This usually happens when the child is a few months old and has gained weight. The final stage is closure of the stoma. This happens once the child's bowel and anus are working well, a few months after the second operation. The three operations are usually completed by the time the child is six to nine months old. PSARP is a major procedure; it may also require an additional abdominal incision and for the patient to be turned from prone to supine. A flexible reinforced tube should be used, and adequate peripheral vascular access for fluid replacement and transfusion should be sited. An arterial line should be considered if the patient has additional comorbidities. If the spine is anatomically normal, an epidural provides good perioperative analgesia.

## Abdominal Tumours

General surgery is an important component of the multidisciplinary care of children with solid tumours. The common tumours presenting to general surgeons are shown in Table 20.1.

## Neuroblastoma

Neuroblastoma is one of the most common abdominal tumours in children. It usually presents around 2 years of age and is rare after the age of 10 years. Neuroblastoma arises from cells of the sympathetic nervous system, commonly in the adrenal gland, although paraspinal, thoracic, pelvic and cervical primaries may occur. Children usually present with non-specific symptoms of fever, weight loss, fatigue and bone pain. An abdominal primary is present in two-thirds of cases. Metastases to the liver, lymph nodes, bone and bone marrow are common at presentation. Urinary catecholamines, vanillylmandelic acid (VMA) or homovanillic acid (HVA), are raised in 90%, but unlike phaeochromocytoma, persistent hypertension is uncommon. Children with orbital secondaries may present with bilateral 'black eyes', and growth of a paraspinal tumour may present with neurological symptoms due to cord compression. There is an associated paraneoplastic syndrome associated with random eye movements and myoclonic jerks which may not resolve as the tumour is treated. Children less than 18 months may be asymptomatic and present with an incidental finding of thoracic neuroblastoma.

Prognosis depends on age at presentation, tumour biology and tumour spread. The overall survival is only around 65% at five years from presentation, although low-, intermediate- and high-risk groups can be identified. Neuroblastoma is chemosensitive, and most children undergo several cycles of chemotherapy preoperatively, using agents such as cyclophosphamide, doxorubicin, carboplatin and etoposide, followed by surgical excision of residual tumour. Children with high-risk disease may undergo radiotherapy, myeloablative chemotherapy with stem-cell rescue or immunotherapy (see Chapter 37). Infants younger than six months may present with a small primary, with metastatic spread to the skin, liver and bone marrow. This distinct condition is associated with spontaneous resolution without treatment (stage 4S disease).

## Wilms Tumour

Wilms tumour (nephroblastoma) has a similar incidence to neuroblastoma but a much better prognosis. Children usually present with a large, painless abdominal mass, although they may present with pain, occasionally requiring fluid resuscitation, if there is bleeding into the tumour. Tumours may be bilateral, and there may be pulmonary metastases or, in some cases, extension of the tumour into the inferior vena cava (IVC). Five to ten per cent of children have acquired von Willebrand disease and may require treatment with desmopressin (DDAVP) or cryoprecipitate prior to surgery. There is an association between Wilms tumour and Beckwith–Wiedemann

**Table 20.1** Abdominal tumours in children in England 2001–2015

| | Mean number of cases per year | Total number of cases registered 2001–2015 | Percentage total of all cases of malignancy registered |
|---|---|---|---|
| Neuroblastoma | 85 | 1,268 | 6 |
| Wilms tumour | 81 | 1,208 | 5.6 |
| Soft tissue tumours | 91 | 1,369 | 6.4 |
| Germ cell tumours | 47 | 704 | 3.3 |
| Hepatoblastoma | 18 | 267 | 1.25 |

*Source:* Childhood Cancer Statistics, England Annual Report 2018. Public Health England Available at: www.gov.uk/phe.

syndrome. Hypertension is uncommon and is due to compression of the renal artery causing elevated renin levels. It is unusual to require specific antihypertensive agents preoperatively or intraoperatively in these children.

In contrast to neuroblastoma, 90% of children with Wilms tumour have a good prognosis, with five-year survival around 85%. In the United States, surgery may be undertaken before chemotherapy, but in Europe the preference is for treatment with several cycles of chemotherapy using agents such as vincristine, actinomycin-D and doxorubicin, followed by nephrectomy (or heminephrectomy in bilateral Wilms), and radiotherapy in high-risk cases. Children with residual tumour in the IVC after chemotherapy may require surgery on cardiopulmonary bypass. Children who relapse and receive high-dose chemotherapy and/or radiotherapy may be susceptible to late adverse effects of treatment, particularly second neoplasms and cardiomyopathy.

## Anaesthesia and Surgery for Children with Abdominal Tumours

Children with abdominal tumours may present for diagnostic and staging procedures such as CT, MRI, bone marrow and trephine or in some cases tumour biopsy. Most children require long-term intravenous access insertion for chemotherapy. Neuroblastoma cells take up $I^{123/131}$-meta-iodobenzylguanidine (MIBG), which is the basis of MIBG scans to identify primary tumour and metastatic disease in neuroblastoma.

Surgery for tumour excision can be long and difficult, and there is the potential for high fluid requirements and major blood loss. Neuroblastoma commonly encases major vessels such as the aorta and IVC, and Wilms tumours may be very vascular, particularly if the child has not received prior chemotherapy. Preoperative imaging should be reviewed.

If the patient has received preoperative chemotherapy with anthracyclines such as doxorubicin, a recent echocardiogram should be reviewed.

Children usually have a tunneled central line in situ. Intravenous access suitable for rapid transfusion is necessary, and children should be cross-matched with at least two units prior to theatre. Bleeding may occur from the IVC, so vascular access in the upper body is required. Invasive monitoring should be used. Serial arterial blood gases will help guide fluid and blood replacement. Appropriate warming is required, and a urinary catheter should be inserted before laparotomy to allow for accurate measurement of urine output. If possible, an epidural should be sited for intra- and postoperative use, although this is contraindicated in children with paraspinal neuroblastoma or coagulopathy. Most children do not require postoperative ventilation and can be cared for in a high-dependency ward. Fluid balance should be closely monitored, and laboratory blood results reviewed (full blood count, electrolytes). If an epidural has not been used, an NCA/PCA will be necessary; a background infusion may also be required for the first postoperative night.

### Key Points

- Congenital abnormalities requiring general surgery are often associated with cardiac and other pathologies which should be identified as part of preoperative assessment.
- All children having major surgery should have a multidisciplinary team meeting as part of their preoperative care planning.
- Multimodal analgesia should always be provided, and regional anaesthesia should be used where possible as part of the perioperative analgesia plan.

## Additional Reading

Greaney D, Everett T. Paediatric regional anaesthesia: updates in central neuraxial techniques and thoracic and abdominal blocks. *BJA Education* 2019; 19(4):126–34.

McCann ME, De Graff JC, Dorris L. Neurodevelopmental outcome at 5 years of age after general anaesthesia or awake-regional anaesthesia in infancy (GAS): an international, multicentre, randomised, controlled equivalence trial. *Lancet* 2019; 393(10172):664–77.

Whyte SD, Ansermino JM. Anesthetic considerations in the management of Wilms tumor. *Pediatric Anaesthesia* 2006; 16:504–13.

Chapter 21

# Anaesthesia for ENT Surgery in Children

Reema Nandi

## Introduction

Ear, nose and throat (ENT) procedures are amongst the most common operations in children. They present numerous challenges to the anaesthetist, including the shared airway, increased incidence of perioperative respiratory adverse events (PRAE), high incidence of postoperative nausea and vomiting, emergence delirium, numerous day-case procedures, high turnover lists and comorbidities with anaesthetic implications. Airway surgery can be particularly challenging for the anaesthetist and surgeon alike and requires careful preparation, excellent communication and close teamwork as well as a high-level of expertise and flexibility.

## Preoperative Assessment

Preoperative assessment of children undergoing ENT procedures should include information about sleep disordered breathing (SDB), recent upper respiratory tract infections (URTIs) and congenital syndromes, in addition to the usual assessment.

### Obstructive Sleep Disordered Breathing

Obstructive SDB has become the most common indication for adenotonsillectomy. It is a syndrome of upper airway dysfunction during sleep, characterised by snoring and/or increased respiratory effort secondary to upper airway resistance and pharyngeal collapsibility. It is of significance because it is associated with an increased risk of laryngospasm, airway obstruction and oxygen desaturation perioperatively. Children who will benefit from adenotonsillectomy are those with upper airway obstruction whilst awake; abnormal sleep study in combination with SDB symptoms, such as snoring; conditions predisposing to SDB, such as mandibular hypoplasia; SDB and complex conditions, such as Down syndrome, Prader–Willi syndrome; or sickle cell disease associated with obstructive SDB. Notably, obstructive sleep apnoea (OSA) is also associated with an increased sensitivity to the respiratory depressant effect of opioids, which should be used with caution in severe OSA, and their effects monitored postoperatively. Rarely, severe OSA can result in hypoxia, which may lead to pulmonary vasoconstriction, right ventricular hypertrophy and right heart failure requiring high-dependency unit (HDU) management pre- and/or postoperatively.

SDB is measured objectively using polysomnography (PSG) and its severity is determined by the apnoea-hypopnoea index (AHI). The AHI is the number of mixed, obstructive and central apnoeas and hypopnoeas per hour of total sleep and can be predictive of the need for admission and level of postoperative monitoring required. Mild obstructive sleep apnoea syndrome (OSAS) is frequently diagnosed with obstructive AHI one to five episodes per hour, moderate OSAS with obstructive AHI >5–10 episodes per hour and severe OSAS with obstructive AHI >10 episodes per hour. There is little consensus about the admission criteria for children with SDB and OSA, especially in those requiring adenotonsillectomy, and different centres will have their own guidelines for suitability of procedure in their institution and monitoring and admission. A significant practical consideration with the PSG is that it requires an overnight stay in hospital and has limited availability as a result. It is important to remember that severe OSA in small children can limit growth and development, and undue delay of surgery because of poor availability of 'objective' quantification of OSA can be very detrimental. A pragmatic approach is therefore advocated, including history from parents, evidence of failure to thrive and poor growth and general development. Surgery should not be delayed unduly because of the lack of preoperative OSA assessment with PSG. Home-based sleep apnoea testing devices are being investigated as alternatives for the assessment of OSA in children and may assist in risk stratification and better use of resources. This includes the McGill score, which can also be used to stratify the severity of OSA. It ranges from 1 (normal or inconclusive) to 4 (severely abnormal) according to the number of clusters and the depth of desaturation events seen in overnight oximetry. Compared to full polysomnography, the McGill score has a high positive predictive value and a low negative predictive value. The current European Respiratory Society and American Academy of Pediatrics guidelines suggest that an abnormal overnight oximetry based on McGill criteria can accurately detect OSA of at least moderate severity, but a negative result does not exclude OSA with certainty. Children with severe OSA may still develop airway obstruction after surgery due to surgical swelling and the effects of anaesthesia and should be monitored for the first night. According to recent guidelines, clinicians should arrange for overnight, inpatient monitoring of children after tonsillectomy if the child is under three years old or has severe obstructive sleep apnoea (AHI $\geq$10 obstructive events/hour, oxygen saturation nadir $<$80%, or both).

## Upper Respiratory Tract Infections (URTIs)

Children requiring ENT procedures often present with mild to moderate URTIs, and the decision whether to proceed with surgery can be difficult. The airway remains hyperreactive over two weeks after a respiratory tract infection and puts the child at increased risk of a PRAE, such as oxygen desaturation, bronchospasm and laryngospasm. Delaying surgery for two weeks after the resolution of systemic symptoms of URTI, such as fever and malaise, is recommended. A pragmatic approach is required, however, and surgery often proceeds despite the presence of mild URTI without systemic symptoms, as the purpose of the operation, such as a tonsillectomy, is to address the underlying cause of the infections or alleviate their consequences. Some steps, such as less instrumentation of the airway and the use of propofol and total intravenous anaesthesia (TIVA), can be taken to mitigate the risk of the two- or threefold increase in PRAE. Propofol induction and TIVA reduces airway reactivity, laryngospasm, bronchospasm and emergence coughing.

## SARS COVID-19

There have been several publications with guidelines and recommendations for the perioperative management and planning of ENT care in children during the SARS CoV-2 pandemic (COVID-19). Some ENT procedures carry a high risk of generating aerosols (aerosol-generating medical procedures, or AGMP), which need to be taken into consideration when deciding how to care for the patient and to protect the team. Local policies and procedures, which are usually guided by community prevalence, will dictate how each hospital manages issues such as preoperative testing prior to surgery.

## Congenital Anomalies

The commonly encountered congenital, syndromic or genetic anomalies associated with ENT procedures include trisomy 21, craniosynostoses and hemifacial microsomia, children with cleft lip and/or plate and cardiac anomalies. Coagulopathies, although rare, should be considered as they can cause severe morbidity in ENT procedures.

## Myringotomy and Grommet Insertion

Myringotomy with or without grommet insertion is a common and quick day-case procedure for the treatment of persistent middle ear effusions (glue ear) and recurrent otitis media.

The usual preoperative assessment should be conducted, paying particular attention to URTIs, which are common in children undergoing this procedure.

Intraoperatively, the airway can usually be maintained with a supraglottic airway device (SAD) with the child breathing spontaneously. Myringotomy can be very stimulating, and this should be pre-empted with a small dose of intravenous opioid, such as 1 mcg $kg^{-1}$ fentanyl IV. Ondansetron and dexamethasone should be used for antiemesis, and IV paracetamol and a non-steroidal anti-inflammatory drug (NSAID) are useful adjuncts for analgesia.

Analgesic requirements postoperatively are variable, but opioids are usually not required.

## Adenotonsillectomy

Adenotonsillectomy is the most performed operation in children, and the primary indication is now SDB or OSA rather than recurrent tonsillitis. Surgery is usually undertaken as a day case in children over the age of three years without other comorbidities.

Standard preoperative assessment should be made with particular attention to the severity of OSA, as discussed in the section 'Obstructive Sleep Disordered Breathing', and screening for high-risk features that might predict a PRAE, which have an estimated incidence of up to 40% in this population. Previous studies have recommended HDU admission for patients with high-risk features, but recent literature does not support this practice. Patients should be assessed in the postanaesthetic care unit (PACU) for signs of airway obstruction, desaturation or prolonged oxygen requirement and then triaged accordingly.

## Anaesthesia Management for Children Undergoing Adenotonsillectomy

Children undergoing ENT surgery do not often require preoperative sedation, and it should be used with caution in patients with OSA.

A gas induction is commonly used in younger children. If intravenous induction is planned, topical anaesthetic cream should be applied. The airway may become difficult to maintain in severe OSA, particularly at light planes of anaesthesia. The use of a Guedel airway and the application of continuous positive airway pressure (CPAP) is important and will help to maintain the airway until anaesthesia is deepened. After obtaining intravenous access, the airway can be maintained with an oral south-facing Ring-Adair-Elwin (RAE) tracheal tube (TT), micro cuff endotracheal tube (ETT) or flexible SAD. There are some advantages of using a laryngeal mask airway (LMA), such as less pain postoperatively and improved emergence with less coughing and potential for bleeding. However, there is a greater risk of displacement of the SAD than a TT during surgery, particularly in smaller children. This can be especially problematic at the time of placement of the tonsillar gag, which can obstruct any artificial airway. The anaesthetist must be aware of this and alert the surgeon to any airway concerns. Maintenance can be with volatile or TIVA. TIVA has been shown to decrease postoperative nausea and vomiting (PONV) and may also reduce emergence delirium (ED) and PRAE, although these benefits have not been quantified.

There are several techniques for tonsillectomy, and studies continue to debate which is optimal.

Coblation (cold ablation) is a relatively new and increasingly popular tonsillectomy technique because it is associated with a reduction in postoperative pain and intraoperative bleeding. Coblation is operated at surface temperatures (40–70°C) much lower than those of more traditional techniques, minimising the painful damage of surrounding healthy tissue. This reduces postoperative pain and speeds up recovery. Studies suggest that coblation decreases delayed haemorrhage and postoperative pain and does not worsen intraoperative bleeding and reactionary haemorrhage in children undergoing tonsillectomy compared to the more traditional bipolar technique. Coblation also has improved outcomes with respect to tonsillar tissue recovery, reduced thermal damage, reduced need for analgesia and faster return to normal diet. Bipolar diathermy is another technique that has similar pain and morbidity rates to other tonsillectomy techniques like cold dissection tonsillectomy, but it provides significant advantages such as shorter operative time and lower blood loss levels.

Adenotonsillectomy is a painful procedure usually requiring opioids intraoperatively. Care should be taken in children with OSA as they are more sensitive to the respiratory depressant effects of opioids. Small doses of intraoperative morphine (0.05 mg $kg^{-1}$) or fentanyl (1–2 mg $kg^{-1}$) are usually well tolerated. The use of the coblation technique has reduced postoperative pain and made management easier to some extent.

Dual antiemetics of IV ondansetron 0.15 mg $kg^{-1}$ and IV dexamethasone 0.15 mg $kg^{-1}$ are recommended as routine for tonsillectomy and adenoidectomy by the Association of Paediatric Anaesthetists of Great Britain and Ireland. Dexamethasone should be used in all cases unless contraindicated, as there is good evidence for its analgesic properties as well as prophylaxis for PONV.

## Analgesia Following Adenotonsillectomy

The management of posttonsillectomy pain can be challenging and is often inadequate. Tonsillectomy has been identified as one of the most painful surgical procedures, and pain remains poorly managed in clinical practice. The degree of pain is often underestimated as the surgery is minimally invasive and pain assessment in children can be difficult. It involves a unique type of tissue trauma, the exposure of the healing wound to movement of the pharynx during ingestion, the risk of bleeding and limitations in the choice of drugs in children. Despite numerous studies comparing and combining analgesics to find the most effective postoperative regimen, there is still no consensus on the best treatment strategy.

The Procedure-Specific Postoperative Pain Management (PROSPECT) Working Group is an international collaboration of surgeons and anaesthetists working to formulate procedure-specific recommendations for pain management after common but potentially painful operations. The recommendations are based on a procedure-specific systematic review of randomised controlled trials using a standardised methodology. For tonsillectomy, randomised controlled trials published in the English language up to November 2019 assessing postoperative pain using analgesic, anaesthetic or surgical interventions were identified. Approximately one-third (226 of 719) of the potentially eligible randomised control studies met the inclusion criteria.

## PROSPECT Recommendations: Analgesia Following Tonsillectomy

- The basic analgesic regimen should include paracetamol and NSAIDs administered preoperatively or intraoperatively and continued postoperatively.
- A single dose of dexamethasone IV is recommended for its analgesic and antiemetic effects.
- Preoperative gabapentinoids, intraoperative ketamine (only in children) and dexmedetomidine are recommended in patients with contraindications to the basic analgesic regimen.
- Analgesic adjuncts such as intraoperative and postoperative acupuncture and postoperative honey are recommended.
- Opioids should be reserved as rescue analgesics in the postoperative period.

Previously, postoperative analgesia included codeine. Its use has stopped due to concern for codeine 'ultra-metabolisers' within the population being overdosed with standard dosing of codeine with resultant apnoea.

There is much interest in the use of dexmedetomidine during adenotonsillectomy to reduce opioid requirements and postoperative emergence delirium. The data are inconclusive. The PROSPECT Working Group identified eight studies concerning IV dexmedetomidine in paediatric patients. Any analgesic benefit is unclear, but none of these studies assessed the benefit of adding dexmedetomidine on top of a basic analgesic regimen. Dexmedetomidine was associated with less agitation after sevoflurane-based anaesthesia in two studies.

## Postoperative Management Following Adenotonsillectomy

In children with severe OSAS, a nasopharyngeal airway can be inserted by the surgeon under direct vision at the end of surgery before the child is woken up. Keeping this in situ for the first post-operative night helps to bypass upper airway oedema caused by surgery. This is particularly helpful in syndromic children and children with sickle cell disease. The use of NPAs has reduced the requirement of postoperative paediatric intensive care unit (PICU) in children with severe OSA and complex comorbidities.

## Postoperative Complications Following Adenotonsillectomy

Nine per cent of children less than four years old have an unplanned admission following adenotonsillectomy, commonly because of vomiting. Postoperative primary haemorrhage (within six hours) is uncommon but is a life-threatening complication requiring emergent operative management with considerations that include full stomach, soiled airway and hypovolemic shock.

Intravenous access must be left in place in case of immediate postoperative bleeding. Early signs of important blood loss include:

- Pallor
- Slow capillary refill (>1 second)
- Tachycardia

Restlessness, confusion and hypotension are late signs and suggest significant blood loss. Large amounts of blood may be swallowed, leading to an underestimate of losses. A full blood count, clotting screen and blood cross-match should be performed. Ideally, fluid resuscitation should be undertaken before returning to theatre to mitigate the effect of anaesthesia in a hypovolaemic child.

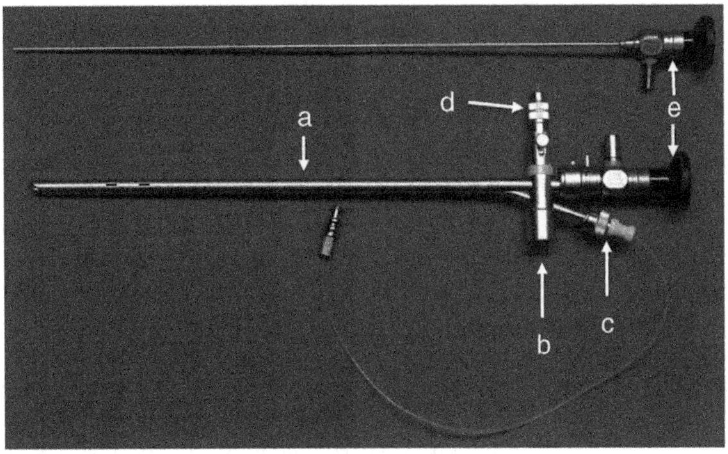


**Figure 21.1** Storz ventilating bronchoscope and Hopkins rod.
Notes:
(a) Centre channel, through which Hopkins rod can be passed.
(b) Port for anaesthetic gas flow; (c) suction channel; (d) light source attachment; (e) Hopkins rod. The lower image shows the bronchoscope with the Hopkins rod inserted.

In addition to hypovolaemia, anaesthesia is problematic because the child may have a stomach full of blood and active bleeding may make laryngoscopy and intubation difficult. There is little agreement on the safest technique of anaesthesia for a bleeding tonsil, and the anaesthetist should use the technique they are comfortable with. A rapid sequence induction with pre-oxygenation and cricoid pressure is advocated by some, whilst others prefer an inhalational induction with sevoflurane in oxygen, starting in a head-down, lateral position.

During the operation, further fluid and blood should be given as required, and near patient testing can help guide transfusion requirements. Before termination of anaesthesia, a wide bore orogastric tube can be passed to empty the stomach. Extubation should be in a lateral, head-down position with the child awake.

## Diagnostic and Therapeutic Endoscopy

Diagnostic and therapeutic microlaryngoscopy and bronchoscopy (MLB) is an important part of paediatric ENT surgery. It allows visualisation of the larynx, trachea and proximal bronchi. The indications include, but are not limited to, patients with stridor, unresolving and recurring pneumonitis, persistent atelectasis, persistent cough, tracheoesophageal fistula, airway trauma, tumours and suspicion of foreign body.

MLB may involve the use of a suspension laryngoscope and operating microscope or more commonly a Storz ventilating bronchoscope (Figure 21.1) with a Hopkins rod telescope that is passed through it.

### Diagnostic Endoscopy

MLB is often performed in children with mild to moderate airway obstruction.

An understanding of the likely pathology and the underlying medical condition helps to optimise anaesthesia for these investigations, which can be challenging at times. Many common abnormalities of the paediatric airway are dynamic (e.g. laryngomalacia, tracheomalacia and vocal cord palsy). To make a diagnosis, the surgeon needs a larynx that is still and unobstructed by a tracheal tube, with the patient breathing spontaneously. The depth of anaesthesia may need to be varied rapidly, as accurate assessments of dynamic pathology need the patient to be almost awake but not coughing or prone to laryngeal spasm.

### Preoperative Preparation

Signs of upper airway obstruction include stridor, sternal depression and/or indrawing of the supraclavicular, intercostal and subdiaphragmatic areas. These signs are evident when the airway is significantly reduced (by 70%) and can be magnified because of the very compliant chest wall in infants. Inspiratory stridor indicates obstruction at or above the larynx whilst hoarseness suggests vocal cord involvement. Biphasic stridor (inspiratory and expiratory) is heard with obstruction above or below the vocal cords. Expiratory stridor alone is a symptom of intrathoracic obstruction.

The preoperative investigations required are determined by history and examination and may include chest X-ray, lateral neck X-ray, barium swallow and echocardiography. Previous tracheal intubation may have given rise to airway pathology such as cricoarytenoid fixation, subglottic stenosis (SGS) or tracheal stenosis, whilst surgery may have resulted in injury (e.g. recurrent laryngeal nerve palsy during ligation of a patent ductus arteriosus). A full medical history should be obtained, as children with airway pathologies often have complex histories and may have undergone many medical interventions.

Historically, patients have been premedicated with an anticholinergic agent with the idea that reduction of secretions may reduce the incidence of coughing, breath-holding and laryngospasm. There are no data to support this, and this practice is no longer considered essential.

## Anaesthesia

The challenge for anaesthetists is maintaining adequate depth of anaesthesia without tracheal intubation whilst avoiding apnoea, hypoxaemia and hypercapnia, often in children with comorbidities and complex medical histories.

The onset of oxygen desaturation during endoscopy is age dependent. Virtual modelling of healthy children who were 1 month, 1 year, 8 years and 18 years has shown that oxygen desaturation occurs in the order of age, with the 1-month-old neonate desaturating first, followed by the 1 year old, 8 year old and then the 18 year old. This modelling was conducted with open and obstructed airways, and repeated with preoxygenation periods of 0, 1 and 3 minutes. The rate of oxygen desaturation from 90% to 40% was approximately the same for all ages (~33%/minute for an obstructed airway, and ~26%/minute for an open airway). Preoxygenation delayed the onset of oxygen desaturation in all age groups, but the benefit of preoxygenation was least in the one-month neonate. In the absence of preoxygenation and an open airway, a one-month-old neonate desaturated in only 6.6 seconds compared to 33.6 seconds for the eight-year-old child. This difference can be explained by the physiology of the neonate, as they have a larger minute ventilation to functional residual capacity (FRC) ratio, a high metabolic rate and low maximal $SaO_2$ compared to older children.

## Induction of Anaesthesia

Sevoflurane in 100% $O_2$ is commonly used for gas induction. Nitrous oxide can be used in carefully selected patients as the second gas effect can be helpful to speed up the process of gas induction. It is important to maintain spontaneous respiration during induction and maintenance of anaesthesia in children with airway obstruction. Muscle relaxants should be avoided until reliable bag mask ventilation is possible.

In children with severe airway obstruction, it can be challenging to undertake a gas induction and maintain anaesthesia with inhalational agents as the obstructed airway can impede the delivery of the inhalational agent. Induction can be slow and particularly difficult in lighter planes of anaesthesia when obstruction can become worse due to reduction of tone in the airway. The author prefers to have IV access in situ in difficult cases so anaesthesia can be rapidly deepened if necessary and/or other rescue medication can be administered rapidly. Traditionally, IV induction has been avoided in airway obstruction for fear of apnoea and subsequent difficulty in maintaining or establishing an airway. However, careful and judicious use of IV agents like propofol does not necessarily result in apnoea and has the benefit of separating the mode of delivery of anaesthesia from the area of pathology, the obstructed airway. In addition, propofol and TIVA are associated with reduced airway complications and smoother wake-up.

CPAP is often required to maintain the airway and oxygenation once the child with the obstructed airway is anaesthetised. Positive pressure helps to overcome the loss of tone after induction of anaesthesia and splint the airway open. It is particularly important in smaller infants and babies where tidal breathing can impinge on FRC, resulting in relatively rapid airway collapse and desaturation. It can take several minutes to deepen anaesthesia so that laryngoscopy can be tolerated in a child with an obstructed airway using an inhalational agent alone. If not already in situ, intravenous access is obtained as rapidly as possible. The cords are sprayed with topical anaesthesia. There is a risk of laryngeal spasm if spray is attempted at an inadequate depth of anaesthesia, so depth of anaesthesia should be carefully assessed before this is attempted. It can be helpful to administer a small bolus of propofol pre-spray to prevent laryngospasm. Lidocaine (to a maximum of 5 mg $kg^{-1}$, or 160 mg) is sprayed onto the glottis, vallecula and trachea. The author prefers to limit the dose of lidocaine used around the larynx to 2 ml of 1% lidocaine. This seems to be as effective as higher doses and concentrations of lidocaine as the cords are exquisitely sensitive to topical lidocaine application. Using a low dose of lidocaine on the cords means that additional lidocaine can be used elsewhere in the airway if necessary, such as around the carina, whilst remaining within safe dose limits. A nasopharyngeal airway, usually a RAE tube half a size smaller than a tube suitable for the airway, is passed through the nose into the posterior pharyngeal space, ideally under the same laryngoscopy as the cord spray. This is used to supply oxygen and/or inhalational agent to maintain anaesthesia. One hundred per cent oxygen is used to maintain oxygenation. The risks of desaturation can be significant, particularly in babies where oxygen consumption is high and FRC is reduced, resulting in decreased oxygen storage capacity. The author's preference is to maintain anaesthesia using TIVA, as this separates delivery of anaesthesia from the airway, which can be frequently compromised. It requires some experience to avoid hypoventilation or apnoea, but the airway is easier to manage once this technique has been perfected. Close monitoring is essential to detect hypoxia and hypoventilation as well as excessively light anaesthesia. At the end of the examination, anaesthesia is stopped, 100% oxygen is continued and the larynx is observed until the patient is virtually awake.

## Maintenance of Anaesthesia

Anaesthesia can be maintained using inhalational agents namely sevoflurane or TIVA or a combination of both. TIVA, with a combination of propofol (200–400 mcg $kg^{-1}$ $min^{-1}$) and remifentanil (0.05–0.15 mcg $kg^{-1}$ $min^{-1}$) by infusion, or propofol and alfentanil by intermittent injection. Using TIVA means that the maintenance of anaesthesia is independent of the airway, which is an advantage where intermittent obstruction by the surgeon can lead to light anaesthesia and patient movement. TIVA also usually results in a better recovery than with volatile agents, particularly in children over two years, but should be used with caution if there is concern that the airway cannot be adequately maintained (although in the author's experience this is very unusual).

Intermittent boluses of propofol and alfentanil by hand (propofol 10–20 mg $kg^{-1}$ $h^{-1}$ and alfentanil 20–30 mcg $kg^{-1}$ $h^{-1}$) can be very effective, as it allows rapid titration of anaesthesia to the stimulus being applied. It does require careful observation of the surgical procedure and awareness of the requirements of different interventions. For example, balloon dilation of the trachea is very stimulating, and it is difficult to avoid coughing. Application of topical lidocaine can be helpful, using a pre-emptive bolus of propofol with alfentanil. Too much IV agent can result in apnoea, and if there is desaturation the surgery will have to be stopped. The anaesthetist and surgeon should be prepared for this eventuality, and tracheal tubes of various sizes should be available and ready to be placed urgently if desaturation occurs.

As oxygenation is so critical and at times challenging, alternative forms of oxygenation have been sought. Transnasal humidified oxygenation and ventilatory exchange (THRIVE) has been used as an adjunct in airway surgery, and in the appropriate population group can allow improved oxygenation and surgical conditions using flow rates of 2 l $kg^{-1}min^{-1}$. The Optiflow (Fisher and Paykel Healthcare™) is a heated humidified high-flow delivery system. The nasal cannulas are specifically designed for this purpose, to withstand high flows of gas. The cannulas are made of soft silicon and are designed with skin applicators for the face to improve patient comfort during prolonged use. Adult flow rates of 70 l $min^{-1}$ have been described for THRIVE. Recommended paediatric flow rates appear in Table 21.1.

An early report of 20 infants less than three months old undergoing tracheal intubation with Optiflow™ found that the benefit seemed to depend on whether the child was sick or healthy. Oxygen saturation remained normal throughout the intubation for 12 healthy children with normal lungs, but five of the eight sick children desaturated. The use of Optiflow™ during paediatric anaesthesia is still novel compared to the extensive experience in paediatric intensive care. Potential applications during paediatric anaesthesia might include Optiflow™ for preoxygenation, tracheal intubation, laryngeal and other upper airway surgery, endoscopy and anaesthesia recovery.

**Table 21.1** Suggested flow rates for children receiving heated humidified high-flow nasal cannula (HHHFNC) oxygen/air (personal communication from Associate Professor Andreas Schibler, Mater Research Institute, University of Queensland, Brisbane, Australia)

| Weight (kg) | Flow rate (l $kg^{-1}$ $min^{-1}$) |
|---|---|
| 0–15 | 2 |
| | **Flow rate (l $min^{-1}$)** |
| > 15–30 | 35 |
| > 30–50 | 40 |
| > 50 | 50 |

## Apnoeic Oxygenation

There is much interest in the use of apnoeic oxygenation for MLB to optimise oxygenation and operating conditions. The concept of delivering oxygen to apnoeic patients was first described by Holmdahl in 1956. It was recognised that, during apnoea, oxygen is taken up by the blood from the FRC at a rate that exceeds the outflow of carbon dioxide. This occurs because of the relatively high solubility of carbon dioxide in the blood. Flow rate differential then occurs between oxygen removal from the alveoli and carbon dioxide excretion. This generates a negative pressure gradient of −20 cm $H_2O$, creating bulk flow of oxygen from the upper airway to the alveoli. Oxygen can be delivered from the nose, face mask, pharynx or trachea at varying flow rates and inspired concentrations. However, the effectiveness of apnoeic oxygenation varies depending on the delivery technique and the age and physical status of the patient. With preoxygenation and apnoeic oxygenation through a tracheal tube, normal oxygen saturations can be maintained for 10 minutes in children, but infants may desaturate after only 3 minutes of apnoea. In a study by Cook et al. of 28 children and infants, $PaO_2$ decreased at 4.1 kPa $min^{-1}$ or 30 mmHg, which is three times faster than an adult. A similar study by Kernian et al. demonstrated that, after preoxygenation and apnoeic oxygenation with 0.1 l $kg^{-1}$ $min^{-1}$ through a tracheal tube, oxygen desaturation was prevented for 3 minutes. In a control group breathing air, oxygen desaturation occurred after 116 seconds in patients who were 3–10 kg; 147 seconds if weight was 10–20 kg and 217 seconds if the child weighed >20 kg.

A limitation of this technique is the steady increase in $PaCO_2$ of 0.4–0.8 kPa $min^{-1}$ due to absent ventilation and clearance of carbon dioxide. Over time, this can cause respiratory acidosis and an associated spectrum of complications.

## Diagnostic Bronchoscopy

Most diagnostic ENT bronchoscopies are undertaken using the Hopkins rod, and anaesthesia continues as described in the preceding sections. If a full bronchoscopic examination is needed, a Storz ventilating bronchoscope is used. A side arm allows attachment of an anaesthetic T-piece for administration of 100% oxygen with or without volatile agent (see Figure 21.1). Once the Hopkins rod is in place, a closed system exists, allowing ventilation to occur in the annular space between the telescope and the surrounding bronchoscope. A suction catheter can also be passed through another side arm on the instrument. Resistance is high in the smaller bronchoscopes, significantly increasing the work of breathing, particularly for infants. Furthermore, resistance increases with the length of the instrument; at 3 l $min^{-1}$ flow rates, the resistance of a 30 cm 3.5 bronchoscope is four times that of a 20 cm model. Assisted ventilation may be needed, especially for infants. Resistance to expiration is high, and air trapping can occur unless a long expiratory phase is employed. It may be necessary to remove the telescope temporarily and allow unobstructed ventilation through the empty bronchoscope.

Fibreoptic endoscopy can be used in the diagnosis of upper airway obstruction, more commonly by respiratory physicians or interventional radiologists. Anaesthesia is best conducted with a SAD or face mask using a bronchoscopic swivel mount, which has a small self-sealing hole through which the fibrescope is passed. A diagnostic bronchogram may be performed at the same time.

## Complications during Bronchoscopy

The most common complications are related to oxygenation and ventilation. Frequently patients may become hypoxic or hypercapnic, which may lead to bradycardia, cardiac arrhythmias and arrest. Barotrauma can occur (e.g. pneumothorax, pneumomediastinum) from inadequate egress of air from insufflation of oxygen during bronchoscopy. Introduction of the laryngoscope, the Hopkins telescope or bronchoscope can damage the teeth, gingiva or surrounding soft tissue. Downward force should not be placed onto the maxillary teeth with the bronchoscope.

When passing the bronchoscope, gentle manoeuvring around the soft tissue of the posterior pharyngeal wall and epiglottis is important to avoid laceration and/or laryngeal fracture. In addition, there may be damage to the arytenoids or vocal folds when traversing this area. Ensuring that the bronchoscope passes through abducted vocal cords, posteriorly and at a 90-degree angle can help to minimise laryngeal trauma. Placing the bronchoscope into the subglottic region and trachea can trigger a vagotonic response and bradycardia, which is typically more pronounced in children <6 months of age.

Significant trauma from the bronchoscope itself or from the therapeutic intervention could potentially induce a pneumothorax. If a pneumothorax is suspected, all operating room staff should be made aware of the situation and a chest drain inserted, the urgency of which will be determined by the condition of the child.

## Loss of Airway during Diagnostic Investigation

On occasion the loss of tone associated with the onset of anaesthesia may result in airway decompensation, requiring CPAP to preserve respiration. This manoeuvre may be insufficient, especially in patients with small and/or obstructed airways. An array of tracheal tubes of varying sizes should be readily available in case of emergency. In extremis, a tracheal tube can be loaded onto the Hopkins rod and the surgeon can intubate under direct vision. The key is to be very vigilant and proactive and to not let saturations drop below a predetermined level (e.g. 95%) before intervention is undertaken. This is particularly important in babies and small children who have limited oxygen reserves and high oxygen consumption. Many patients undergoing these investigations or interventions are ex-prems or children with recurrent aspiration who may have poor lung function. Constant vigilance and a proactive approach are key to prevent desaturations.

## Specific Conditions Identified by Diagnostic Endoscopy or Bronchoscopy Laryngomalacia

This is the most common cause of stridor in infancy. Stridor can be present within a few days of birth but rarely requires immediate intervention. Infants may have inspiratory stridor with marked sternal recession and tracheal tug. Feeding difficulties are common in more severe cases. The airway obstruction is due to collapse of the supraglottic structures on inspiration. The natural history of the condition is to resolve by two years of age, but in severe cases with marked stridor, recession and impaired growth due to feeding difficulties, surgery to divide the aryepiglottic folds or remove excess arytenoid mucosa can be undertaken and is usually successful. This is performed after airway examination under spontaneous ventilation with oxygen delivered either via a nasopharyngeal airway or via the suspension laryngoscope and anaesthesia provided by TIVA/target-controlled infusion (TCI).

## Tracheomalacia and Tracheobronchomalacia

These conditions cause collapse of the airway on expiration. Symptoms may be intermittent and include expiratory wheeze, stridor and severe episodes of cyanosis and reflex apnoeas sometimes called 'dying spells'. The presentation is usually during the first year of life. It may be due to underlying deficiency or weakness of the tracheal rings, caused by extrinsic compression commonly from a vascular anomaly, or seen in babies after repair of tracheooesophageal fistula. Diagnosis is made by bronchoscopy and/or bronchogram with spontaneous ventilation maintained. The level of positive end expiratory pressure (PEEP) required to maintain airway patency can be measured during the bronchogram. In the acute situation, airway management is not usually difficult, and positive pressure ventilation stabilises the child.

Surgical options depend on the aetiology of the problem and include correction of the vascular anomaly, aortopexy or, occasionally, airway stenting. In the case of cartilaginous weakness, prolonged positive pressure airway support may be needed, sometimes via a tracheostomy.

## Vocal Cord Palsies

These may be present from birth or develop after thoracic surgery or neurological injury. Unilateral cord palsy often causes relatively mild symptoms of stridor and a whispery cry but may be a cause of failed extubation after cardiac surgery. Bilateral cord palsy will cause much more severe symptoms of stridor with marked sternal recession and tracheal tug. If acute intervention is required, PEEP applied during induction acts as a dynamic splint to maintain a wider airway. Treatment options depend on the severity of symptoms; tracheostomy may be required for bilateral vocal cord palsy.

## Therapeutic Endoscopy

A wide range of therapeutic operations can be performed on the airway, often in patients with significant airway obstruction. Maintenance of anaesthesia by volatile agents or TIVA, as described previously, is indicated. Paracetamol and a NSAID should be given as analgesia.

$CO_2$ laser is rarely used in the paediatric airway due to an increased propensity to scarring in the airway. The usual precautions for the use of a potassium titanyl phosphate (KTP) laser should be undertaken. The inspired oxygen concentration should be reduced when using the KTP laser to reduce the risk of airway burns. Laser surgery should only be undertaken in properly equipped theatres, and all staff should wear appropriate eye protection. Viral papillomas are occasionally lasered. High-volume theatre air scavenging is important, as vaporised viral particles may be released, and theatre staff should wear masks.

## Specific Conditions Treated by Therapeutic Endoscopy Laryngeal Papillomas

These are benign proliferations of squamous epithelium usually caused by the human papilloma virus types 6 and 11. The usual site is the larynx, but they can occur anywhere in the tracheobronchial tree (see Figures 21.2 and 21.3). The onset of symptoms is often very slow, with progressive dyspnoea sometimes treated as asthma and hoarse voice or aphonia. These children usually require anaesthesia as a planned procedure for airway investigation or for surgery but may present acutely with severe respiratory distress and stridor with an airway almost completely obstructed by florid cauliflower-like growths.

Anaesthesia can be induced using gas or slow IV injection, which has the advantage of separating the anaesthesia from the obstructed airway. This makes induction more predictable, but it should be undertaken slowly and with caution so that spontaneous ventilation is maintained. The treatment is by surgical debulking usually with spontaneous ventilation, so topical lidocaine is required. Intubation is avoided if possible to reduce the chance of seeding papilloma further down the airway.

Anaesthesia is maintained either with gas via a nasopharyngeal airway or with TIVA. Adjuvant treatments such as intralesional injections of the anti-viral cidofovir are sometimes used.

The condition is recurrent in some cases, requiring numerous procedures over many years to maintain an airway. Afflicted children are often distressed because of repeated general anaesthetics and may require premedication despite some airway compromise. In future, countries where the quadrivalent human papilloma virus vaccine is given to prevent cervical cancer could see a significant reduction in the incidence of laryngeal papillomatosis.

## Airway Cysts

Congenital supraglottic cysts are uncommon but may present with stridor from birth, sometimes requiring immediate intervention. Although at times very large, they are fluid filled and compressible and can sometimes be pushed aside by a tube

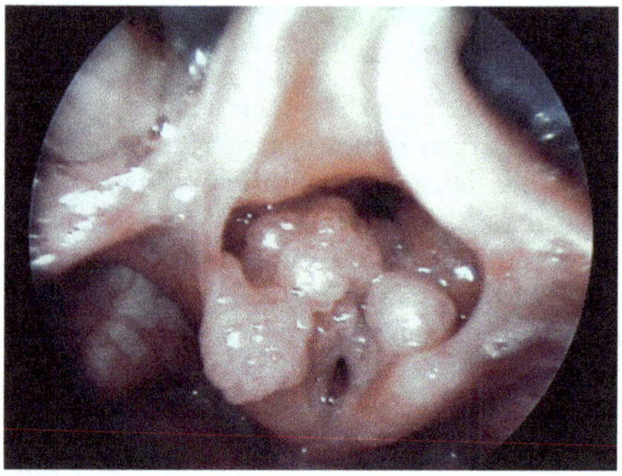

**Figure 21.2** Laryngeal papillomas causing partial airway obstruction.
*Source:* With thanks to Dr S. Bew.

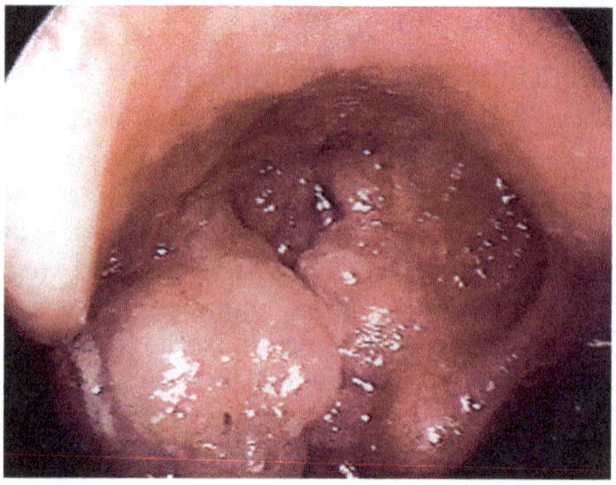

**Figure 21.3** Laryngeal papillomas causing severe airway obstruction.
*Source:* With thanks to Dr S. Bew.

with a stylet allowing intubation. Occasionally the whole larynx is obscured, and the cyst may need aspiration under direct laryngoscopy to reveal the larynx. The cysts are then marsupialised to prevent recurrence.

Subglottic cysts are usually seen in infants who have been intubated previously, often as neonates. They probably result from subglottic trauma, although the period of intubation does not need to be prolonged. These infants may present with biphasic stridor or audible harsh breathing sounds and respiratory distress several months after discharge from the neonatal unit. Subglottic cysts can be excised using grabbing forceps and/or sickle knife.

### Postanaesthesia Care

Meticulous observation in the PACU is essential following diagnostic or therapeutic endoscopy. Airway oedema because of intervention or instrumentation is common, and children may develop respiratory distress with stridor on recovery. All patients undergoing therapeutic endoscopy and those in whom instrumentation may have been difficult should receive dexamethasone (250 mcg $kg^{-1}$ initial dose, thereafter 100 mcg $kg^{-1}$ 8 hourly).

Stridor in the PACU may also require nebulised adrenaline (1:1,000, 5 ml). The ECG should be monitored during administration of nebulised adrenaline, which should be stopped temporarily if the heart rate is >190 beats per minute.

## Airway Emergencies

### Acute Airway Emergencies

The most common infective conditions are acute viral laryngotracheobronchitis (croup), acute epiglottitis and bacterial tracheitis.

### Epiglottitis

The incidence of this condition fell steeply in 1992 after the introduction of routine vaccination against *Haemophilus influenzae type b* and is now only seen very occasionally in unvaccinated children, in cases of vaccine failure or when other organisms cause epiglottitis. Epiglottitis presents with rapidly progressive fever, dysphagia, drooling, tachypnoea and stridor, typically in children between one and six years of age. Classically these children adopt a tripod posture, leaning forward on their hands to maintain their airway.

The child can be toxic and very unwell and should be kept in a comfortable position with oxygen delivered as tolerated, which is often more effective with the parent holding the mask. The child should be kept as calm and comfortable as possible, as distress can result in further airway compromise. Nebulised adrenaline may reduce swelling and improve the chance of successful intubation. Anaesthesia can be by gas or very slow IV induction with the child in the sitting position. Spontaneous ventilation should be maintained. The larynx may be very difficult to identify with all supraglottic structures red, swollen and distorted (see Figure 21.4). The movement of secretions or a bubble of gas from the larynx may help identification. Intubate with a tube smaller than expected for age. The child should remain intubated on PICU until a leak develops round the tube.

### Croup or Laryngotracheobronchitis

This is an upper respiratory infection usually caused by the parainfluenza virus. Symptoms are slower in onset than in epiglottitis and are characterised by a barking cough.

The subglottis is narrowed by swelling, which can be seen on an anterior-posterior neck X-ray as a loss of the normal shouldered appearance of the air column, giving the appearance of an inverted *V* known as the steeple sign (see Figure 21.5).

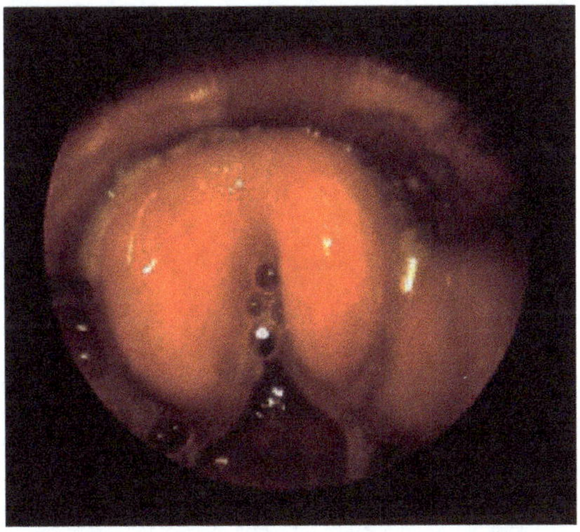

**Figure 21.4** Endoscopic view of the epiglottis in epiglottitis. *Source:* Reprinted from Hammer J. Acquired upper airway obstruction. *Paediatric Respiratory Review* 2004; 5:29, with permission from Elsevier.

(a)

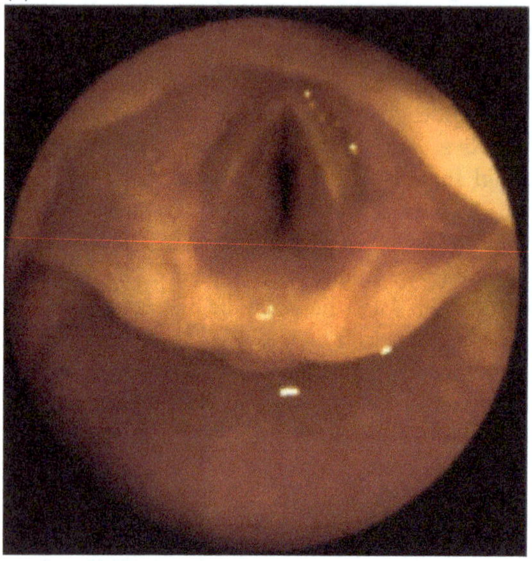

(b)

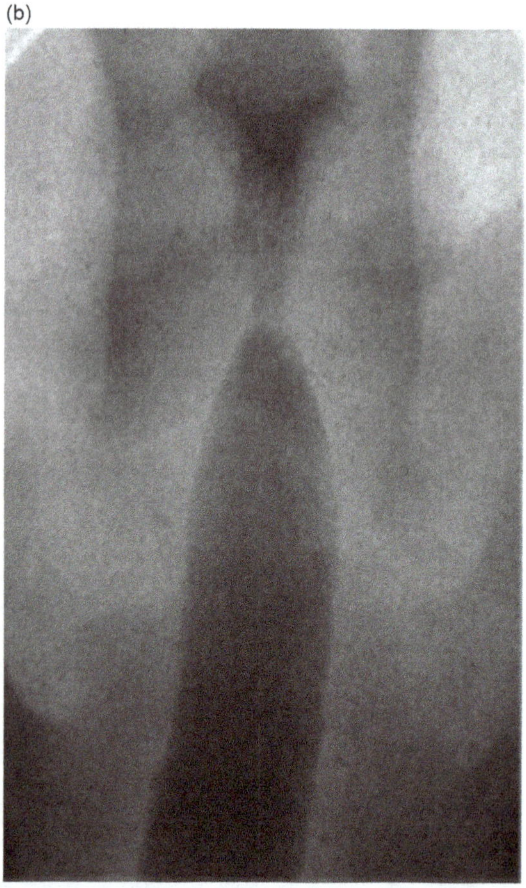

**Figure 21.5** Endoscopic view of the larynx in croup (a). Radiological presentation of subglottic oedema in viral croup (b), compared with normal (c).
*Source:* Reprinted from Hammer J. Acquired upper airway obstruction. *Paediatric Respiratory Review* 2004; 5:26, with permission from Elsevier

(c)

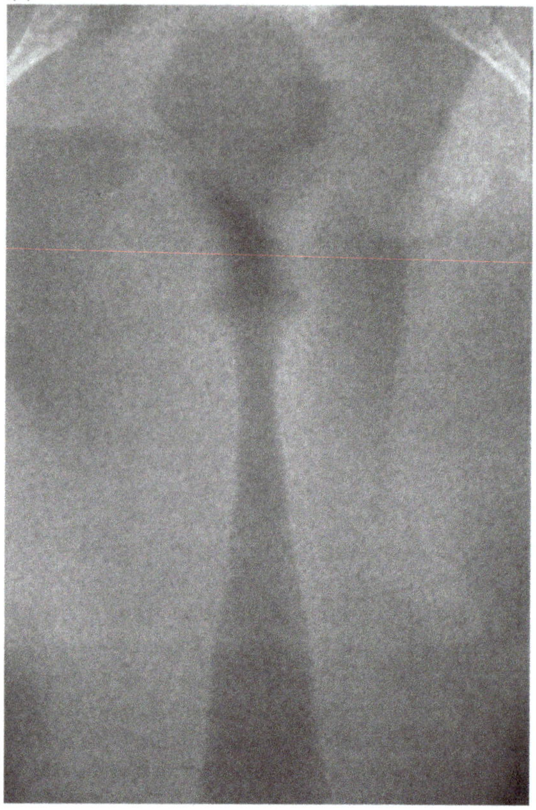

**Figure 21.5** *(cont.)*

Mild croup is common in the winter, but only a very small proportion of cases require hospital admission. Most respond to medical treatment with inhaled budesonide or intravenous dexamethasone and nebulised adrenaline. Humidification of inspired gases is also widely used. A small number of children do not respond to medical treatment and gradually deteriorate, becoming exhausted and requiring intubation.

Although there will be inflammation of the supraglottic tissues and excess secretions, the laryngoscopy is not usually difficult, although a smaller tracheal tube than expected for age will be needed.

## Bacterial Tracheitis or Pseudomembranous Croup

In some centres, this is now a more common cause of PICU admission than croup. The initial presentation is often croup-like, but the child is toxic and rapidly deteriorates with cough, fever and stridor. An anteroposterior (AP) neck X-ray may also show the 'steeple' sign. The most common organism is

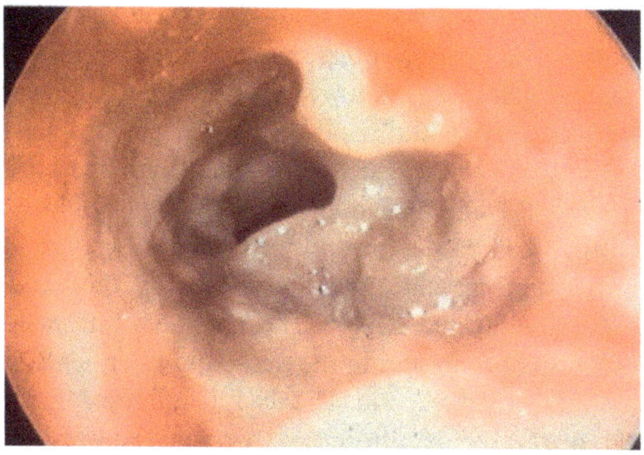

**Figure 21.6** Endoscopic view of the trachea in bacterial tracheitis.

*Staphylococcus aureus*, which causes inflammation and thick mucopurulent secretions (see Figure 21.6). The tracheal tube may become obstructed by secretions or sloughing of the tracheal epithelium, and the child will require frequent suctioning or occasionally rigid bronchoscopy to remove the pseudomembranes. The course on PICU may be complicated by sepsis and pneumonia, and the duration of intubation is usually longer than in croup.

## Retropharyngeal Abscess

This is caused by lymphatic spread of infection from sinuses, teeth or middle ear into the space between the posterior pharyngeal wall and the prevertebral fascia. It is mainly seen in young children and presents with fever, sore throat, neck pain and swelling with limitation of movement and drooling. These children are usually stable enough for a CT scan. Larger abscess collections will require surgical drainage.

Stridor is not often a major feature, but the intubation can be very difficult, with copious secretions and tissues distorted by the bulging pharyngeal wall.

Attempts to pass a tube or bougie can rupture the abscess, with the risk of airway soiling and the laryngeal view becoming obscured by purulent secretions.

## Removal of an Inhaled Foreign Body

Inhalation of a foreign body usually occurs between the age of one and three years; it is more common in males. The episode is often witnessed; an episode of choking is usually followed by a bout of coughing. Hoarseness and/or stridor suggest that the foreign body is impacted in the larynx, whereas passage into the trachea or main bronchi may cause wheeze or unilaterally reduced breath sounds. Rarely, an object causes a complete glottic or subglottic obstruction, which is rapidly fatal. Partial obstruction is caused by objects lodged in or around the laryngeal inlet. The initial choking or coughing episode is followed by biphasic stridor and a change in the voice or cry, which may become hoarse. An object with sharp edges may cause pain on swallowing, causing infants to drool. Most children will present immediately with marked respiratory distress.

If it is radio opaque, the foreign body may be seen on chest X-ray (CXR), but the majority are radiolucent. Inspiration and expiration films are required as hyperinflation may be seen on the affected side, but a normal CXR does not exclude the diagnosis. In later presentations, collapse and consolidation may be seen distal to the obstruction.

The approach to anaesthesia is as for diagnostic bronchoscopy. Atropine premedication, gaseous induction using oxygen and an inhalational agent with topical anaesthesia are satisfactory. If there is respiratory distress, urgent bronchoscopy is indicated; otherwise, the procedure should wait for an appropriate starvation period. A smooth technique using deep anaesthesia and avoiding coughing is essential. Intubation should be avoided if the foreign body is in or near the larynx, whilst positive pressure ventilation is best avoided if the foreign body is in the trachea or creating ball-valve obstruction. A 30 cm ventilating bronchoscope with Hopkins rod and grasping forceps is used. Application of topical adrenaline (1:10,000) to the area of impaction is useful to reduce oedema and facilitate removal of the foreign body.

Ventilation may need to be gently assisted if the bronchoscope is in a main bronchus for a prolonged period. Side holes in the Storz bronchoscope assist proximal ventilation. Once the object is firmly grasped in the forceps, the whole instrument is slowly removed from the airway under vision, ensuring that the foreign body does not fall out of the forceps. Once the bronchoscope has been removed, anaesthesia is maintained by mask whilst awaiting reinsertion of the bronchoscope to confirm full removal. When withdrawing the bronchoscope with the foreign body, the danger is loss of the object either in the trachea or larynx, which may cause total obstruction to ventilation.

Should this occur, the bronchoscope should be reinserted to push the object into the distal airway so that satisfactory ventilation can be re-established.

## Choanal Atresia

Choanal atresia is a membranous or bony occlusion of the posterior nares with an incidence of 1:8,000 births. It may be unilateral, when presentation is often delayed. Bilateral obstruction causes acute respiratory distress in neonates as they are obligate nasal breathers. An oral airway and an orogastric tube should be inserted and taped to the face, whilst surgery is undertaken within 24 hours. Other anomalies are common (e.g. CHARGE syndrome), and thorough preoperative assessment including echocardiography is needed.

In choanal atresia, surgery involves dividing the membrane obstructing the posterior nares. Where there is bony occlusion, a passageway is drilled, and this can cause significant bleeding despite intraoperative use of topical adrenaline. There should be a preoperative group and save serum. A standard technique for neonatal anaesthesia can be used, with muscle relaxant, tracheal intubation (RAE tracheal tube), positive pressure ventilation and analgesia (paracetamol and fentanyl). A throat pack is not used as it will obstruct the surgical view. Patency of the new nasal passageway is ensured by the insertion of nasopharyngeal stents made from standard tracheal tubes. These require regular suctioning and are left in situ for eight weeks. Restenosis is common, and patients may return for further surgical correction.

## Anaesthesia for Tracheostomy

Tracheostomy is indicated for congenital or acquired airway obstruction, to facilitate long-term respiratory support or in the presence of a neurological abnormality. Anticholinergic premedication can be useful if there are a lot of secretions. Inhalational induction can be with sevoflurane in oxygen or a slow IV induction used. Relaxants should be avoided unless reliable manual ventilation can be achieved. Some patients (e.g. those with Pierre Robin sequence) may be impossible to intubate. In these patients, anaesthesia is maintained using oxygen, a volatile agent and spontaneous respiration or judicious use of TIVA whilst the airway is maintained using an LMA or face mask.

Once the airway is secured, muscle relaxants, positive pressure ventilation and a volatile agent can be given. Respiratory obstruction may occur during surgery, and hand ventilation permits early detection. The patient is positioned with the head extended using a sandbag under the shoulders; strapping is passed around the chin and secured to the operating table, thereby stabilising the head. Lidocaine 1% and 1:200,000 adrenaline is infiltrated at the site of incision in the neck, and the trachea is identified by dissection. The second and third tracheal rings are identified, and two stay sutures are inserted, one on either side of the planned tracheal incision. These sutures are taped to the chest at the end of the operation and are not removed until the first tube change at one week. They are vital for postoperative safety; if the tracheostomy tube falls out, these sutures are used to pull the trachea to the surface to facilitate tube reinsertion.

Before the tracheal incision is made, 100% oxygen is given and the proposed tracheostomy tube and connector is checked. Standard tracheostomy tubes (Portex, Shiley or Bivona) with 15 mm connectors are used. Once the trachea has been incised, the tracheal tube is withdrawn into the upper trachea and the tracheostomy tube is inserted. The anaesthesia circuit is connected, and ventilation is checked by auscultation of the chest and capnography to confirm correct placement of the tracheostomy tube. At the end of surgery, the head is taken out of extension, and tracheostomy tapes are passed around the neck to secure the tube.

Postoperatively, a CXR is taken to confirm correct tube placement and to exclude a pneumothorax. Warmed humidified air/oxygen, using elephant tubing and tracheostomy mask, is given to neonates and infants; cold humidity is used for older children. This is combined with regular sterile suctioning with saline irrigation (1–2 ml) to ensure that crusting and blockage do not occur. A spare tracheostomy tube, tapes and dilators are kept with the patient. Humidification can usually stop after the first tube change, and a 'Swedish nose' is used instead.

## Open Operations on the Larynx

### Subglottic Stenosis (SGS)

This may be congenital, but more often develops postintubation and can occur at any age after even a brief period of intubation. Children may present with biphasic stridor, dyspnoea on exertion and croupy cough, or after failed extubation in the PICU. In some patients, the symptoms and signs may be very subtle. An infant who is not yet mobile may show only minimal subcostal recession and, rather than stridor, have soft biphasic respiratory sounds.

It is important to maintain spontaneous ventilation whilst the airway is assessed under anaesthesia, as it may be extremely difficult to ventilate through a very narrow airway, and the high pressures cause gastric distension. If intubation is required either to secure a safe airway or for a tracheostomy, it can be very difficult to pass a tube. It may be possible to pass a straight 5 Fr bougie and corkscrew in a size 2 tracheal tube, but at times even this is too big. A Cole tube is more rigid and may be useful in this situation. Repeated attempts to pass a tube will rapidly lead to oedema and worsening obstruction. A tracheostomy should be performed whilst spontaneous ventilation and face mask anaesthesia is still possible. Definitive treatment of SGS is by anterior cricoid split, laryngotracheal reconstruction or cricotracheal resection.

## Anterior Cricoid Split

This operation is used in children with SGS, often those unable to be extubated in the PICU but who are otherwise well with no pulmonary disease. Head positioning is the same as for a tracheostomy; the trachea is dissected, after which the cricoid cartilage and the first and second tracheal rings are divided in the midline anteriorly. Anaesthesia with tracheal intubation, a muscle relaxant, opioid and ventilation by hand is appropriate. Following the split, a nasotracheal tube of a larger size is passed with the tube tip positioned just distal to the lowest divided ring; this acts as a tracheal stent for 5–10 days.

Patients are cared for in the PICU, where meticulous attention to the tracheal tube is needed. Tracheal tube blockage or accidental extubation are very hazardous as attempts at reintubation can result in the bevel of the tracheal tube being pushed through the anterior tracheal wall to create a false passage. If extubation occurs, nasotracheal reintubation should not be attempted in the PICU as the angle of tracheal tube passing through the larynx from the nose encourages anterior perforation through the surgical division. The airway should be supported with a face mask to achieve oxygenation and orotracheal intubation attempted. Afterwards the patient can be returned to theatre for nasotracheal intubation in controlled circumstances. At 5–10 days, extubation is attempted whilst using steroid cover.

## Laryngotracheal Reconstruction

This may be performed as a single-stage or two-stage procedure with a tracheostomy. It involves a similar approach to the cricoid split but opens the larynx anteriorly and posteriorly if required. Harvested rib cartilage is interposed into the anterior and posterior split, thereby increasing the diameter of the airway. If performed as a single-stage procedure, with no covering tracheostomy, the anaesthetic and PICU considerations are the same as those for the cricoid split, including the caveat regarding reintubation. If a posterior graft is needed, a sterile cuffed flexometallic tracheal tube or cut-down RAE tube is placed by the surgeon in the trachea distal to the graft site; ventilation is continued in this manner until just before the anterior graft is ready to be placed. At this point, a larger nasotracheal tube is passed with the tip positioned just below the graft site by the surgeon under direct vision. Wet neurosurgical patties can be used to pack around this tube to create a temporary seal for intermittent positive pressure ventilation (IPPV). The patient is returned to the PICU for care, as described earlier. Patients tolerate nasotracheal tubes well, and after the first 24–48 hours only minimal sedation is needed.

Laryngotracheal reconstruction is also performed as a two-stage procedure, the first stage being a tracheostomy. At the second stage, anaesthesia is induced through the pre-existing tracheostomy; maintenance is with an opioid, muscle relaxant and volatile agent. Intravenous fluids are given and continued postoperatively, and a nasogastric tube is passed. To manage the airway, a cuffed flexometallic tracheal tube or cut-down RAE tracheal tube is inserted through the tracheostome, after which the anaesthetist should check for equal ventilation. The tube is secured by surgical suture just below the tracheostome. Care is needed during the operation as surgical manipulation can move the tube, resulting in extubation or bronchial intubation; the cuff can also be pierced by surgical suturing. Should this happen, the surgeon will need to assist with tube positioning. Wet neurosurgical patties will create a temporary seal if the cuff ruptures.

A stent is placed in the trachea to support the grafts, after which the anterior larynx is closed. The flexometallic tube is removed after careful tracheal suctioning, a tracheostomy tube is reinserted, and the patient is awoken to be returned to the ENT ward. Humidified oxygen is given via a tracheostomy mask. A CXR is required to exclude a pneumothorax, which may occur following rib harvest. Analgesia is with paracetamol, an NSAID and morphine patient- or nurse-controlled analgesia (PCA/NCA). A local anaesthetic infusion through an epidural catheter placed in the site of rib harvest can afford useful pain relief for up to 72 hours.

### Cricotracheal Resection

Short segment tracheal resection can be performed for Grade III and IV SGS. The patient will already have a tracheostomy, and the approach to anaesthesia is the same as the two-stage laryngotracheal reconstruction. A segment of trachea is excised, and a new cricotracheal anastomosis is made. Difficulties with the temporary cuffed flexometallic tube are even more likely in this operation. More complex slide tracheoplasties are used for patients with long-segment tracheal stenosis; these require cardiopulmonary bypass and are highly specialised operations.

## Non-airway ENT Surgery

### Middle Ear Surgery

Exploration of the middle ear requires the anaesthetist to consider:

- Control of bleeding
- Preservation of the facial nerve
- Avoidance of graft displacement

Procedures include:

- Mastoidectomy
- Myringoplasty
- Cochlea implantation

### Minimising Blood Loss

Bleeding can be of arterial origin secondary to a hyperdynamic circulation with a high cardiac output, hypertension and tachycardia. Control of heart rate and cardiac output will minimise this loss. Venous ooze secondary to raised internal jugular venous pressure may be caused by poor patient positioning, partial airway obstruction during spontaneous respiration, abdominal compression or raised mean intrathoracic pressure with IPPV or PEEP.

Strategies to minimise blood loss during middle ear surgery are presented in Table 21.2. These involve controlled hypotension which may be defined as a reduction of systolic blood pressure to 80 to 90 mmHg, a reduction of mean arterial pressure (MAP) to 50–65 mmHg or a 30% reduction of baseline MAP. Total intravenous anaesthesia has revolutionised anaesthesia for middle ear surgery. The blood pressure cuff should be sited on the arm opposite to the operation to avoid interference with readings by surgical activity. The remifentanil infusion is stopped 15 minutes before the end of surgery, and a long-acting opioid, paracetamol and NSAID are given. A postoperative antiemetic should be prescribed, as PONV can be problematic after middle ear surgery.

### Preservation of the Facial Nerve

The tympanic segment of the facial nerve is at risk during middle ear surgery; facial nerve monitoring is used, based upon electromyography, and requires neuromuscular function. Neuromuscular blockers are thus avoided.

### Avoiding Graft Displacement

Nitrous oxide ($N_2O$), being more soluble than nitrogen, diffuses in and out of body cavities more quickly than nitrogen. When the middle ear has been closed by a myringoplasty, termination of $N_2O$ will result in a negative pressure being applied to the graft. Using TIVA or avoiding $N_2O$ is ideal.

### Surgery for Congenital Ear Defects

Children with congenital defects of the external ear present for the insertion of osseointegrated temporal screws for an artificial pinna or bone-anchored hearing aid; reconstructive surgery to form an external ear is also undertaken (see Chapter 28). Many of these defects are associated with Treacher Collins and Goldenhar syndromes, both of which present difficulty for tracheal

**Table 21.2** Strategies to minimise blood loss during middle ear surgery

| Strategy | Method | Comment |
|---|---|---|
| Smooth induction of anaesthesia avoiding tachycardia or hypertension | Calm, relaxed patient | Sedative premedication if required<br>Avoid anticholinergic medication |
| Avoid coughing or straining on intubation | Establish TIVA before intubation | Use remifentanil to facilitate intubation, 0.5–1 mcg $kg^{-1}$ over 1 min: Propofol loading dose<br>Use topical laryngeal anaesthesia 1 mg $kg^{-1}$ |
| Keep the venous pressure low | Patient's head up tilted to 15–20° positioning | Avoid excessive head turning as it may obstruct the contralateral internal jugular vein |
| Ventilation strategy | Aim for normocapnia | Slow respiratory rate<br>No PEEP<br>Long expiratory time |
| Aim for a systolic blood pressure of 80 mmHg | Analgesia: infiltration with lidocaine and adrenaline1:200,000<br>Anaesthesia (TIVA): remifentanil 0.1–0.5 mcg $kg^{-1}$ $min^{-1}$<br>Propofol 2%<br>Manual control or target control.<br>Propofol manual control: 13/11/9 mg $kg^{-1}$ $h^{-1}$<br>Reduce at 10 min intervals until 9 mg $kg^{-1}$ $h^{-1}$ maintenance | Titrate to desired blood pressure |

intubation. Anaesthesia for these operations can usually be managed using a flexible LMA, which obviates the need for intubation. It is essential to be satisfied with the performance of the LMA with the head in the operative position before surgery commences.

## Head and Neck Tumours

Extensive dissection may be required in some head and neck masses. Anaesthesia management includes potentially difficult intubation, appropriate monitoring, compensation for heat loss and preparation for rapid transfusion if needed, as in any major surgical intervention.

## Juvenile Nasopharyngeal Angiofibroma

Juvenile nasopharyngeal angiofibroma (JNA) is a highly vascularised and histologically benign tumour of the nasal cavity and paranasal sinuses, with aggressive behaviour and locally invasive growth patterns. It comprises 0.05% of head and neck tumours and predominantly occurs in young boys, with a mean age of presentation of 15 years. The best treatment to date remains surgical removal of the tumour. Preoperative embolisation is used for virtually all cases of JNA, resulting in reduction of intraoperative bleeding; occlusion of surgically inaccessible arterial feeding vessels; decreased operative time; and improved surgical visualisation, identification and protection of adjacent structures. This results in a significant reduction of overall surgical complications and is the standard of care in most centres. The anaesthetist must be prepared for significant blood loss. Large bore cannulae, tranexamic acid, cross-matched blood available and remifentanil infusion are advised.

## Ex-Utero Intrapartum Treatment

The ex-utero intrapartum treatment (EXIT) procedure is performed by a multidisciplinary team during caesarean section. It is indicated when the neonate's airway is at significant risk of severe obstruction immediately after birth. The technique allows the fetus to be partially delivered and the airway to be controlled whilst placental perfusion is maintained. It was originally used in 1989 to deliver a fetus with a large anterior neck mass. It then became part of the antenatal treatment of congenital diaphragmatic hernias. In this condition, it was discovered that prenatal obstruction of the trachea using surgical clips could allow expansion and maturation of fetal lungs. The EXIT procedure allowed removal of the tracheal clips prior to delivery whilst the fetus remained well oxygenated on placental bypass.

The EXIT procedure is now indicated for other fetal conditions where airway obstruction is a significant risk immediately after birth. These conditions include giant fetal neck masses, lung or mediastinal tumours, congenital high airway obstruction syndrome (CHAOS) and EXIT to extracorporeal membrane oxygenation (ECMO) for certain congenital cardiac conditions and congenital cystic adenomatoid malformation. Recently, EXIT-to-airway for severe micrognathia has been added to this list. An EXIT procedure provides the opportunity to maintain oxygenation for up to 60 minutes prior to placental separation. This window of opportunity can be used to safely intubate the airway prior to delivery.

### Key Points

- Extreme vigilance is essential during procedures on the airway.
- Diagnostic microlaryngoscopy and bronchoscopy requires spontaneous ventilation to be maintained. This necessitates good topical anaesthesia of the larynx.
- Postoperative vomiting occurs commonly during ENT surgery, and antiemetics should be administered in all cases.
- TIVA is the most appropriate mode of anaesthesia for middle ear surgery.

## Further Reading


Cook TM, Wolf AR, Henderson AJ. Changes in blood-gas tensions during apnoeic oxygenation in paediatric patients. *British Journal of Anaesthesia* 1998 September; 81(3):338–42. doi: 10.1093/bja/81.3.338.

Dick JR, Wimalasundera R, Nandi R. Maternal and fetal anaesthesia for fetal surgery. *Anaesthesia* 2021 April; 76(Suppl 4):63–8.

Din T, Abdalla T, Chiesa-Estomba C et al. YO-IFOS guidelines for pediatric ENT surgery during COVID-19: an overview of recommendations. *Laryngoscope* 2021 August; 131 (8):1876–83. doi: 10.1002/lary.29335. Epub 2020 Dec 25. PMID: 33325043 Review.

Hardman JG, Wills JS. The development of hypoxaemia during apnoea in children: a computational modelling investigation. *British Journal of Anaesthesia* 2006 October; 97 (4):564–70.

Mitchell RB, Archer SM, Ishman SL et al. Clinical practice guideline: tonsillectomy in children (update). Executive summary. *Otolaryngology – Head and Neck Surgery* 2019 February; 160 (2):187–205. doi: 10.1177/0194599818807917.

Zubair A, Sutton L, Murkin C et al. The changing face of paediatric airway endoscopic surgery: an 8-year single surgeon review. *International Journal of Pediatric Otorhinolaryngology* 2022 May; 156:111104. doi: 10.1016/j.ijporl.2022.111104. Epub 2022 Mar 15.

Chapter 22

# The Compromised Paediatric Airway*

Nadine Dobby

## Introduction

The incidence of a difficult paediatric airway is rare with risk of difficult laryngoscopy estimated at 1.35%. Familiarity with the differences in anatomy and physiology, thoughtful planning, clear communication and a thorough knowledge of specialised paediatric airway equipment are essential. Anaesthetists will be required to provide airway stabilisation for either elective surgical situations in a child with a known difficult airway or to establish a definitive airway in a child in an emergency with most likely a normal airway. An unpredicted difficult pediatric airway is extremely rare.

A compromised airway can be considered to occur when a trained anaesthetist experiences difficulty with face mask ventilation, difficulty with tracheal intubation or both. A Cormack and Lehane grade 3 or 4 airway is considered difficult, though other abnormalities can compromise the airway even when the grading is less.

The causes of difficulty are largely infections or congenital abnormalities (see Table 22.1). Infections often present acutely and in children with no other comorbidity. Children with a known difficult airway may present for planned investigations or surgery but may also present acutely with symptoms exacerbated by respiratory infection. Congenital abnormalities associated with dysmorphic features, macroglossia, limited submandibular space (retrognathia, micrognathia, mandibular hypoplasia) and limited neck or temporomandibular joint (TMJ) mobility all lead to difficult bag mask ventilation, difficult intubation or both.

Even maintaining the airway in a normal neonate or infant under anaesthesia can prove a challenge for the inexperienced practitioner, further highlighting the need for knowledge of the anatomy and paediatric airway equipment and the difficulties likely to be encountered. It is only with knowledge and experience that clear formulation of a plan can be put in place to avoid complications and achieve successful intubation.

A major recent study found that occurrence of complications is associated with more than two tracheal intubation attempts, a weight of less than 10 kg, short thyromental distance and three direct laryngoscopy attempts before an indirect technique is attempted. All these factors will be exacerbated when associated with an inexperienced operator unaware of the likely challenges of a paediatric airway with little experience of using specialised paediatric airway equipment.

## Features of the Paediatric Airway

It is easy for management of a normal airway to spiral out of control if one does not realise that the prominent occiput of an infant tends to cause neck flexion and the tongue is relatively large. These factors contribute to airway obstruction, as pharyngeal tone is lost. Simple techniques such as chin lift (avoiding compression of the structures of the floor of the mouth), application of continuous positive airway pressure (CPAP) and insertion of a Guedel airway (if the child is adequately anaesthetised) are useful. The supraglottic airway (SGA) has an important role in managing the difficult airway in children of all ages.

The upper airway mucosa is loosely adherent to the submucosa in infants and prone to oedema, except over the vocal cords and laryngeal surface of the epiglottis. Laryngeal oedema from repeated intubation attempts may convert a difficult intubation into an impossible one. The diameter of the airway at the cricoid in neonates is only 4–5 mm, and even 1 mm of oedema, for instance from infection, results in significant reduction in

* Many thanks to Dr Stephanie Bew, who wrote the first edition of this book chapter, much of the content of which has been used in this revised update.

**Table 22.1** Common causes of upper airway obstruction in children

| Congenital | | Acquired | |
|---|---|---|---|
| *Choanal atresia* | | *Infections* | Croup (laryngotracheobronchitis)<br>Epiglottitis<br>Bacterial tracheitis |
| *Craniofacial malformations* | Pierre Robin syndrome<br>Treacher Collins syndrome<br>Goldenhar syndrome<br>Midfacial hypoplasia | | Quinsy<br>Ludwig's angina<br>Diphtheria |
| *Macroglossia* | Down syndrome<br>Beckwith–Wiedemann<br>Mucopolysaccharidoses | *Physical obstruction* | Foreign body<br>Trauma<br>Adenotonsillar hypertrophy<br>Thermal or chemical burns |
| *Larynx* | Laryngomalacia<br>Laryngeal web<br>Laryngeal cleft<br>Vocal cord palsy<br>Subglottic stenosis<br>Haemangioma | | Postintubation oedema<br>Postoperative oedema<br>Angio-oedema<br>Acquired laryngeal or subglottic stenosis<br>Rheumatoid arthritis<br>Tumours<br>Cysts |
| *Tracheal* | Tracheomalacia<br>Tracheal stenosis<br>Vascular rings | *Neurogenic* | Lymph nodes<br>Depressed consciousness<br>Nerve palsy |

cross-sectional area and an increase in resistance (Poiseuille's law). The cartilaginous structures of the chest wall are compliant in infants and young children, and increased respiratory effort causes sternal and subcostal recession with decreased mechanical efficiency. The metabolic rate and oxygen consumption are high, the functional residual capacity is relatively small and the diaphragm has fewer fatigue-resistant fibres, all limiting respiratory reserve. The infant with severe respiratory infection is easily exhausted, and airway obstruction leads to rapid desaturation.

In some cases, progression to severe airway compromise is rapid, and immediate intervention is required. In others, problems may develop over days or weeks, or the child may present for elective surgery unrelated to the airway. In any situation, it is important to assess the airway carefully, to formulate a clear plan, including contingency plans should the first one fail.

## Assessment of the Airway

The diagnosis of a narrow or compromised airway may be obvious, for instance in a child with a known congenital condition or a child who presents with loud stridor or marked respiratory distress. Sometimes the signs may be very subtle, and it is easy to underestimate the degree of airway compromise. This is particularly the case where there is a slowly worsening fixed narrowing when there is often minimal stridor and little sign of increased work of breathing at rest. An example of this is the child with subglottic stenosis or airway complications of caustic ingestion.

Airway assessment in terms of the typical measurements in adults (Mallampati grade, thyromental and sternomental distances) have not been validated in children, and the paediatric population may not be keen to comply in any case. Instead, assessment of the airway requires a careful clinical history, from often well-informed parents, and examination to obtain an indication of the likely cause and whether the problem is supraglottic, glottic, subglottic or lower down the respiratory tract. Investigations are rarely helpful or appropriate in the acute situation but may have a role in the stable child.

## History

In addition to the normal anaesthetic history, questions should be targeted at airway problems.

Is this a previously normal airway? Consider previous airway problems or airway surgery and previous episodes of intubation and ventilation, especially for ex-premature infants. Even short periods of intubation can lead to the development of subglottic stenosis or cysts that may not cause any issues until the next intubation attempt. Previous cardiac surgery or repair of a tracheoesophageal fistula can make vocal cord palsy or tracheomalacia more likely.

Pay attention to previous respiratory problems such as asthma, especially if diagnosed at a particularly young age, atypical or not responding to treatment.

Have the parents heard stridor or other respiratory noise? Has there been a witnessed coughing or choking episode suggestive of an inhaled or swallowed foreign body?

Ask the questions:

---

**Is the noise constant or intermittent; what are the effects of positioning or exertion? Is it getting worse or better?**

**Ask about the onset and duration of the problem.**

**Are there any exacerbating or relieving factors?**

---

In addition, ask if the parents have noticed a change to the child's voice or cry; weakness, hoarseness or aphonia suggest a laryngeal pathology.

Airway obstruction should also be considered. Question the parents regarding the presence of snoring, periods of apnoea and what position the child adopts for sleeping. A child with an obstructed airway may adopt odd positions to help maintain their airway during normal sleep. Children who obstruct their airways during sleep will almost certainly obstruct on induction of anaesthesia, and the anaesthetist should be prepared to manage this.

It is useful to assess respiratory reserve by asking if the child can keep up with their peers in the playground and during sport. For infants, ask about feeding and thriving. A child who is using up too much energy to breathe or struggling to breathe will not feed well or gain weight and may be requiring nasogastric feeds.

## Examination

In the case of a compromised airway, examination may be best done from a distance so as not to cause further distress and deterioration.

Are they expected size for age?

- If small, are they an ex-premature infant, or is faltering growth due to chronic airway obstruction?
- Note BMI, which may lead to rapid desaturation in obese children, especially since you may not be able to effectively preoxygenate.

Look at the child's position:

- Are they maintaining a tripod position or extended neck to optimise their airway?
- Do they have torticollis? This may suggest neck pain associated with a retropharyngeal abscess.

Look at the pattern of breathing:

- Signs of increased work of breathing: tracheal tug, sternal recession, subcostal recession, head bobbing, nasal flaring, grunting and tachypnoea are concerning.
- Further deterioration of the child is evidenced by signs of hypoxaemia or hypercapnia such as tachycardia, pallor, peripheral or central cyanosis, agitation and confusion. Rapid intervention is needed before apnoeas (signalling total exhaustion) commence.
- Other signs such as prolonged expiration may suggest laryngeal or subglottic narrowing, whereas drooling suggests pain or inability to swallow due to epiglottitis, laryngeal foreign body or a retropharyngeal abscess.

Listen to the breathing:

- Abnormal breath sounds often indicate the site of airway narrowing. The loudness of the stridor does not, however, relate to the severity of obstruction; a child with a critically obstructed airway may be almost silent.
- Stridor: a high-pitched sound on inhalation or exhalation
    - Inspiratory stridor is classically associated with a narrowing above the cords.
    - Expiratory stridor is associated with narrowing below the vocal cords or an intrathoracic problem.
    - Biphasic stridor is associated with narrowing at or just below the cords.
- Stertor: heavy snoring inspiratory sound
    - Obstruction at the tongue base or larynx
- Croupy cough
    - Subglottic pathology

- Hoarse cry or breathy voice
  - Vocal cord pathology

In assessing the airway, a great deal of useful information can be gained even from a distance. Determine whether laryngoscopy or face mask ventilation are likely to be challenging; syndromic facies, retrognathia and micrognathia (most obvious when the child is viewed in profile) increase the likelihood of difficulty.

Check for adequate mouth opening, examine the teeth and the tongue and consider whether the oral cavity will allow access for a standard laryngoscope, videolaryngoscope or an SGA Also assess neck flexion and extension.

Examine the chest to check for any problem that is potentially reversible, such as bronchospasm or infection. Decreased respiratory reserve may cause rapid desaturation during induction of anaesthesia. In addition, pyrexia and increased metabolic rate and oxygen consumption may also exacerbate this.

Remember to assess venous access, as this may be difficult in the ex-premature infant or any child who is unwell.

## Monitoring

Pulse oximetry is well tolerated and allows continuous monitoring of heart rate as well as oxygen saturation. In an acutely unwell child, the respiratory rate must be checked frequently. Increased rate suggests increased work of breathing; a marked decrease in rate suggests exhaustion. Frequent documentation of these observations will highlight the trends and allow faster recognition of deterioration, which may require urgent intervention to secure the airway.

## Investigations

Investigations and imaging are often inappropriate in an acutely compromised child. Attempts to take a sample for blood gas analysis or site a cannula may cause agitation and crying, increase turbulent airflow, worsen respiratory distress or precipitate complete airway obstruction. In a stable child, anteroposterior (AP) and lateral soft tissue neck X-rays may be helpful in diagnosis, for example in croup or retropharyngeal abscess. In children with a chronic problem, MRI and CT scans or a barium swallow to look for tracheal compression may be helpful. Increasingly, ENT surgeons are using awake nasendoscopy in children. These investigations may give detailed information about the size and site of narrowing. Children with obstructed breathing during sleep may have a sleep study or overnight oximetry recording.

## Management: Acute Airway Compromise

In acute airway compromise, medical management will sometimes resolve the problem or avoid the need for immediate intubation. The use of inhaled or intravenous steroids and nebulised adrenaline in the treatment of croup reduces the duration of illness and the need for intubation (dexamethasone 600 mcg $kg^{-1}$ PO to a maximum of 8 mg or nebulised budesonide 2 mg; nebulised adrenaline 0.5 ml $kg^{-1}$ 1:1,000 solution to a maximum of 5 ml). These treatments may also 'buy time' and stabilise the child whilst preparations are made to secure the airway. Occasionally, inhaling a helium–oxygen mixture (heliox, usually 21% O2 in helium) is helpful in reducing work of breathing and preventing exhaustion and may allow time for steroids to act.

## Planning Management of Acute Airway Problems

Based on your assessment, decide what difficulties you anticipate and how you will manage these with the skills and equipment available. It is likely that more hands will be required, so call for help early. Two experienced anaesthetists are often needed along with a skilled anaesthetic assistant and a surgeon capable of performing a rigid bronchoscopy and tracheostomy. The familiar environment of an anaesthetic room or theatres with the staff and equipment you need to safely manage the situation is often most suitable but must be balanced against the risk of transferring the child with an unsafe airway from the ward or emergency department.

Parental presence can help to keep the child calm and cooperative, but you must clearly discuss the risks and plan in detail with them and the child without causing distress.

Parents need to know what problems you anticipate, what to expect in the anaesthetic room, and how they can help their child. If appropriate, the possibility of death, disability and tracheostomy need to be discussed, including plans for postoperative care on the intensive care unit. It may be useful to have the parents present for induction, but be aware of time spent trying to remove parents from the anaesthetic room at this critical moment and assign someone who will swiftly but gently escort them away.

Prepare your 'Plan A' airway management and for contingency plans, as these may need to be employed in light of changing circumstances. Having decided what equipment you require, you must check it personally, ensure that it is all working and that you have it in a range of appropriate sizes.

Cognitive skills, teamwork and clear communication are essential to success. A team brief and WHO checklist should be undertaken to ensure the correct team is present, to communicate the roles and responsibilities of the team members and to ensure the whole team understands the plans.

Only rarely in paediatrics is the airway secured awake, either by fibreoptic intubation or tracheostomy under local anaesthetic. Children, particularly those most likely to have a difficult airway, are unlikely to cooperate, and this can result in a chaotic and uncontrolled situation. In most acute cases where the exact pathology and degree of narrowing is unknown, general anaesthesia is required.

Induction of anaesthesia can be inhalational or intravenous, depending on the anaesthetist's preference and experience. The aim of induction in a compromised airway is to achieve anaesthesia whilst maintaining spontaneous respiration. Intravenous induction agents should be used cautiously; tolerance can be unpredictable, causing apnoeas and deterioration of the situation. If the anaesthetist is comfortable performing an inhalational induction with sevoflurane in oxygen, generally it will allow a more gradual deepening of anaesthesia and continuation of respiration. Apnoeas can also occur with this technique once the child is deep, but the operator should be able to monitor respiratory depth and effort more easily and reduce sevoflurane early enough to prevent apnoea. Each case needs individual assessment of whether to insert a cannula before induction or whether this would cause distress and worsening of symptoms. Similarly, the application of full monitoring prior to induction may not be appropriate, but pulse oximetry is generally well tolerated. If the child is adopting a particular position to optimise their airway, anaesthesia should be induced in this position. Atropine was once used as standard in these cases, either 20 mcg $kg^{-1}$ after intravenous access is obtained or orally pre-induction (20–30 mcg $kg^{-1}$), but this requires over an hour to be effective. It is no longer used routinely, but in cases with copious secretions, atropine can prove useful.

Be prepared to wait some time to achieve the required depth of anaesthesia, particularly when the airway is extremely narrow and there is little gas moving with each breath. If in doubt, wait a little longer and keep assessing the respiratory pattern and depth. The operator must be careful to maintain a patent airway but not cause pain or stimulation whilst doing so, as this may lead to laryngospasm. An oropharyngeal airway may be used to assist achieving airway patency, but this should only be placed once the anaesthetist is sure of adequate depth of anaesthesia. A nasopharyngeal airway may be used and is often better tolerated in lighter planes of anaesthesia, but it should be well lubricated, as bleeding from insertion will only add to the risk of laryngospasm and impair laryngoscopy.

To achieve control of the airway and allow depth of anaesthesia to be reached, gentle, basic airway opening manoeuvres such as chin lift and jaw thrust are used. Application of CPAP via face mask is almost always helpful, acting as a dynamic splint to increase the airway diameter, decrease atelectasis and reduce thoracoabdominal asynchrony. If holding the airway is difficult, immediately convert to a two-person technique with one anaesthetist holding the face mask to gain a good seal and the other maintaining CPAP. Aim for 5–10 cm of CPAP but beware that too much pressure can cause gastric distension. If this does occur, the stomach may be deflated with an oro- or nasogastric tube. If holding a face mask continues to be difficult but the child is anaesthetised, you can consider placing a supraglottic airways device (SGA) as an interim step before attempting intubation.

Opinion varies regarding the use of neuromuscular blocking drugs (NMBDs) in these cases. Some would prefer to achieve adequate depth of anaesthesia and perform direct laryngoscopy without NMBDs to prevent a 'cannot intubate, cannot ventilate' situation. Others argue that it is possible to take over the child's ventilation when the child is deeply anaesthetised, giving the operator confidence that they can ventilate should they give an NMBD and intubation fails. In addition, it is argued that an NMBD should be given to provide the best conditions for intubation on the first attempt.

Intubation in difficult circumstances should be undertaken by the most experienced anaesthetist. Remember that you may need a much smaller tracheal tube than expected for age. If you do not get a good view or cannot pass a tube at the first attempt, return to face mask ventilation or insert an SGA. Think carefully about how you will proceed.

Recent publications show that in a difficult paediatric airway, first-attempt success rates at intubation with direct laryngoscopy are extremely low at around 3% compared to a success rate of 55% with fibreoptic bronchoscopy, and 55% with video laryngoscopy. The complications were associated with more than two intubation attempts.

Therefore, carefully consider whether there any point in repeating laryngoscopy with the same laryngoscope. Is it likely that a shoulder roll, bougie, stylet or different sized tracheal tube will achieve intubation?

After two unsuccessful attempts at direct laryngoscopy, the operator should change technique. The choice of technique depends on the equipment available and the skills and experience of the anaesthetist.

## Advanced Techniques for Managing the Airway

### Indirect Laryngoscopy

There is a range of video larygoscopes/endoscopes available, including the McGrath®, Airtraq®, Glidescope® and C-MAC™. C-MAC and McGrath have specific paediatric airway blades which are useful in these situations. There is a learning curve associated with each, so practice on elective surgical lists should take place.

There are situations, however, when an indirect laryngoscope alone will not affect intubation and then more advanced techniques are required.

Flexible endoscopy:

A flexible fibreoptic scope is another option depending on availability and experience. If the child is breathing spontaneously, anaesthesia and oxygenation can either be maintained with a circuit attached to a short tracheal tube used as a nasopharyngeal airway or using a face mask or angle piece with a fisheye through which you can insert your fibreoptic scope. If the patient has been paralysed, intravenous anaesthesia will be required.

**Table 22.2** Minimum tracheal tube sizes for different sized endoscopes

| Endoscope diameter | Minimum tracheal tube size |
|---|---|
| 2.2 mm | 2.5 |
| 2.8 mm | 3 fits tightly, ideally 3.5 |
| 3.7 mm | 4 fits tightly, ideally 4.5 |

Flexible endoscopy can be performed via the nasal or oral route. In a difficult paediatric airway with an anterior larynx, the nasal route is likely to be easier; the nasal anatomy is easy to follow, with fewer angles to be navigated by the scope. The nose should be prepared with a local anaesthetic agent and vasoconstrictor before starting. Even a small amount of blood can obscure the view.

Be aware of the endoscopes available in your hospital and the correctly sized tracheal tubes which can be preloaded onto them (see Table 22.2).

### Combined Technique: Indirect Laryngoscope with Endoscopy

An additional method is to use a videolaryngoscope combined with a fibreoptic scope acting as a manoevreable bougie. This method can quickly secure the airway but does require two skilled anaesthetists who are familiar with the equipment and technique (Figure 22.1). The first anaesthetist operates the videolaryngoscope to obtain an optimal view of the larynx whilst a second anaesthetist operates the endoscope with a tracheal tube preloaded onto the scope.

### Fibreoptic Intubation via an SGA

A further method is to use an SGA as a conduit for fibreoptic intubation using a guidewire and airway exchange catheter. This is especially useful if there is no availability of small fibreoptic scopes.

This technique was originally described using the classic LMA™ (cLMA), which is made from silicone so that the fibreoptic scope usually passes smoothly between the epiglottic bars. If a disposable SGA is used, you may encounter resistance

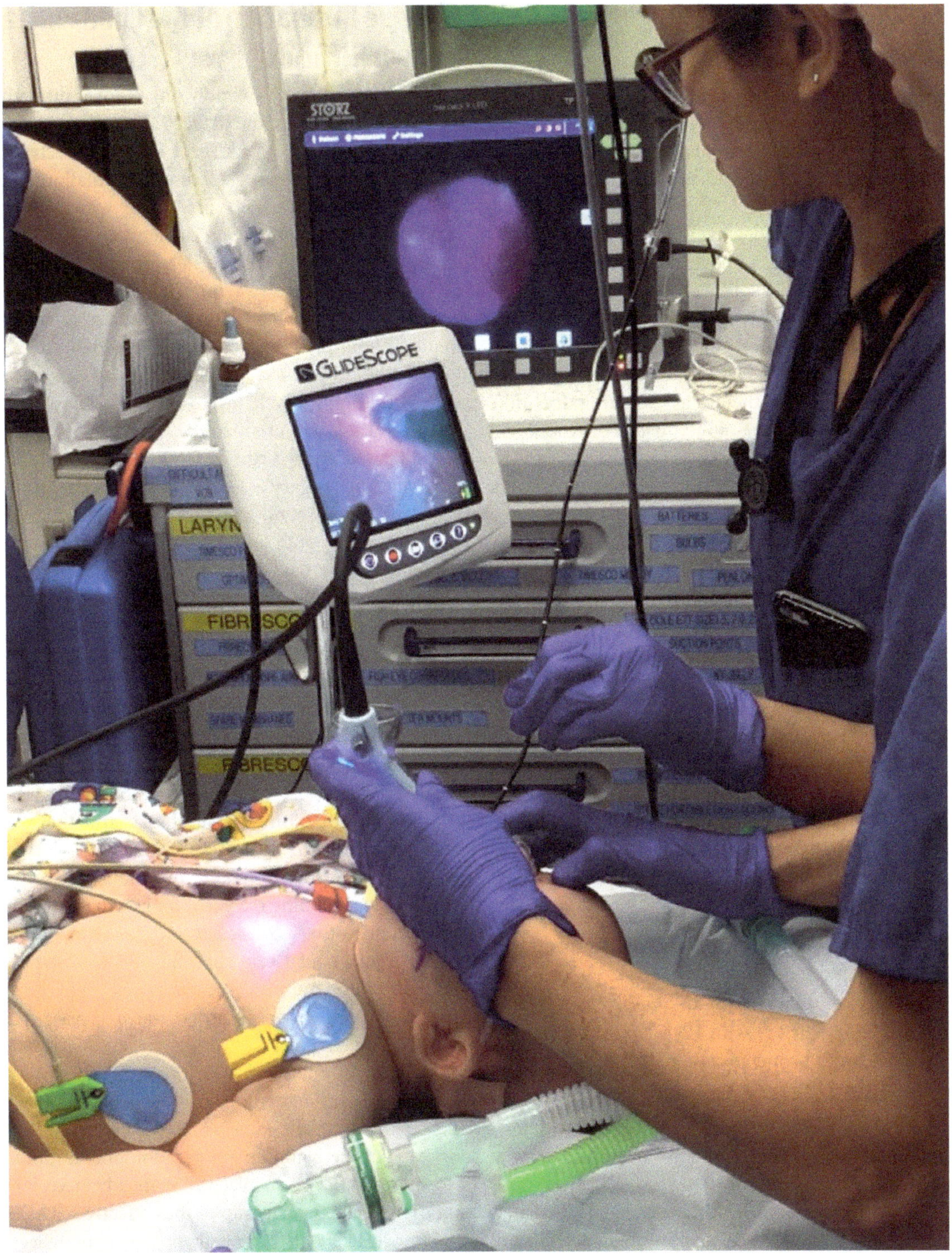


**Figure 22.1** Combined videolaryngoscope–fibreoptic scope technique. One operator uses a videolaryngoscope to visualise the larynx, whilst a second operator uses the fibreoptic scope as a manoevreable bougie.

passing the fibreoptic scope through the epiglottic bars, and it is better to remove them before starting or to use a Fannin SGA. It is essential to check meticulously that any bars that are removed are identified and disposed of well away from the equipment trolley.

The larynx is usually easily visualised or the scope can be manipulated past the epiglottis to get a view. Once the scope is positioned above the larynx, topical lidocaine 1% (3 mg $kg^{-1}$) is applied via the suction port either using an epidural catheter or a 5 ml syringe containing the topical anaesthetic plus a few millitres of air to spray the larynx. Alternatively, a muscle relaxant may be administered and ventilation maintained via the SGA.

A J-tipped guidewire can then be passed through the suction port and into the distal trachea, and the fibreoptic scope removed.

An 8 Fr paediatric airway exchange catheter is railroaded over the guidewire and the wire removed. It is easier to intubate over the stiff airway exchange catheter, as inserting the tube over the guidewire alone usually results in oesophageal intubation. A capnograph can be attached to the airway exchange catheter to check for $CO_2$.

The SGA is removed, leaving the airway exchange catheter in place. The tracheal tube can now be inserted over the airway exchange catheter and the position checked in the usual way.

There are occasions where intubation is not possible. There may be a mass obstructing the airway or unrecognisable anatomy. The airway may be too narrow for the smallest tube, or the difficult intubation equipment may not be successful. Multiple repeated attempts at laryngoscopy and intubation will cause oedema and bleeding.

In these situations, maintain spontaneous ventilation and consider the following options:

- Wake the child up. This may not be possible with the child with acute airway compromise but should always be considered.
- Secure the airway with an SGA.
- Secure the airway with ENT surgical support and a rigid bronchoscope or tracheostomy.

It may be necessary to allow the surgeons to remove a mass or aspirate a cyst under spontaneous ventilation or proceed to a surgical airway using only a face mask or SGA.

Effective decision-making is crucial. Repeated attempts at laryngoscopy and intubation will only cause further complications. The airway may already be narrow and inflamed, and the situation can rapidly spiral out of control. Discussion should occur between anaesthesia, intensive care, ENT surgery and the local paediatric transport service; communication will need to be clear and concise.

## Elective Intubation of the Child with a Known Difficult Airway

Elective intubation of a child with a known difficult airway requires the same detailed assessment as for acute airway compromise. There is a wide spectrum of difficulty, from easy face mask ventilation but difficult laryngoscopy, to airways in which every aspect of management is challenging. Previous anaesthetic records may be helpful but must not be relied on, as the airway may change as the child grows. Parents often have extremely useful information about previous anaesthetic experiences.

Ideally, informed discussion and consent should take place well in advance of the surgery in the setting of a preoperative assessment clinic. A multidisciplinary team meeting may be required to ensure the surgery is worth the risk of anaesthesia. The parents and child should have a clear explanation about anticipated difficulties and strategies for managing the airway and discussions regarding the possibility of an emergency or planned tracheostomy should take place. The possibility of waking the child up if the airway cannot be safely managed must also be emphasised.

Many of the known difficult airways in children are associated with anatomical abnormalities as part of a syndrome such as Pierre Robin sequence. In general, it is not difficult to maintain oxygenation after induction of anaesthesia, and there is time for controlled intubation using a videolaryngoscope or flexible fibreoptic technique. In some children, maintaining oxygenation may be very difficult, and other cofascemorbidities can make airway management very challenging. For instance, children with mucopolysaccharidoses may have limited oxygen reserve, cardiac valve disease, an unstable neck and copious airway secretions, as well as being anatomically difficult to fit mask airways and perform laryngoscopy. The options for airway management are the same as for the compromised airway, but the planning, preparation and communication should be in place well in advance. The option to wake the child up in these elective cases is also more likely to be possible. Two experienced anaesthetists should be present.

## Extubation and Continuing Care of Children with Airway Compromise

A child undergoing a difficult intubation requires a plan for extubation. Many children will need to remain intubated in the intensive care unit for a period whilst airway oedema and infection resolve, and they may require a further airway examination under anaesthesia before extubation. Some will require tracheostomy either permanently or until all foreseen surgical procedures have taken place. In some children, natural growth may be needed for development of a safer airway.

Preparation for extubation should include checking for a leak around the tracheal tube, this is not always possible to hear but if present can give some confidence that airway swelling has settled. Dexamethasone 0.25 $mg.kg^{-1}$ IV should be used whenever possible to reduce oedema. It is best administered intraoperatively and continued in the lead-up to extubation.

Patients should be completely off sedation and awake with minimal secretions. They may be extubated on the intensive care unit, or at times returning to the theatre suite may be appropriate. The plan for extubation should be as clear as the plan for intubation and the team and equipment for reintubation should be fully prepared and present.

It is best to extubate the child in an upright position and apply positive end expiratory pressure (PEEP) with a face mask immediately after the tracheal tube has been removed. A nasopharyngeal airway inserted before waking can also be considered and is well tolerated in an awake child. Any patient previously receiving CPAP or BIPAP will most likely benefit from extubation directly to their preoperative machine and settings.

Placement of a guidewire through the tracheal tube, into the trachea and taped in place after extubation has been described with the thought that if emergency reintubation is required, a small airway exchange catheter can be passed over the wire and a tube railroaded over. In paediatric practice, this is uncommon, and the wire is unlikely to remain in the correct place once the child is extubated unless they are extremely compliant.

Difficult airways in children are uncommon, and elective intubations of children with known difficult airways are important opportunities for teaching and mutual sharing of experiences and knowledge. It is important to document findings, with a clear description of how difficulties were managed. Parents also need to be informed, as the child may present subsequently at a time and place where the anaesthetic records are not available. Giving the family an airway letter or airway 'passport' detailing relevant history to carry with them is useful for future hospital visits.

## Difficult Airway Guidelines and 'Cannot Intubate, Cannot Ventilate' Scenarios

The Association of Paediatric Anaesthetists of Great Britain and Ireland and the Difficult Airway Society have published a series of algorithms for difficult airways in children: difficult mask ventilation in a child 1 to 8 years of age; unanticipated difficult intubation; and cannot intubate and cannot ventilate (see www.apagbi.org.uk/publications/apa-guidelines). In children with compromised airways, oxygenation is often difficult, but it is rarely impossible. If the situation does deteriorate to 'can't intubate, can't oxygenate', hypoxia and bradycardia will rapidly ensue and a transtracheal airway must be achieved immediately. In a small infant, the options are very limited, and there is little evidence in the literature to guide practice.

## Transtracheal Techniques

Cricothyroidotomy as a rescue technique is very rarely required in children, and surgical tracheostomy may be a safer option. However, paediatric ENT support is not available in every hospital where children are anaesthetised, and occasionally an anaesthetist may need to insert a transtracheal airway with a patient in extremis.

In the small infant, the cartilages of the larynx are difficult to palpate and identify, and the cricothyroid membrane measures only 2.6 × 3 mm. In a neonate or small infant, the cricothyroid membrane is so closely related to the mandible that it is virtually impossible to access at the required angle even with the neck in full extension. These rescue attempts are highly unlikely to be successful.

An 18 G intravenous catheter can be inserted between the tracheal rings if the cricothyroid membrane cannot be identified. The catheter should be inserted with a syringe attached to the end of it, and the operator should continually aspirate as they insert. As soon as air is easily and successfully aspirated, further forward movement of the needle should be stopped and the cannula advanced into the trachea, the needle should be removed and air aspiration should be checked again. Oxygenation can be achieved by jet ventilation, but only if a device with adjustable pressure and flow is available. Start at low pressure (0.4 bar) and slowly increase to see the chest rise. Exhalation must occur through the natural airway, so the rate of jetting needs to be very slow. If you do not have a jet ventilation device, then the connector from a 3 mm tracheal tube will fit into the hub of an intravenous cannula, which then allows connection with any standard bag valve device.

In the older child, cannula cricothyroidotomy or a percutaneous cricothyroidotomy may be performed as in an adult, the latter allowing insertion of a small tracheostomy tube. Several manufacturers make devices in paediatric sizes. Positive pressure ventilation is possible through these tubes.

**Key Points**

- An unanticipated paediatric difficult airway is rare, but getting the basics wrong can cause an easy airway to become difficult. Be aware of the pitfalls of managing the paediatric airway.
- Gain knowledge and experience of at least one advanced airway technique in paediatrics. Practice with equipment as regularly as possible on elective lists.
- Call for appropriate help early, including a second consultant anaesthetist, and prepare your team well.
- Have a clear plan and aim for the highest quality of communication both within your team and with the family involved.

## Further Reading


Adewale L. Anatomy and assessment of the pediatric airway. *Paediatric Anaesthesia* 2009; 19:(suppl 1):1–8.

Black AE. Management of the difficult airway. In: Bingham R, Lloyd-Thomas A, Sury M, eds. *Hatch and Sumner's Textbook of Paediatric Anaesthesia*, 3rd ed. Hodder Arnold. 2008. 315–29.

Bruce IA, Rothera MP. Upper airway obstruction in children. *Paediatric Anaesthesia* 2009; 19:(suppl 1): 88–99.

Cote CJ, Hartnick CJ. Pediatric transtracheal and cricothyrotomy airway devices for emergency use: which are appropriate for infants and children? *Paediatric Anaesthesia* 2009; 19:(suppl 1): 66–76.

Fiadjoe J et al. Normal and difficult airways in children: 'whats's new' – current evidence. *Paediatric Anaesthesia* 2019 23 December; 30(3): 257–63.

Fiadjoe J, Nishisaki A. Airway management complications in children with difficult tracheal intubation from the Pediatric Difficult Intubation (PeDI) registry: a prospective cohort analysis. *Lancet* 2016 1 January; 4 (1):P37–48.

Habre W, Disma N. Incidence of severe critical events in paediatric anaesthesia (APRICOT): a prospective multicentre observational study in 261 hospitals in Europe. *Lancet Respiratory Medicine* 2017 May; 5(5):412–25.

Royal College of Anaesthetists and the Difficult Airway Society. 4th National Audit Project: Major Complications of Airway Management in the United Kingdom. Report and Findings. Chapter 21: Children. 2011 March.

Chapter 23

# Anaesthesia for Cleft Lip and Palate Surgery in Children*

Ravi Shihurkar, Agnes Watson and Philip Cunnington

## Introduction

Successful anaesthesia for cleft lip and palate surgery requires an understanding of the cleft condition, associated abnormalities and the surgery involved. Close cooperation with the surgeon is vital to manage the child's airway during and after surgery. The aim is to provide balanced anaesthesia and optimum analgesia, so a child starts feeding and is able to return to normal activities as soon as possible after surgery.

## Incidence, Type of Cleft and Embryology

Cleft lip and palate is a common congenital abnormality with an incidence of one in 700 live births, with around 1,100 affected children born in the United Kingdom each year. It encompasses two distinct conditions: cleft lip with or without cleft palate making up 55% of cases, and isolated cleft palate making up 45% of cases (Figure 23.1). The embryological abnormality is a failure of fusion at four to eight weeks of fetal life of the five facial prominences that form the facial structures. The medial nasal process and lateral maxillary process fuse to form the upper lip and front of the mouth. The embryonic palatal shelves fuse to form the palate– the primary palate anterior to the incisive foramen and the secondary palate posterior to this.

## Cleft Lip with or without Cleft Palate

In cleft lip with or without cleft palate (CL +/–P), the anomaly can be a cleft lip alone (CL), a unilateral cleft lip and palate (UCLP) or bilateral cleft lip and palate (BCLP). The condition varies in severity from a small notch caused by a defect in the muscle of the upper lip, called a microform cleft lip, to a wide bilateral cleft lip and palate. Cleft lip is termed complete if it goes to the nasal sill and incomplete if not. A scheme for surgical classification is shown in Figure 23.2.

Cleft lip is more often left-sided and has a male preponderance. It is more common in Chinese people than Caucasians and less common in the African-Caribbean population. The aetiology is both genetic and environmental. The presence of cleft lip with or without cleft palate in a first-degree relative increases the risk of a cleft in a pregnancy to 3–4%. Environmental factors that have been implicated are maternal diabetes, alcohol, folic acid deficiency and drugs, including phenytoin, corticosteroids and diazepam.

## Isolated Cleft Palate

Isolated cleft palate (iCP) is less common, accounts for 45% of clefts and has a female preponderance. The genetic risk of recurrence depends on the risk of recurrence of any associated syndrome.

The cleft may be of the soft palate or extend into the hard palate (Figure 23.2). A submucous cleft palate (SMCP) is a defect in the musculature of the soft palate; the palate may look normal, or there may be a bifid uvula or central lucency of the soft palate. A submucous cleft may present with speech abnormality or nasal regurgitation of food.

## Velopharyngeal Incompetence without Cleft Palate

A cleft service may encounter several children who do not have a cleft palate but who are referred with velopharyngeal incompetence (VPI). This condition is due to a relative mismatch between the palate and pharynx whereby speech sounds resonate in the nasal space producing, amongst other

* We wish to thank Mr Loshan Kangesu and Mr Amir Sadri for their advice regarding surgical management.

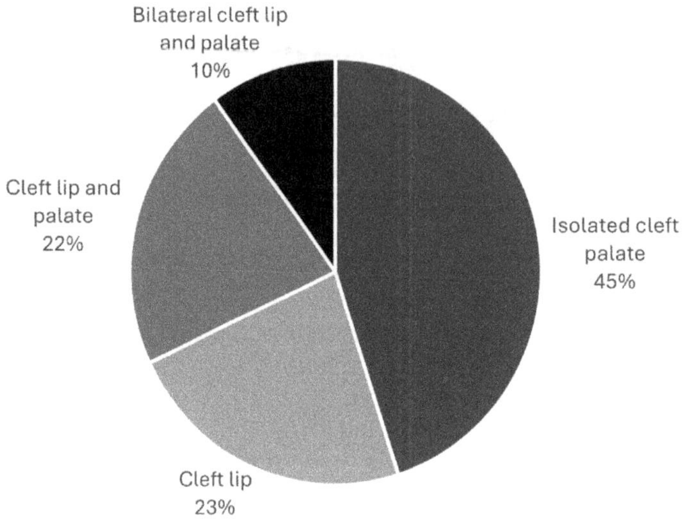


**Figure 23.1** The relative incidence of the common cleft types in the United Kingdom.

features, hypernasal speech. These children as a group are more complex. They are more likely than the cleft population to have associated syndromes, such as 22q deletion, other anomalies, feeding issues or learning difficulties. They may have an SMCP or a seemingly normal palate, and the VPI may be due to a large pharynx or neuromuscular weakness or poor coordination within the muscles responsible for speech.

## Association between Cleft Conditions and Other Congenital Abnormalities

There is an association between cleft conditions and other congenital abnormalities, especially iCP, which should be borne in mind during anaesthetic assessment. Infants with clefts are more likely to be born preterm with low birth weight. Up to 150 different congenital syndromes have been associated with clefts, and some of the more commonly occurring syndromes are listed in Table 23.1. Syndromes causing mandibular hypoplasia (micrognathia) result in airway problems, and those with associated cardiac defects are of particular relevance to the anaesthetist. Reviews of children with clefts have quoted an incidence of congenital heart disease from 3.7% to 15%, much higher than that in the general population.

### Pierre Robin Sequence

Pierre Robin sequence (PRS) is a combination of cleft palate, micrognathia and glossoptosis (posterior displacement of the tongue) and is present in 20–30% of children with isolated cleft palate. It may be associated with airway obstruction from the neonatal period through to early infancy in severe cases. Disease severity is classified as type 1–3. Babies with type 1 PRS have mild symptoms, and any airway obstruction may be relieved by side-to-side positioning rather than nursing supine. Babies with type 2 PRS have associated feeding difficulties requiring nasogastric feeding. Babies with type 3 PRS have moderate respiratory distress and are managed in the United Kingdom with a nasopharyngeal airway. A minority will require tracheostomy. Airway and feeding problems resolve with age as mandibular growth occurs.

### 22q11.2 Deletion Syndrome

22q deletion syndrome (previously called velocardiofacial or Di George syndrome) is caused by a microdeletion on chromosome 22. It usually occurs as a new mutation, although in some cases there is autosomal dominant inheritance.

It is the syndrome most commonly associated with clefts, and children may present with isolated cleft palate or submucous cleft palate, causing velopharyngeal incompetence and hypernasal speech. There is a wide spectrum of associated abnormalities, including cardiac defects (interrupted aortic arch, truncus arteriosus, tetralogy of Fallot or pulmonary atresia with VSD), typical facial characteristics of a broad nose and

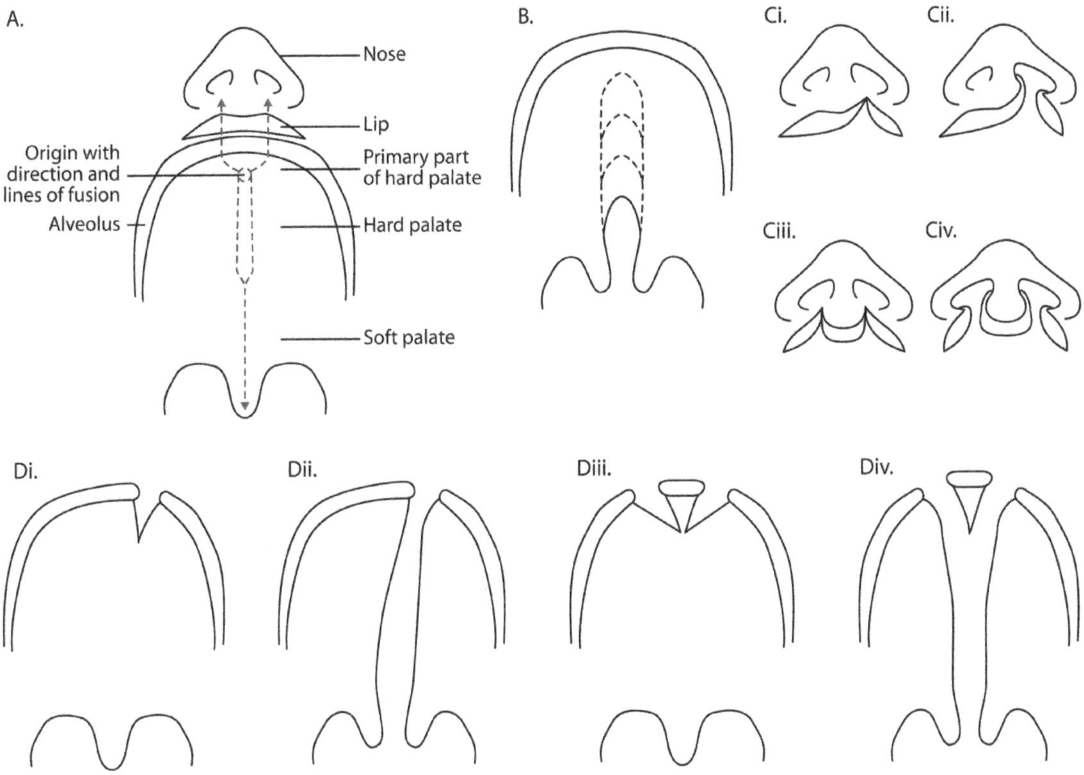


| | Left | Right | Midline |
|---|---|---|---|
| Lip | | | * |
| Alveolus | | | * |
| Hard palate | | | |
| Soft palate | N/A | N/A | |

*Very rare

**Figure 23.2** Surgical classification of cleft lip with or without cleft palate. Diagnostic findings are recorded in the grid.
Key:
A. Normal anatomy of nose, lip and alveolus and hard and soft palate with the lines of fusion emanating from the incisive foramen.
B. Differing extent of isolated cleft palate.
C. Cleft lip variants: Ci = left unilateral incomplete cleft lip; Cii = left unilateral complete cleft lip; Ciii = bilateral incomplete cleft lip; Civ = bilateral complete cleft lip.
D. Cleft palate variants: Di = left unilateral cleft of alveolus and primary hard palate; Dii = left unilateral cleft of alveolus, hard and soft palate; Diii = bilateral cleft of alveolus and primary hard palate; Div = bilateral cleft of alveolus, hard and soft palate.
*Source:* Reprinted from Demircioglu M, Kangesu L, Ismail A et al. Increasing accuracy of antenatal ultrasound diagnosis of cleft lip with or without cleft palate, in cases referred to the North Thames London Region. *Ultrasound in Obstetrics and Gynaecology* 2008; 31:649 copyright ISUOG, with permission from John Wiley and Sons.

long face, hypotonia in infancy, defective thymic development and learning disabilities.

## Multidisciplinary Care: The Cleft Team

The care of a child with a cleft requires a multidisciplinary approach from a team ideally involving specialist cleft nurses; plastic, maxillofacial and ENT surgeons; orthodontists; speech therapists; dieticians; paediatricians; geneticists; and clinical psychologists. In the United Kingdom, resources have now been concentrated into 11 specialist cleft centres following a review of services in 1998 by the Clinical Standards Advisory Group

**Table 23.1** Common syndromes associated with cleft lip and/or palate

| Name of syndrome (affected chromosome) | Clinical features |
|---|---|
| 22q11.2 deletion syndrome (velocardiofacial, Di George syndrome) | Isolated cleft palate or submucous cleft, cardiac defects, defective thymic development, learning disability, characteristic facial appearance |
| Pierre Robin sequence | Cleft palate, micrognathia and glossoptosis |
| Stickler (12q13.11–q13.2, 1p21, 6p21.3) | Collagen disorder, micrognathia, eye abnormalities, hearing loss, joint problems, characteristic facial appearance |
| Van der Woude (1q32–q41) | Cleft lip, lower lip pits, missing teeth. Autosomal dominant |
| Treacher Collins (5q32–q33.1) | Micrognathia, ear abnormalities, deafness, abnormal lower eyelids |
| Hemifacial microsomia (Goldenhar) (14q32) | Vertebral and cardiac abnormalities |
| Down (trisomy 21) | Macroglossia, cardiac defects, atlanto-axial instability, learning disability |
| Edwards (trisomy 18) | Cardiac defects, micrognathia, renal malformations. Often fatal in infancy |
| Patau (trisomy 13) | Developmental delay, microcephaly, micrognathia, cardiac defects. Often fatal in infancy |
| Ectodactyly ectodermal dysplasia and clefting syndrome (7q11.2–q21.3, 3q27) | Disordered temperature control with hypohidrosis, malnutrition, respiratory tract infections |

(CSAG). The goals of treatment are to enable the baby to develop into a confident child who becomes a socially integrated adult with normal speech and hearing, minimal facial disfigurement and normal dentition.

Timely detection has steadily improved in the United Kingdom over last 10 years, and nearly 85% of babies born with clefts are diagnosed antenatally or within 24 hours of birth. Over 70% of cleft lips are picked up on the 20-week anomaly scan, and support from the cleft team can be arranged at this stage. In other cases, diagnosis and referral are made after birth. Paediatricians are advised to make a visual inspection of the palate (rather than digital examination) during routine postnatal screening to exclude cleft palate. After diagnosis, assessment of feeding, facial appearance, speech, hearing and dentition is necessary to plan treatment.

Feeding difficulties are common for babies with cleft palate as they will not be able to suck effectively; the baby will have to work hard to feed and will be slow to put on weight. Parents are advised to use a special feeding bottle. Nasogastric feeding is sometimes necessary if oral feeding is unsuccessful, or if the baby presents for surgery with severe failure to thrive. Babies may also have uncoordinated swallowing and problems with reflux of milk. Most infants with isolated cleft lip are able to breastfeed successfully.

Hearing assessment is important in older infants, as the Eustachian tube does not open properly. Secretory otitis media is common, and grommets may be required at the time of cleft palate surgery.

Expert surgical care is the cornerstone of successful management. Repair of cleft lip is undertaken after three months of age and involves correction of the lip and nasal deformity (flattened alar margin and loss of nasal tip prominence on the cleft side and a displaced septum). Closure of the palate before the age of 13 months is recommended for optimum speech development. Late repair in older children or adults produces poorer results. The aim of surgery is to close the cleft palate and ensure good function of the soft palate without affecting normal maxillary growth. If the palate is short or does not function properly, air escapes through the velopharyngeal orifice during speech (VPI), which impairs phonation and causes hypernasal speech. The function of the normal soft palate is shown in Figure 23.3.

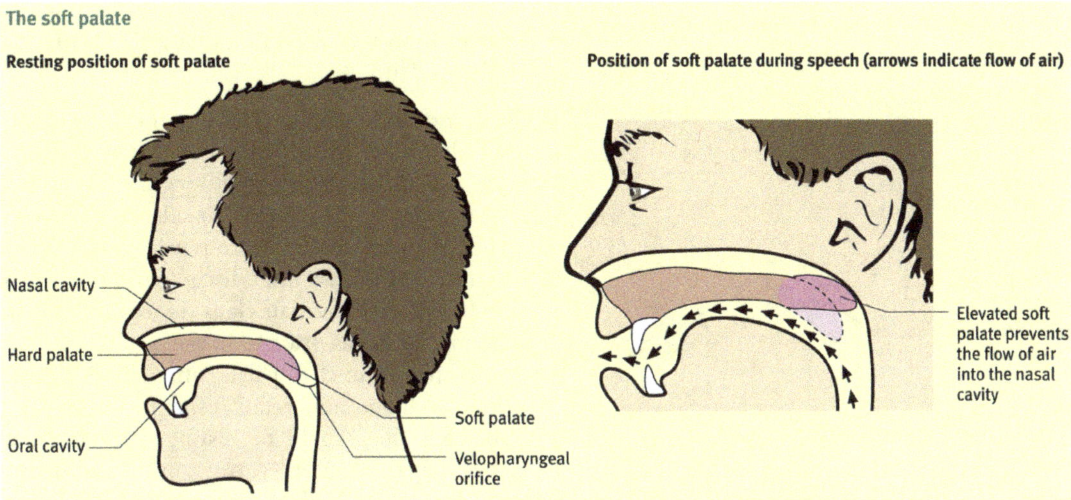


**Figure 23.3** The position of the soft palate at rest and during speech.
*Source:* Reprinted from Mosahebi A, Kangesu L. Cleft lip and palate. *Surgery (Oxford)* 2006; 24:34–7, with permission from Elsevier.

Later orthodontic surgery may be required to repair an alveolar defect to facilitate normal eruption of secondary teeth. Towards early adulthood, when facial growth has ended, surgery may be undertaken to improve bite, improve the airway or change the appearance of the nose.

Depending on the type of cleft, the child may require one procedure or multiple operations from infancy to early adulthood. The surgical procedures and the typical age at surgery in the North Thames Cleft Network are described in Table 23.2. Ongoing support for the family by the cleft team is essential, and in the United Kingdom, there are also national groups such as the Cleft Lip and Palate Association (CLAPA) that have played an important role in the design of patient-centred services.

**Table 23.2** Timing of surgery in the North Thames Cleft Service

| Age at surgery | Potential surgical procedures |
|---|---|
| 3–6 months | Primary cleft lip and nose repair and anterior palate |
| 9–12 months | Primary cleft palate repair +/– grommets |
| 1 year | Second-stage lip repair for bilateral cleft lip |
| 3 years onwards | Lip +/– nose revision |
| 3 years onwards | Secondary speech surgery – re-explore palate, buccinator flaps, pharyngoplasty, autologous fat transfer |
| Any age | Repair of palatal fistula |
| Any age | Primary repair of submucous palate |
| 9–10 years | Alveolar bone graft |
| 17–20 years | Maxillary osteotomy |
| 17–20 years | Rhinoplasty |

## Primary Repair of Lip and Palate

The quality of primary surgery is thought to determine the outcome of speech and facial growth. The practice in the North Thames Cleft Service is to undertake primary repair of cleft lip, nose and anterior palate (if required) at 3–6 months and primary repair of the palate at 9–12 months. Closure of the lip and palate during the neonatal period has been advocated previously but adds additional risk and appears to confer no surgical benefit.

Repair of the lip involves repositioning of the orbicularis and perioral muscles and correction of the nasal deformity. The anterior palate, if involved, can be closed at the same time, mobilising the periosteum of the septum, called a vomerine flap, to cover the defect.

The aim of palate repair is to close the defect, ensuring good function of the soft palate and the

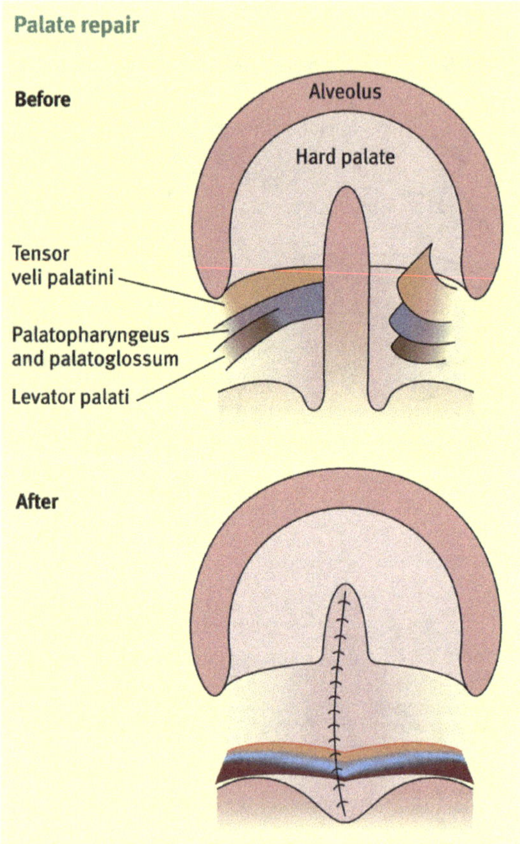


**Figure 23.4** Primary cleft palate repair – muscles of soft palate are realigned transversely.
*Source:* Reprinted from Mosahebi A, Kangesu L. Cleft lip and palate. *Surgery (Oxford)* 2006; 24:34–7, with permission from Elsevier.

least effect on maxillary growth. Closure of the palate is performed using an operating microscope to dissect the soft palate muscles and realign them transversely to the back of the soft palate (Figure 23.4). Lateral releasing incisions through the mucosa may be performed to reduce tension on the midline repair. Grommets may be inserted at the same time as palatal surgery, if required.

## Preoperative Assessment

Prior to surgery, infants should be well, thriving, gaining weight and following centile lines. Twelve per cent of babies with cleft are born prematurely compared to 7% in the general population. The historic guide of '10s' advocated by Wilhelmsen and Musgrave in 1966 was a useful guide for infants having lip repair. The infant should be:

Over 10 lb (4.5 kg)
Over 10 weeks old with a haemoglobin $>10$ g dl$^{-1}$
WCC $<10 \times 10^9$ dl$^{-1}$

Review of postoperative complications has identified that feeding difficulty, oesophageal reflux, poor weight gain and respiratory tract infections are associated with higher incidence of wound dehiscence and need for re-repair surgery. Our practice is to have multidisciplinary assessment led by general paediatricians to optimise these systemic concerns prior to surgery.

Infants with cleft palate often have chronic nasal discharge and reflux of milk through the nose, but this should be distinguished from an active upper respiratory tract infection. Infants who are unwell with mucopurulent nasal secretions or raised temperature are best postponed, as they are at much higher risk of airway complications perioperatively.

It is important to identify potential airway problems and other associated abnormalities (see Figure 23.5).

Airway assessment includes questioning regarding a history of obstructive symptoms and looking for micrognathia (best viewed in lateral profile). Severity of obstructive symptoms can be investigated with overnight oxygen saturation monitoring and polysomnography. Infants with severe micrognathia, most commonly associated with Pierre Robin sequence, may have a nasopharyngeal airway (NPA) in situ to relieve obstruction. They may have grown sufficiently so that the NPA is no longer needed but may still be required in the immediate postoperative period.

Infants with suspected cardiac abnormalities, such as those with low oxygen saturation readings or a heart murmur, require an echocardiogram and formal cardiology assessment. Healthy infants scheduled for simple lip repair do not require any routine blood tests. Those who are failing to thrive, are clinically anaemic or are having a bilateral lip repair require baseline haemoglobin measurement.

## Anaesthesia and Airway Management

Premedication in infants is not generally required. Inhalational induction of anaesthesia with sevoflurane in 100% oxygen is recommended to ensure good oxygenation and allow assessment of the airway whilst maintaining spontaneous ventilation. Infants with micrognathia may develop airway obstruction as they lose pharyngeal tone;

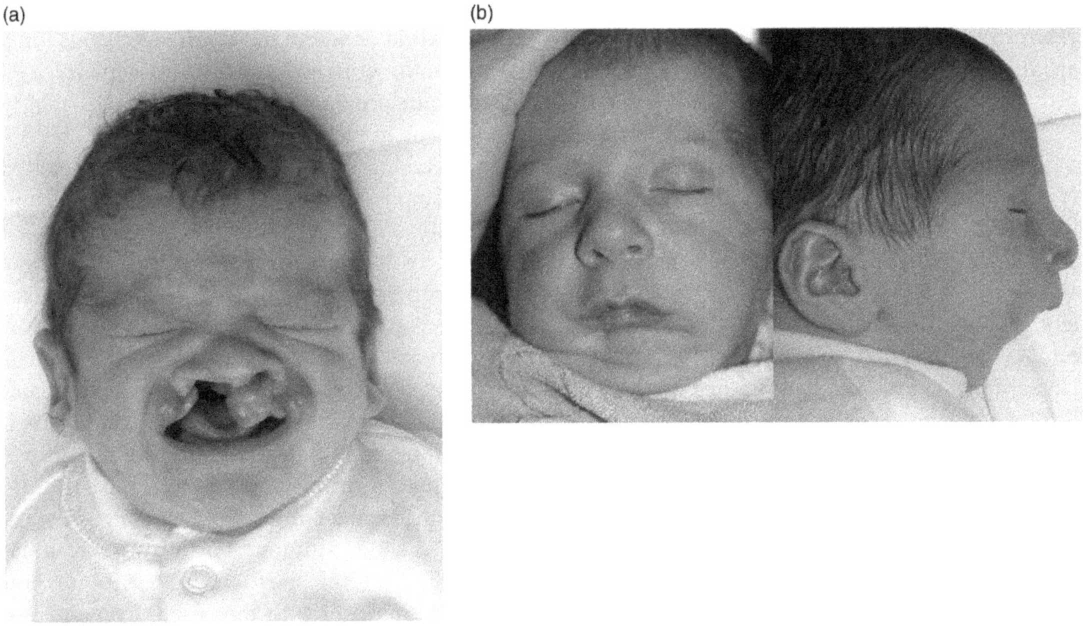

**Figure 23.5** Factors predicting difficult intubation. (a) Wide bilateral cleft lip and palate with protruding premaxilla. (b) Micrognathia in an infant with Pierre Robin sequence.
*Source:* Reprinted with permission from Sesenna E, Magri AS, Magnani C et al. Mandibular distraction in neonates: indications, techniques and results. *Italian Journal of Pediatrics* 2012; 38:7, www.ijponline.net/content/pdf/1824-7288-38-7.pdf).

this can usually be relieved by repositioning, use of continuous positive airway pressure or insertion of a nasal or oral airway. It is an early indicator of the need for a nasopharyngeal airway postoperatively. After intravenous access is secured, a non-depolarising muscle relaxant can be administered after the ability to inflate the lungs is confirmed. If there is difficulty, spontaneous breathing should be maintained.

Most infants will be easy to intubate. A preformed south-facing cuffed tracheal tube fixed in the midline provides a stable airway and aids surgical access. Difficult laryngoscopy is seen in approximately 5–8% of cases. Factors that predict a grade 3 or 4 Cormack and Lehane view at laryngoscopy are a wide bilateral cleft with protruding premaxilla or micrognathia in an infant under six months of age (Figures 23.5a, b). It is helpful that these factors are all readily identifiable preoperatively. Children with Pierre Robin sequence generally become easier to intubate as they become older, but this is not the case for children with other syndromes such as Treacher Collins or hemifacial microsomia.

Should difficulty be encountered with intubation, a variety of aids can be employed. Simple manoeuvres include pressure over the larynx and use of a gum elastic bougie or a stylet. Videolaryngoscopy has the obvious advantage of clearer visualisation of anatomy and helps in shared situational awareness for the airway team. Hyperangulated blades facilitate viewing the anterior larynx, although intubation of the trachea often needs shaping the tube with a stylet. Care should be taken to avoid the flange of the laryngoscope blade slipping into the cleft or injuring the premaxilla (in BCLP) as it is supplied by an end artery. More advanced techniques depend on the equipment available and the experience of the anaesthetist. A fibreoptic scope can be used alone or using a laryngeal mask airway as a conduit. The tracheal tube may be railroaded over the scope or a guidewire placed via the suction channel. An airway exchange catheter is then railroaded over the guidewire and the tracheal tube passed over this (see Chapter 22 regarding difficult airways in children).

It is rare that intubation is not possible (less than 1% of cases). Surgery should be postponed in this situation, as the child may become easier to intubate with age, and access for the surgery will be improved. Plans for difficult airway management can be made, including tracheostomy if necessary.

Routine use of a throat pack to reduce soiling of the airway with blood is now questioned. With increasing use of cuffed tracheal tubes, careful suctioning and meticulous haemostasis, several centres have stopped using throat packs, thereby avoiding the risk of mucosal injury, sore throat, oedema and retained throat pack.

Anaesthesia should be maintained with a volatile agent. Dexamethasone is administered to reduce airway oedema, and surgeons may request tranexamic acid to reduce operative blood loss and aid surgical view. Analgesia may be achieved with a variety of analgesic techniques such as intermittent boluses of fentanyl (1–3 mcg $kg^{-1}$) or remifentanil infusion (0.1–0.2 mcg $kg^{-1}$ $min^{-1}$). Lateral releasing incisions are particularly painful. Effective analgesia will contribute to smooth anaesthesia and may avoid the need for further muscle relaxation.

During surgery, the infant is positioned with the head in a neutral position on a head ring. Ensuring correct tube length is crucial. Note that the tracheal tube tip may move up towards the larynx if the head is extended (conversely, down towards the carina if the head is flexed). Fixation of the tube in the midline is important to facilitate symmetric and aesthetic repair of cleft lip. Water-resistant transparent dressings aid tube fixation following skin preparation with cleaning solution. A mouth gag is inserted during cleft palate repair. The tracheal tube must be checked by hand ventilation or by assessing airway pressures when the gag is opened to make sure that the tube is not compressed. The gag time should be limited to two hours to avoid development of tongue oedema secondary to impaired perfusion. The anaesthetist must be constantly alert to possible disconnection of the circuit near the patient end, and to accidental extubation when the gag is adjusted or removed. Clear surgical drapes allow for easy visualisation of the patient, breathing circuit and tracheal tube position.

Total anaesthetic and surgical time ranges from 90 minutes for a simple lip or palate repair to up to three hours for a bilateral lip repair. Pressure areas should be protected, the infant warmed and temperature monitored to avoid overheating. Blood loss is usually not significant, although there is often more bleeding associated with a vomerine flap repair or if lateral release incisions have been performed.

## Extubation and Postoperative Airway Management

Upper airway obstruction may occur in some infants after palate repair, particularly those with micrognathia or where the repaired palate is long. It is due to obstruction of the nasopharyngeal space by the oedematous palate and is particularly problematic in young infants who are still obligate nose breathers. The infant should be extubated when completely awake, after direct inspection and suction of the pharynx and documented removal of the throat pack. Signs of airway obstruction include sternal and subcostal recession, decreasing oxygen saturation and stertor. Residual anaesthetic effect, opioids and blood or secretions can contribute to upper airway obstruction. Other important causes to exclude are a swollen tongue, if the gag has been in place for a long time, or a retained throat pack.

The obstructed child should be managed with 100% oxygen, continuous positive airway pressure and/or careful insertion of an NPA or oral airway, taking care with the surgical repair. The NPA can be fashioned from a tracheal tube or a preformed nasal airway, usually 0.5 mm diameter smaller than that used to intubate the trachea. Tube length can be estimated by measuring from tip of the nostril to the tragus of the ear. If obstruction is not relieved by the NPA, reintubation may be required. In infants with micrognathia, particularly for those with Pierre Robin sequence who are likely to develop airway obstruction postoperatively, it is better for the surgeon to place the NPA electively at the end of surgery whilst the child is still anaesthetised. This minimises damage to the surgical repair and ensures the correct length of the NPA, that is, with the tip of the NPA just protruding from behind the soft palate. If the NPA is too short, it will be ineffective; if it is too long, it will irritate the larynx and the baby will not settle postoperatively due to coughing.

Any baby that is dependent on an NPA needs to be monitored closely postoperatively in a level 2 high-dependency area, and the NPA needs to be suctioned regularly to make sure that it remains patent. A spare NPA of the same dimensions should be immediately available at the bedside in case of accidental dislodgement or blockage of the existing one. Intravenous dexamethasone is useful to help to reduce surgical oedema (first dose 250 mcg $kg^{-1}$ IV; three further doses 100 mcg $kg^{-1}$ IV 8 hourly). Positioning the baby in the lateral or sitting position may help airway patency. Tongue sutures are seldom used. The NPA can usually be removed after 24 hours.

## Analgesic Management

Multimodal analgesia should be used so that the infant is comfortable but not over-sedated at extubation. There are a wide variety of analgesic techniques available, and our current practice in the North Thames Cleft Network will be described.

Infants undergoing cleft lip repair are managed with infraorbital nerve blocks with bupivacaine, performed using an intraoral approach. Blocks are performed prior to the start of surgery by the anaesthetist or the surgeon. The surgeon will also infiltrate the surgical field with local anaesthetic containing adrenaline 1:200,000 to reduce blood loss and aid surgery. Intravenous paracetamol is given intraoperatively, with regular paracetamol and ibuprofen PO postoperatively. The anterior palate is not anaesthetised by the infraorbital nerve block, and children who undergo vomerine flap repair at the same time as lip repair receive a loading dose of morphine during surgery (50–100 mcg $kg^{-1}$ IV). These children may also require oral morphine for breakthrough pain in the postoperative period, as for cleft palate repair.

Cleft palate repair is a more painful procedure. All children receive a combination of IV paracetamol, rectal diclofenac and morphine administered towards the end of surgery (100 mcg $kg^{-1}$ IV). Our practice is for the surgeon to infiltrate the palate with bupivacaine 0.25% and adrenaline 1:200,000, maximum 0.8 ml $kg^{-1}$, to provide pain relief and to reduce blood loss. Bilateral suprazygomatic maxillary nerve blocks placed before the start of surgery have been shown to be effective in reducing opioid consumption. Anatomical landmarks are used to guide the injection, and confirmation of local anaesthetic spread can be obtained with ultrasound. Clonidine 1–2 mcg $kg^{-1}$ IV is a useful adjunct to provide analgesia without respiratory depression for children older than six months undergoing cleft palate repair.

The use of a validated pain score such as FLACC allows objective assessment of pain in the postoperative period and guides analgesic use. If the infant does not settle with a feed or comforting in the recovery room, increments of morphine (20 mcg $kg^{-1}$) are given. On the postoperative ward, regular oral paracetamol and ibuprofen are given, with oral morphine for breakthrough pain as required (morphine 100 mcg $kg^{-1}$ PO).

## Perioperative Fluid Management

It is our practice to administer an intraoperative fluid bolus of 20 ml $kg^{-1}$ of Hartmann's solution to replace deficit and for maintenance requirements. Additional Hartmann's is given as required, but blood loss is usually small, and transfusion is seldom required.

Infants are encouraged to feed postoperatively, and after lip repair most will manage well. After palate repair, some infants require short-term intravenous fluid until feeding is established. Alternatively, a nasogastric tube can be placed at the end of primary palate surgery to enable top-up feeding and to meet maintenance fluid requirements postoperatively via the enteral route. This avoids the need for monitoring urea and electrolytes and cannulation in the postoperative period and allows for the regular administration of oral analgesia.

## Postoperative Care

Postoperative bleeding after palate repair is rare but may require blood transfusion and return to theatre. Anaesthesia management is similar to that of bleeding post tonsillectomy – the infant will need fluid resuscitation, there will be blood in the airway, intubation may be difficult, residual anaesthesia must be taken into account and there may be a full stomach due to swallowed blood.

Infants who undergo uncomplicated cleft lip surgery are usually discharged from hospital after one night, although term infants having lip repair without vomerine flap may be managed as a day case if there are no other concerns. A two-night stay is usual for infants having palate repair. Absorbable sutures are increasingly being used for lip repair, eliminating the need for removal of sutures under general anaesthesia or oral sedation.

## Secondary Cleft Surgery

Children may present for a variety of secondary procedures in childhood (see Table 23.2). Children for secondary procedures may become increasingly anxious about anaesthesia. Discussion about their concerns, giving choice for method of induction and using different distraction and coping techniques can help. Sedative premedication may be useful.

Secondary procedures on the lip and nose are undertaken to improve cosmetic appearance or improve nasal airway patency. Anaesthetic technique is generally similar for primary lip repair, although revisions in older children and adults can be performed using a laryngeal mask. Palate re-exploration may be undertaken to improve palatal length (and hence function) or to repair a palatal fistula. Principles are as for primary palate repair.

Alveolar bone graft is performed for children with a defect in the alveolus to provide a base for the eruption of the permanent teeth. Bone is taken from either the iliac crest or tibia. For details of anaesthesia for maxillofacial procedures, please refer to Chapter 24.

Secondary speech surgery may be carried out after investigation by videofluoroscopy and nasal endoscopy performed by speech therapists. Children are usually over three years old, and the procedure involves improving apposition of soft palate to posterior pharyngeal wall by using one or more of the following techniques:

- Repositioning muscles of soft palate – re-repair or Furlow Z-plasty
- Lengthening of the soft palate with buccinators myomucosal flaps
- Pharyngoplasty, of which there are three broad types: Hynes, sphincter (Orticochea) or midline superior posterior pharyngeal flaps

## Buccinator Flaps

This operation increases the length of the palate by rotating buccinator myomucosal flaps from the inner cheek into the junction between the hard and soft palate. The donor sites on each cheek are closed directly. The trachea should be intubated with a pre-formed south-facing tracheal tube. Good pain relief is important with a combination of local anaesthetic infiltration, paracetamol, an NSAID and morphine. Intravenous clonidine is a useful adjunct. Postoperatively, regular simple analgesics are given, with rescue analgesia provided by oral morphine.

This is a painful procedure, and some children are particularly reluctant to take oral fluids postoperatively. It is useful to pass a nasogastric tube perioperatively to provide a route for analgesia administration and postoperative feeding and fluid intake until the child is eating and drinking. After three weeks, the muscle flaps have vascularised, and the flap pedicles are divided under general anaesthesia.

## Pharyngoplasty

A Hynes pharyngoplasty involves mobilising local flaps from the posterior wall of the pharynx to produce a bulge at the junction of the nasopharynx and oropharynx that can then oppose the end of the soft palate to provide palatal competence. In the Orticochea pharyngoplasty, palatopharyngeus myomucosal flaps are positioned lower down on the posterior oropharyngeal wall, and the posterior tonsillar pillars are sutured to the posterior pharyngeal wall. This procedure purportedly utilises the sphincter action of the muscle in the flaps, helping to seal the velopharyngeal orifice during speech. Another form of pharyngoplasty consists of a posterior pharyngeal flap sutured onto the soft palate. Two lateral nasopharyngeal ports are thus created. The choice and exact nature of surgical procedure is individualised depending on the anatomy and the dynamic physiology of a patient.

Conduct of anaesthesia is similar to primary palate repair and requires tracheal intubation. The procedure is painful, and multimodal analgesia should be used with care so as not to cause oversedation with opioids. The operation, by its nature, produces a degree of upper airway obstruction, particularly in the immediate recovery period. Close monitoring is required, including monitoring of oxygen saturation. Dexamethasone may reduce local oedema. The passage of a nasopharyngeal airway is contraindicated, as this will cause damage to the surgical site. After Orticochea or posterior pharyngeal flaps, nasal intubation for future surgery is absolutely contraindicated.

Postoperative haemorrhage may occur as a complication of pharyngoplasty, owing to bleeding from the posterior pharynx. Particular care should be taken with children with 22q deletion who have more medial carotid arteries lying close to the pharyngeal flap donor site. Occasionally, bleeding may necessitate transfusion and/or return to theatre. The child will need fluid resuscitation and careful induction of anaesthesia to avoid aspiration.

Obstructive sleep apnoea occurs more frequently after posterior pharyngeal flap surgery than other techniques and may persist for up to three months postoperatively. Severe obstruction can be life-threatening, and death has been reported in the literature. The child may require reintubation and return to theatre to reverse the surgery.

## Transoral Robotic Cleft Surgery (TORCS)

This technique shows some promise and may be carried out in the future in UK settings. The learning curve for this technique is steep, and all anaesthetic concerns of robotic surgery in a shared airway apply, in particular, the challenges of managing airway emergencies requiring rapid disengagement of robot arms. Infrastructure upgrade and further experience are needed before it becomes a mainstream technique.

### Key Points

- There are two distinct cleft conditions: cleft lip with or without cleft palate (Cl+/−P) and isolated cleft palate (iCP).
- Many children with cleft will have associated abnormalities, more commonly in those with isolated cleft palate; of particular importance are airway problems and cardiac defects.
- Depending on the type of cleft, children may require only one operation for correction or several procedures throughout childhood. A multidisciplinary approach is essential.
- Most children will be easy to intubate for primary repair. Children under six months with micrognathia or a wide bilateral cleft may be more difficult to intubate.
- Cleft palate repair is managed with multimodal analgesia, including opioids, taking care to avoid over-sedation.
- Upper airway obstruction following cleft palate repair should be anticipated. It is more common in infants with micrognathia and can be managed with a nasopharyngeal airway.
- Pharyngoplasty surgery may be complicated by postoperative upper airway obstruction and bleeding.

## Further Reading


Cleft Registry and Audit Network. CRANE Database 2020 Annual report. 2020. Available at: www.crane-database.org.uk/content/uploads/2020/12/CRANE-2020-Annual-Report_V1.pdf. Accessed 8 July 2021.

Cole A, Lynch P, Slator R. A new grading of Pierre Robin sequence. *Cleft Palate Craniofacial Journal* 2008; 45:603–6.

Losee JE, Kirschner RE. *Comprehensive Cleft Care*, 2nd ed. Thieme Medical Publishers Inc.; 2015.

Mets EJ, Chouairi F, Torabi SJ, Alperovich M. Predictors of adverse events following cleft palate repair. *Journal of Craniofacial Surgery* 2019; 30:1414–8.

Obayah GM, Refaie A, Aboushanab O, Ibraheem N, Abdelazees M. Addition of dexmedetomidine to bupivacaine for greater palatine nerve block prolongs postoperative analgesia after cleft palate repair. *European Journal of Anaesthesiology* 2010; 27:280–4.

Oberhofer HM, Breslin N, Heindel H, Ching J. Analgesic efficacy of intraoperative nerve blocks for primary palatoplasty. *Journal of Craniofacial Surgery* 2021; 32:594–6.

Xue FS, Zhang GH, Li P et al. The clinical observation of difficult laryngoscopy and difficult intubation in infants with cleft lip and palate. *Paediatric Anaesthesia* 2006 March; 16:283–9.

Chapter

# 24 Anaesthesia for Dental and Maxillofacial Surgery in Children*

Jamuna Navaratnarajah

## Introduction

Commonly performed dental and maxillofacial surgical procedures in children include:

- Dental extractions
- Dental restorations
- Dental exposure and bonding
- Alveolar bone grafts

These will all be considered in more detail in this chapter, together with the management of dento-facial infection and maxillofacial trauma in children. Although sedation and local anaesthetic techniques have been used successfully for dental procedures in children, there will always be a requirement for general anaesthesia for dental and maxillofacial surgery. Many of these procedures are performed in a day-case setting, although inpatient care is sometimes required. The process of general anaesthesia involves preoperative assessment, patient preparation, intraoperative management and postoperative care. Recent guidance recommends that all paediatric dental patients referred for general anaesthesia should be assessed by dental practitioners who are skilled and trained in the treatment of children.

Local anaesthetic techniques are used to supplement postoperative analgesia and to provide haemostasis and will be outlined at the end of this chapter.

## General Principles

Although anaesthetic assessment of patients presenting for dental surgery often takes place on the same day, this should occur ideally during a separate hospital consultation. This can be done either as a telephone appointment or, if there are more complex medical issues or a need for a full airway assessment, through a hospital visit to a specific preoperative assessment clinic:

- Preoperative assessment involves obtaining a comprehensive medical and anaesthetic history, performing a physical examination and reviewing the results of appropriate clinical investigations.
- Parents and carers should be informed of the risks of general anaesthesia and offered alternative treatment where indicated. Written consent should also be taken for the procedure.
- Management strategies for the uncooperative child should be discussed preoperatively.
- In all cases, the child should be adequately fasted. Applying a topical local anaesthetic cream makes intravenous cannulation easier, and sedative oral premedication may also be indicated in some children.
- The availability of anaesthetic, monitoring and resuscitation equipment should comply with national guidelines such as those published by the Association of Anaesthetists of Great Britain and Ireland.

Induction of anaesthesia may be achieved using either the intravenous or inhalational method, with intravenous access obtained at the earliest possible opportunity. Intraoperatively, the main considerations are maintenance of the airway whilst allowing adequate surgical access. The airway device employed is usually determined by the procedure to be carried out. Suitable airway options include flexible supraglottic airway devices (SGA) or tracheal tubes that can be either oral or nasal.

Good communication between the surgeon and the anaesthetist is vital as the airway is shared. The potential for blood or debris in the pharynx should also be considered.

Throat packs are often indicated and must be removed at the end of the procedure before the child's emergence from anaesthesia. Recent

* Many thanks to Dr Lola Adewale, who wrote the first edition of this book chapter, much of the content of which has been used in this revision.

guidelines advise that both visual and documented evidence should be provided whenever a throat pack is inserted. A clearly established protocol should also be in place to ensure that the throat pack is always removed and that this is witnessed and documented.

Adequate perioperative analgesia should always be administered, with antiemetic agents as indicated. At the end of the procedure, suction of the oropharynx should be performed under direct vision where possible. The patient may then be placed in the left lateral position with head-down tilt unless this is contraindicated. In the period immediately following general anaesthesia for dental or maxillofacial surgery, the child should be managed in the postanaesthetic care unit by a designated member of staff who is trained in both basic and advanced paediatric resuscitation techniques. Supplemental oxygen should be administered until the child is fully awake.

Paediatric dental patients may suffer from conditions that have major anaesthetic implications, such as cardiac disease or epidermolysis bullosa. These will require appropriate modifications to the anaesthetic technique used.

The complications of general anaesthesia for dental and maxillofacial surgery may be minor or major. Minor complications include:

- Postoperative nausea, retching and vomiting, with the latter occurring particularly in association with swallowed blood
- Damage to teeth or soft tissues adjacent to the operative site
- Injury to the neck caused by intraoperative positioning
- Postoperative cough and sore throat following tracheal intubation or because of irritation from the throat pack

Major complications include complete respiratory obstruction from inhalation of foreign material or cardiac arrest secondary to arrhythmias.

## Dental Extractions

When complete, the primary dentition consists of 20 teeth, whereas there are 32 permanent teeth. The most commonly used dental identification system divides the dental arch into four quadrants. All primary central incisors are designated tooth 'A' and followed posteriorly in alphabetical order so that all primary second molars are designated tooth 'E'. All permanent central incisors are designated tooth '1' and are followed posteriorly in numerical order to tooth '8', which is the third molar or 'wisdom tooth'.

Dental extractions are commonly required in children who suffer from dental caries or trauma as well as those who are undergoing orthodontic treatment regimes. Extractions may also be indicated when there are certain dental anomalies such as impacted teeth. Often if a tooth is impacted, the tooth may be extracted to encourage the permanent tooth to erupt. On occasion, a permanent tooth must be extracted, or exposed and bonded if it is in a decent position.

The main indications for general anaesthesia for dental extractions in children are:

- Contraindication to local anaesthesia
- Previous failure of local anaesthesia or sedation
- Lack of patient cooperation owing to immaturity
- Presence of neurodevelopmental disorders, including global developmental delay, autism spectrum disorder, communication disorders, learning disabilities and attention deficit hyperactivity disorder (ADHD)
- Diagnosis of advanced decay
- Requirement for multiple extractions
- Complex surgical procedures

Most dental extractions in children are performed as a day-case procedure or as outpatients; the general principles of day-case anaesthesia should apply for both these patient groups. However, outpatient general anaesthesia requires additional consideration and meticulous patient selection. Conditions requiring special consideration include coagulation disorders or anti-coagulant therapy, syndromes associated with increased anaesthetic risk, haemoglobinopathies and severe behavioural abnormalities.

Preapplication of a topical local anaesthetic cream is useful when intravenous induction of anaesthesia is planned. Preoperative oral analgesia is sometimes prescribed (usually paracetamol and/or ibuprofen). Oral/buccal midazolam or intranasal dexmedetomidine may also be required for the anxious child.

Induction of general anaesthesia is commonly achieved intravenously using propofol, or via the inhalational route using sevoflurane. Regardless of the method of induction, intravenous access is essential in all cases and must be obtained at the earliest opportunity. Anaesthesia may then be maintained using sevoflurane or propofol. A flexible SGA can be suitable in most circumstances, but tracheal intubation may be necessary particularly in patients who require extensive treatment. If not given preoperatively, paracetamol is administered intraoperatively alongside fentanyl and antiemetics.

Complications related to general anaesthesia for dental extractions include potential airway obstruction caused by the position of the throat pack or mouth prop or the presence of blood or debris. Dislocation of the temporomandibular joint may also occur.

Tachyarrhythmias are uncommon but can follow the use of local anaesthetic agents containing adrenaline, which are usually administered by the dental practitioner and may be injected into the buccal fold of the gum adjacent to the tooth to be treated. Lingual and mental nerve blocks may also be performed intraorally to provide more extensive anaesthesia to the lower incisors. Infraorbital nerve blockade will anaesthetise the upper jaw.

Additional oral analgesia may be required prior to the patient being discharged home.

## Dental Restorations

Restorative dental treatment is performed in children to limit or repair the damage caused by dental caries. Such procedures are often performed in children with learning disabilities, who may require extensive treatment necessitating tracheal intubation via the nasal route. This provides unobstructed access to all four quadrants of the mouth and also facilitates the assessment of tooth alignment and occlusion.

## Dental Exposure and Bonding

Palatal impaction of maxillary canine teeth is a problem that is frequently encountered in paediatric orthodontic clinical practice. It is possible for any tooth to be impacted, and management requires a joint surgical and orthodontic approach. A commonly adopted treatment strategy is surgical exposure of the impacted tooth, followed by bonding of an orthodontic bracket with a miniature gold chain attached to it. Following this, the child will see their orthodontist, who will attach a rubber band to institute a gentle eruptive pulling force on the impacted tooth.

In children, the surgery usually occurs under general anaesthesia most commonly as a day-case procedure. The general principles of day-case general anaesthesia apply with the additional considerations of managing the airway whilst allowing adequate surgical access.

Tracheal intubation is usually required, most commonly via the oral route, with the possibility of direct laryngoscopy being complicated by irregularly spaced dentition. A south-facing oral Ring-Adair-Elwin (RAE) tube is useful. Flexible laryngeal masks have also been successfully used for this procedure. A throat pack is required to protect the airway from soiling.

Before commencing the procedure, the dental surgeon will usually infiltrate an adrenaline-containing local anaesthetic solution, which improves haemostasis and contributes to peri- and postoperative analgesia.

An adequate analgesic regimen is usually provided by paracetamol administered either preoperatively via the oral route or intraoperatively via the intravenous route, together with a non-steroidal anti-inflammatory agent administered in the postoperative period. Opioid analgesics are rarely required, although antiemetic therapy should be routinely administered intraoperatively.

## Alveolar Bone Grafts

Surgical repair of a cleft lip or palate in infancy does not usually involve correction of the alveolar cleft defect. This may result in residual oronasal fistulae with disruption of the maxillary alveolus. Alveolar cleft bone grafts unite the alveolar segments and help to prevent collapse and constriction of the dental arch. Support is then provided for teeth adjacent to the cleft and for those that will erupt into the area of the cleft. The graft also leads to closure of the oronasal fistula, augmentation of the alveolar ridge and the creation of a solid foundation for the lip and alar base of the nose.

The alveolar cleft graft is usually performed as an inpatient procedure when the child is between the ages of 6 and 10 years. General anaesthesia is induced via either the intravenous or inhalation route, with tracheal intubation using an oral RAE tube. Bone is then removed from the patient's iliac crest and placed in the alveolar cleft. The surgical procedure is associated with a small risk of bleeding and requires adequate intravenous access with the administration of intravenous fluids perioperatively.

An intraoperative opioid is routinely required, together with paracetamol and a non-steroidal analgesic. This is supplemented by infiltration of local anaesthetic into both the oral cavity and the iliac crest. Postoperative analgesia may be enhanced if a catheter is placed by the surgeon into the iliac wound site and used postoperatively for the intermittent or continuous administration of local anaesthetic solution. Children undergoing this procedure are usually able to tolerate postoperative oral analgesia, including oral morphine.

Dexamethasone and ondansetron are usually administered, together with antibiotics.

## Management of Dentofacial Infection

Dentofacial infection is either acute or chronic. Acute infection usually presents as an emergency with pain, pyrexia and often a red swollen face. Chronic infection may present as a buccal sinus or a mobile tooth. The management of dentofacial infection involves removal of the cause together with local drainage and debridement intraorally or extraorally as required.

Dental abscesses are usually localised, but cellulitis and oedema may occur because of spread of infection via lymphatics and tissue planes. Limited mouth opening may be caused by pain or spasm (trismus) of the masseter or pterygoid muscles. Pus may also be present within the airway. If the infection spreads into the retropharyngeal space, securing the airway safely can be difficult.

The anaesthetic considerations are as for dental extractions. Antisialagogue agents administered at induction are sometimes useful to control excessive secretions. If problems with the airway are anticipated, an anaesthetic technique that maintains spontaneous ventilation should be considered. It is important to have an airway management plan in place prior to induction of anaesthesia. This may include the use of videolaryngoscopes and other specialised airway equipment. It is usually possible to achieve adequate mouth opening after induction of anaesthesia; occasionally, however, nasal fibreoptic tracheal intubation is required.

## Maxillofacial Trauma

Facial trauma in very young children is commonly the result of falls or accidents, but children may also be victims of assault or road traffic collisions. It is important to recognise and report any suspicion of non-accidental injury. Blunt trauma tends to cause greater damage to the soft tissues and supporting structures, whereas high-velocity or sharp injuries cause subluxations and fractures of the teeth.

General anaesthesia is often required for the suturing of facial lacerations and the management of maxillofacial fractures. However, each child should be assessed on an individual basis. A cooperative child may be able to have a laceration closed with local anaesthetic alone. Consideration should be given to the possibility of associated injuries that may involve the head, neck, chest and spinal cord. The child should be assessed for head and neck injury and appropriate measures instituted before any maxillofacial intervention. There is also the potential for airway obstruction, aspiration of gastric contents and intraoral haemorrhage.

Management of maxillofacial fractures may require long surgical procedures that are sometimes associated with significant blood loss. There is also a risk of bradycardia due to the oculocardiac reflex. Fractures of the zygomatic arch are associated with limited mouth opening. This is because the fracture can impinge on the temporalis muscle, one of the muscles of mastication. Maxillary fractures are often even more serious and are associated with significant head injury (Table 24.1).

Nasal fractures are no longer treated with surgery as commonly as before. Often the bones will heal themselves and are not open to the environment, and therefore pose minimal risk of infection.

## Local Anaesthesia in Paediatric Dentistry

Local anaesthesia (LA) is used to supplement general anaesthesia for dental and maxillofacial surgery in children. It has a dual purpose. When used with adrenaline, the objective is to aid haemostasis; it also has a longer duration of action, therefore acting as an adjunct to analgesia given intraoperatively. LA is administered by the dental surgeon, the agents most used being lidocaine 2% with adrenaline 1:80,000 in the majority of patients, or prilocaine 3% with felypressin (octapressin). The latter is used when the patient has a history of cardiac issues and adrenaline needs to be avoided.

**Table 24.1** Classification of midfacial fractures

| Fracture | Type of injury |
|---|---|
| Le Fort I | Fracture separating inferior portion of maxilla horizontally, extending from piriform aperture of nose to pterygoid maxillary suture area. |
| Le Fort II | Fracture involving separation of maxilla and nasal complex from cranial base, zygomatic orbital rim area and pterygoid maxillary suture area. |
| Le Fort III | Complete separation of midface at level of naso-orbital ethmoid complex and zygomaticofrontal suture area. Fracture extends through orbits bilaterally. |

The techniques for providing LA in children are similar to those used in adults. However, owing to the reduced bone density of the maxilla and mandible in children, there is more rapid diffusion and absorption of LA solution with a faster onset and shorter duration of block.

The upper teeth receive their sensory nerve supply from the superior alveolar (dental) nerves, which are branches of the maxillary division of the trigeminal nerve. The peripheral fibres of these nerves can be blocked effectively at the apical foramina of the tooth by injection of local anaesthetic into the sulcus adjacent to the tooth requiring anaesthesia. The infraorbital nerve, a terminal branch of the maxillary nerve, can be blocked at the infraorbital foramen, which lies just below the inferior orbital margin, approximately halfway along its length. It can be reached from the upper labial sulcus opposite the canine tooth. The block will also include branches of the anterior superior alveolar nerve and will provide anaesthesia to the anterior maxilla and upper lip. The buccal and labial soft tissues are anaesthetised by LA infiltration to these areas. Anaesthesia of the hard and soft palate requires injection directly into the palate.

The lower teeth receive their sensory nerve supply from the inferior alveolar (dental) nerve, a branch of the mandibular division of the trigeminal nerve. This may be blocked before it enters the mandibular foramen on the medial aspect of the ramus, just behind the lingula, providing anaesthesia to the bone of the mandibular body and the pulps of the lower teeth on that side of the mouth. This also blocks the mental nerve, a branch of the inferior alveolar nerve, which provides sensation to the lower lip and chin on that side.

There may be incomplete anaesthesia of the central incisor, as there can be some crossover supply from the contralateral inferior dental nerve. The mental nerve alone can be blocked at the mental foramen, providing anaesthesia to the soft tissues of the labial gingivae, the lower lip and chin. Diffusion of anaesthetic agent via the mental foramen will reach the incisive branch which supplies the pulps of the lower first premolar, canine and incisor teeth. There is some communication with the nerve supply on the opposite side. A periodontal ligament injection may be necessary in older children to achieve adequate anaesthesia of a single mandibular tooth.

As with any use of local anaesthetic agents, the possibility of LA toxicity due to accidental intravascular injection should be anticipated. Convulsions, cardiac arrhythmias and hypotension may occur. All members of staff should be aware of the management protocol for LA toxicity, including the availability of intravenous lipid emulsion solution (see Chapter 15, Box 15.1). Tachycardia and arrhythmias may also be associated with adrenaline-containing solutions. Hypersensitivity reactions to local anaesthetics are very rare, although allergic reactions to preservative agents have been described.

### Key Points

- Thorough preoperative assessment and patient preparation is essential, particularly prior to outpatient general anaesthesia.
- Management of the airway requires careful consideration as it is a shared airway.
- A throat pack is required for most procedures, and there must be an established theatre protocol to ensure it is removed after the surgical procedure.
- Local anaesthetic techniques contribute to the provision of adequate postoperative analgesia.

## Further Reading

Adewale L, Morton N, Blayney M. Guidelines for the Management of Children Referred for Dental Extractions under General Anaesthesia. 2011. Available at: http://udps-srb.org/wp-content/uploads/2015/10/Main-Dental-Guidelines.pdf. Accessed 24 March 2024.

Athanassoglou V, Patel A, McGuire B et al. Systematic review of benefits or harms of routine anaesthetist-inserted throat packs in adults: practice recommendations for inserting and counting throat packs. *Anaesthesia* 2018; 73(5):612–8. https://doi.org/10.1111/anae.14197.

Royal College of Anaesthetists. Guidelines for the Provision of Anaesthesia Services for ENT. Oral Maxillofacial and Dental Surgery. 2021. Available at: www.rcoa.ac.uk/gpas/chapter-12. Accessed 24 March 2024.

Chapter 25

# Anaesthesia for Craniofacial Surgery in Children

David de Beer

## Introduction

Craniofacial surgery encompasses the management of congenital and acquired anomalies of the cranium and face. This ranges from single suture craniosynostosis to complex multi-sutural craniofacial and orbital dysostoses, encephalocoeles and craniofacial clefts (Figure 25.1). The surgery may be highly complex and is often protracted, but when conducted within the multidisciplinary setting of a specialist craniofacial unit, the incidence of serious complications is fortunately low.

Optimal perioperative management of these patients is dependent on a multidisciplinary team approach that includes thorough preoperative assessment and preparation, meticulous intraoperative planning, anticipation and proactive management of intraoperative complications and a high level of postoperative care within an appropriate setting.

## Craniosynostosis

Craniosynostosis is a congenital condition in which premature fusion of one or more of the cranial sutures occurs, leading to cranial deformity and possible compromised intracranial volume. Craniosynostosis occurs in approximately one in 2,500 live births and can be an isolated finding (non-syndromic synostosis) or part of a multi-system syndrome (syndromic synostosis).

## Non-syndromic Synostosis

Non-syndromic (simple) synostosis is the most common form of craniosynostosis, accounting for approximately two thirds of cases. It results from the premature fusion of a single cranial suture, most commonly the sagittal, coronal and metopic sutures. The resulting skull deformity depends on the suture involved (Table 25.1).

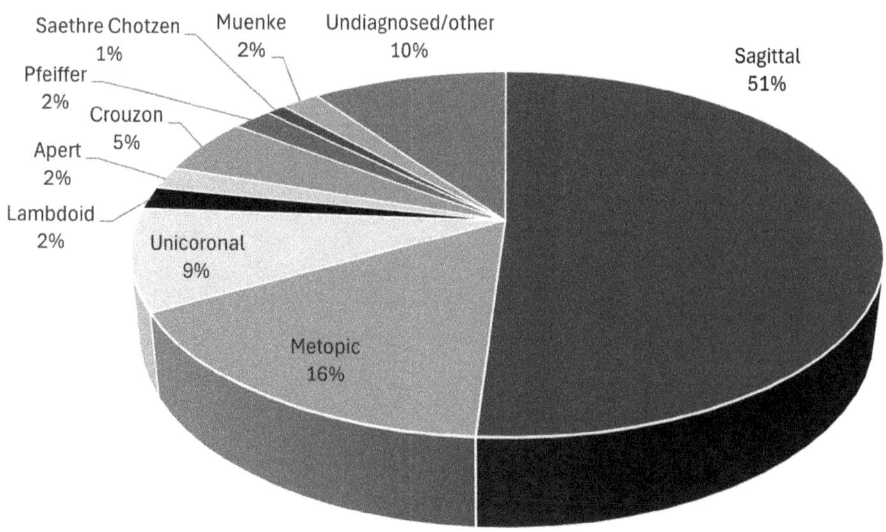


**Figure 25.1** Distribution by diagnosis amongst children undergoing major/ complex major cranial vault surgery. *Source:* Great Ormond Street Hospital (GOSH) for Children data for 2020–2021.

**Table 25.1** Classification of craniosynostosis

| Suture | Problem | Solution |
|---|---|---|
| Sagittal<br>*1:5,000*<br>*M:F = 2.5–4:1* | Elongated and narrow head<br>*Scaphocephaly* | <6 m: spring-assisted cranioplasty<br>>18 m: total calvarial remodelling<br>(± Melbourne modification) |
| Metopic<br>*1:7,000–15,000*<br>*M:F = 1.8–2.8:1* | Broad triangular forehead<br>*Trigonocephaly* | Fronto-orbital remodelling/ advancement |
| Unicoronal<br>*1:10,000*<br>*F:M = 1.6–3.6:1* | Unilateral forehead flattening<br>Contralateral bossing<br>*Anterior plagiocephaly* | Fronto orbital remodelling/ advancement |
| Bicoronal<br>*1:150,000*<br>*M:F = 1:1.5* | Short, broad head<br>*Brachycephaly* | Fronto orbital remodelling/ advancement (if *not* associated with maxillary hypoplasia) |
| Lambdoid<br>*1:200,000*<br>*F > M* | Unilateral occipital flattening<br>Contralateral bossing<br>*Posterior plagiocephaly* | Posterior vault expansion/remodelling |

Non-syndromic synostosis is usually an isolated anomaly, and there are no associated skeletal defects or other anomalies. Indications for surgery are primarily aesthetic, although raised intracranial pressure (ICP), which occurs in 14% of patients with single suture synostosis, is a functional indication for surgery.

## Syndromic Craniosynostosis

Syndromic (multi-sutural) craniosynostosis affects the skull vault and facial skeleton and constitutes up to a third of all cases. The coronal and/or lambdoid sutures are usually affected, often in combination with other sutures. It is a genetically heterogeneous disorder, with most cases showing autosomal dominance and involving mutations in several genes, predominantly the fibroblast growth factor receptor (FGFR1–3) and TWIST 1 genes. Associated malformations are common, and involvement of the facial skeleton often leads to functional problems, including raised ICP, which occurs in approximately half of patients with multi-sutural synostosis, airway obstruction, exorbitism, feeding difficulties and behavioural and psychological problems. There are several craniofacial associated syndromes (Table 25.2), the most common ones being:

- Apert syndrome
- Crouzon syndrome
- Pfeiffer syndrome
- Muenke syndrome
- Saethre–Chotzen syndrome

## Timing of Surgery

Craniofacial surgery may be classified according to the region of the craniofacial skeleton involved, the degree of complexity and whether it is performed using an open or minimally invasive technique (Table 25.3).

The ideal timing of surgery varies between institutions, individual surgeons and whether the procedure is to be performed using an open or minimally invasive technique. To achieve lasting results, definitive surgery should ideally be delayed until the period of maximum growth of the affected area is complete. Earlier surgical intervention is performed for minimally invasive procedures, where success is dependent on the presence of pliable bones, or to treat an urgent functional problem such as raised ICP, airway obstruction and exorbitism. Consideration should also be given to the potential psychological impact the deformity has on the child, and waiting for the ideal time to perform reconstructive surgery may not be acceptable to the patient or their parents.

## Preoperative Assessment

Two groups of patients present for craniofacial surgery: non-syndromic patients with simple craniosynostosis and syndromic patients with

**Table 25.2** Craniofacial associated syndromes

| Syndrome | Gene mutation | Synostosis | Features |
|---|---|---|---|
| Apert<br>*1:65,000–1:100,000* | FGFR-2<br>AD or sporadic | Multisutural (bicoronal) | • Maxillary hypoplasia/hypertelorism ± cleft palate (dental crowding)<br>• Proptosis<br>• Hearing impairment<br>• Choanal stenosis/atresia<br>• Cervical vertebral fusion (C5/C6)<br>• Complex syndactyly, broad thumb<br>• Cardiac defects (~10%)<br>• Developmental delay |
| Crouzon<br>*1:30,000–60,000* | FGFR-2<br>(FGFR-3)<br>AD or sporadic | Multisutural (bicoronal ± lambdoid) | • Maxillary hypoplasia/hypertelorism<br>• Proptosis, strabismus<br>• Cervical spine abnormalities<br>• Arnold–Chiari malformation<br>• No hand/feet anomalies<br>• Mostly normal intellect |
| Pfeiffer<br>*1:100,000* | FGFR-1<br>FGFR-2<br>AD or sporadic | Multisutural<br>Type 1: bicoronal<br>Type 2: cloverleaf skull<br>Type 3: no cloverleaf deformity | • Maxillary hypoplasia/ hypertelorism (± cleft palate)<br>• Proptosis, ptosis<br>• Syndactyly, broad thumbs /toes<br>• Multiple other abnormalities (tracheal, cardiovascular, intestinal)<br>• Developmental delay (Type II, III) |
| Muenke<br>*1:30,000* | FGFR-3<br>AD | Unicoronal<br>Bicoronal | • Maxillary hypoplasia (mild)/ hypertelorism<br>• Macrocephaly<br>• Proptosis, ptosis<br>• Epilepsy (~10%)<br>• Syndactyly (mild)<br>• Sensorineural hearing loss<br>• ± Developmental delay |
| Saethre–Chotzen<br>*1:25–50,000* | TWIST-1<br>AD | Coronal<br>± metopic | • Facial asymmetry, high forehead<br>• Maxillary hypoplasia/ hypertelorism ± cleft palate<br>• Deviation of nasal septum, convex 'beaked' nasal ridge<br>• Ptosis, strabismus<br>• Syndactyly, clinodactyly of 5th finger, broad big toe<br>• Mostly normal intellect |

*Notes:*
AD = autosomal dominant.
FGFR = fibroblast growth factor receptor.

multi-sutural synostosis and craniofacial dysostoses. In the latter group, a thorough preoperative assessment is essential, with a particular focus on assessment of the airway. Preoperative investigations should be tailored to the patient's clinical status and the proposed surgical procedure. As a minimum, baseline haematological tests should be performed. Other investigations may include sleep studies in patients with obstructive sleep apnoea (OSA) and visual evoked potentials in those at risk of raised ICP (pattern reversal may precede papilloedema or other signs of raised ICP). The

**Table 25.3** Classification of craniofacial procedures

| Complex major surgery |
|---|
| **Craniofacial/midface**<br>• Monobloc frontofacial advancement for anterior-posterior and vertical anomalies<br>• Frontofacial bipartition for three-dimensional anomalies of the skull, face and orbits<br>• Orbital box osteotomy for lateral or vertical orbital anomalies |
| **Major surgery** |
| **Cranial vault/ transcranial**<br>• Fronto-orbital remodelling/advancement for metopic and coronal synostosis<br>• Total calvarial remodelling (± Melbourne modification) for sagittal synostosis<br>• Posterior vault expansion for lambdoid synostosis |
| **Subcranial**<br>• Le Fort osteotomies (commonly Le Fort III) |
| **Cranial vault**<br>• Spring-assisted cranioplasty for sagittal, lambdoid synostosis<br>• Endoscopic-assisted suturectomy for metopic, unicoronal, sagittal synostosis |

appropriate volume of blood should be cross-matched and ready for use prior to surgery. This should be guided by the hospital's Maximum Surgical Blood Order Schedule (MSBOS), but one unit of packed red cells are usually adequate for major procedures and two to four units for complex major procedures.

## Airway Assessment

Craniofacial abnormalities are often associated with airway problems, and up to half of patients with syndromic craniosynostosis will present with some degree of supraglottic airway compromise secondary to maxillary hypoplasia. This ranges in severity from mild nasal obstruction to severe OSA. Patients with moderate to severe symptoms require a preoperative sleep study. Symptomatic airway obstruction is managed preoperatively with nasal prong airways or nasal continuous positive airway pressure (CPAP). Surgical options include adenotonsillectomy, uvulopharyngo-palatoplasty or, in the most severe cases, tracheostomy.

Physical appearance may be an unreliable predicter of a potentially difficult airway in some craniofacial patients. Whilst the airway of some syndromic patients with maxillary hypoplasia may look challenging, they rarely present any difficulty at laryngoscopy. On the contrary, syndromic patients whose physical appearance has been improved through corrective surgery may be difficult to intubate due to maxillary advancement and reduced temporomandibular joint movement. The presence of a rigid external distraction (RED) frame may also make laryngoscopy awkward if not impossible.

## Indications for Tracheostomy

A minority of syndromic patients with severe airway obstruction and OSA may present for surgery with a tracheostomy in situ. The decision to perform a covering tracheostomy is made on an individual patient basis following a multidisciplinary team discussion with members of the craniofacial, ENT and anaesthetic teams and the patient (if appropriate) and their parents. Indications for a covering tracheostomy include:

- Severe and deteriorating upper airway obstruction, including life-threatening OSA.
- Patients less than two years of age scheduled for complex major surgery, such as frontofacial advancement
- Patients undergoing extensive facial osteotomies where reintubation may be difficult

When a decision is made to perform a covering tracheostomy, it is best done as a separate procedure at least two weeks prior to the scheduled craniofacial surgery. This ensures the presence of a well-formed tracheostome and avoids the potential risk of iatrogenic tension pneumothorax developing due to positive pressure ventilation during prolonged complex major surgery. A tracheostomy may also be associated with an increased risk of surgical infection, and subsequent decannulation may be challenging.

## Premedication

If intravenous induction of anaesthesia is planned, a topical anaesthetic cream should be applied preoperatively to potential cannulation sites to facilitate cannulation. Patients who are anxious or those with significant behavioural problems may benefit from preoperative psychological preparation with or without the use of sedative premedication.

Caution should be exercised when using sedative premedication in children with severe airway obstruction or raised ICP, although this may be necessary in some cases and is generally well tolerated. Anti-embolism compression stockings (TED™) should be applied in older patients and in those undergoing prolonged surgery.

# Conduct of Anaesthesia

## Induction

Induction of anaesthesia may be achieved using an inhalational or intravenous technique, the technique chosen depending on the preference of the patient, parent and anaesthetist. Inhalational induction may be preferable where a difficult airway is anticipated. Prior to induction of anaesthesia, standard monitoring should be applied, with a pulse oximeter being an absolute minimum.

## Airway Management

Following induction of anaesthesia, maintenance of the airway may be challenging in patients with syndromic craniosynostosis. Relaxation of the upper airway compounds pre-existing supraglottic airway obstruction, and it may be difficult to achieve an adequate face mask seal due to facial asymmetry, maxillary hypoplasia and exorbitism. Use of a soft-seal face mask, rotated through 180° if necessary, combined with simple airway manoeuvres and adjuncts, may be necessary to achieve adequate mask ventilation. Application of CPAP via a close-fitting face mask will also help in alleviating upper airway obstruction.

Difficult laryngoscopy is unusual in patients with midface hypoplasia, although children who have previously had corrective surgery may be more difficult to intubate. For these cases, a full range of intubation equipment, including a laryngeal mask airway, should be readily available in theatre.

The choice of tracheal tube is dependent on the type of surgery. A pre-formed south-facing Ring-Adair-Elwin (RAE) orotracheal tube is suitable for patients undergoing surgery in the supine position. A reinforced orotracheal tube with secure facial strapping is required for patients undergoing surgery in the prone position. Where intraoral surgical access is required, a reinforced orotracheal tube secured with circum-mandibular wiring is preferred at our institution. The tracheal tube should be optimally positioned to avoid accidental extubation or inadvertent bronchial intubation. This may best be achieved by deliberate endobronchial intubation followed by withdrawal of the tube until breath sounds can be auscultated bilaterally. The tube should be taped securely and the position rechecked with the head in flexion and extension. Patients presenting for surgery with a tracheostomy in situ should have the tracheostome intubated with a reinforced tube secured to the anterior chest wall.

## Intravascular Access

At least two appropriately large bore cannulae should be sited for complex surgery and complex major surgery. This may be challenging in syndromic patients with syndactyly or other limb abnormalities, but ultrasound has made this task much easier. The long saphenous vein is a particularly useful vessel, as it allows cannulation with a relatively wide bore cannula that is easily accessible intraoperatively. All children undergoing major and complex major craniofacial surgery require an arterial line to facilitate continuous arterial blood pressure monitoring and serial measurement of haemoglobin and blood gases. A femoral central venous line and monitoring of central venous pressure (CVP) is useful in patients undergoing prolonged complex major surgery.

Antibiotic cover is administered after induction of anaesthesia and prior to the commencement of surgery. Local policies should dictate the choice of antibiotics.

## Maintenance

Maintenance of anaesthesia is achieved using a balanced technique involving a volatile inhalational agent such as isoflurane or sevoflurane delivered in a mixture of oxygen in air with fentanyl or a remifentanil infusion for analgesia. A total intravenous technique using propofol may be considered in older children. In addition to intravenous opioids, multimodal analgesia includes the preoperative infiltration of a tumescent solution containing triamcinolone acetate, lignocaine, levobupivacaine, hyaluronidase and adrenaline (up to 7 ml $kg^{-1}$) and administration of intravenous paracetamol. Intravenous morphine (up to 0.1 mg $kg^{-1}$) is titrated towards the end of surgery, especially if remifentanil has been used intraoperatively.

## Intraoperative Monitoring and Patient Positioning

Standard monitoring includes electrocardiogram (ECG), oxygen saturation ($SpO_2$), end-tidal carbon dioxide ($ETCO_2$), invasive blood pressure, central and peripheral temperature and peripheral nerve function. Measurement of central venous pressure may be useful in patients undergoing prolonged major or complex major surgery. Maintenance of normothermia is essential and is best achieved using a forced-air warming blanket and fluid warming device with careful monitoring to avoid the risks of inadvertent hyperthermia. As the duration of surgery may exceed six hours, meticulous attention should be paid to patient positioning:

- For most craniofacial procedures, the supine, head-up (semi-Fowler's) position is used to reduce cerebral venous congestion.
- Prone positioning is used for sagittal spring cranioplasty, posterior vault expansion and total calvarial remodelling. In this position, it is important to ensure that the abdomen is free to allow unrestricted diaphragmatic movement with ventilation and avoid venous congestion.
- In all cases, pressure points should be adequately padded to avoid cutaneous or peripheral nerve injury.
- The eyes should be well lubricated and adequately protected. This may be difficult in patients with marked exorbitism in whom suturing of the palpebral fissures may be required (tarsorrhaphy).

## Management of Blood Loss

Extensive blood loss and massive transfusion may be unavoidable and remains the greatest risk to infants and children undergoing complex major craniofacial surgery. Haemorrhage may arise from the extensive scalp incision, bone edges or less commonly from extradural venous or sinus tears. Intraoperative blood loss may be rapid and can easily exceed a patient's estimated blood volume, especially in infants and young children. Accurate assessment of blood loss may be difficult due to loss onto surgical drapes and gowns as well as dilution by irrigation fluid used for the surgical power tools.

Intravascular volume replacement and transfusion requirements must therefore be guided by careful monitoring of the following parameters:

- Vital signs: ECG/heart rate, arterial blood pressure and waveform, capillary refill time, core–peripheral temperature gradient, central venous pressure, urine output
- Acid-base status (pH, BE, $HCO_3$, lactate)
- Haemoglobin concentration and haematocrit
- Coagulation parameters and platelet count

The goals of intraoperative fluid management are to maintain a normal circulating volume, an appropriate haemoglobin concentration, normal electrolyte balance and normoglycaemia. Of paramount importance is the avoidance of hypovolaemia and maintenance of adequate organ perfusion. This is best achieved through meticulous matching of transfusion volumes and blood loss using a combination of balanced salt solution (e.g. Hartmann's solution) and packed red cells to maintain an acceptable haemoglobin concentration. As fluid dynamics can change very rapidly, a proactive approach should be adopted, with all fluids being warmed prior to infusion. Transfusion practice also depends on the experience of the anaesthetist, and whilst blood loss is often underestimated, the risks of over-transfusion remain, especially in infants and young children. In addition to intravenous fluids, vasopressors (e.g. phenylephrine) may be required in the management of intraoperative hypotension.

## Reducing Allogeneic Blood Transfusion

Despite donor blood being extensively tested and monitored, allogeneic blood transfusion is not without risk from viruses, reactions or the incorrect blood being transfused. Complications associated with the massive transfusion of allogeneic blood, including metabolic acidosis, hyperkalaemia, hypocalcaemia and coagulopathy, may also be associated with significant morbidity. Strategies should therefore be employed to avoid or at least reduce the use of allogeneic blood.

### Preoperative Measures

- Iron deficiency anaemia should be treated with iron supplements.
- Recombinant erythropoietin therapy should be applied. Preoperative elevation of haemoglobin with erythropoietin has been shown to reduce

transfusion requirements in children undergoing craniofacial surgery, but an unfavourable cost-benefit ratio limits its usefulness, and it is not used in patients undergoing craniofacial surgery at the author's institution.
- Preoperative autologous blood donation is not used routinely in children in the United Kingdom.

## Intraoperative Measures

- Patient positioning (supine, head-up semi-Fowler's position).
- Scalp infiltration with an adrenaline-containing tumescent solution.
- Meticulous surgical technique should be used with particular attention to incremental or marginal losses at each stage of surgery and use of fibrin sealants or fibrin glue.
- Antifibrinolytics (e.g. tranexamic acid) are commonly used for major and complex major surgery and have been shown to reduce blood loss and the requirement for blood transfusion in children undergoing craniosynostosis surgery. The optimal dose is still a matter of debate, but at the author's institution a loading dose of 10–15 mg $kg^{-1}$ is administered, followed in some cases by an infusion of 5 mg $kg^{-1}$ $h^{-1}$.
- Intraoperative cell salvage can be a safe and effective means of reducing intraoperative allogeneic blood use. The newer blood salvage machines have relatively fast processing times and low processing volumes and provide a continuous supply of washed red cells in proportion to the rate at which the patient is bleeding. Despite this, cell salvage alone is often inadequate for infants undergoing craniofacial surgery. The overall efficacy of red cell recovery by cell salvage is dependent on the ability to recover the blood lost in a useable form. This comprises suction losses as well as blood loss to surgical swabs. Washing the blood-soaked swabs in a normal saline/heparin solution can increase the amount of recoverable blood by 30–50%.
- Induced hypotension may be beneficial in the older child undergoing midfacial advancement but has not been widely adopted owing to the increased risk of intraoperative venous air embolism (VAE) and rapid blood loss. There are several agents that may be used to achieve moderate intraoperative hypotension, a commonly used combination being remifentanil and clonidine. The use of induced hypotension in infants and young children undergoing craniosynostosis repair is controversial and is not practised at the author's institution.
- Acute normovolaemic haemodilution is limited by the child's relatively small circulating blood volume and so has limited value.

At the author's institution, preoperative optimisation of iron levels where possible, meticulous attention to patient positioning (particularly when in the prone position with avoidance of venous congestion) and surgical technique and the use of tranexamic acid and intraoperative cell salvage for complex major cases are routinely used.

## Postoperative Measures

- Lower the transfusion threshold in otherwise healthy children (currently 70 g $l^{-1}$ at the author's institution in haemodynamically stable children with no pre-existing cardiac disease).
- Iron supplements may be used. Oral iron therapy may be given to children with a low haemoglobin. Intravenous iron therapy is not used at the author's institution.
- Postoperative cell salvage involves the collection of blood from surgical drains followed by reinfusion, with or without a wash cycle. Although there have been concerns about the safety of transfusing unwashed red cells, postoperative cell salvage is commonly used in orthopaedic surgery. Despite the potential benefits, postoperative cell salvage is not currently used for craniofacial surgery in the United Kingdom.

## Management of Dilutional Coagulopathy

Dilutional coagulopathy may occur in patients undergoing complex major craniofacial surgery. The intraoperative use of Octaplas, a pooled plasma solution (10–15 ml $kg^{-1}$), should be determined by the extent of blood loss, clinical evaluation and serial measurement of coagulation parameters. If blood loss persists in the presence of a low fibrinogen level ($<0.8$ g $l^{-1}$), use of a highly concentrated source of fibrinogen such as cryoprecipitate (5–10 ml $kg^{-1}$) may be required. In the author's experience, platelets are rarely required, although they may be necessary in some complex major cases in the presence of demonstrable thrombocytopenia ($<50 \times 10^9\ l^{-1}$).

## Intraoperative Complications

Intraoperative complications are fortunately uncommon but may include:

- Unintentional extubation, endobronchial intubation or severing of the tracheal tube pilot balloon.
- Acute bradycardia secondary to the oculocardiac reflex. This may occur in response to orbital manipulation and responds in most cases to immediate cessation of the stimulus. Occasionally a vagolytic such as glycopyrrolate or atropine is required.
- VAE. Use of the head-up position places patients at increased risk for VAE. The incidence of VAE during surgery for craniosynostosis has been reported as high as 83%, although only 1–2% were clinically significant with haemodynamic compromise. At the author's institution, capnography is used to monitor for clinically significant VAE, and the incidence of haemodynamically significant VAE is fortunately very low.
- Sudden major blood loss resulting in hypotension and impaired organ perfusion. This responds to fluid resuscitation in most cases, although a vasopressor such as phenylephrine is often necessary.
- Significant metabolic acidosis. Children undergoing craniofacial surgery may develop a varying degree of intraoperative metabolic acidosis as evidenced by an increased base deficit. This occurs despite the patient being haemodynamically stable and clinically well perfused and is most likely the result of hyperchloremic acidosis. In the author's experience, the base deficit usually reverts to baseline over a period of approximately 12 hours.

# Postoperative Care

Most children undergoing major and complex major craniofacial surgery can be extubated at the end of surgery. Following a period of stabilisation on the recovery ward, further postoperative care should be provided on a neurosurgical high-dependency unit where invasive monitoring can be continued. Admission of a patient to the intensive care unit for mechanical ventilation is uncommon at the author's institution but may occasionally be required in the event of an unexpected or significant intraoperative complication.

Bilateral nasopharyngeal airways are routinely used in children at risk of postoperative upper airway obstruction following complex major surgery, such as frontofacial advancement. These remain in situ for up to five days or until such time as the facial oedema has resolved. To reduce the potential for further facial oedema within the initial 24–48 hours postoperatively, patients are nursed in a head-up position. Frost sutures (between the lower eyelid and eyebrow) may also be used in this group of patients to protect the cornea.

## Fluid Management

Fluid losses may continue into the initial postoperative period, and meticulous attention should be paid to postoperative fluid management with ongoing monitoring of haemodynamic parameters, drain losses and coagulation profile. A falling haematocrit in association with minimal drain losses should alert one to the possibility of an intracranial haemorrhage. This constitutes an emergency for which an immediate neurosurgical opinion should be sought.

## Pain Management

It is important that adequate pain control is achieved prior to transfer of a patient to the neurosurgical high-dependency unit. This may involve the titration of further doses of intravenous morphine in the recovery ward. Thereafter, satisfactory analgesia can be achieved in most patients with a combination of regular intravenous paracetamol (15 mg $kg^{-1}$ every six hours), oral morphine (0.1–0.2 mg $kg^{-1}$ every four hours) as required and a non-steroidal anti-inflammatory drug (e.g. ibuprofen, diclofenac) once the clotting profile has normalised. Intravenous morphine delivered via a patient- (PCA) or nurse-controlled analgesia (NCA) device is used for patients following complex major surgery. It may also be used following some major procedures (e.g. fronto-orbital remodelling) but may be associated with an increased incidence of nausea and vomiting and delayed mobilisation.

Postoperative nausea and vomiting are common following craniofacial surgery, and dual antiemetic therapy should be used.

## Specific Craniofacial Procedures

### Minimally Invasive Surgery

Minimally invasive approaches to the surgical management of craniosynostosis is gaining wider acceptance, and early suturectomy with some form of distraction to passively reshape the head has become an accepted treatment for single-suture craniosynostosis. Surgical techniques include spring-assisted cranioplasty, commonly performed for sagittal synostosis and for posterior vault expansion. More recently, endoscopic suturectomy with helmet therapy (ESCH) has emerged as a successful treatment for metopic, unicoronal and sagittal synostosis. Minimally invasive surgery offers many advantages over traditional open techniques, including shorter operative times, less blood loss, fewer transfusions and a reduced length of hospital stay.

### Spring-Assisted Cranioplasty

Dynamic distraction with steel springs is increasingly being used in the management of sagittal and lambdoid craniosynostosis. Spring-assisted cranioplasty is the treatment of choice for sagittal synostosis at the author's institution and is increasingly being used for posterior vault expansion.

### Spring-Assisted Sagittal Cranioplasty

Spring-assisted cranioplasty involves performing a small craniectomy straddling the sagittal sinus, approximately halfway along the fused suture, followed by two parasagittal osteotomies. Two titanium springs are then placed across the defect to gradually separate the bones (Figure 25.2). Surgery should be performed between three and six months of age as the development of frontal bossing in late infancy precludes the use of this technique. Spring removal is typically undertaken three months later through the same incision as a day-case procedure.

This minimally invasive procedure has had an enormous impact on the surgical management of infants with sagittal synostosis, and it has several advantages over the traditional open technique. A quantitative analysis of 100 consecutive cases at the author's institution showed a reduced operating time (~1 h vs 2–3 h), smaller scar with minimal dural dissection, minimal blood loss, reduced blood transfusion (9% vs ~ 95%), rapid recovery and shorter hospital stay (one night vs three nights) compared with alternative treatment strategies.

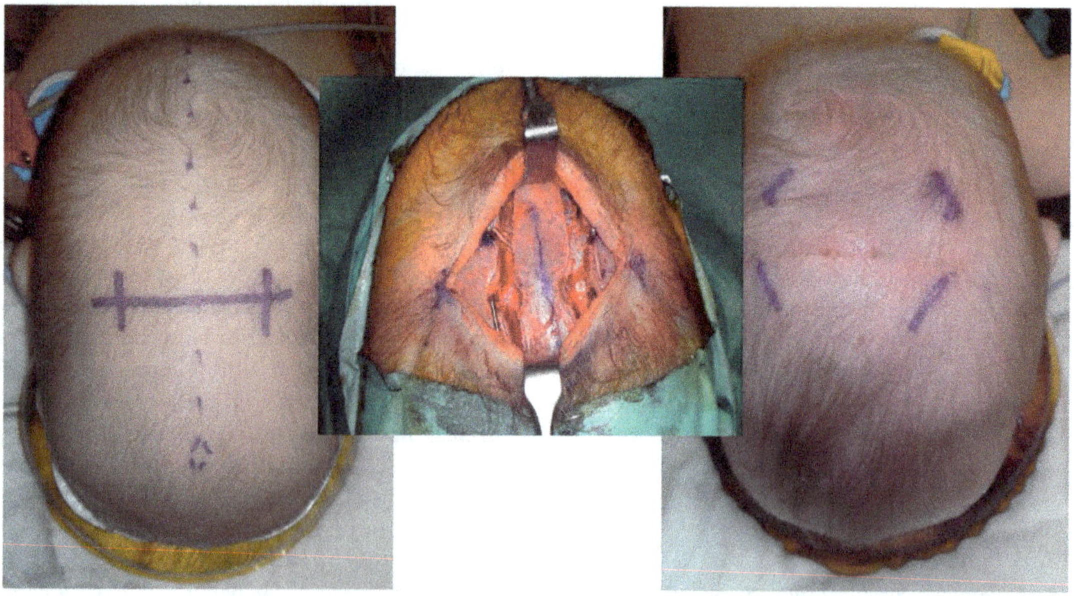

**Figure 25.2** Operative technique for sagittal spring cranioplasty demonstrating 'sphinx' positioning and location of scalp incision (left), location of parasagittal osteotomies and springs (centre) and residual postoperative scar post spring removal (right).

## Anaesthetic Considerations

- Patient position: modified prone with neck extension ('sphinx position')
- Surgical approach: small transverse incision
- Surgical duration: one hour
- Reinforced orotracheal tube with full neurosurgical strapping
- Peripheral venous cannula × 1
- Arterial line not essential

## Spring-Assisted Posterior Vault Expansion

Spring-assisted posterior vault expansion is also commonly performed at the author's institution. Although it has some advantages over the traditional surgical technique, spring cranioplasty has not had quite the same impact as it has for sagittal synostosis. The procedure remains of similar duration to the traditional open technique, and although blood loss may be less, the risk of significant and rapid blood loss remains.

## Anaesthetic Considerations

- Patient position: modified prone position with neck extension ('sphinx position')
- Surgical approach: bicoronal incision
- Surgical duration: three to four hours
- Reinforced orotracheal tube with full neurosurgical strapping
- Peripheral venous cannulae × 2
- Arterial line essential

## Endoscopic Suturectomy for Craniosynostosis with Postoperative Helmeting (ESCH)

ESCH is increasingly being used in the treatment of single-suture synostosis in the United Kingdom. The procedure involves the early surgical removal of the affected cranial suture with postoperative guidance of remaining brain growth using helmet orthoses.

At the author's institution, a recent retrospective cohort study of 18 patients (mean age 4.6 months [range 2.5–7.8 months]) showed this to be a safe and well-tolerated technique for the treatment of metopic, unicoronal and sagittal synostosis with low morbidity (one surgical complication, suture abscess), transfusion requirement (2 of 18) and short hospital stay (median length one night).

## Anaesthetic Considerations

- Patient position: supine/modified prone with neck extension ('sphinx position')
- Surgical approach: small transverse incision
- Surgical duration: one hour
- Reinforced orotracheal tube with full neurosurgical strapping
- Peripheral venous cannula × 1
- Arterial line not essential

## Open Surgery

### Fronto-orbital Remodelling/Advancement

Fronto-orbital remodelling/advancement is currently the surgical procedure of choice for unicoronal, bicoronal and metopic synostosis. These forms of craniosynostosis affect the forehead and upper part of the eye sockets, producing a characteristic triangular deformity of the frontal bone with lateral forehead deficiency (trigonocephaly) in metopic synostosis, flattening of the ipsilateral forehead with bossing of the contralateral side (frontal plagiocephaly) in unilateral craniosynostosis and a skull that is short in the anterior–posterior dimension (brachycephaly), tall vertically (turricephaly) and wide in bicoronal synostosis. Fronto-orbital remodelling/advancement involves a bifrontal craniotomy with release of the affected suture(s) and simultaneous supraorbital and frontal reconstruction. The ideal timing of surgery varies between institutions and surgeon preference; advocates for early reconstruction (typically 9–12 months of age) claim that greater bony pliability results in a more favourable result, whilst those who prefer to delay surgery until 12–18 months of age do so to reduce the chance of recurrence.

## Anaesthetic Considerations

- Patient position: supine, head up
- Surgical approach: bicoronal incision
- Surgical duration: three to four hours
- Pre-formed south-facing RAE orotracheal tube
- No eye covering (eye ointment only)
- Peripheral venous cannulae × 2
- Arterial line essential
- Intraoperative cell salvage may be useful for redo surgery

## Total Calvarial Remodelling

Sagittal craniosynostosis is the most common form of synostosis and results in a skull shape that is typically long and narrow (scaphocephaly). The timing of reconstructive surgery is paramount to both the nature and extent of the surgical procedure performed. If surgery is performed within six to eight months of birth when the cranial bones are still very pliable, a spring-assisted sagittal cranioplasty is performed. This is the preferred technique at the author's institution, but a more extensive strip craniectomy involving a combination of wide sagittal craniectomy with plication of the vertically divided parietal bones is still performed in some centres.

Correction of sagittal synostosis in older children involves total calvarial remodelling. This is a more extensive procedure involving reconstruction of at least the anterior two thirds if not all the calvarium. The modified 'Melbourne' technique allows remodelling of both the anterior and posterior cranium. This involves an intraoperative change in patient position from the prone to supine position, during which meticulous care is required to avoid unintended dislodgement of the airway, arterial line or cannulae.

### Anaesthetic Considerations

- Patient position
  Anterior two-thirds procedure: modified prone with neck extension ('sphinx position')
  Modified Melbourne procedure: combined modified prone and supine
- Surgical approach: bicoronal incision
- Surgical duration: total calvarial remodelling three to four hours; modified 'Melbourne' technique five to six hours
- Reinforced orotracheal tube with full neurosurgical strapping
- Peripheral venous cannulae × 2
- Arterial line essential
- Intraoperative cell salvage may be useful for redo total calvarial remodelling

## Posterior Calvarial Vault Expansion/ Remodelling

Posterior vault expansion/remodelling is performed to treat raised ICP, which can be related to craniosynostosis (multi-sutural or unilateral lambdoid synostosis), abnormal venous drainage, OSA or hydrocephalus. Posterior vault expansion can be performed as an open procedure involving the removal and reshaping of the posterior skull with bone grafting, or more commonly by spring cranioplasty. As posterior vault expansion is used to treat raised ICP, it may be performed at any age, although this typically occurs at 6 months of age and usually before 10 years of age. There is a risk of significant bleeding with this procedure whether it is performed using an open or minimally invasive technique.

### Anaesthetic Considerations

- Patient position: modified prone with neck extension ('sphinx position')
- Surgical approach: bicoronal incision
- Surgical duration: three to four hours
- Reinforced orotracheal tube with full neurosurgical strapping
- Peripheral venous cannulae × 2
- Arterial line essential
- Intraoperative cell salvage may be useful for redo surgery

## Monobloc Frontofacial Advancement and Facial Bipartition with or without Distraction Osteogenesis

Monobloc frontofacial advancement and bipartition have an important role to play in the management of syndromic synostosis. They can be used to reverse the associated facial deformity seen in children with Apert, Crouzon and Pfeiffer syndromes and to treat functional problems such as raised ICP, severe exorbitism with or without globe subluxation and upper airway obstruction. Monobloc frontofacial advancement addresses all these functional issues in a single procedure. The operation combines transcranial frontal advance and extracranial Le Fort III midfacial advance with the frontal bones and maxilla being brought forward in one piece either immediately at surgery or more slowly by distraction using a RED frame (Figure 25.3). The RED frame comprises a halo device which is attached to the mobilised facial skeleton through a combination of cranial pins, rods and wires. Postoperative distraction (~1.5 mm/day) is achieved by progressively shortening the wires. The distractor is removed under general anaesthesia once the midface has advanced the required distance and following a consolidation period of six weeks.

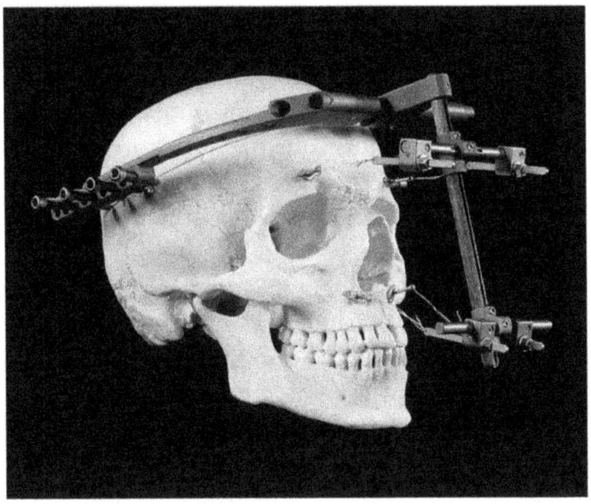

**Figure 25.3** A rigid external distractor (RED) in situ.

A facial bipartition occurs naturally as part of a midline facial cleft. A midline split can also be created surgically as an extension of a monobloc frontofacial advancement to correct frontonasal dysplasia, facial dysostoses and orbital hypertelorism (horizontal dystopia). Following mobilisation of the maxilla and orbits, removal of a midline segment of bone and extension of the central osteotomy down to the incisors allows rotation of the two hemifacial segments together, thereby narrowing the interorbital distance and expanding the maxilla. It also corrects any down-going slant to the eyes, which is a feature of Apert syndrome.

Both procedures may be associated with high morbidity, especially in young infants and children. Timing of surgery is crucial, and the procedure should ideally be delayed until skeletal maturity has been achieved at approximately 12 years of age. Indications for early frontofacial advancement include severe upper airway obstruction, ocular exposure or subluxation and raised ICP.

## Orbital Box Osteotomy

Orbital box osteotomy is used in the treatment of hypertelorism and vertical orbital dystopia, particularly when lateral movement of a single orbit is required. It involves making a 360° osteotomy around one or both orbits, thereby allowing them to be moved medially either upwards or downwards. As the osteotomy extends between the orbital floor and the roots of the permanent dentition, this procedure should only be performed once puberty has been reached.

## Anaesthetic Considerations

- Patient position: supine head up.
- Surgical approach: combined intraoral and transcranial (bicoronal) incisions.
- Surgical duration: six to eight hours.
- Reinforced orotracheal tube with circum-mandibular wiring. In patients with a tracheostomy in situ, a reinforced tracheal tube is placed via the tracheostome and secured to the anterior chest wall.
- A throat pack is essential to protect the airway from blood and bony fragments and assist with securing the tracheal tube.
- Eye ointment and temporary tarsorrhaphies are used to protect the eyes intraoperatively (replaced with Frost sutures for 48 hours postoperatively).
- At least two large bore peripheral venous cannulae.
- Femoral central venous line is recommended, especially in the younger child.
- Arterial line is essential.
- Urinary catheter.
- Intraoperative cell salvage.
- Care should be taken to ensure that all pressure points are padded, and these should be rechecked during the procedure.
- Anti-embolism compression stockings (TED™) for older teenagers with mechanical deep venous thrombosis (DVT) prophylaxis system (e.g. Flowtron).
- Bilateral nasopharyngeal airways and a nasogastric tube are inserted at the end of surgery.
- It is usual practice at the author's institution to extubate all patients at the end of surgery if surgery has been uneventful, the patient is haemodynamically stable and there is no respiratory compromise.
- As the RED frame is bulky, it may impede access to the airway, making reintubation very difficult. If there are any postoperative airway concerns, the halo may be placed with delayed fitting of the suspension frame.

## Removal of the RED Frame

In the older child, removal of a rigid external distractor is a relatively simple procedure involving disconnection of the halo device followed by removal of the cranial pins. The situation is very different in infants, owing to the insertion of titanium mesh sheets to prevent penetration of the skull by the cranial pins. This necessitates removal of the distractor and sheets via a bicoronal incision.

The presence of a RED frame may make airway management difficult, so it is important to ensure that the necessary tools and expertise to remove the frame are readily available prior to induction of anaesthesia. In cooperative children, the suspension frame may be removed prior to induction of anaesthesia. If this is not feasible, the face mask may have to be inverted and then changed for a laryngeal mask airway once the patient is anaesthetised, as the frame's wires and bars make conventional placement of a face mask impossible. Laryngoscopy and intubation may also be difficult if not impossible, and for procedures other than removal of the frame where intubation is deemed necessary, it is advisable that the surgeon remove the wires and bars.

### Key Points

- Craniosynostosis results from the premature closure of one or more cranial sutures and can occur in isolation or as part of an associated syndrome.
- Preoperative evaluation should focus on any comorbidities and the possibility of difficult airway management. Children who have undergone previous corrective surgery may be difficult to intubate, despite the lack of any history of difficult laryngoscopy.
- Successful perioperative management is dependent on understanding the proposed surgical procedure and the anticipation and prompt treatment of the many potential complications that may arise.
- Blood loss and major transfusion remain the greatest risk to infants and children undergoing complex major craniofacial surgery. Blood loss, which may be dramatic or insidious, and dilutional coagulopathy should be managed proactively.
- Intraoperative cell salvage is useful in reducing the need for allogeneic transfusion, particularly in prolonged major or complex major surgical cases.
- Most patients can be extubated at the end of surgery, with postoperative care being continued on the neurosurgical high-dependency unit (HDU) with continued invasive monitoring.

## Further Reading


Halim J, Silva A, Budden C et al. Initial UK series of endoscopic suturectomy with postoperative helmeting for craniosynostosis: early report of perioperative experience. *British Journal of Neurosurgery* 2020; 26:1–6.

Jones B, Dunaway D, Hayward R. Surgery. In: Hayward R, Jones B, Dunaway D, Evans R, eds. *The Clinical Management of Craniosynostosis.* Cambridge University Press. 2004; 374–401.

Mallory S, Bingham R. Anaesthesia for craniosynostosis surgery. In: Hayward R, Jones B, Dunaway D, Evans R, eds. *The Clinical Management of Craniosynostosis.* Cambridge University Press. 2004; 355–73.

Murad GJA, Clayman M, Segal MB, et al. Endoscopic-assisted repair of craniosynostosis. *Neurosurgical Focus* 2005; 19(6):E6.

O'Hara J, Ruggiero F, Wilson L et al. Syndromic craniosynostosis: complexities of care. *Molecular Syndromology* 2019; 10:83–97.

Pearson A, Matava CT. Anaesthetic management for craniosynostosis repair in children. *BJA Education* 2016; 16 (12):410–6.

Proctor MR, Meara JG. A review of the management of single suture craniosynostosis, past, present, and future. *Journal of Neurosurgical Pediatrics* 2019; 24 (6):622–31.

Rodgers W, Glass GE, Schievano S et al. Spring-assisted cranioplasty for the correction of nonsyndromic scaphocephaly: a quantitative analysis of 100 consecutive cases. *Plastic and Reconstructive Surgery* 2017; 140(1):125–34.

Chapter 26

# Anaesthesia for Neurosurgery in Children

Amaki Sogbodjor and Su Mallory

## Introduction

Neurosurgery is a rapidly evolving field with innovative techniques and novel procedures frequently being developed. The children undergoing these procedures are often complex and have a range of cognitive abilities demanding a tailor-made approach to their care. An understanding of normal development and neurophysiology is key to delivering an anaesthetic appropriate for both patient and procedure.

This chapter addresses some of the challenges faced by the paediatric neuroanaesthetist, with specific attention being paid to some of the more common and complex procedures.

## Anatomy and Physiology

In the neonate, the calvarium is composed of ossified plates covering the dura, which are separated by fibrous sutures and two fontanelles. The posterior fontanelle closes during the second or third month, whilst the anterior fontanelle usually closes between 10 and 18 months. Both fontanelles fully ossify in the second decade. These fontanelles and non-fused sutures can separate up to early adolescence, providing some protection from a chronic increase in intracranial pressure (ICP). When ICP is acutely elevated, the compliance of the cranium is limited by the dura mater. A clinical assessment of intracranial pressure in infancy can be made by examination of the fontanelles.

## Intracranial Pressure

Intracranial pressure in neonates and infants is normally in the range 0–6 mmHg. It increases until adulthood when values of 7–17 mmHg are normal. Brain tissue, blood and cerebrospinal fluid (CSF) are contained within the cranium in the proportions 80%, 10% and 10% respectively. Intracranial pressure may be increased by cerebral oedema, intracranial masses and rises in cerebral blood or CSF volumes. As the skull is essentially a closed box, ICP rises rapidly once compensatory mechanisms have been exhausted. Clinical signs of increased ICP include vomiting, irritability, drowsiness, bulging fontanelles, 'sun-setting eyes' (downward gaze) and increased head circumference. If ICP continues to rise, the Cushing reflex of systolic hypertension, bradycardia and respiratory irregularity occurs, which are signs of imminent brainstem coning, coma and death. ICP can be affected by surgery and anaesthesia, and a clear understanding of the many factors involved is essential knowledge for those undertaking neuroanaesthesia.

## Cerebral Blood Flow and Perfusion Pressure

Much of neuroanaesthesia is directed towards controlling ICP. Central to this is the ability to manipulate cerebral blood flow (CBF) which is related to cerebral blood volume (CBV) and in turn to ICP. CBF varies with age (see Table 26.1) and is affected by a number of additional factors, some of which can be manipulated by the anaesthetist in order to reduce ICP when this is indicated.

Cerebral blood supply is coupled to the cerebral metabolic rate. Autoregulation, vasoconstriction or vasodilation of the cerebral vasculature

**Table 26.1** Cerebral blood flow: normal range at different ages

| Age | Cerebral blood flow (ml $min^{-1}$ 100 $g^{-1}$) |
|---|---|
| Neonate | 40–42 |
| 6 months to 3 years | 90 |
| 3–12 years | 100 |
| Adult | 50 |

changes cerebral blood supply to meet the metabolic demands of the tissue. Metabolic demands are increased in conditions such as sepsis or seizures. Here blood flow increases, leading to a rise in cerebral blood volume and consequently ICP. In conditions of decreased metabolic activity such as hypothermia, the reverse is true, and blood flow decreases. Cerebral metabolic rate is higher in children than in adults, as is the demand for both glucose (child 6.8 mg $min^{-1}$ 100 $g^{-1}$, adult 5.5 mg $min^{-1}$ 100 $g^{-1}$) and oxygen (infant 5.8 ml $min^{-1}$ 100 $g^{-1}$, adult 3.5 ml $min^{-1}$ 100 $g^{-1}$). In the presence of oxygen, the substrate for cerebral metabolism is glucose. There are limited stores of glucose and glycogen in cerebral tissue, so normal cerebral blood flow is essential to maintain glucose and oxygen levels. The high metabolic rate in infants and children increases the impact of any interruption in cerebral blood supply.

Cerebral perfusion is controlled by autoregulatory mechanisms within the normal range of mean arterial pressure (MAP). If excessive hypo- or hypertension, hypoxia, hypercapnia or cerebral ischaemia occurs, these mechanisms fail, and cerebral perfusion becomes dependent on systolic blood pressure. Where there is anaemia or haemodilution, leading to decreased blood viscosity, then viscosity autoregulation also plays a role. Lower viscosity increases oxygen delivery and vasoconstriction occurs. Here CBV decreases, although CBF is constant.

Cerebral perfusion pressure (CPP) is defined according to the formula:

$$CPP = MAP - (ICP + CVP)$$

where MAP is mean arterial pressure, ICP is intracranial pressure and CVP is central venous pressure.

Volatile anaesthetic agents inhibit autoregulation via dose-dependent cerebral vasodilation. In children, this impairment of autoregulation is presumed to be due to the lower MAP. When CPP falls below this lower limit, autoregulation is impaired, and CBF falls in proportion with MAP. Sick neonates have impaired autoregulation, and CBF in this group is highly dependent on systolic pressure. Fluctuations in MAP may explain the occurrence of intraventricular haemorrhage in this patient group. The effects of carbon dioxide on CBF appear to be the same as in adults, but a linear relationship exists between $PaCO_2$ and CBF in sick neonates; hyperventilation has been demonstrated to restore autoregulation in this group. Cerebral steal may occur in some circumstances; hypercapnia results in vasodilation of normal vessels and diversion of blood away from abnormal vessels, for example in tumours or ischaemic areas. Inverse steal may occur in the presence of hypocapnia; normal vessels become constricted, and there is preferential flow to the abnormal vasculature, which is less able to regulate flow.

Control of $PaCO_2$ is an essential tool for the reduction of CBF and therefore ICP. In raised ICP, the interventions that can help to reduce it are mild hyperventilation, moderate hypothermia, cessation of seizure activity, osmodiuresis, increasing sedation/depth of anaesthesia, a head-up tilt, treatment of sepsis and haemodilution. Hypoxia, vasodilators and high concentrations of volatile agent as well as pathological changes (tumour, abscess, trauma) will also adversely affect autoregulation, potentially increasing CBF and consequently ICP.

### Cerebrospinal Fluid

CSF surrounds the brain, circulating nutrients, removing waste, supporting structures and offering some protection against trauma. CSF is mainly produced by the choroid plexus. It flows from the lateral ventricles through the foramen of Monro into the third ventricle, then through the cerebral aqueduct of Sylvius to the fourth ventricle and out via the foramina of Luschka and the foramen of Magendie to the subarachnoid space, where it is absorbed by the arachnoid villi. Furosemide or acetazolamide can be used to reduce CSF production in an effort to control ICP. The contribution of these interventions to ICP regulation is very small, and manipulations of CBF and CBV have far greater impact. CSF production is relatively constant in children and adults, but there is a lower storage capacity for CSF in children, so disturbed CSF reabsorption has a far greater effect.

## Conduct of Anaesthesia for the Neurosurgical Patient

### Preoperative Management

Inclusion of a neurological assessment is essential. Signs of raised ICP, altered conscious level and focal findings should be noted. Vomiting due to raised ICP may cause dehydration and electrolyte imbalance. Brain stem lesions can be associated with bulbar palsies that may result in aspiration with pulmonary consolidation. Some children have multi-system disease, such as ex-premature infants (chronic lung disease), those with cerebral abscesses (e.g. cyanotic heart disease) and those with major spinal defects (renal disease).

Preoperative investigations should include a full blood count for all patients and electrolytes in those with a history of vomiting or a ventricular drain. Neurosurgery in children can be associated with significant blood loss if sinuses or dilated veins from raised ICP are disrupted. Blood must be cross-matched for children undergoing craniotomy. A clotting screen may be required as anticonvulsant treatment can cause coagulopathy.

Sedative premedication is avoided in children with significantly raised ICP, as further elevation of ICP due to hypercapnia may be catastrophic. Atropine or glycopyrrolate can reduce oral secretions, the pooling of which, especially in the prone or the sitting position, may result in reduced adhesion of tracheal tube fixation tape. Their use has the added benefit of providing a degree of protection against bradycardia.

## Induction of Anaesthesia

General anaesthesia remains the norm for craniotomy in children, although awake craniotomy has been reported in adolescents. Induction may be inhalational or intravenous. A thorough explanation and understanding of the process of induction will ideally help assure a calm patient and family, as the anaesthetist needs to be mindful of the ICP at this time. An intravenous technique might have to be adapted to avoid upset should cannulation prove difficult:

- Sevoflurane has become the volatile agent of choice for gas induction in children. It causes cerebral vasodilation, but this may have less effect on the intracranial pressure than an intravenous induction accompanied by crying or breath-holding.
- If intravenous induction is preferred and feasible, then propofol is commonly used.
- A non-depolarising muscle relaxant is used, such as atracurium or vecuronium.
- Suxamethonium may be used if a rapid sequence induction is indicated, although there is a theoretical risk of raising ICP.

Surges in arterial pressure at laryngoscopy should be prevented using fentanyl or remifentanil, and the airway should be secured with an armoured tracheal tube of appropriate size to avoid undue leak and hypoventilation. Consider nasal intubation if advantageous for prone position or post-operative management on the intensive care unit. Satisfactory bilateral lung ventilation should be assessed with the head in a neutral position and then once more in its position for surgery. Cerebral venous obstruction should be avoided by careful patient positioning, 'head-up' tilt and taping rather than tying the tracheal tube. The tape must be moisture-proof, as surgical prep solutions or blood can jeopardise its security. Prophylactic antibiotics are indicated for most neurosurgery, and it is imperative that their administration is appropriately timed.

## Intraoperative Monitoring

Routine monitoring includes electrocardiogram (ECG), non-invasive blood pressure (BP), pulse oximetry, capnography, temperature probes (both central and peripheral) and a peripheral nerve stimulator. Capnography also vitally alerts the anaesthetist to the occurrence of venous air embolism (VAE). All major cases require direct arterial pressure measurement to maintain BP close to baseline. If central venous pressure monitoring is required for assessment of intraoperative fluid balance, the most appropriate route is via the femoral vein. This avoids potential obstruction of cerebral venous drainage and raised ICP. Two peripheral cannulae are required in case rapid fluid resuscitation is necessary. Urinary catheters are not used routinely but are indicated in patients at risk of diabetes insipidus, those undergoing prolonged surgery or where large blood loss is anticipated.

The large surface area to volume ratio of paediatric patients makes temperature control difficult. It is essential to monitor body temperature and to maintain it between 36°C and 36.5°C using patient warming devices and fluid or blood warmers.

If the patient's temperature rises, all warming devices should be switched off, and this is usually sufficient to reduce temperature.

Hypothermia has a cerebral protective effect, and temperature reduction can allow surgery to continue in cases where cerebral perfusion is compromised. Moderate hypothermia of 34–36°C post-ischaemia has neuroprotective benefits without the additional risk of cardiac arrhythmias and metabolic changes.

Post-ischaemic neurological function and cerebral histopathology appear to be detrimentally affected by 1–2°C increases in temperature; hyperthermia should therefore be avoided.

Postoperative hyperpyrexia, which is more likely after craniopharyngioma resection and hypothalamic, pontine and midbrain manipulations, should be treated urgently, especially if the temperature exceeds 40.5°C

## Anaesthetic Agents

Balanced anaesthesia should be maintained, with 0.5–1.0 minimum alveolar concentration (MAC) of sevoflurane or isoflurane in air/oxygen. Nitrous oxide should be avoided when ICP is critically raised, or there is a risk of venous air embolism. The ideal agent for neuroanaesthesia should maintain cerebrovascular autoregulation, allow the continued coupling between CBF and metabolism, avoid an increase in CBV or ICP, have no impact on the electroencephalogram (EEG) and have both neuroprotective and anticonvulsant potential.

Volatile agents at low dose cause cerebral vessels to constrict by suppressing metabolism. Sevoflurane has been demonstrated to have the most favourable profile as it is the least vasoactive volatile agent. This results in less vasodilation for the same depth of anaesthesia, with little or no effect on autoregulation, CBV and ICP below 1 MAC. Its fast elimination also allows neurological status to be assessed more reliably in the immediate postoperative period. With increasing concentrations of volatile agent, vasodilatory effects predominate, and whilst ICP may only increase marginally, the effects on CPP are clinically significant owing to a decrease in MAP. Whilst sevoflurane causes less suppression of somatosensory-evoked potentials than isoflurane, it significantly attenuates motor-evoked potentials.

Propofol, in contrast, does not impair autoregulation; it decreases CBF and ICP and has a lesser effect on somatosensory and motor-evoked responses. This makes it an attractive option in instances when intraoperative neuromonitoring (IONM) is required, and total intravenous anaesthesia (TIVA) is now the preferred technique in these circumstances.

Neuromuscular blocking agents (NMBA) can also be problematic, as their action may be prolonged in patients taking anti-epileptic medication. NMBA use after intubation is precluded when IONM is needed.

## Ventilation

Mild to moderate hyperventilation ($PaCO_2$ approx. 3.8–4.2 kPa) will cause vasoconstriction, reducing cerebral blood volume, and is useful when ICP is elevated. Cerebral ischaemia has been described if $PaCO_2$ is allowed to fall below 3.5 kPa, although paediatric patients are less prone to focal ischaemia due to healthier blood vessels.

Control of the fractional inspired oxygen is important, and the anaesthetist should aim for normoxia. Hypoxia increases the risk of ischaemia and subsequently leads to an increase in CBF. Conversely, hyperoxia promotes excitotoxic damage through the generation of oxygen free radicals.

## Analgesia

The intraoperative analgesic of choice has traditionally been fentanyl, which, unlike alfentanil and sufentanil, does not increase CBF or ICP. Unless the procedure is prolonged or postoperative ventilation is planned, the maximum dose should not exceed 7–10 mcg $kg^{-1}$. Remifentanil is now widely used, as its short duration of action enables easy titration in response to surgical stimulus and facilitates rapid recovery from anaesthesia. Supplementation with alternative analgesia on cessation of a remifentanil infusion prior to emergence is essential. On completion of surgery, muscle relaxation is reversed with neostigmine and glycopyrrolate if necessary. Children should be extubated when breathing well with a normal end-tidal carbon dioxide. Excessive coughing can be avoided by a deep extubation if it is possible.

## Fluid Replacement and Haemodynamic Parameters

In a normal brain, osmotic forces produce fluid fluxes. A fall in osmotic pressure of 5–10 mOsmol $kg^{-1}$ may result in cerebral oedema. A balanced fluid such as Hartmann's solution can be used for intraoperative fluid maintenance in neurosurgery, but where large volumes are required this mildly hypo-osmolar solution is not ideal and normal saline may be preferable. Hyperglycaemia is associated with adverse outcomes in head injuries, and blood sugar should be monitored regularly. Glucose-containing infusions should be used cautiously and only when indicated.

It is difficult to measure blood loss accurately in neurosurgery, and the relatively large head size of children results in proportionately larger blood loss compared with adults. An assessment of blood loss can be made by reviewing haemodynamic parameters, in particular heart rate and arterial pressure. Massive blood transfusions may be required for some neurosurgical procedures in small children and are generally well tolerated provided clotting, blood gases and potassium levels are checked regularly. Rapid and large transfusion of blood carries several risks in the infant and is discussed in Chapter 14. The use of antifibrinolytics such as tranexamic acid should be considered when blood loss is a risk.

Optimal surgical conditions are associated with a relatively slow heart rate, and this can be achieved with deep anaesthesia and normovolaemia. Induced hypotension should be used with great caution. Remifentanil facilitates intraoperative haemodynamic control, and when necessary its hypotensive effects may be offset using $\alpha 1$ agonists such as phenylephrine. Acute rises in ICP can usually be managed with moderate hyperventilation and mannitol. Dexamethasone may be used to decrease cerebral oedema but should be used with caution in the presence of infection such as cerebral abscess.

## Postoperative Management

The majority of patients do not require postoperative ventilation. The decision to ventilate a patient may be made preoperatively where specific indications exist, or intraoperatively if surgery has been unexpectedly prolonged, the patient has been cardiovascularly unstable or if there is a neurosurgical indication. Patients who are slow to wake up may require radiological imaging in the immediate postoperative period.

Patients undergoing craniotomy require high-dependency care postoperatively. Direct arterial pressure monitoring should be maintained for 24 hours, and cardiorespiratory function, fluid balance and neurological status should be monitored. Analgesia for these patients includes regular intravenous paracetamol and an opioid, with the addition of an NSAID if no contraindication exists. Oral morphine is often used postoperatively, but reduced doses may be necessary to avoid undue reduction in conscious level or pupil size. Patient- or nurse-controlled intravenous morphine analgesia is useful, particularly for patients who have had posterior fossa craniotomy or spinal surgery. Antiemetics should be administered to mitigate postoperative nausea and vomiting.

# Specific Considerations

## Acute Head Injury

The force required to produce a skull fracture in a child is large, so an associated brain injury is more likely than in an adult. Rapid increase in ICP from cerebral oedema and subdural haematoma may necessitate urgent surgical intervention. Secondary injury; scalp lacerations resulting in large blood loss; facial injuries causing airway compromise; and additional thoracic, abdominal or limb injuries need to be considered. This is particularly true for cervical spine injuries which can occur in children without radiological evidence.

## Brain Tumours

Tumours may be vascular lesions, and some are suitable for preoperative embolisation of large feeding vessels to reduce operative blood loss. Neurosurgery for tumours is still not without significant risk of morbidity and mortality. The majority of brain tumours in children occur in the posterior fossa. Surgery performed with the child in the sitting position provides excellent surgical access, improved cerebral venous drainage, decreased blood loss, lowering of ICP and improved postoperative recovery, including preservation of cranial nerve function. This position provides an anaesthetic challenge, as there is increased risk of VAE, and it can be associated with cardiovascular instability, pneumocephalus, compression injuries due to pressure on neurovascular structures and quadriplegia due to spinal cord infarction. Hypotension is unusual in the paediatric population provided the patient is adequately fluid loaded.

Posterior fossa syndrome is a unique postoperative complication of this procedure. It consists of several components, including ataxia, nerve palsies, hemiparesis, irritability and cortical blindness. It is often associated with symptoms of cerebellar mutism, resulting in loss of speech and occasionally loss of the ability to eat or drink. Recovery over time is variable and has been reported to take anything from days to years. The cause remains debated, but focal decrease in cerebral blood flow is considered most probable.

## Venous Air Embolus

VAE is uncommon, but the consequences can be significant in children. The problem is amplified in neonates and babies whose heads are proportionally larger and sit higher than the heart when lying supine. This pressure differential is exaggerated in the sitting position. If it occurs, VAE can be catastrophic in those with congenital heart disease such as a patent foramen ovale. Nitrous oxide should not be used in cases where there is a risk of VAE.

Diagnosis of VAE can be made using several methods, including oesophageal stethoscope, precordial Doppler or transoesophageal echocardiography. Capnography is used in many units to monitor for VAE; the alarm limits are set close to the end-tidal carbon dioxide level ($ETCO_2$), so that the anaesthetist is immediately alerted if the $ETCO_2$ falls. Significant emboli are those which cause a fall in blood pressure of more than 10%, or changes in heart rate and in particular arrhythmias. If VAE is suspected, immediate management is to flood the surgical site with fluid to seal the veins, provide 100% oxygen, administer jugular venous compression and resuscitate with fluid to raise the venous pressure and limit the embolus size. Head-down tilt or even CPR may become necessary, and the anaesthetist should know how to release the child from the sitting position should this uncommon event occur.

## Craniopharyngioma

Craniopharyngioma is a slow-growing cystic suprasellar tumour arising from remnants of the craniopharyngeal duct. It has benign histology, but insidious growth may produce significant mass effect, including progressive neurological and endocrine deterioration as the tumour expands into the hypothalamus, optic nerves and pituitary stalk. These children are often either small owing to growth failure or obese because of hypothalamic dysfunction. The major problems in the perioperative period are likely to be related to blood loss or diabetes insipidus (DI), the latter due to failure of antidiuretic hormone (ADH) secretion from the posterior pituitary. Involvement of the endocrinology team is essential as these patients may be on steroids, and synthetic vasopressin (DDAVP) may be required in the perioperative period to control DI.

CVP monitoring, arterial access and an indwelling catheter are essential, as measuring perioperative urine specific gravity and plasma osmolality will be needed to assess DI. There is also an increased incidence of seizures and hyperpyrexia requiring treatment after craniopharyngioma surgery.

## Epilepsy surgery

There are two major types of surgery for intractable epilepsy:

- Excision of a specific seizure focus (e.g. temporal lobe resection)
- Interruption of neural transmission (e.g. corpus callosotomy)

Developmental delay and behavioural issues as well as coexisting disease make anaesthesia for patients with epilepsy a challenge. Anaesthetic agents can display pro- and anticonvulsant properties depending on the dose being administered. Less than 1 MAC sevoflurane minimises the effects on the EEG and facilitates mapping of the lesion. The patient's anticonvulsant medications may produce a number of side effects, including sedation, altered drug metabolism (both enhanced and inhibited), platelet abnormalities, liver dysfunction, metabolic acidosis and increased risk of idiosyncratic drug reactions. An increased tolerance to neuromuscular blockade and opioid analgesia is of particular relevance in these cases. Children with refractory epilepsy on a ketogenic diet will need acid–base balance and blood glucose monitored throughout the perioperative period.

Significant advances have been made in paediatric epilepsy surgery. Awake craniotomy techniques have been used in older children to minimise intraoperative iatrogenic injury. This approach requires multidisciplinary team input and careful patient selection. The implantation of a vagal nerve stimulator is another contemporary treatment which inhibits seizure activity with minimal side effects. Laser ablation may also be employed to destroy seizure foci located within deep structures of the brain. This technique involves the stereotactic-guided insertion of a laser catheter via a burr hole to enable thermal destruction of the epileptogenic focus, thus negating the need for craniotomy. The procedure requires a series of transfers between the operating theatre, CT and MRI scanners and requires strict adherence to standard laser and MRI precautions.

## Neural Tube Defects

Exposed neural tube defects, such as encephalocele or myelomeningocele in neonates, should be repaired as an emergency. Early surgery may be indicated for large lesions, or where there is a risk of rupture and meningitis. In other instances, surgery can be deferred until all investigations, including imaging, have been completed.

Traditionally, intubation has been in the left-lateral position, but the supine position can be used if the lesion is protected adequately from pressure. A Montreal mattress (Figure 26.1) with the head and body supported and the defect in the central space of the mattress is ideal. Surgery is usually performed in the prone position, and care is needed to ensure the eyes are free from pressure and to avoid inferior vena caval compression, which causes engorgement of the paraspinal veins. Haemangiomas in the surrounding tissues may increase surgical blood loss. Long procedures in the prone position also place the patient at risk of airway and tongue oedema. Intraoperative opioids are avoided or minimised unless postoperative ventilation is planned. Wound infiltration with 0.25% bupivacaine is a useful adjunct.

## Hydrocephalus

Hydrocephalus can be acquired (e.g. intrauterine infection, meningitis, tumour, haemorrhage) or congenital (e.g. Arnold Chiari malformation, myelomeningocele) with these patients presenting for surgery as neonates. Ventriculo-peritoneal (VP) shunt insertion is the usual treatment for this condition. In the premature infant, coexisting inguinal hernias may have to be repaired to prevent CSF accumulating in the hernial sacs. The peritoneal route is avoided if there is intra-abdominal pathology that may require surgical intervention in the future. Ventriculo-atrial shunts are rarely used and are potentially complicated by bacterial endocarditis. Alternatively, a ventriculo-pleural shunt may be used, but this is usually reserved for cyst or subdural fluid drainage.

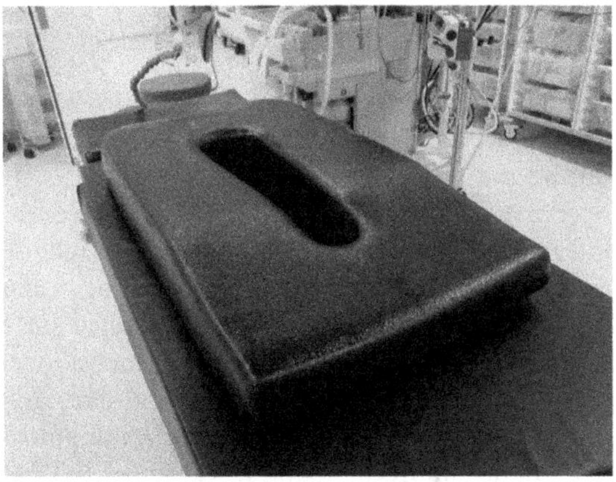

**Figure 26.1** Montreal mattress.

Many infants requiring a VP shunt will have received neonatal intensive care and will be less than 44 weeks postgestation at surgery. A subgaleal shunt may be indicated in particularly small neonates for whom a VP shunt would be too large. This procedure presents the anaesthetist with all the problems associated with surgery in the ex-premature neonate (see Chapter 19). Exposure of skin surfaces and the surgical field preparation make temperature control difficult. Although blood loss is minimal, there is a potential risk of air embolism with catheter insertion, and excessive drainage of CSF can result in cardiac instability.

# Spinal and Craniocervical Surgery

## Congenital Abnormalities

Abnormalities in the lumbar region include dermal sinus tracts or tethered filum terminale. They present with minimal clinical features, but a dermal pit or hair tuft may be apparent. Dermal sinus tracts predispose to meningitis and may present with progressive paraplegia. Tethered filum terminale may present with leg weakness or bowel and bladder symptoms. These abnormalities are usually avascular, and intraoperative transfusion is rare. An anaesthetic technique, such as TIVA, should be used to facilitate spinal monitoring when required. The patient is positioned prone with all the accompanying risks that this may present.

## Spinal Tumours

Extramedullary spinal tumours arise from abnormal embryogenesis or as metastases. Intramedullary tumours, most commonly astrocytomas or ependymomas, are a greater surgical challenge as they involve the spinal cord itself. IONM is usually required, and anaesthesia will need to facilitate it.

Spinal tumours are often extremely vascular, and despite optimal positioning and induced hypotension, patients can require large-volume transfusions. Surgical manipulation of the spinal cord may be associated with arrhythmias and hypotension. This is especially true in the thorax, and suboptimal anaesthesia may exacerbate this picture.

## Instability of the Craniocervical Spine

This can be acquired or congenital. Congenital cases may be associated with inherited disorders such as Down syndrome, Morquio syndrome and pseudoachondroplasia. Atlanto-axial subluxation (Figure 26.2) may be posterior but is much more commonly anterior.

Subluxation creates a kyphosis over C2. The spinal cord, tethered by the dentate ligament, is compressed primarily by the dens. Flexion is more hazardous than extension, with sudden flexion causing cord contusion.

Instability of the craniocervical spine in patients presenting for corrective surgery presents several significant problems. The main problem initially is inducing anaesthesia and intubation prior to fixation of the neck in a halo jacket or surgery. Intubation is usually achieved by standard techniques, but the neck must be held in line by an assistant, who prevents flexion or extension. In adult practice, videolaryngoscopy or awake fibreoptic intubation (FOI) is often the first choice for securing the airway; at the author's institution, asleep FOI is the method of choice where difficulty is anticipated. Cricoid pressure is contraindicated.

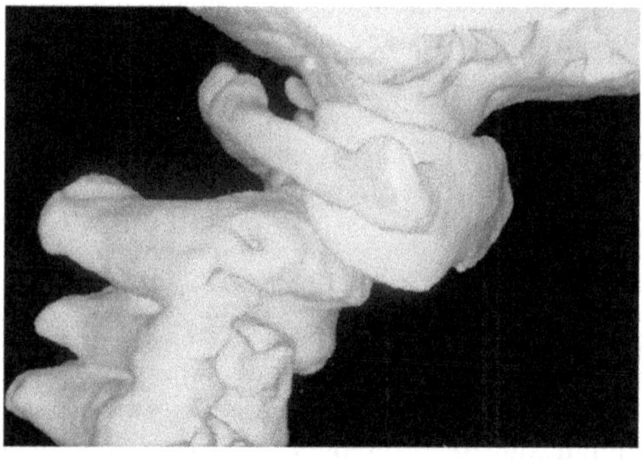

**Figure 26.2** Atlanto-axial subluxation.

Depending on the lesion, the surgical approach will either be posterolateral or transoral. With the latter approach, the child remains intubated postoperatively until all oral swelling has settled, usually within 24–48 hours. Once the child is in the halo jacket, it is essential to appreciate that the previous laryngoscopic view is altered by the fixation position, and intubation may no longer be straightforward. The standard laryngoscope handle normally clashes with either the lateral rods or the top of the jacket, and therefore a polio handle is advantageous. The option of FOI should always be available when anaesthetising a child in a halo jacket, although many procedures can be performed safely with a supraglottic airway device (SAD). A SAD not only provides an airway but may also facilitate intubation where indicated.

## Stereotactic Surgical Techniques

Stereotactic surgery allows precise mapping and access to small, deep-seated lesions of the brain, with decreased neurological morbidity. In the past, the application of the stereotactic headframe in children required general anaesthesia and involved moving the anaesthetised patient between CT scanner and operating theatre. These devices have now been superseded by frameless stereotaxy, for which general anaesthesia is still required, but movement of the anaesthetised patient between different clinical areas is not. External markers on the patient's scalp act as reference points for a pair of cameras above the operating field, which feed back the position of the tip of a chosen surgical tool to a 3D computer-generated image. Intraoperative MRI may also be used to improve the precision of tumour resection and epilepsy surgery. The development of a dedicated suite incorporating an MRI scanner and operating theatre is a costly endeavour, but it enables contemporaneous imaging providing information about the anatomical changes which have occurred during the resection and avoids a separate postoperative scan and general anaesthetic. Procedures integrating MRI are time consuming and require extra care with patient positioning and thermoregulation. Airway access is limited once the headframe is in place and the anaesthetist must be ready and equipped to remove it if necessary. The requirement for MRI-compatible equipment (e.g. non-reinforced endotracheal tube [ETT]), and monitoring introduces additional complexity.

All personnel involved must be familiar with MRI safety, and a dedicated procedural checklist should be used.

## Neuroendoscopic Techniques

Neuroendoscopy is a helpful technique in the treatment of several disorders, including hydrocephalus, cyst puncture and periventricular tumour biopsy. Its indications and applications continue to expand. The procedure requires minimal anaesthesia once the burr hole has been made. The patient's age and clinical state usually guide the choice of anaesthetic technique for this minimally invasive procedure. Video facilities allow the anaesthetist as well as the surgeon to view the surgery as it proceeds, and this improves communication. Patient positioning varies, and access can be limited. Invasive monitoring may be used for prolonged cases or where there is a patient-specific indication.

## Third Ventriculostomy

Third ventriculostomy is an alternative to a VP shunt. It involves fenestration of the floor of the third ventricle, allowing it to communicate with the basal cisterns facilitating reabsorption of CSF. It is relatively contraindicated in individuals with abnormal ventricular anatomy, ventricular haemorrhage or a history of meningitis. Endoscopic ventriculostomy eliminates the risk of shunt-related complications and decreases the necessity for repeated operations after VP shunt insertion.

Complications of third ventriculostomy include haemorrhage, particularly injury to the basilar or perforating arteries (which can result in intraoperative death) and transient or permanent sequelae from midbrain manipulation (variable cardiovascular instability, bradycardia and asystole). Increases in ICP due to pre-existing disease, irrigation fluid or bleeding are also possible, and hypertension and tachycardia may offer the most reliable clue to the development of significantly raised ICP rather than the classic Cushing reflex.

Altered mental state, cranial nerve palsies, vomiting and aspiration, syndrome of inappropriate antidiuretic hormone (SIADH) and ventriculitis may all complicate recovery. Electrolyte imbalance postoperatively has been attributed to several factors including irrigation fluid, disturbance of the hypothalamic nuclei and hormonal imbalance.

## Endoscopic Transphenoidal Surgery

Endoscopic transphenoidal surgery can be used for removal of various lesions, including pituitary tumours and craniopharyngiomas. Surgical access to the pituitary gland is achieved without brain retraction, and the associated morbidity and mortality are decreased.

A preoperative endocrine assessment as for patients with pituitary tumours should occur. It is useful to insert central venous access at induction, as these patients may require repeated blood tests to monitor endocrine function postoperatively.

Cardiovascular instability may be encountered on application of nasal epinephrine at the start of the procedure, and there is potential for intraoperative haemorrhage.

On extubation, the airway may be jeopardised in obligate nasal breathers by pharyngeal blood, gastric blood and nasal packs. Acute haematoma may present with sudden blindness, ophthalmoplegia, hypotension and decreased conscious level.

## Revascularisation Surgery/Extracranial–Intracranial Bypass

Children presenting for this procedure have Moyamoya disease, a progressive chronic occlusive cerebrovascular disease. It usually presents in childhood with symptomatic stenosis of the arteries of the circle of Willis and the internal carotid arteries. These children may have had transient ischaemic attacks or strokes, indicating significantly compromised cerebral blood flow. Medical treatment consists of anti-platelet therapy with aspirin in most cases.

The anaesthetist's aim is to avoid ischaemia and its sequelae. Preoperative fluids will maintain hydration for surgery. Patient distress needs to be minimised, and premedication is advisable.

Normocapnia should be maintained intraoperatively, as hyperventilation reduces cerebral blood flow and can precipitate an ischaemic event; carbon dioxide retention may cause 'steal' from compromised vessels by areas of healthy vasculature. Normocapnia is also of importance in the postoperative period and adequate analgesia provided to avoid crying and hyperventilation.

Normothermia, normovolaemia and normotension are also essential during recovery. Careful perioperative control of these parameters helps avoid hyperperfusion injury. Hyperperfusion of previously hypoperfused regions of the brain where autoregulation is no longer functioning can be detrimental, resulting in nausea, vomiting, seizures, haemorrhage and permanent neurological deficit.

## Conclusion

Paediatric neuroanaesthesia is complex. It requires knowledge of neuroanatomy, neuropathology and pharmacology as well as an insight into what is practical for the patient. Some of the points to consider are summarised in Table 26.2. With suitable planning and preparation, the perioperative period can be managed to optimise the outcome for the patient and their family.

**Table 26.2** Considerations for paediatric neurosurgery

| Procedure | Preoperative considerations | Intraoperative considerations | Postoperative considerations |
|---|---|---|---|
| Acute head injury | Time critical<br>Secondary damage<br>Airway compromise<br>C-spine stabilisation<br>Blood loss<br>Limb/organ injury | Fluid management<br>Blood loss<br>ICP | May require HDU/ICU |
| Sitting craniotomy | Oral secretions and stability of ETT | VAE<br>Cardiovascular instability<br>Pneumocephalus | HDU<br>Cord infarction<br>Posterior fossa syndrome |
| Craniopharyngioma | Increased BMI<br>Endocrine review<br>DDAVP | Risk of DI<br>Central monitoring/ urinary catheter | Risk of DI<br>Endocrine follow-up |
| Epilepsy surgery | Developmental delay/<br>behavioural issues<br>Coexisting disease<br>Medication effects (coagulopathy) | Idiosyncratic drug reactions<br>Altered drug metabolism<br>Intraoperative monitoring (EEG effects) | Increased risk of seizures |
| Stereotactic surgical techniques | Universal MRI precautions | Limited airway access<br>Intraprocedure transfers<br>Temperature control | May need HDU |
| Neural tube defects | Timing of procedure<br>Neonates/ex-premature infants<br>Intubation position | Prone position<br>Blood loss<br>Temperature control | May require ICU |
| Hydrocephalus | Coexisting conditions<br>Prematurity | Temperature control VAE<br>Cardiac instability with CSF drainage | May require ICU |

**Table 26.2** *(cont.)*

| Procedure | Preoperative considerations | Intraoperative considerations | Postoperative considerations |
|---|---|---|---|
| Spinal surgery | Instability of C-spine<br>FOI may be required<br>Halo/jacket in situ<br>Associated syndromes | Neurophysiological monitoring<br>Prone position<br>Arrhythmias/ hypotension<br>Blood loss | Halo/jacket in situ<br>+/– altered laryngoscopic view<br>May require ICU |
| Transphenoidal surgery | Endocrine review | Cardiovascular instability<br>Blood loss<br>+/– central monitoring | Airway management (pharyngeal blood/ nasal packs)<br>Acute haematoma |
| EC–IC bypass | Premedication<br>Associated disease process<br>Anti-platelet therapy<br>+/– preoperative fluids | Maintain normocapnia/ normotension/ normothermia | Maintain normocapnia/ normotension/ normothermia<br>Adequate analgesia |

**Key Points**

- Paediatric neuroanaesthesia sometimes requires compromise between theory and practicality.
- Knowledge of neurophysiology and the ability to manipulate it is key.
- Preoperative assessment must pay particular attention to the symptoms and signs of raised ICP.
- Extreme vigilance is required where VAE is a risk.
- Provision for appropriate postoperative care is essential.

## Further Reading


Baykan N, Isbir O, Gercek A et al. Ten years of experience with pediatric neuroendoscopic third ventriculostomy. *Journal of Neurosurgical Anesthesiology* 2005; 17(1): 33–7.

Engelhard K, Werner C. Inhalational or intravenous anaesthetics for craniotomies? Pro inhalational. *Current Opinion in Anaesthesiology* 2006; 19(5):504–8.

Harrison EA, Mackersie A, McEwan A et al. The sitting position for neurosurgery in children: a review of 16 years' experience. *British Journal of Anaesthesia* 2002; 88(1):12–7.

Szabo EZ, Luginbuehl I, Bissonnette B. Impact of anaesthetic agents on cerebrovascular physiology in children. *Paediatric Anaesthesia* 2009; 19(2):108–18.

Chapter 27

# Anaesthesia for Ophthalmic Surgery in Children

Ian James and Hannah Lewis

## Introduction

Ophthalmic surgery is undertaken across the entire paediatric age range, from the newborn with a congenital cataract to the teenager with a lens dislocation. The most common procedures are listed in Table 27.1. In contrast to adults, children undergoing eye surgery will nearly always require general anaesthesia. Many of these children are ASA class 1 and will be managed as routine day cases. In others, the eye problem may be associated with a congenital or metabolic abnormality, and anaesthesia may not be so straightforward.

**Table 27.1** Procedures that may require general anaesthesia

| | |
|---|---|
| **Examination of the eye** | - General examination<br>- Measurement of intraocular pressure<br>- Retinoblastoma follow-up |
| **Extraocular procedures** | - Steroid injection of haemangioma |
| *On the lids and orbit* | - Excision of meibomian cysts<br>- Excision of orbital dermoids/tumours<br>- Ptosis surgery<br>- Tarsorrhaphy |
| *On the nasolacrimal system* | - Syringing and probing of ducts<br>- Insertion of Crawford tubes<br>- Dacryocystorhinostomy (DCR) |
| *On the eye* | - Squint surgery<br>- Episcleral dermoid excision<br>- Enucleation/evisceration<br>- Laser surgery/cryotherapy |
| **Intraocular procedures** | - To reduce intraocular pressure<br>  - Goniotomy<br>  - Trabeculectomy<br>- Lensectomy ± artificial lens insertion<br>- Vitreoretinal surgery<br>- Corneal grafting<br>- Intravitreal injection<br>- Eye trauma |

## Preoperative Assessment

It is important to establish potential anaesthetic difficulties in those patients whose eye problem is part of a syndrome. This may be limited to developmental delay but may on occasion pose significant airway difficulty.

Most congenital cataracts are idiopathic; some are hereditary. Occasionally they occur after intrauterine infection with rubella, cytomegalovirus or toxoplasma with attendant associated anomalies. Congenital cataracts can also be associated with a chromosomal abnormality (e.g. Down syndrome), the Pierre Robin sequence and Stickler syndrome (an inherited connective tissue disorder of collagen associated with airway problems similar to Pierre Robin, with micrognathia and cleft palate). Neonatal cataracts are also a feature of Hallerman–Strieff syndrome, which, although very rare, is associated with a particularly difficult airway. Squints and glaucoma may be seen in other syndromes in which there may be major airway and intubation difficulties, such as the craniosynostoses or the mucopolysaccharidoses (see Table 27.2).

Other disorders that are associated with eye lesions requiring surgery include homocystinuria, Marfan syndrome and the phakomatoses.

Homocystinuria is a metabolic disorder in which hypoglycaemia and thromboembolic episodes occur readily. Patients may have dislocated lenses that require extraction. It is recommended that an intravenous glucose infusion is started preoperatively to ensure adequate hydration and prevent catabolism in these children. Patients may be on low-dose aspirin or other anti-thrombotic medication, which should be continued in the perioperative period to minimise the risk of thromboembolic episodes.

**Table 27.2** Syndromes with eye disorders and airway difficulties

| Syndromes associated with airway difficulty | Associated eye disorders |
|---|---|
| Mucopolysaccharidoses | Corneal clouding, glaucoma |
| Craniosynostoses<br>- Crouzon, Apert, Pfeiffer | Squints, cataracts, glaucoma, proptosis |
| Craniofacial syndromes<br>- Goldenhar, Treacher Collins, Smith Lemli Opitz, Pierre Robin | Nasolacrimal duct obstruction, lid colobomas, squints, cataract, glaucoma |
| Hallerman–Strieff | Neonatal cataracts |
| Stickler | Cataracts, glaucoma, retinal detachment |

Dislocated lenses also occur in patients with Marfan syndrome, a disorder caused by a deficiency of the structural protein fibrillin. Cardiac abnormalities such as mitral regurgitation, mitral valve prolapse and aortic root dilatation are common in these children, although most have no cardiovascular symptoms; many will be on β-blockers. Hypertension should be avoided. There is a small risk of spontaneous pneumothorax in these patients, and particular care must be taken with patient positioning due to their hypermobile joints.

The congenital phakomatoses are neuro-oculo-cutaneous disorders and may have ocular lesions that require surgery. This group includes Sturge–Weber syndrome, neurofibromatosis and tuberous sclerosis, disorders that are associated with seizures and cardiac lesions, and in von Hippel–Lindau disease with phaeochromocytoma. These patients will require careful preoperative assessment and management.

## General Principles of Anaesthesia

Most children undergoing eye surgery are otherwise healthy day-case patients. Some will have very poor vision, and particular care is necessary in approaching and handling children who may not be able to see or be fully aware of what is happening. Many children, particularly those with glaucoma, cataracts or retinoblastoma, may need to undergo multiple procedures over several years. They too will need sympathetic handling as they can develop periprocedural anxiety.

Premedication and induction are a matter of personal and patient preference. Spontaneous ventilation via a face mask will suffice for simple eye examinations, although it is more convenient to use a supraglottic airway device (SAD) to allow the ophthalmologist unrestricted access to the eyes. Spontaneous ventilation with a SAD is also satisfactory for most extraocular cases and non-surgical procedures such as laser treatment. Although most orbital dermoids are superficial and simple to excise, some can be very deep and may require extensive surgery behind the globe. It is important to discuss the exact nature of these with the surgeon, as the anticipated length of surgery and the potential for bleeding may influence airway management.

The surgeon will usually require a 'quiet' eye for intraocular procedures, which is best achieved using paralysis and controlled ventilation. Because of the inaccessibility of the airway when the face is covered with sterile drapes, a secure airway is essential. The lower incidence of coughing at the end of a procedure associated with a SAD offers some advantage over a tracheal tube. It should be borne in mind, however, that the surgeon's and their assistants' hands are perilously close to the airway, particularly in small infants, and can dislodge a poorly secured SAD. If there is any doubt about the security or position of a SAD, a tracheal tube should be used. A pre-formed oral RAE tracheal tube is generally used, but the fixed length of the endotracheal portion of these tubes is often too long in infants and can result in endobronchial intubation. It is possible to insert some form of padding under the curve of the tube at the lips to prevent this. This can be bulky, and it is our practice to use a reinforced, flexible tracheal tube in infants under six months to ensure proper tube position.

A dilated pupil is necessary for many ophthalmic procedures. The mydriatic agents most used perioperatively are the parasympatholytic drug cyclopentolate 0.5% or 1%, or the sympathomimetic drug phenylephrine 2.5%. These are normally administered preoperatively, but occasionally adequate pupillary dilatation is not achieved. Further drops can be applied once the child is asleep. Rarely, the surgeon will inject subconjunctival mydricaine, a mixture of adrenaline, atropine and procaine, to improve pupillary dilatation. It is prudent to avoid a high concentration of volatile agent in this scenario and to avoid hypercapnia to minimise the risk of dysrhythmias should there be systemic absorption of the mydricaine. On occasion, the surgeon may apply phenylephrine to the eye during surgery; systemic absorption via the lacrimal duct can lead to alarming hypertension and tachycardia, although this usually settles very rapidly.

Most surgical procedural pain involving the eye and orbit is well managed with intravenous paracetamol, topical anaesthetic agents and postoperative analgesia with oral paracetamol and a non-steroidal analgesic such as ibuprofen. Strabismus surgery, evisceration of the eye, cryotherapy and vitreoretinal surgery are associated with more severe perioperative pain, and an opiate such as fentanyl 1–2 mcg $kg^{-1}$ should be administered intraoperatively.

A regional block, often used in adult practice, may reduce opioid requirement as well as lower the incidence both of postoperative nausea and vomiting (PONV) and the oculocardiac reflex (OCR). A sub-Tenon block is regarded as the safest option in paediatrics because of the low risk of the severe complications of globe perforation and retrobulbar haemorrhage associated with intraconal (retrobulbar) and extraconal (peribulbar) blocks. An injection of less than 5 ml of local anaesthetic should be sufficient and avoids significant increases in intraocular pressure (IOP). Lidocaine 1% or 2% or bupivacaine 0.25% or 0.5% are suitable options. As the injection of local anaesthetic can increase IOP, blocks are generally avoided in conditions where increased IOP is already a concern. A scleral buckle (for retinal detachment) can make insertion of the block difficult and spread unreliable as a consequence of scar tissue. In children with retinoblastoma, a block is not recommended due to the risk of extraocular tumour seeding.

The successful and safe use in children of intraconal and extraconal blocks have been described for vitreoretinal surgery and laser treatment for retinopathy of prematurity (ROP) but are not widely used.

Many ophthalmic procedures in young children are quite short and there can be problems with emergence delirium, particularly if sevoflurane has been used. The intraoperative administration of a small dose of fentanyl, dexmedetomidine or clonidine may help to ameliorate this.

## The Oculocardiac Reflex

The OCR is a well-recognised occurrence during squint surgery, featuring in approximately 60% of cases. It is also encountered during enucleation, vitreoretinal surgery and orbital surgery. The OCR is evoked by pressure on the globe or by traction on the extrinsic eye muscles. It is generally believed that the OCR occurs most commonly when the medial rectus muscle is manipulated, but traction on any of the extraocular muscles can evoke it. The reflex is mediated through trigeminal afferent and vagal efferent pathways leading to bradycardia, which may be profound. The bradycardia reverts almost immediately once the stimulus is removed, and it is unusual to see a more serious rhythm disturbance, but rarely sinus arrest or major dysrhythmias may occur. Children with a positive OCR appear to be more likely to develop PONV than those with no obvious reflex, leading to suggestions that preventing the OCR may reduce the incidence of PONV (see Table 27.3). Blocking the afferent limb of the reflex using a sub-Tenon block at the start of surgery may be one way of achieving this. Administering atropine 10 mcg $kg^{-1}$ at induction and accepting the resultant modest tachycardia is another effective strategy. The administration of atropine is especially helpful if propofol, which has a bradycardic effect, is used for induction or maintenance of anaesthesia.

**Table 27.3** Oculocardiac reflex

| |
|---|
| - Common during squint surgery, particularly with traction on medial rectus muscle |
| - Also occurs in enucleation, vitreoretinal surgery, pressure on globe and surgery on maxilla |
| - Results in bradycardia, rarely sinus arrest |
| - Reverts when muscle traction released |
| - Associated with increased PONV |
| - Best prevented with IV atropine at induction |

# Specific Procedures

## Eye Examination under Anaesthesia (EUA)

General anaesthesia for EUA is necessary in very young children and some older children who are too uncooperative to allow an adequate examination when awake. This can be carried out satisfactorily using a face mask, although a SAD is preferable when the examination is likely to be lengthy, or where it is necessary to use the operating microscope. As many of these children require regular examinations and repeated anaesthetics, it is essential that induction is managed in as sympathetic a manner as possible.

## Measurement of Intraocular Pressure

Special consideration is required if IOP is to be measured, as most anaesthetic agents reduce IOP. It is a concern that IOP will be lowered to such an extent by injudicious anaesthesia that a high IOP may be masked, potentially compromising treatment and vision. Some anaesthetists therefore use ketamine, which does not reduce IOP. When it is not possible to obtain venous access, a dose of 5–10 mg $kg^{-1}$ ketamine intramuscularly will result in a child who is still enough to permit a thorough eye examination within a few minutes. It is essential to ensure that the airway is well maintained. Ketamine may lead to a slight increase in IOP, although there are conflicting reports about this, but it is probably safer to have a falsely high IOP than a falsely low one that might result in IOP treatment being delayed (see Table 27.4).

Most paediatric anaesthetists are reluctant to use intramuscular ketamine, and an alternative technique is to undertake an inhalation induction using sevoflurane. The ophthalmologist should be close by during induction and ready to measure the IOP as soon as the child stops moving and whilst the eyes are still central (i.e. before the 'excitation' phase of general anaesthesia). It is important to try to limit the sevoflurane concentration to minimise the fall in IOP. Care must be taken to ensure that the face mask does not encroach upon the eye as this may elevate IOP.

**Table 27.4** Intraocular pressure (IOP)

- Normal IOP is between 10 and 22 mm Hg.
- IOP depends on the balance between the production of aqueous humour (mainly from the ciliary body in the posterior chamber) and its drainage via a trabecular meshwork to the canal of Schlemm in the anterior chamber.
- Venous drainage from the eye is valveless. Any increase in venous pressure (for example, from coughing or straining) leads to an immediate rise in IOP by altering the volume of the choroid and by impeding aqueous drainage via the canal of Schlemm.
- Arterial pressure has little effect on IOP

Both techniques are acceptable. As these children are likely to have repeated measurements over many months or years to assess efficacy of treatment, the more important issue is to ensure that the same technique is used when comparing IOP measurements over time. IOP measurements should be taken before laryngoscopy or SAD insertion, even though the latter does not appear to raise IOP significantly.

## Nasolacrimal Duct Obstruction

Children with blocked nasolacrimal ducts, usually caused by membranous obstruction, often present within the first year of life. Initial treatment involves probing of the punctum of the duct in the eyelid with a small blunt needle and irrigation with 1–2 ml of saline, sometimes with a dye such as fluoroscein in it. This is a short procedure and can be safely managed with a SAD. It is helpful to place a fine suction catheter in the nasal cavity to aspirate the irrigation fluid. Where a simple probing has failed, a Crawford tube or other fine silicone catheter may be passed through the duct into the nose and secured in place for a few weeks. This may be preceded by a dacryocystogram (DCG) in which about 1 ml of radio-opaque dye is injected into the duct and the course of the duct confirmed radiographically. Rarely, the surgeon will manipulate or 'fracture' the inferior turbinate to relieve any obstruction at the lower end of the duct. A very small amount of saline or blood may appear in the nose or nasopharynx, which should be suctioned before removal of the SAD.

When the duct is completely blocked, usually by bony obstruction, a dacryocystorhinostomy (DCR) may be undertaken. This involves surgical exposure of the lacrimal sac below the medial canthus and the creation of a new opening from it through the bony upper lateral aspect of the nose into the nasal cavity. This can result in modest amounts of blood trickling into the nasopharynx, so airway protection with a tracheal tube is recommended. A mild head-up tilt and a modest degree of hypotension are helpful in minimising bleeding. Application of a topical vasoconstrictor to the nasal mucosa, such as xylometazoline or lidocaine with phenylephrine, may be beneficial. DCR can be painful, and opioid analgesia (e.g. fentanyl) is indicated.

Minimally invasive DCR utilising an endoscopic laser is now performed in some centres; a similar anaesthetic technique will be necessary.

Throat packs have previously been recommended in DCR to reduce respiratory complications from aspirated blood and to prevent PONV due to blood entering the stomach. A recent evidence-based consensus statement recommends against the routine insertion of throat packs in adults by anaesthetists because of the well-recognised complications and the lack of evidence of benefit. Studies in paediatrics have also demonstrated no difference in complications when throat packs are not used in ENT and maxillofacial surgery. The rationale for routine throat pack insertion should be questioned, and they should only be inserted for carefully selected cases.

The pharynx should be suctioned under direct vision to remove any clot or debris prior to extubation.

### Squint Surgery

Squint correction is the most common ophthalmic surgical procedure in children. It is usually performed on a day-case basis, but there is a high associated incidence of PONV which occasionally results in unplanned overnight admission. Squint surgery is also associated with the OCR (see the section 'The Oculocardiac Reflex'). There is reportedly an increased incidence of malignant hyperpyrexia in patients with a squint. Although this is rare, a high index of suspicion should be maintained for this; succinylcholine should be avoided, and temperature monitoring should be used.

A spontaneous ventilation technique with a SAD is commonly employed during squint surgery. Hypercarbia has been shown to double the incidence of significant bradycardia, and some surgeons prefer a completely immobile eye, so controlled ventilation may be more suitable. Atracurium is associated with a greater incidence of OCR than pancuronium, but the shorter duration of action of atracurium makes this a more appropriate choice. Rocuronium appears to attenuate the OCR and is a suitable alternative.

Squint surgery is one of the most painful ophthalmic procedures, but the use of intraoperative opioids risks an increased incidence of PONV. The use of morphine in preference to the shorter-acting opioids fentanyl and alfentanil has been demonstrated to reduce moderate to severe post-operative pain in squint surgery. This does not result in increased PONV if appropriate antiemetic prophylaxis is administered.

Use of a sub-Tenon block also reduces post-operative pain. Tenon's capsule is the fascial layer that extends from the limbus, fusing posteriorly to the optic nerve, separating the globe from orbital fat. Sensation of the eye is provided by ciliary nerves that cross the episcleral space after emerging from the globe. Strabismus surgery on the extraocular muscles is carried out within this space, so instilling local anaesthetic here can be very effective. This can be done at the start or end of the procedure, but the advantage of administering it at the start is less stimulation of the OCR and PONV, by blocking the afferent limb of the reflex.

Diclofenac 0.1% or oxybuprocaine 0.4% eye drops also provide useful analgesia following squint surgery. If these are administered selectively to the operative site by the surgeon prior to suturing the conjunctiva, the problems associated with an insensate cornea can be minimised.

Adequate postoperative analgesia can usually be achieved satisfactorily using topical anaesthesia, paracetamol and a non-steroidal analgesic such as diclofenac or ibuprofen. Where analgesia is inadequate, as it may be for the more painful myopexy repair or repeat surgery, ketorolac has been shown to be effective. On occasion, it may be necessary to administer stronger analgesia such as an opioid.

In some older, cooperative children, the surgeon may place an adjustable suture as part of the technique. Fine adjustments to the repair can be made, using topical anaesthesia, when the patient is awake. In some patients with strabismus, a minute quantity of botulinum toxin, a neuromuscular blocking agent, is injected directly into one or more extraocular muscles. This is often done using electromyography (EMG) control, so use of intravenous neuromuscular blocking drugs should be avoided.

### Vomiting Following Strabismus Surgery

Nausea alone is difficult to quantify in children, who generally have a higher incidence of post-operative vomiting than adults. PONV is a well-recognised complication following strabismus surgery, particularly in children over the age of two years, with studies showing that more than half of

**Table 27.5** Squint surgery

| |
|---|
| - Commonest paediatric ophthalmological surgical procedure |
| - Watch out for oculocardiac reflex |
| - High incidence of PONV – give antiemetics |
| - More painful than generally recognised |
| - Sub-Tenon block is very helpful, especially if performed at start of surgery |
| - Malignant hyperthermia (MH) risk – but very rare |

children undergoing strabismus surgery will be sick if no preventative measures are taken. Vomiting may not start until several hours after surgery, and parents should be warned about this at the preoperative assessment (see Table 27.5).

The precise mechanism for the increased incidence of vomiting following squint surgery remains unknown but may well be part of an oculo-emetic reflex, involving the ophthalmic division of the trigeminal nerve and the vomiting centre in the medulla. Local anatomic factors probably play a part, as different surgical techniques affect the incidence of vomiting. In particular, the Faden myopexy technique of squint repair has a significantly higher incidence of PONV than the simpler muscle recession/resection technique.

Many different strategies have been suggested to reduce the incidence of vomiting following squint surgery, with varying success. These include the use of anticholinergic agents (e.g. dimenhydrinate), dexamethasone, clonidine, antiemetics (e.g. metoclopromide, droperidol or ondansetron) and utilising the putative antiemetic properties of propofol either for induction or as part of a total intravenous anaesthesia (TIVA) technique. These publications have been comprehensively reviewed (see 'Further Reading').

Unfortunately, it is not possible to compare the studies relating to strabismus surgery and PONV satisfactorily because they involve very different underlying anaesthetic techniques and have often not taken into account different surgical techniques. It is clear, however, that 5-$HT_3$ (serotonin) antagonists have led to a significant reduction in the incidence of PONV and should be administered intraoperatively. Ondansetron alone is very effective, although combination therapy is better, for example using ondansetron 0.1 mg $kg^{-1}$ with dexamethasone 0.15 mg $kg^{-1}$. Dexamethasone is particularly useful in preventing late PONV (>6 hours). It is possible to reduce the incidence of vomiting to less than 10% using a multimodal approach. The 2016 updated APAGBI guidance recommends dual antiemetic prophylaxis intraoperatively with a different agent utilised in recovery if required. Droperidol 25 mcg $kg^{-1}$ and dimenhydrinate 0.5 mg $kg^{-1}$ are the only other two agents, aside from ondansetron and dexamethasone, shown to be effective and licensed in children. Cyclizine and metoclopramide are no longer recommended. A recent systematic review and meta-analysis found oral clonidine premedication at a dose of 4 mcg $kg^{-1}$ to be effective in reducing PONV after strabismus surgery. A secondary outcome was reduced postoperative pain.

### Enucleation/Evisceration

Removal of the whole eye, enucleation, may be necessary because of retinoblastoma or when there is an unsightly blind eye. The surgical technique involves dissection of each of the extraocular muscles off the globe, so the oculocardiac reflex may readily be evoked. Anaesthetic management should be as for strabismus surgery.

In evisceration, the contents of the globe are removed rather than the whole eye, leaving the sclera behind. There are no specific anaesthetic problems, but the procedure can be very painful and appropriate analgesia, including an intraoperative opioid, should be administered.

### Intraocular Surgery

Intraocular surgery in children may be for the management of glaucoma or for cataract extraction with or without an intraocular lens implant. Lens implants are being inserted now even in infants. Congenital cataracts will frequently need surgical removal in the first weeks of life to prevent permanent loss of vision. Neonates are at risk of postoperative apnoea, and arrangements should be made for appropriate postoperative monitoring. Paediatric glaucoma is usually a result of an intrinsic disorder of aqueous outflow. Medical therapy is of limited value, and surgery is usually required to improve aqueous humour drainage to lower IOP.

The principal surgical drainage procedures to treat glaucoma include goniotomy, trabeculotomy and trabeculectomy. An alternative technique is cyclodestruction of the ciliary body using laser cyclophotocoagulation or cryotherapy to reduce aqueous humour production. These procedures can be painful and require good analgesia. Protective eye goggles need to be worn by all theatre staff during laser surgery. It is important to be aware that there are several different types of lasers, each requiring different goggles.

It is essential that the eye is motionless during intraocular procedures. Sudden rises in IOP should be avoided to prevent the extrusion of intraocular contents through the incision. Neuromuscular paralysis and controlled ventilation provide optimal operating conditions. Most intraocular surgery is not particularly painful, although a small dose of fentanyl is usually administered. Alternatively, a remifentanil infusion can be used which may obviate the need for paralysis. The combination of paracetamol and diclofenac is usually satisfactory for postoperative pain relief.

It is good practice to try to prevent an increase in IOP at the end of the procedure, caused for example by coughing on the tracheal tube at extubation. This is less critical than it used to be with the advent of very fine suture material allowing complete closure of the ocular wounds. A SAD can be used for intraocular surgery, even in small children, and has the advantage of smoother emergence with less coughing and reduced likelihood of acute IOP elevation than with a conventional tracheal tube. If a SAD is used, it is imperative to ensure that it is perfectly positioned and well secured before proceeding with surgery. If there is any doubt, a tracheal tube should be used.

Anaesthesia can be maintained until neuromuscular blockade has been reversed, the patient is breathing spontaneously and extubation has been performed. A small dose of propofol (0.5 mg $kg^{-1}$) given immediately prior to extubation may be useful in obtaining a smooth extubation. Topical anaesthesia to the airway can be helpful in older children, though this should be avoided in infants, as the simplest way to avoid the elevated IOP associated with crying in the immediate postoperative period is to offer them an early feed.

### Corneal Grafting (Keratoplasty)

Corneal opacities may be congenital or because of scarring from infection, burns or trauma in older children. Penetrating keratoplasty involves replacing all five layers of the cornea with donor cornea (full thickness graft). A more recent technique is a selective anterior lamellar keratoplasty which leaves healthy layers in situ. This may be preferable as it retains the host endothelium and reduces the risk of rejection. Anaesthesia for corneal grafting is like that outlined in the section 'Intraocular Surgery', but it is a longer procedure. It is particularly important to maintain a motionless eye and prevent sudden rises in IOP as a large defect is created over the cornea. There is a high risk of extrusion of intraocular contents. The surgeon may suture a ring around the cornea to support the eye during the procedure. Neuromuscular blockade and controlled ventilation should be used.

Acetazolamide, which reduces aqueous production, or mannitol may be administered intravenously during these procedures to lower the IOP, and it may be beneficial to induce modest hypotension. Acetazolamide can increase the incidence of PONV. The airway is often inaccessible to the anaesthetist and can be secured with either a SAD or tracheal tube (TT). Advantages of a SAD are a smoother emergence with less postoperative coughing causing increased IOP. A TT provides a definitive airway and is more suitable for the longer procedures or if there is any doubt about the SAD position. It is a painful procedure, and intraoperative opioids are warranted. Regional anaesthesia in the form of a sub-Tenon block offers good analgesia and akinesis and reduces PONV and the consequent increase in IOP. Isoflurane appears, in our experience, to produce a quieter eye than sevoflurane.

### Vitreoretinal Surgery

Retinal detachment is a tear in the retina, allowing the leak of aqueous humour which lifts the retina away from the underlying epithelium. It occurs most often secondary to trauma and is sight threatening. Certain predisposing ocular and systemic diseases increase the risk of detachment in children, for example retinoblastoma, ROP or Coats disease. Repair of retinal detachment generally takes place in specialised centres. Cryotherapy or laser therapy can be used to repair smaller retinal tears and to ablate the abnormal vessels in Coats disease. Vitrectomy may be needed in larger tears with the placement of a scleral buckle towards the back of the eye to obtain apposition of the retinal pigment epithelium and the neuroretina. An intraocular gas bubble containing sulphur hexafluoride ($SF_6$) or perfluoropropane ($C_3F_8$) may be injected into the eye to tamponade the detached surfaces together whilst adhesions develop. Nitrous oxide must not be administered when these gases are used, as it will rapidly diffuse into the gas bubble and increase its size. The intraocular gases may remain in the eye for several weeks, and diffusion of nitrous oxide from a subsequent anaesthetic during this period into an existing intraocular gas bubble can result in rapid expansion of the bubble and an acute rise in pressure within the globe. This can cause irreversible ischaemic damage to the retina and optic nerve, so patients and their carers must be given very clear instructions about passing this information on to other anaesthetists should they require further surgery during this time.

Opioid analgesia should be administered perioperatively, as vitreoretinal surgery is painful. A sub-Tenon block has been shown to be effective in providing analgesia for children having vitreoretinal surgery and reduces the incidence of OCR.

## Emergency Eye Surgery

Injuries to the eye are common in paediatrics. They often occur in isolation, but in the context of polytrauma, management of life-threatening injuries takes priority. Orbital floor fractures can trap the extraocular muscles, restricting eye movement and triggering the OCR. This often necessitates timely surgical repair. Trauma that breaches the full thickness of the sclera, cornea or both is known as an 'open' globe injury. Urgent surgery is required to close the wound to reduce the risk of infection and extrusion of ocular contents and to prevent visual loss. This is a true ophthalmic emergency and should be performed within 12–24 hours of injury. Time to ensure fasting status may not be possible. This has been a contentious issue for anaesthesia. The possibility of a full stomach would conventionally dictate a rapid induction-intubation sequence using succinylcholine, but it has been traditionally taught that any acute rise in IOP, such as that caused by succinylcholine, may cause extrusion of ocular contents through even very small wounds, leading to total loss of vision in that eye.

There are in fact no well-documented reports describing vitreous extrusion following the use of succinylcholine, and in those difficult situations where the eye is at risk and regurgitation is a concern, there is no good reason to avoid succinylcholine as part of a conventional rapid sequence induction (RSI). However, rocuronium 1–1.2 mg $kg^{-1}$ is a good alternative and has largely superseded succinylcholine for RSI in the trauma population. The effects can be readily reversed with sugammadex 8–16 mg $kg^{-1}$ if necessary. This avoids the concern, albeit probably theoretical, of increased IOP with succinylcholine use. In small children who are at risk of aspiration, most experts advocate a modified RSI in which atracurium or rocuronium are used, and gentle ventilation is continued to avoid hypoxaemia until laryngoscopy. Premature attempts at intubation should be avoided, as this may provoke coughing, which significantly raises IOP. A nerve stimulator may be helpful in indicating when full neuromuscular blockade has occurred.

Occasionally children will allow removal of a foreign body when awake under local anaesthesia. Proxymetacaine is frequently used, as it causes less stinging and therefore improves compliance.

## Retinopathy of Prematurity (ROP)

Severe ROP still occurs despite meticulous neonatal care and can lead to total blindness. The improved survival of extremely and very preterm babies has resulted in a significant increase in the incidence of ROP. Infants at risk are those less than 31 weeks gestational age and/or less than 1,500 g (see Table 27.6). ROP is characterised by abnormal blood vessel growth in the retina and is classified in five stages, ranging from mild (stage 1) to severe (stage 5). Infants who develop severe ROP (stage 3 or more) are at significant risk of retinal detachment and blindness. The outcome of the disease process can be improved by cryotherapy or, more commonly now, argon laser photocoagulation, which ablates the peripheral retinal vessel proliferation. Treatment needs to be undertaken early in the disease, and so early identification is essential. Eye examinations in at-risk infants should take place between six- and seven-weeks postnatal age and continued every two weeks until the risk has passed.

These premature infants are transferred to theatre for their treatment, and the usual precautions for managing preterm infants should be adopted (see Chapter 19), particularly in relation to temperature and glycaemic control. Many of these infants will have other systemic disorders due to their extreme prematurity, such as bronchopulmonary dysplasia, which may influence both the conduct of anaesthesia and the need

**Table 27.6** Babies at risk for severe ROP

| |
|---|
| - Birth weight ≤1,500 g |
| and/or |
| - Gestational age ≤31 weeks |

for postoperative support, and they will need careful assessment. Laser therapy is better tolerated than cryotherapy, although both often warrant opioid analgesia. This has implications for the postoperative care of these babies, who will be at increased risk of apnoeic episodes following anaesthesia. Appropriate facilities for postoperative monitoring and ventilation must be arranged, and many return to NICU intubated.

Avoiding the risk of transfer to theatre and general anaesthesia is clearly beneficial. In some centres, carefully selected cases can undergo examination and laser treatment on the NICU using sedation combined with a regional technique. Chloral hydrate has been used successfully with a sub-Tenon block for this purpose. Both laser and cryotherapy can be painful and can cause cardiorespiratory instability.

A novel therapy for ROP is intravitreal injection of anti-vascular endothelial growth factor (VEGF) antibodies that work to block the angiogenic factors that stimulate pathological vessel proliferation. Early studies indicate it is well tolerated, and treatment could take place at the bedside on intensive care. Longer-term studies are required to look at safety outcomes.

Retinal detachment is a complication of severe ROP. Endoscopic vitrectomy is a new surgical method that can save some sight. Outcomes are better if performed early. There is a short window of opportunity to undertake this surgery, and cases may present as an emergency. As this is a painful procedure and often long, the majority of cases will return to NICU ventilated.

### Retinoblastoma

This is the most common intraocular malignancy in childhood with an average age of onset under two years old. It can occur sporadically or be inherited. Treatment and screening occur in specialist centres. Children who have a parent with the disease will undergo screening in the form of a regular EUA. In children with the disease, EUA can be as frequent as every one to two months until the child is three years old. Anxiety is common, and premedication may be necessary. There are different treatment modalities depending on the stage of the disease, which is determined by the size and location of the tumour and the chance that treatment will preserve some sight. Local therapies available for small tumours are cryotherapy, laser photocoagulation and plaque irradiation (local radiotherapy). Larger or bilateral tumours require chemotherapy. This can be delivered systemically or using more targeted methods of intravitreal or selective intra-arterial chemotherapy. Enucleation is performed for advanced unilateral disease where it is not possible to save the eye.

Intra-arterial chemotherapy, in which melphalan is injected directly into the ophthalmic artery, has specific anaesthetic considerations. This procedure takes place in an interventional radiology suite in only a few specialist centres in the United Kingdom and is described in detail in Chapter 36.

**Key Points**

- Bradycardia is readily produced by traction on extraocular muscles or pressure on the globe – the oculocardiac reflex.
- Squint surgery is associated with a high incidence of postoperative vomiting.
- A SAD can be used in most ophthalmic procedures but must be safely secured.
- A sub-Tenon block, most easily administered by the surgeon, is useful in many procedures.
- Nitrous oxide should be avoided in vitreoretinal surgery.

## Further Reading

Ali U, Tsang M, Campbell F et al. Reducing postoperative pain in children undergoing strabismus surgery: from bundle implementation to clinical decision support tools. *Pediatric Anesthesia* 2020; 30:415–23.

Farkouh A, Frigo P, Czejka M. Systemic side effects of eye drops: a pharmacokinetic perspective. *Clinical Ophthalmology* 2016; 10:2433–41.

Jean Y-K, Kam D, Gayer S, Palte H, Stein A. Regional anesthesia for pediatric ophthalmic surgery: a review of the literature. *Anesthesia Analgesia* 2020; 130:1351–63.

Lewis H, James I. Update on anaesthesia for paediatric ophthalmic surgery. *BJA Education* 2021; 21(1):32–8.

Vachon CA, Warner DO, Bacon DR. Succinylcholine and the open globe: tracing the teaching. *Anesthesiology* 2003; 99(1): 220–3.

Chapter

# 28 Anaesthesia for Plastic Surgery in Children

Michael Frost

## Introduction

Plastic surgeons treat a range of congenital and acquired conditions in children from birth to adolescence, and paediatric work makes a significant contribution to the plastic surgery caseload. Procedures are classified as 'reconstruction' or 'cosmetic', but this distinction is often blurred in children, as many abnormalities are both unsightly and impair physical function.

Common procedures such as correction of anomalies of the ears, hands and feet will be described in this chapter. Repair of cleft lip and palate is covered in Chapter 23. Urological surgeons undertake hypospadias repair in some centres, and this topic is covered in Chapter 34.

Several skin conditions are amenable to treatment with targeted laser surgery. Modern lasers have allowed many lesions to be treated in childhood, with less scarring, better cosmetic outcomes and reduced need for treatment in later life. Anaesthetists need to understand the principles of lasers, the attendant risks and the precautions required for safe use.

## Preoperative Assessment

Most children undergoing plastic surgical procedures are ASA 1 or ASA 2 and require minimal investigation prior to surgery. Most children can be managed on a day-case basis. A routine plastic surgery list may include infants and adolescents, and key anaesthetic requirements are adaptability and close attention to detail. A friendly and supportive environment is vital, as many children will attend repeated visits, and bad experiences will lead to future anxiety. Time and effort spent building rapport with the parent and child will pay dividends.

## General Principles

Distraction techniques in the anaesthetic room are helpful, and premedication is rarely required. Induction technique depends on the individual anaesthetist's preference, taking the age of the patient into consideration. Success with venous access in small infants is related to skin temperature, and it helps if the child is kept both warm and hydrated. Allowing clear fluids up to an hour prior to anaesthesia is now widely accepted as safe practice, and this in turn facilitates success in cannulation. Pain on injection may be reduced by using 0.5% propofol or by adding 1 ml of 1% lidocaine per 100 mg propofol. A strong light source for transillumination or ultrasound may be used to find hidden veins after inhalational induction.

A supraglottic airway device (SAD) may be used in most plastic surgical procedures. Care should be taken to avoid displacement in infants during surgery involving the face or in cases where the head is likely to be moved, such as during a pinnaplasty procedure. A reinforced SAD may be more stable, but there should be a low threshold to using a tracheal tube in these patients. Care should be taken to protect vulnerable areas such as the eyes and in the application of tourniquets.

Surgical procedures on the limbs are usually performed using a tourniquet to provide a clear surgical field and reduce blood loss. Relative hypotension may be helpful in some procedures; blood pressure of no more than 20% below baseline appears to be safe in healthy older children. It is safer to aim for normotension in infants, as adverse cardiovascular events are more common in this age group (bradycardia, myocardial depression from deep volatile anaesthesia). A combination of remifentanil and sevoflurane allows for good control of blood pressure. Great care must be taken to flush infusion lines at the end of surgery to avoid inadvertent boluses of drugs such as remifentanil.

## Pain Management

Effective pain control is essential for plastic surgery. Apart from humanitarian concerns, inadequate analgesia during surgery leads to labile blood pressure, poor operating conditions, the increased use diathermy and consequent inflammatory pain and further risk of rebound bleeding after surgery. Wound infection is more common if there is a postoperative haematoma. It is important to have a good understanding of the surgery, as surgical stimulation can vary enormously during a plastic surgical procedure.

Multimodal analgesia is especially relevant to paediatric plastic surgery. General anaesthesia should be combined with regional anaesthesia, local block or field infiltration where possible. It is helpful to inject local anaesthetic prior to incision, as this reduces hypnotic and analgesic requirements and improves recovery. If the surgeon is planning a complex procedure, local infiltration may have to be delayed until the end of the procedure to prevent interference with mapping of incisions or finding the right 'plane' in the surgical field. It is also important to anticipate analgesic requirements when the block wears off.

Remifentanil is ideal intraoperatively, as it blocks virtually all surgical stimulation, provides excellent cardiovascular stability, reduces hypnotic dosage and is simple to use in children of all ages. We commonly use a remifentanil infusion in our unit for procedures expected to take an hour or more. An initial bolus of 1 mcg $kg^{-1}$ IV is followed by an infusion, normally at 0.1–0.2 mcg $kg^{-1}$ $min^{-1}$. Morphine 50–100 mcg $kg^{-1}$ IV should be given to provide analgesia postoperatively, particularly where remifentanil is used, and is best given early in the operation. Intravenous paracetamol provides a useful contribution to analgesia. Postoperatively, a combination of ibuprofen and paracetamol should be prescribed regularly, with morphine 200 mcg $kg^{-1}$ orally (80 mcg $kg^{-1}$ in infants) every three to four hours as required.

## Congenital Limb Deformities and Hand Surgery

There is an enormous variety of congenital limb deformities, with most corrective surgery in the upper limb undertaken by plastic surgeons, particularly hand surgery. The aims of surgery are primarily to improve function and secondly to improve appearance. Manual dexterity develops at an early age, so surgery is often undertaken within the first two years, which allows for improved function. There are over 100 recognised syndromes with associated hand abnormalities, but this still only represents a small fraction of congenital hand abnormalities. A classification of upper limb abnormalities proposed by Swanson has been adopted internationally (see Table 28.1):

- Failure of formation
- Failure of differentiation
- Duplication
- Overgrowth
- Undergrowth
- Constriction band syndromes
- Generalised skeletal abnormalities

Correction of many congenital limb deformities involves some form of skin cover, either as a full thickness graft from an area such as the groin or as a split skin graft from the thigh or medial arch of the sole of the foot. This needs to be discussed with the surgeon in advance to allow appropriate preparation and to anticipate analgesia requirements both during and after skin grafting. The child may become cold during long operations if multiple sites are exposed. Standard warming measures should be used with careful monitoring of skin temperature. Be aware that modern convective warming devices can easily lead to overheating of a small child or infant, so always start on a gentle setting and reassess.

Most hand and foot surgery is carried out using a tourniquet to minimise blood loss and to provide a bloodless surgical field. Poor application will make dissection of tissue planes and identification of individual nerves very difficult, so it is vital to check that the tourniquet is the correct size, is functional and has been properly positioned with appropriate padding before draping.

Tourniquets may be used for up to two hours, but long tourniquet times are associated with increased postoperative oedema. In infants, the tourniquet becomes less effective after two hours owing to excellent collateral blood supply via bones, which cannot be occluded. Blood loss should be anticipated when the tourniquet is released if there has been extensive dissection. It is good practice to release the tourniquet briefly and reinflate to allow the surgeon to identify any major bleeding points. After the tourniquet is deflated, it is best to remove it fully to prevent venous congestion.

Regional blockade is ideal for limb surgery and has the added advantage of sympathetic block and vasodilation. This is useful for procedures

**Table 28.1** International classification of upper limb congenital abnormalities

| Type | Example | Notes |
|---|---|---|
| Type I – failure of formation | Hypoplasia of thumb | Failure of formation may be in:<br>• Transverse axis (any level from shoulder to thumb)<br>• Longitudinal axis (pre-axial (radial), central or post-axial (ulnar) |
| Type II – failure of differentiation of parts | • Soft tissue – syndactyly, camptodactyly, trigger finger<br>• Skeletal – clinodactyly<br>• Vascular/neurological | • Two or more digits fused together<br>• Complex syndactyly as part of a syndrome (e.g. Apert) |
| Type III – duplication | • Polydactyly | • Extra digits<br>• May occur as part of syndrome<br>• Pre-axial (thumb)<br>• Central (ring, middle and index)<br>• Post-axial (little finger) most common<br>• 2 in every 1,000 live births |
| Type IV – overgrowth | • Macrodactyly | Localised gigantism, |
| Type V – undergrowth | • Radial hypoplasia<br>• Brachydactyly<br>• Brachysyndactyly | e.g. radial club hand, thumb hypoplasia<br>• Shortness of fingers and toes<br>• Short and fused digits |
| Type VI –constriction band syndromes | • Amniotic band syndrome | • Entrapment of fetal parts (usually a limb or digits) in fibrous amniotic bands whilst in utero |
| Type VII – generalised anomalies | • Atypical cleft hands | |

*Source:* Swanson, AB, Swanson, GD, Tada, K. A classification for congenital limb malformation. *Journal of Hand Surgery American* 1983; 8:693–702.

involving microscopic anastomosis of vessels, such as toe-to-hand digit transfers. Axillary brachial plexus block can be performed using a single injection placed under ultrasound guidance (see Chapter 15).

## Digit Relocation and Transplantation

With a hypoplastic or missing thumb but normal fingers, the usual treatment is pollicisation of the index finger, which involves shortening and rotating the index finger on its neurovascular supply to occupy the position of the thumb. With congenitally short (brachydactyly) or absent digits, microsurgical techniques now allow reconstruction of digits by using one or more toes.

The principal aims of reconstruction are focused on improvement in function. Surgery has the greatest impact when the missing digit is a thumb or where there are several digits missing. The second toe is the most common digit transplanted, as it is relatively long, has a reliable blood supply and has the ability to grow. Removing the second toe does not appear to have a great impact on the function or appearance of the foot. The big toe is rarely used to reconstruct digits, but a partial flap called a 'wrap-around flap' may be created from the pulp and nail of the big toe, with the donor site being covered with a skin graft.

Digit transfer operations take two to three hours. Careful planning is required to make sure all equipment is available and the child is appropriately positioned for microsurgical access. A vacuum bean mattress can be very helpful to reduce the risk of pressure-related injury. Antibiotics should be given five minutes prior to inflation of the tourniquet to allow for good tissue penetration. A peripheral block at the donor site and an axillary plexus block are ideal.

## Syndactyly and Polydactyly

Syndactyly (fusion of digits) and polydactyly (accessory digits) are the two most common congenital abnormalities of the hand. Syndactyly tends to affect the ring and little finger but can affect all fingers. It may vary in severity from a single slightly displaced web to a full fusion up to the tips of the nails affecting many digits with bony abnormalities included. With increasing complexity of syndactyly, there is the additional risk of complex neurovascular arrangements, especially when associated with osseous abnormalities (see Figure 28.1).

With the increased detail provided by modern ultrasound machines, traditional peripheral nerve blocks have effectively been superseded by reliable and anatomically easy to identify blocks performed in the forearm or elbow. For the median nerve, a position midway along the forearm is best, as the nerve is easily identified centrally being away from most of the tendons but also not too deep in the muscle layers. For the radial nerve, placing the probe in the crease of the elbow on the lateral side allows easy access to the nerve. An in-plane technique using a 22G short bevel needle is ideal to judge both the depth and trajectory. The aim is simply to gently float the nerve in a few milliliters of plain local anaesthetic to ensure the needle remains clear of the nerve. The ulnar nerve is generally not so easy to locate using ultrasound but can easily be blocked by inserting 2 ml of plain local anaesthetic under the flexor carpi ulnaris muscle just proximal to the pisiform bone at the wrist.

# Ear Surgery

## Correction of Prominent Ears

This condition is associated with loss of the antehelical fold of cartilage. Surgery aims to correct this to allow the pinna to lie parallel to the head.

Pinnaplasty is usually delayed until the age of four to five years, when the ear cartilage is more rigid. This operation has traditionally been associated with a high risk of postoperative nausea and vomiting (PONV). The use of propofol infusion combined with local anaesthetic infiltration and minimal opioid helps to reduce this risk. Careful attention must be given to bandaging postoperatively to reduce the risk of haematoma, at the same time avoiding excessive pressure on the cartilage of the pinna, which may also increase PONV. A flexible SAD is often used so that the head can be turned easily during the procedure. It is important to ensure the head is not rotated more than 65° from the midline to avoid neck injury, including atlantoaxial dislocation.

## Ear Reconstruction

Approximately one in 6,000 infants are born with microtia. This can be corrected by a two-stage reconstruction using costal cartilage. A tracheal tube should be used for the first stage as it takes several hours, involves rib harvest and has the potential for pneumothorax. After the first stage, a continuous infusion of levobupivacaine using a fine catheter in the costal wound provides good postoperative analgesia for 24 hours. As with

(a)

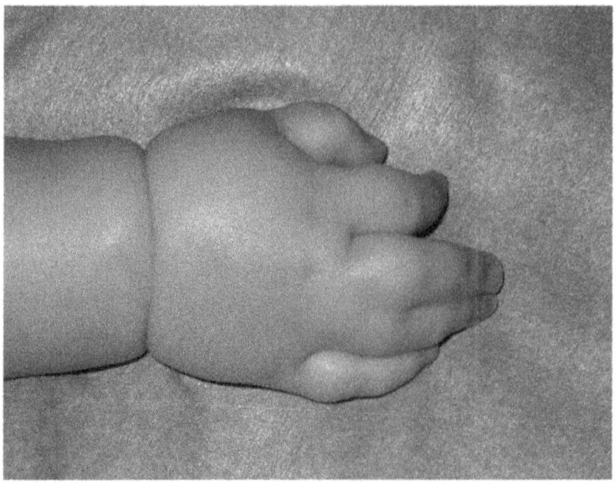

(b)

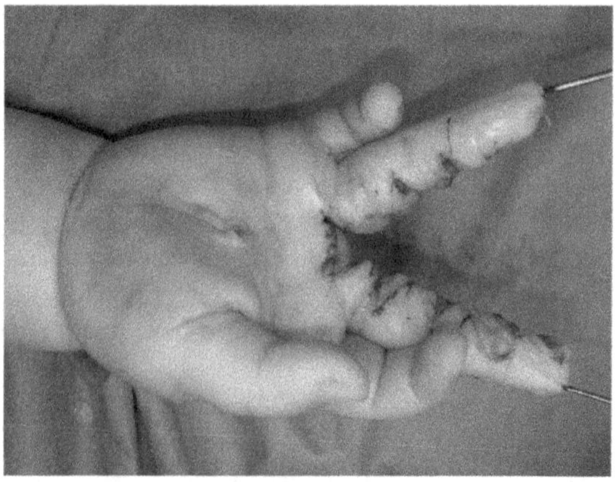

**Figure 28.1** Syndactyly release in a one-year-old infant.

pinnaplasty, attention must be paid to the bandaging of the ears to minimise the risks of graft ischaemia. Mini-vacuum-suction drains are usually inserted to avoid haematoma. The second stage is a shorter procedure but incorporates a skin graft, usually from the thigh.

## Accessory Auricles

Accessory auricles are abnormal segments of ear tissue commonly in the pre-auricular region but sometimes on the cheek and neck. They may contain cartilaginous remnants and require adequate exposure and removal. Surgery is generally performed when the infant is three to six months old.

## Dermoid Cysts

These commonly occur at the outer border of the eyebrow (external angular dermoid cyst). In this location, they are generally superficial and are removed via a small incision adjacent to the eyebrow. Dermoid cysts also occur in the midline of the nose. The problem here is that there may be a sinus with an epithelial lined track extending deeply into the nasal septum and possibly to the base of the skull. Always consider the possibility for the need for deep exploratory surgery and choose a secure airway technique.

## Tongue Tie

Tongue tie release to free up mobility of the tongue is a short procedure commonly performed in infants. A flexible SAD may be used, with a carefully positioned throat pack and local infiltration of the area.

## Poland Syndrome

Poland syndrome comprises congenital breast hypoplasia associated with unilateral absence of pectoralis major muscle and an ipsilateral hand deformity. The aim is to achieve a natural shaped breast and chest wall symmetry. Surgery using tissue expanders and implants is normally carried out in late adolescence.

## Gynaecomastia

Gynaecomastia is excessive breast formation in boys and usually occurs because of oestrogen and testosterone imbalance at puberty. Surgery is undertaken either by liposuction or direct excision via the areolar margin of the breast tissue. Surgical excision is associated with increased postoperative bleeding and haematoma. It is important that the blood pressure is normal prior to closure of the wound so that good haemostasis can be obtained, especially if local anaesthetic with adrenaline has been used. The adrenaline in the infiltration solution will wear off after two hours, which may increase the risk of bleeding and haematoma formation.

## Laser Surgery

Lasers are used to treat a range of congenital and acquired skin conditions, most of which respond well to treatment. The use of lasers presents a variety of challenges in children. Vascular and pigmented lesions such as port wine stains change in their pigmentation as the child gets older, making the lesion more resistant to laser intervention. Lesions are now treated at an earlier age so that fewer treatment sessions are required, with fewer complications as a result.

## Principles of Laser Surgery

Chromophores are pigmented targets that selectively absorb certain wavelengths of light. Laser light is intense monochromatic light, the wavelength of which is determined by the medium (gas, liquid or solid) through which the light passes. Laser irradiation can be used to selectively target chromophores (water, haemoglobin or melanin) in the skin by selecting an appropriate wavelength along with an appropriate pulse and energy setting. The net result is intense localised production of heat in the chromophore resulting in vaporisation in the target tissue. To target specific tissues precisely, it is necessary to consider the thermal relaxation time of the chromophore. This is defined as the time necessary for the target chromophore to cool to half its peak temperature after irradiation. The pulse time of the laser must be equal to or less than this to prevent damage to surrounding tissues and allow time for appropriate cooling and dissipation of energy.

Early laser technology used continuous-wave mode for treating vascular skin lesions and was associated with a high degree of scarring because of uncontrolled heating effects. This led to the development of pulsed dye lasers (PDL), with wavelengths of 585 nm or 595 nm, which have become the mainstay for treatment of vascular lesions in terms of efficacy and low risk of adverse scarring. The PDL emits a laser beam with wavelength close to one of the maximum absorption peaks of oxyhaemoglobin. Transient bruising lasting several days is common after use of PDL lasers. Recent advances include dynamic surface cooling, which increases the efficacy of the laser (e.g. Candela laser) and very short pulse duration, which improves the clinical result and helps minimise adverse effects.

## Laser Surgery and Anaesthesia

The choice of laser and laser settings needs to be adjusted to take account of the smaller vessels in children and the unpredictable nature of scarring. The laser is applied in multiple 'dots' to cover the birthmark and to produce a controlled burn. Wound aftercare is a vital part of the treatment process, and aloe vera is commonly used for cooling the skin. If the treatment results in an open wound, a topical antiseptic such as mupirocin ointment is usually applied.

Each shot of the laser feels like being flicked with an elastic band, so many children will require general anaesthesia. The aim is to keep the patient immobile, warm and well perfused so the surgeon can visualise the vessels at the site of surgery clearly. The airway can generally be managed with a SAD, and it is helpful to avoid tapes to secure the SAD if lasering around the mouth. Analgesia such as fentanyl, paracetamol and ibuprofen should be given, and cool face packs help to reduce discomfort. A stat dose of dexamethasone reduces facial swelling after treatment. Some children will be able to undergo laser treatment with just a topical anaesthetic cream applied an hour before surgery. Whichever method is undertaken, efforts should be made to ensure the experience for the child is pleasant, as four to six treatments may be required at intervals of every six months. Children should avoid sun exposure before, during and after laser treatment as it may decrease the efficacy of the procedure or contribute to postoperative pigmentation changes.

## Laser Safety

Universal safety precautions are mandatory:

- Wet swabs should be used to protect the child's eyes, and staff should wear protective goggles appropriate to the specific laser used.
- The theatre doors should be locked or alarmed and notices displayed to indicate laser treatment in progress.
- The $CO_2$ laser is particularly associated with fires, and stringent fire precautions must be taken.
- Risks include burning holes in drapes or ignition of flammable substances such as tincture of benzoin. It is sensible to reduce the inspired oxygen as low as possible when lasering in the region of the airway. A fire extinguisher must be immediately on hand and wet swabs used to cover potential ignition points.
- Scavenging systems need to be in place, and face masks should be worn when lasers are used to remove viral warts, as an aerosol of vaporised tissue is produced with the potential risk of viral DNA being inhaled.
- There is a potential for electrical injury or an accident from tripping over cables when several lasers are used in the same theatre, and extra vigilance is required.
- Forgetting to change goggles when switching lasers is another potential risk.

## Lesions amenable to treatment by laser surgery

Vascular birthmarks are relatively common in infants and can be separated into two distinct categories:

- Vascular tumours otherwise known as haemangiomas
- Vascular malformations such as port wine stains

It is important to identify the type of lesion correctly as they have quite different natural histories and treatments. Most infantile haemangiomas are uncomplicated and do not require any intervention, as they will naturally involute with time. Some haemangiomas undergo rapid proliferation and may threaten vital structures or have the potential to cause major disfigurement. Lasers can be used to target symptomatic superficial haemangiomas, with specific indications being bleeding, rapid proliferation and ulceration.

The most used laser for this is the PDL (585 nm or 595 nm) targeting oxygenated haemoglobin. For more deeply embedded haemangiomas, the 755 nm alexandrite or the 1064 nm Nd:

YAG laser may be used for higher penetration (see Figure 28.2). A course of treatments over several weeks is often necessary, and residual telangiectasias may require further treatment, again with the PDL laser. Laser therapy for such lesions will invariably involve general anaesthesia for patients in this age group.

Vascular malformations such as port wine stains are less common than infantile haemangiomas and do not undergo rapid growth followed by involution. They tend to grow with the child and become prominent during puberty. Several unusual conditions may be associated with port wine stain

- Glaucoma (port wine stain around the eye)
- Sturge–Weber syndrome (malformation affects superficial vessels of the brain, associated with developmental delay, hemiplegia and seizures)
- Klippel–Trenaunay syndrome (vascular malformation affecting arm or leg, associated with hypertrophy and venous and lymphatic malformations)
- Proteus syndrome (associated with hemihypertrophy, lymphangioma, lipoma and macrocephaly).

The underlying pathology is associated with an increased number of ectactic vessels in the papillary and reticular dermis. They can also be treated by targeting oxygenated haemoglobin in the vascular compartment with the PDL laser. This is effective in reducing the visual impact of lesions by around 80%.

The response to treatment is hugely variable and will depend on the depth of the lesion, with deeper structures being more difficult to treat. Timing of treatment is controversial, but earlier intervention during childhood is generally felt to be helpful, as the laser has more effective penetration in thinner skin and reduces the need for intervention at a later stage. When planning a course of laser treatment, it is helpful to undertake a test patch to show the parents the effect and demonstrate the postoperative bruising associated with the procedure.

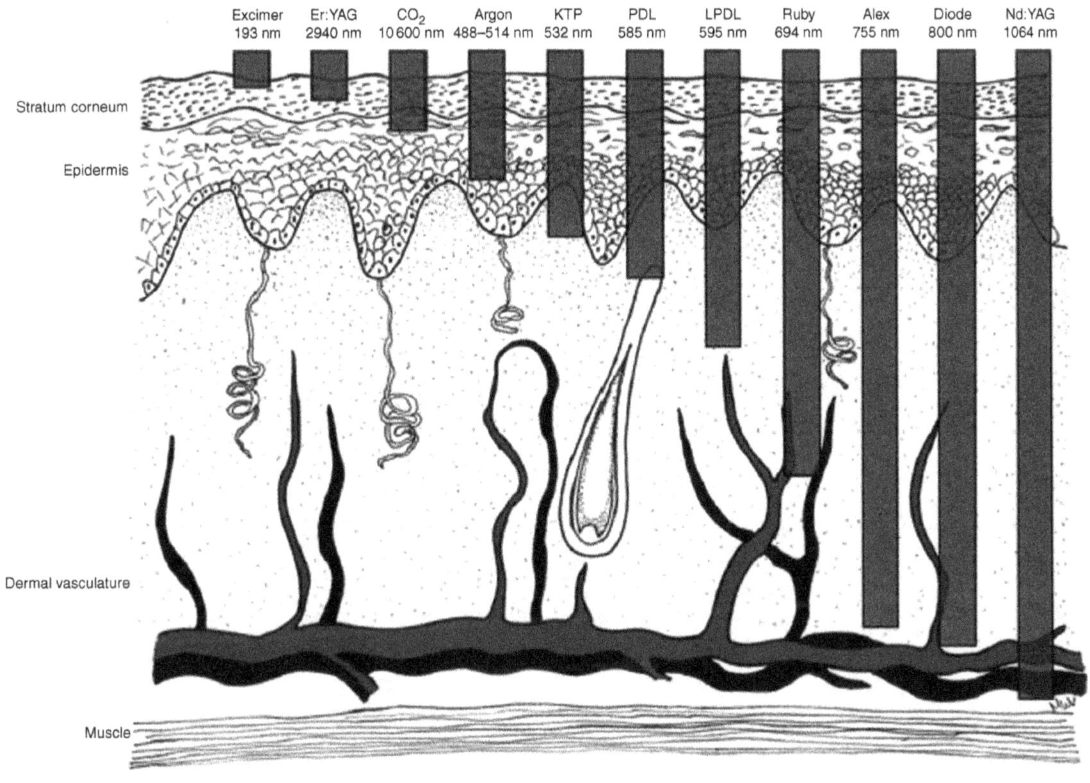


**Figure 28.2** Depth of penetration of different lasers and site of damage in the skin. Er- and Nd-YAG, erbium- and neodymium-doped yttrium aluminium garnet; KTP potassium titanyl phosphate; PDL, pulsed dye laser; LPDL, long-pulse dye laser; Alex, Alexandrite laser.
*Source:* Adapted from figure 1.13 of Dover JS, Arndt KA, Geronemus RG. *Illustrated Cutaneous and Aesthetic Laser Surgery*, 2nd ed. McGraw-Hill. 1999.

Childhood pigmented lesions are amenable to treatment with Q-switched lasers, which have a very short pulse duration but very high peak power. They produce largely non-thermal mechanical damage with shock waves, vaporisation of tissue and destruction of melanin pigment. Ruby (694 nm) and alexandrite (755 nm) laser light are well absorbed by melanin but not haemoglobin. They are effective in the treatment of epidermal lesions such as sebaceous naevus and naevus of Ota and can be used in non-pulsed mode for the removal of hair. If the density of pigment is relatively low, laser surgery is often combined with local anaesthesia infiltration, but if used for depilatory action, then application of ice is usually adequate for pain relief.

## Key Points

- Multimodal analgesia techniques are key to success in paediatric plastic surgery.
- Being skilled in simple peripheral and regional blockage is invaluable to aiding smooth recovery.
- Time invested in preparation to enable a calm cooperative child who is both warm and hydrated pays dividends.
- Use local anaesthesia field infiltration, local blocks or regional blockade where possible.
- Administer long-acting opioids early.
- Good communication between the anaesthetist and surgeon is vital.
- Safety is paramount when undertaking anaesthesia for laser surgery.

Chapter

# 29 Anaesthesia for Orthopaedic and Scoliosis Surgery in Children

Ben Clevenger and Marina George

## Introduction

Anaesthetic requirements for children undergoing orthopaedic surgery can be very varied, ranging from simple to complex. The scope of surgery includes management of acute trauma, disorders of musculoskeletal development and highly specialised operations for congenital, neuromuscular and acquired musculoskeletal conditions. Complexity can be related to the invasiveness of the procedure or an underlying associated medical condition when even minor surgery can be hazardous due to anatomical, physiological or biochemical abnormalities.

This chapter will discuss the general principles of anaesthesia for elective orthopaedic and spinal surgery, common procedures and underlying medical conditions. Anaesthesia for hand surgery is discussed in Chapter 28. Emergency surgery is most commonly associated with trauma, which is discussed in Chapter 39. Regional anaesthesia is increasingly utilised to provide perioperative analgesia, which is described in detail in Chapter 15.

## Preoperative Assessment and Preparation for Elective Surgery

Many patients presenting for orthopaedic surgery have coexisting conditions which influence the focus of examination and investigation.

Examples of coexisting conditions include:

- Cerebral palsy (gait correction, hip surgery, scoliosis surgery)
- Muscular dystrophy (scoliosis surgery)
- Osteogenesis imperfecta (fractures, scoliosis surgery)
- Arthrogryposis (joint contractures, scoliosis surgery)
- Neurofibromatosis (scoliosis surgery, pseudoarthrosis of the tibia)
- VATER/VACTERL association (scoliosis surgery, hand surgery)

Multidisciplinary review is essential preoperatively to assess, investigate and optimise and for health professionals, patients and carers to discuss risk. Orthopaedic patients often require repeat surgery and prolonged hospital admissions. Care should be individualised, and negative experiences minimised. Attention should be paid to the presence of muscle spasm and use of anti-spasmodics. Postoperative muscle spasm may be severe in an immobilised limb and should be anticipated and well managed. Patients with coexisting cardiac disease are particularly high risk, and all members of the multidisciplinary team must be involved in their preoperative assessment.

## Cardiorespiratory Disease

Children with syndromes associated with cardiac disease require detailed review including electrocardiogram (ECG), echocardiogram and cardiology assessment. Diseases of the skeleton leading to thoracic cage deformities, scoliosis and restrictive lung disease can progress to pulmonary hypertension and cor pulmonale, and these children also require specialised review. The risks and benefits of surgery in such patients should be explored carefully using a multidisciplinary approach, with postoperative ventilation and critical care planned if required. Discussions regarding significant risks such as long-term ventilation, the need for tracheostomy and potential mortality must take place during the assessment process, prior to planned surgery.

## Obstructive Sleep Apnoea

Obstructive sleep apnoea (OSA) is common in children with hypotonic neuromuscular diseases, obesity and associated craniofacial abnormalities. Sleep studies should be considered in patients with symptoms of OSA to evaluate the need for respiratory support and plan the level of postoperative care. These patients are likely to have increased sensitivity to sedative premedication and opioid analgesia.

## Airway Assessment

Assessment of the airway must take into account the potential for difficult mask ventilation and/or difficult tracheal intubation and/or cervical instability. For example, conditions such as achondroplasia and osteogenesis imperfecta may lead to craniocervical instability, placing the spinal cord at risk during tracheal intubation.

## Preoperative Blood Tests

Preoperative blood tests will be guided by the history, examination and planned surgery. Blood transfusion is rarely required for peripheral orthopaedic surgery, as tourniquets are used routinely and many of these children will not require any preoperative blood tests.

Major pelvic and femoral operations, including pelvic osteotomy and total hip replacement, require full blood count, urea and electrolytes and blood group and antibody screen as a minimum. Coagulation testing should be undertaken for major tumour surgery such as hemipelvectomy, sacrectomy and femoral replacement as well as for spinal surgery. Abnormalities of the coagulation screen should lead to individual clotting factor assays.

Iron deficiency is common. Treatment of pre-existing anaemia will reduce the risk of transfusion. Correction of nutritional deficiencies is straightforward, but occasionally erythropoietin is indicated in chronic disease. Vitamin D deficiency is common and frequently associated with orthopaedic conditions. Vitamin D and parathyroid hormone (PTH) levels should be measured and severe deficiencies treated.

Many children take anticonvulsants, which need to be continued in the perioperative period. Children taking these should have liver function tests monitored.

## Venous Thromboembolism

Deep venous thrombosis (DVT) is uncommon in children, but all patients should have a DVT risk assessment. Risk factors include central venous catheter insertion, cancer, known thrombophilia (antiphospholipid syndrome, factor V Leiden, protein C, S or antithrombin III deficiency), obesity, significant medical comorbidities, oral contraceptive pill use, previous DVT, prolonged immobility, lower-limb fractures and pelvic, hip or spinal surgery and age. DVT prophylaxis is not normally required in pre-pubertal children unless there are specific risk factors, even after major surgery. Post-pubertal children are at higher risk and require good hydration, early mobilisation and mechanical compression methods to be used. Pharmacological prophylaxis with low molecular weight heparin (LMWH) should be considered and discussed with the surgeon in patients with multiple risk factors.

## Pre-anaesthesia Checks

Wrong site surgery is a 'never event' and is a significant risk in orthopaedic surgery. There must be a special focus on pre-induction checks during the sign-in phase of anaesthesia, particularly when checking the consent for surgery and surgical site marking. Ionising radiation is commonly used during orthopaedic surgery, so the possibility of pregnancy must be excluded in female patients after menarche or over the age of 12 years.

## Anaesthesia Techniques

### Inhalational Induction

Medical factors favouring inhalation induction include management of a difficult airway or difficult venous access. In certain circumstances, the use of volatile agents is contraindicated. This can be absolute, as for malignant hyperthermia susceptibility (MHS), or relative where there is insufficient clinical evidence to guarantee safety, as in the case of the muscular dystrophies (see the section 'Muscular Dystrophy'). MHS is a specific autosomal dominant inherited disorder, and there are only a few rare diseases linked to MHS. These are:

- Core myopathies (particularly central core disease)
- King–Denborough syndrome
- Brody disease

Children with these conditions should all receive a 'trigger-free' anaesthetic. No other diseases have a proven association with MHS.

## Neuromuscular Blocking Agents

Neuromuscular abnormalities are common in patients presenting for orthopaedic surgery. Suxamethonium should be avoided and can never be considered safe in this group of patients due to the risk of hyperkalaemia and cardiac arrest. If neuromuscular blockade is required, a judicious dose of a non-depolarising agent should be used (taking into account the severity of the neuromuscular condition).

Continued neuromuscular blockade after intubation is contraindicated if motor nerve function needs to be monitored. For example, during limb lengthening surgery, percutaneously applied wires and struts may cause nerve damage. This risk is minimised if a motor response can be detected if a nerve is inadvertently irritated. It is essential to monitor motor evoked potentials (MEPs) during scoliosis surgery.

## Maintenance of Anaesthesia

Anaesthesia can be maintained using volatile agents or total intravenous anaesthesia (TIVA) using propofol and remifentanil. The aim is to provide safe operating conditions, facilitate spinal monitoring where indicated, provide good analgesia, achieve rapid recovery and minimise complications such as postoperative nausea and vomiting (PONV).

## Antibiotics

Antimicrobial prophylaxis is indicated if metalwork is to be implanted, with the choice of agent directed by local policy. Antibiotics should be administered prior to skin incision and as soon as possible after induction so that tissue concentrations can be maximised – this is most important when a tourniquet is used.

## Analgesia

Multimodal analgesia is central to optimal pain management. Local anaesthetic blocks should be used whenever possible, use of opioids kept to a minimum and deep anaesthesia avoided in vulnerable patients. Intraoperative ketamine and clonidine reduce opioid requirements. Clonidine may be added to local anaesthetics to enhance single-shot caudal blocks when indicated. Regular paracetamol and non-steroidal anti-inflammatory drugs (NSAIDs) should be given postoperatively unless there are contraindications. Oral opioids are usually adequate for soft tissue surgery, but IV opioids are often required postoperatively for bone-disrupting surgery, ideally by means of a nurse-controlled or patient-controlled analgesia (NCA or PCA) device.

Local anaesthetic infiltration can be used for simple procedures, however patients undergoing more complex surgery would benefit from single shot or continuous peripheral nerve blocks. The use of high-frequency ultrasound and appropriately sized probes can provide high-resolution images of neurovascular structures, tissue planes and needle position. The following regional techniques are effective:

| | |
|---|---|
| **Shoulder surgery:** | Interscalene block |
| **Upper-limb surgery:** | Supraclavicular, infraclavicular and axillary brachial plexus blocks |
| **Lower-limb surgery:** | Caudal |
| | Epidural |
| | Femoral nerve block: anterior thigh and medial aspect of the knee |
| | Popliteal and saphenous nerve block: lower leg |
| | Ankle block: foot surgery |

It is essential to monitor for nerve injury and compartment syndrome postoperatively if continuous epidural infusions are used. If removing the catheter at the end of surgery, consider elective top-up of the block prior to catheter removal.

Bladder catheterisation should be considered if an epidural is used, for prolonged surgery and in the presence of lower-limb plaster casts. Catheterisation will prevent acute postoperative urinary retention but also simplify patient care and prevent soiling of plaster casts.

## Use of Non-steroidal Anti-inflammatory Drugs (NSAIDs) in Orthopaedic Surgery

Animal and human studies suggest that fracture healing and ossification is reduced by NSAIDs, probably owing to their effects on cyclo-oxygenase-2 and mesenchymal cell differentiation, but this is controversial and not all studies are consistent. There is no evidence from studies in children that NSAIDs have a detrimental effect upon bone healing, and the analgesic benefit of short-term NSAIDs frequently outweighs any theoretical risk. If bone healing is a major concern, NSAIDs should be limited to the first 48 hours postoperatively.

## Positioning

Pre-existing neurological deficits, contractures, deformities and fractures should be carefully documented. Meticulous positioning is essential to avoid intraoperative damage. Each joint should be carefully padded to provide support to prevent pressure sores and accidental dislocation in children with contractures. The prone position is discussed further in the section 'Scoliosis Surgery'.

## Tourniquets

Pneumatic tourniquets are placed whenever indicated. Inflation pressures are determined by systolic blood pressure. Lower-limb inflation pressures should be set at approximately 150 mmHg above systolic and upper-limb 100 mmHg above systolic pressure. Adequate skin padding under the tourniquet is essential, and the site must be protected from any ingress of irritant fluids such as skin cleaning fluid. Inflation times should be limited to 75 minutes and simultaneous bilateral inflation avoided. Inflation times above 90 minutes lead to a progressive rise in core temperature. Tourniquets must be used with caution in children with sickle cell disease, with careful exsanguination of the limb prior to inflation.

# Specific Orthopaedic Conditions

## Developmental Dysplasia of the Hip

Congenital or developmental dysplasia of the hip (DDH) occurs in approximately four in 1,000 live births, with females more often affected than males. Prolonged displacement of the femoral head from the acetabulum can lead to permanent dislocation, dysplasia and eventual osteoarthritis if left undetected. Treatment should begin in the neonatal period and aims to reduce the dislocation and optimise the position of the femoral head in the acetabulum, thus promoting healthy growth. This can be achieved non-invasively by traction or closed reduction with application of a hip frog plaster (hip spica). Invasive procedures are needed in difficult cases; this may involve adductor tendon releases (to improve mobility and relocation of the femoral head), open reduction of the joint, femoral rotational osteotomy to improve femoral head engagement and acetabular procedures to improve the coverage of the femoral head.

### Anaesthetic Management

Major hip surgery may result in significant blood loss. Often the exact nature of the surgical intervention is not known until after further examination and arthrogram under anaesthesia. Insertion of a regional block can be delayed until the surgical procedure to be performed is confirmed. Single-shot caudal or lumbar epidural are effective intraoperatively for all invasive procedures, although opioids are often required to cover skin incisions over the iliac crest by the end of extensive procedures. Opioid NCA/PCA will be required postoperatively. Postoperative immobilisation is often achieved using a hip spica – this limits the use of a lumbar epidural catheter, as there is minimal access to the lumbar spine. The legs need to be raised to reduce swelling postoperatively and a postoperative haemoglobin level checked. Capillary refill and distal pulses should be examined regularly to detect circulatory compromise.

### Application of Hip Spica

A hip spica is an extensive hip plaster cast that is the cornerstone of treatment to maintain hip position in smaller children. The patient must be suspended on a casting table during application. Control of the airway may be difficult in this position, and even if undertaken as a sole procedure, intubation should be considered. Moving the patient onto the spica table is stimulating and may reveal a lighter plane of anaesthesia than expected, particularly if the spica is applied at the end of a long procedure and the surgical site is covered by a regional block; take care to maintain an appropriate depth of anaesthesia at the end of surgery. Application of a hip spica can take 40 minutes, and it can be challenging to keep the child warm. Double nappies are used to avoid soiling of the cast and should be in place before the child wakes up. Urinary catheterisation simplifies immediate postoperative care after extensive surgery.

## Congenital Talipes Equinovarus

Congenital talipes equinovarus (CTEV), or club-foot, is a common congenital deformity occurring in approximately one in 1,000 live births. Most cases are idiopathic but can be associated with neuromuscular abnormalities. Early treatment is by soft tissue manipulation and serial casting. Percutaneous Achilles tendon lengthening or soft tissue release may be required to aid correction, and in later stages osteotomy may be needed. Rarely, the correction is achieved by application of an external frame and gradual correction.

### Anaesthetic Management

Occasionally the patient will need to be positioned prone. A caudal epidural block is standard practice, and if an osteotomy is performed, regional techniques, including popliteal and saphenous nerve blocks, can be used. Parenteral opioids will be required postoperatively. Any procedure involving the stretching of muscles combined with postoperative casting will be associated with postoperative muscle spasm. Severe intermittent cramping pain that is unresponsive to opioids may become apparent as the caudal recedes. Spasm responds to oral diazepam, and this should be prescribed preoperatively rather than pursuing increasing doses of opioids.

## Limb Lengthening

Simple limb length imbalance can be corrected via epiphysiodesis (fusion of the growth plate) or require complex operations for limb lengthening via the Ilizarov method. The latter procedure involves complex osteotomies, distraction and fixation with an external fixation frame, which can be gradually extended. There is a high risk of compartment syndrome, particularly with tibial lengthening, and therefore regional anaesthetic techniques are usually avoided to facilitate postoperative neurovascular monitoring. However, these are painful procedures which require multimodal analgesia, usually with postoperative PCA/NCA opioids.

## Cerebral Palsy

Cerebral palsy results from central nervous damage caused either antenatally or in the immediate perinatal period. It is characterised by motor dysfunction, which can be classified into spastic (most common), dyskinetic, ataxic or mixed. The clinical picture is highly variable. Some patients may have normal intellect masked by communication difficulties; during the preoperative visit, it is essential to enquire about levels of comprehension and not to make assumptions that will alienate the child. The Gross Motor Function Classification System (GCMFS) is used to categorise the child's motor function and ranges from level 1, where children can walk and perform gross motor skills, to level 5, where children require a wheelchair for all movement and are limited in maintaining antigravity head and trunk posture.

The area of the brain affected will dictate any associated problems. Epilepsy occurs in about 40%, and intellectual or cognitive problems are common. Swallowing and feeding problems are frequent and can result in malnutrition and recurrent chest infection. These patients are at risk of developing chronic respiratory insufficiency. Gastro-oesophageal reflux is common, and many have anti-reflux procedures, often with a gastrostomy. Enthusiastic feeding can rapidly develop into obesity with little appreciation of the underlying lack of muscle mass. Difficult venous access is common. Scoliosis is common and can further impact upon respiratory function. Many children have had ventriculo-peritoneal shunts inserted for the treatment of hydrocephalus, and damage to these systems must be avoided. Latex allergy occurs with greater frequency in this group of patients.

Orthopaedic surgery is aimed at improving function, mobility and reducing pain. The simplest procedure is injection of botulinum toxin into the spastic muscles combined with postoperative physiotherapy and splinting. This is usually performed as a day-case procedure, even for the most high-risk patients. Hip surgery can be performed to reduce painful dislocation or enhance function by rotational femoral osteotomy to realign the limb. Fixed flexion deformities require extensive soft tissue releases and casting to maintain the correction.

### Anaesthetic Management

Gastro-oesophageal reflux and respiratory impairment are common, so in all but minor procedures the child should be intubated and ventilation controlled. In the absence of a gastrostomy, the placement of a nasogastric tube simplifies the postoperative administration of anticonvulsant therapy. Difficult venous access increases the need for central access; care must be taken to avoid damage to ventriculo-peritoneal drainage systems. Temperature regulation is often disordered, and in severe cases the basal metabolic rate so low that severe hypothermia may occur rapidly. Pain assessment is difficult in the postoperative period owing to general irritability and poor communication. Muscle spasm must be managed aggressively, and the early use of oral diazepam is encouraged. Opioids must be used when indicated, although atypical responses are common. There is a fine balance between the safe provision of analgesia and respiratory compromise, and postoperative respiratory infections are common and can be life threatening. High-dependency care is frequently required to manage postoperative analgesic and respiratory requirements safely.

## Muscular Dystrophy

The dystrophinopathies include Duchenne muscular dystrophy and the less common Becker muscular dystrophies. Progressive muscle weakness leads to respiratory failure and cardiomyopathy that can progress to circulatory failure. Recent advances that have extended survival and reduced morbidity include non-invasive ventilatory support, steroids and a variety of cardiovascular drugs. Scoliosis is common and the decision to proceed to surgery must be balanced against the risks of surgery in this group of patients.

TIVA should be used in muscular dystrophy patients and exposure to volatile agents avoided. Volatile agents and suxamethonium are associated with anaesthesia-induced rhabdomyolysis (AIR), hyperkalaemia and cardiac arrest, although this is rare. This metabolic derangement is distinct from malignant hyperthermia (MH) and can first appear on emergence from anaesthesia with the onset of spontaneous movement.

Blood loss during surgery is increased due to impaired contraction of arteriolar smooth muscle. Poor cardiac function and respiratory reserve require expert management.

## Osteogenesis Imperfecta

Osteogenesis imperfecta (OI) is a group of rare autosomal-dominant inherited connective tissue disorders with four major variants which result in increased bone fragility. Bones are osteoporotic and easily fractured, and joints are hypermobile and frequently dislocated. Surgery is usually indicated for the treatment of fractures and scoliosis. Airway management, positioning and blood pressure measurement can result in fractures. The risk of fractures from tourniquets is high. Suxamethonium should be avoided because of unpredictable effects of fasciculations, but OI is not associated with MH. Some OI patients have a bleeding diathesis due to defective platelet aggregation, and bleeding is increased from exposed abnormal bone matrix, which can be severe and difficult to control.

## Arthrogryposis Multiplex Congenita

Arthrogryposis multiplex congenita (AMC) describes the condition of congenital non-progressive symmetrical joint contractures arising from a variety of causes of fetal immobility. Neurogenic causes are present in the vast majority and often associated with a reduction in muscle mass. The involvement of the temporomandibular joint may limit mouth opening and, if combined with micrognathia, may make intubation difficult. Vascular access can be extremely difficult owing to the abnormal and featureless appearance of the limbs. There is a common association with congenital heart disease. Surgery is often needed to correct lower-limb deformities to improve posture and joint mobility and for scoliosis. Intraoperative temperature monitoring is essential, since patients cool rapidly due to low muscle mass, but they may also develop a hypermetabolic state, distinct from malignant hyperthermia, which can require active cooling. There are reports of a similar hypermetabolic state in osteogenesis imperfecta.

## Sarcoma

Sarcomas arise from connective tissue and comprise both soft tissue and bone tumours. Approximately 60 malignant bone tumours are diagnosed in children annually in England whilst soft tissue sarcomas account for approximately 6% of paediatric malignancies. Osteosarcoma and Ewing sarcoma mostly affect children and young adults. Benign bone tumours include osteochondromas, bone cysts (simple and aneurysmal), fibrous dysplasia, Langerhans cell histiocytosis and non-ossifying fibromas.

Osteosarcoma is the most frequent primary cancer of bone and accounts of over 10% of solid cancers in adolescents. It usually arises in the metaphysis of long bones, most commonly around the knee, and there is suggestion of an association with rapid bone growth and the pubertal growth spurt.

Ewing's sarcoma is a round cell tumour that most frequently involves the long bones, pelvis, ribs and vertebral column. It is the second most common primary malignant bone tumour in children and adolescents. All forms are of high grade, and approximately 26% of patients with Ewing's sarcoma have metastatic disease at presentation. Multidisciplinary treatment involving preoperative neoadjuvant combination chemotherapy, surgery, postoperative adjuvant chemotherapy and radiotherapy is usually required.

Many of the chemotherapy treatment regimens for sarcoma are cardiotoxic and require baseline and surveillance echocardiography. Preoperative blood tests are essential to examine renal, liver and haematological side effects of chemotherapy. Neoadjuvant chemotherapy can result in patients presenting for major surgery with anaemia and neutropenia, and the timing of surgery needs to be considered to permit recovery and appropriate treatments, including the use of granulocyte colony stimulating factor and transfusion.

The range of surgeries for sarcoma is wide, including limb salvage operations, massive resections (e.g. hemipelvectomies or sacrectomies) and amputation. Such operations require multidisciplinary planning and preoperative preparation of the patient and parents for the effects of chemotherapy and surgery and the subsequent recovery and need for further chemotherapy. Limb amputation carries additional psychological challenges to the child and family and requires preoperative preparation with psychologists, nurse specialists and prosthetists.

Anaesthetic management of major resection surgery requires planning for major haemorrhage and postoperative pain management. Central venous access, invasive blood pressure monitoring and rapid infusion and warming systems should be utilised. Cell salvage is not routinely employed due to the theoretical risks of metastasis. Central neuraxial and regional anaesthesia is used as routine, with the use of postoperative parenteral analgesia. Patients are routinely managed in a high-dependency environment postoperatively.

## Scoliosis Surgery

Scoliosis is an abnormal lateral curvature of the spine and can be classified into congenital, idiopathic (infantile, juvenile, adolescent) and acquired. Congenital scoliosis arises as a result of failure of fetal vertebral formation, segmentation or a combination of both. It is commonly associated with other abnormalities and often progresses rapidly at an early age. The major causes of acquired scoliosis are neuromuscular diseases, particularly cerebral palsy and the muscular dystrophies.

Surgical treatment is indicated when the degree of curvature or its rate of acceleration puts other organs at risk or when pain intervenes. The type of surgical intervention depends upon the reason for the scoliosis and the child's skeletal maturity. Before skeletal maturity, the aim is to allow growth whilst controlling the progression of the curve. In older children, when truncal growth has slowed down the aim is to correct the deformity and prevent any further progression with a definitive procedure. The most common procedures requiring anaesthesia are posterior spinal surgery, anterior spinal surgery, insertion of growing systems and application of plaster jackets.

The largest group requiring surgery comprises adolescents with idiopathic scoliosis. These patients are fit and healthy; pre-assessment should concentrate on imparting information and the detection of anaemia. This group of patients is ideal to include in enhanced recovery after surgery programmes. At the other end of the spectrum are patients with progressive end-stage neuromuscular disease, where multidisciplinary discussions are required to focus on the potential benefits and the risks of surgery.

All patients requiring scoliosis surgery should attend a pre-assessment clinic. Multidisciplinary involvement is mandatory. Pre-assessment allows for the detection and optimisation of any underlying disease and secondary morbidity. Risks of anaesthesia need to be discussed openly and can sometimes limit the surgical options. Postoperative care needs to be planned and the likelihood of elective postoperative ventilation evaluated.

### Preoperative Assessment

A thorough assessment is required, including a full history of previous procedures under general anaesthetic; in particular, any potential difficulties with airway management, potential for airway obstruction, cervical spine instability and risks of induction using volatile anaesthetic drugs should be assessed.

Respiratory function is the critical area of focus. Many children find it difficult to cooperate with formal assessment of respiratory function. Frequent chest infections, poor cough or symptoms suggestive of sleep apnoea warrant further investigation, which may include blood gas analysis, respiratory function tests and, most usefully, sleep study analysis. Sleep studies monitor continuous $SpO_2$ and transcutaneous $CO_2$ and provide useful information as to the need for postoperative respiratory support. Respiratory investigations can also be used to monitor the progression of neuromuscular disease and guide preoperative intervention and the need for of non-invasive respiratory support. The increased use of home ventilation has increased the number of patients being offered surgery despite advanced respiratory disease.

Cardiomyopathy may be a feature of the muscle pathology leading to scoliosis, or a structural cardiac anomaly may be part of an associated syndrome. Severe chest wall deformity rarely leads to primary cardiac insufficiency. Severe pulmonary disease can lead to elevated pulmonary vascular resistance and right ventricular dysfunction. Previous cardiac surgery itself may predispose to scoliosis by disrupting chest wall growth secondary to damage to the ribs and sternum. The severity of cardiac disease can be masked in wheelchair-bound patients by lack of activity, and surgery can produce unique stresses that may result in acute decompensation. A recent ECG and echocardiogram are required. Children with progressive neuromuscular disease may require a cardiac MRI scan before surgery to give an objective measure of cardiac and myocyte function.

Nutrition needs to be optimised preoperatively and any feeding difficulties resolved. Supplementary enteral feeding may need to be started. Similarly, patients with a raised body mass index should be managed to reduce the risks of perioperative morbidity, including wound infections. Anaemia and vitamin D deficiency should be investigated and fully treated before embarking upon major surgery.

Epilepsy is common, and therapy should be continued over the perioperative period with a management plan for breakthrough seizure activity, including conversion to alternate intravenous therapies should there be a significant postoperative ileus delaying medication absorption. Patients often take steroids, cardiac medications and contraceptive therapies, and they may need specialist perioperative plans.

### Spinal Cord Injury and Monitoring

Spinal cord damage is a prime concern during scoliosis surgery. Injury can be caused by direct mechanical trauma or vascular insufficiency. Mechanical trauma can be caused by malpositioning of instrumentation or due to compression or stretch of neural structures during spinal manipulation. Vascular insufficiency may result from disruption of the arterial blood supply during spinal manipulation or vascular spasm following an insult.

Monitoring of spinal cord function intraoperatively is essential. This is achieved using monitoring of somatosensory evoked potentials (SSEPs) and transcranial motor evoked potentials (MEPs) and occasionally by performing a 'wake up' test. Surface and needle electrodes are placed on the scalp, neck and limbs once the patient is asleep to elicit and record evoked potentials. SSEPs monitor the main sensory pathways, the dorsal columns, that make up the posterior third of the cord, which are supplied by two spinal arteries. MEPs monitor the main motor pathways, the corticospinal tracts, within the anterior cord, which, although making up two thirds of the spinal cord, are only supplied by a single spinal artery and as a result is more susceptible to ischaemia.

Additional modalities such as free-running or triggered electromyelography may be utilised to detect pedicle breaches or malpositioning of screws. Electroencephalography (EEG) may be recorded to observe ongoing cortical activity and gauge the depth of anaesthesia. A neuromonitoring specialist monitors these modalities continuously throughout the procedure.

Evoked potentials (SSEPs and MEPs) are suppressed by all types of anaesthetic agents to some extent, so optimisation of anaesthesia is required. MEPs are more severely suppressed by inhalational agents than TIVA, so for robust neuromonitoring, TIVA is recommended. Since MEPs monitor muscle activity, neuromuscular blockade should be avoided intraoperatively. As a consequence of transcranial stimulation, muscle contraction occurs, so a bite block is essential to prevent injury to the tongue and mouth, as well to protect the tracheal tube.

Baseline waveforms are obtained once the patient is positioned and must be deemed adequate for monitoring prior to the start of surgery. In some circumstances, pre-positioning baselines may be beneficial. Clear communication between anaesthetic, surgical and neuromonitoring staff is always vital so that significant neuromonitoring changes are identified promptly. This allows appropriate interventions to be made in a timely fashion to reduce the risk of permanent neurological deficit.

Common events resulting in neuromonitoring changes are:

- Insertion of instrumentation, for example screws or cages
- Manipulation of the spine, such as rod insertion and curve correction
- Periods of cardiovascular instability

Neuromonitoring can also be of benefit in detecting peripheral nerve compromise due to patient positioning, such as compression of the brachial plexus or ulnar nerve at the elbow, which can often be resolved by simple repositioning of the affected limb.

## Posterior Spinal Surgery

Posterior spinal surgery is increasingly performed as the sole procedure to correct scoliosis due to technological advancements in the equipment used and improved neuromonitoring. Spinal fixation is usually achieved by attaching a pair of suitably curved rods to the bony spine. Previously this was achieved with a combination of pedicle screws in the lumbar region and laminar hooks or wires in the thoracic and cervical region. Currently most procedures use screws inserted into the pedicles throughout the spine to provide a more robust attachment. This enables the bony spine to be manipulated to a greater degree, achieving more correction and restoring trunk symmetry and balance. Ongoing advances include the use of image guidance and robotics.

### Anaesthetic Management

The technique for induction of anaesthesia can be as preferred, but the needs of intraoperative spinal monitoring will dictate further management. TIVA is required for successful motor monitoring, and neuromuscular blockade can only be used to aid intubation. High-dose intraoperative opioids provide optimal conditions, and propofol/remifentanil-based TIVA is a common choice.

### Analgesia

Pain relief intraoperatively is best provided by high-dose, short-acting opioids, usually fentanyl or a continuous infusion of remifentanil. Postoperatively, pain control requires a multimodal technique. Paracetamol should be given regularly along with regular NSAIDs if excessive bleeding has not occurred. Large doses of opioid will be required postoperatively via NCA/PCA initially with background infusions. Other strategies include the use of ketamine, clonidine, diazepam, regional techniques and intraoperative spinal opioid administration. Postoperatively, the patients usually have to lie supine for 12 hours to tamponade the wound and reduce bleeding.

The two major concerns for anaesthesia in posterior spinal surgery are high anticipated blood losses and surgery in the prone position.

### Blood Loss

Blood losses can be life-threatening. Bleeding occurs from the traumatic detachment of muscle from the spine and from bone. For definitive spinal fixation to occur, the periosteum of the bony elements must be removed and the interarticular joints need to be disrupted. This, combined with bleeding from the pedicle marrow, provides a vast area over which bleeding can occur. Higher blood losses are expected with increased tissue disruption, longer lengths of surgery, fusion into the pelvis and the development of coagulopathy. In extreme cases, haemostasis is only achieved by judicious premature surgical closure of the wound. Blood should be immediately available for all but limited posterior procedures.

Venous access is dictated by anticipated blood loss. Two large-bore peripheral cannulae are desirable. A system for rapid infusion should be available, preferably with integrated warming. Central venous access is indicated when large losses are expected and peripheral access is limited, when coexisting disease adds complexity or when extended postoperative venous access is required. Intraoperative arterial access is desirable in all but the most limited cases, as blood pressure can change rapidly owing to fluid loses and occasionally as a result of spinal cord disruption. It is an essential guide to spinal perfusion pressures. Blood pressure should be controlled intraoperatively to reduce blood losses. Profound hypotension may compromise cord perfusion, and if spinal monitoring detects deterioration, this needs to be aggressively reversed. Urinary catheterisation is standard to assess fluid balance and will be required in the initial postoperative period.

Blood loss during surgery is reduced by maintaining normothermia and controlled hypotension, avoiding hypertension and administering antifibrinolytics (e.g. tranexamic acid). Blood salvage should be routine, using an automated cell saver for suction blood, and to collect the blood rinsed out of swabs in physiological saline. In many cases, blood transfusion can be avoided, provided postoperative anaemia is acceptable. Massive blood transfusion leads to coagulopathy, which should be anticipated and actively treated to prevent escalation. Cord injury can occur during periods of hypotension, and cord monitoring should be used to assess adequacy of resuscitation.

### Prone Positioning

The aim of safe prone positioning is to ensure that all tubes and lines remain secure, baseline physiological parameters are maintained and that the risk of nerve/tissue injury and blindness is kept to a minimum. Airway control in the prone position needs to be secure. Reinforced flexible tracheal tubes are ideal, and placement of a bite guard reduces possible damage to lips, tongue and tracheal tube. A nasogastric tube is necessary to decompress the stomach and can be retained into the postoperative period; a nasopharyngeal temperature probe is placed to assess core temperature. Positioning the patient prone requires time, coordination with the theatre team and familiarity with the equipment available to support the body. Vascular access must be secure, the abdomen must remain unrestricted, the head must be well supported in a neutral position without pressure on the orbits or nose and all peripheral pressure points must be padded. The arms must drape comfortably, without undue compression or extension that may lead to brachial plexus or peripheral nerve injury. The simplest way to assess posture is to replicate it on oneself to judge the degree of comfort and then modify as appropriate. Responsibility for positioning should be clear; logically, the anaesthetist should control positioning of the upper body as a minimum. A fenestrated warm-air body warmer enhances the ability to maintain normothermia, and clear drapes improve the ability to continuously assess the patient's position.

### Postoperative Care

All patients should be managed in a high-dependency unit (HDU) environment postoperatively. Elective admission to the paediatric intensive care unit (PICU) will depend on patient factors and the extent of surgery. The presence of severe behavioural issues, neuromuscular disease or cardiorespiratory disease will necessitate a period of elective ventilation so that stability can be established prior to extubation. Patients undergoing extensive combined anterior–posterior spinal surgery should electively be admitted to PICU for postoperative ventilation, even in the absence of underlying medical concerns. Occasional unplanned PICU admission may be necessary if massive blood loss has occurred.

## Anterior Spinal Surgery

Anterior spinal surgery is usually performed to release the spine and enhance its flexibility to achieve a better degree of correction from the following definitive posterior fusion. The problems of anterior surgery are related to those of thoracotomy and therefore one-lung ventilation and postoperative pain relief. Surgery often involves a thoracoabdominal incision in the lateral position with disruption to the diaphragm. This type of surgery is inappropriate in patients with severe coexisting disease and significant respiratory impairment.

The conduct of anaesthesia is again influenced by spinal cord monitoring. A standard tracheal tube is adequate, as exposure of the spine is by lung retraction, and ventilation/perfusion mismatch rarely causes significant changes in oxygenation. Of greater concern is retraction resulting in compression of major blood vessels or mediastinal shift. For this reason, invasive arterial monitoring is essential. Blood loss is usually well controlled, and transfusion is rarely required. Central venous access is only required if peripheral access is difficult or if there is complicating coexisting disease.

Optimal pain relief in the postoperative period is essential to prevent lung collapse and infection. Coughing is inhibited by wound pain and irritation from the chest drain. Intraoperative infiltration of the intercostal nerves can be performed by the surgeon. Epidurals and other regional techniques can also be used. A multimodal approach to analgesia is used, with regular paracetamol, NSAIDs and opioid PCA/NCA that can be augmented with ketamine. Postoperative ventilation is rarely required, as patient selection implies that respiratory reserve is adequate, but patients should be nursed in an HDU environment.

## Thoracoscopic Spinal Surgery

There is increasing interest in thoracoscopic spinal surgical procedures such as vertebral body tethering (VBT). This involves anterior screws being inserted into the spine followed by a flexible plastic cord connected to these screws via a thoracoscopic approach. The cord is tensioned during the operation to provide an initial correction, whilst tethering limits growth on the outside of the curve to allow gradual correction of the scoliosis as the patient grows. This surgery necessitates one lung ventilation facilitated by a double-lumen tracheal tube or use of a bronchial blocker. Anaesthetic considerations are otherwise as for conventional anterior spinal surgery.

## Growing Systems

Spinal fixation with a definitive fusion cannot take place whilst the spine is still growing. Growing systems provide dynamic stabilisation and correction of scoliosis in younger patients and permit further growth over time. With traditional growing rods, two rods are attached posteriorly with limited attachment to the spine. They overlap and their overall length can be increased by distraction over years. These remain in place until definitive posterior fixation is feasible. Blood loss is not a major issue since there is only limited exposure of the spine, but spinal cord monitoring is necessary, so it will influence the conduct of anaesthesia. The surgery for further distractions involves even less exposure, but again spinal monitoring will dictate anaesthetic technique.

## Plaster Jacket Application

The use of plaster jackets offers a non-surgical management of scoliosis in young patients where significant growth is yet to occur. The programme requires repeated general anaesthetics as truncal growth is rapid in the early years. The child must be intubated and the tracheal tube fixed securely, as the application requires significant movement and precarious positioning with limited monitoring and access to the patient. The fixed thoracoabdominal jacket will impede ventilation, and an aperture must be cut as soon as possible to allow abdominal movement.

## Wound Debridement for Wound Infection

Wound infection is a devastating and life-threatening complication after scoliosis surgery, owing to the amount of implanted material and underlying poor medical condition of many patients. Antimicrobial agents are continued routinely postoperatively until the wound becomes dry. Patients presenting for exploratory surgery with wound infection must be managed aggressively. Superficial infections may be connected to deep extensive lesions producing widespread tissue necrosis. Debridement can result in massive blood loss, and this must be anticipated. Long-term venous access is required to provide access for antimicrobial agents and often to supplement nutrition.

**Key Points**

- Children presenting for elective orthopaedic surgery may have associated medical conditions, and a careful history should be taken, particularly to identify associated neuromuscular disorders.
- Multimodal analgesia should be used, and regional anaesthetic techniques are of benefit.
- Procedures involving muscle stretch and casting may be associated with postoperative muscle spasm.
- All children undergoing scoliosis surgery should be assessed preoperatively in a multidisciplinary clinic. The perioperative major concerns are bleeding and spinal cord function.
- TIVA is the anaesthesia technique of choice to facilitate spinal cord monitoring in scoliosis surgery.

## Further Reading

Grover H, Walsh P, Sanders B, Shirley C. Updated ANS/BSCN Guidelines for Neurophysiological Recordings of the Spinal Cord during Corrective Spinal Deformity Surgery. British Society for Clinical Neurophysiology. 2018. Available at: www.bscn.org.uk/data/files/Guidelines/IOM_guide2.pdf. Accessed 9 May 2021.

Katz JA, Murphy GS. Anesthetic consideration for neuromuscular diseases. *Current Opinion in Anaesthesiology* 2017 June; 30 (3):435–40.

Lerman J, Perioperative management of the paediatric patient with coexisting neuromuscular disease. *British*

*Journal of Anaesthesia* 2011; 107 (Suppl 1):i79 –89.

Orphan Anesthesia. Anaesthesia Recommendations for Osteogenesis Imperfecta. 2019. Available at: www.orphananesthesia.eu/en/rare-diseases/published-guidelines/osteogenesis-imperfecta/881-osteogenesis-imperfecta-2/file.html. Accessed 9 May 2021.

Schieren M, Defosse J, Böhmer A, Wappler F, Gerbershagen MU. Anaesthetic management of patients with myopathies. *European Journal of Anaesthesiology* 2017; 10:641–9.

Chapter 30

# Anaesthesia for Thoracic Surgery in Children*

Valentine Woodham and James Ip

## Introduction

Anaesthesia for thoracic surgery in children poses different problems from those encountered in adult practice. It is a low-volume specialty largely confined to specialist paediatric hospitals. Anaesthesia may be required for a heterogeneous range of conditions, will frequently be of an urgent or emergency nature and can very often be challenging. This chapter will cover the management of congenital and acquired lung abnormalities, intrathoracic masses, intrapleural collections and pectus surgery. Patient positioning, surgical retraction of the lung and underlying disease processes all contribute to the demands placed on the paediatric thoracic anaesthetist. Thoracotomy for cardiac surgery (e.g. coarctation repair) is covered in Chapter 31 and thoracotomy for oesophageal anomalies is covered in Chapter 18.

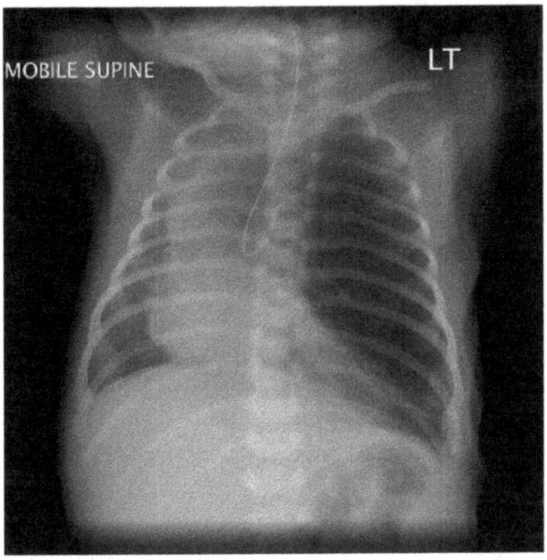


**Figure 30.1** Chest X-ray showing congenital lobar emphysema.

## Congenital Abnormalities of the Lung

### Congenital Lobar Emphysema (CLE)

This condition is due to bronchial cartilaginous dysplasia that generates a ball-valve effect resulting in pathological emphysematous accumulation of air within the affected lobe. It is associated with poor deflation of that lobe. Usually a single lobe is affected, most commonly the left upper. There is a spectrum of disease which usually presents in the neonatal period. Presentation may be that of a coincidental X-ray finding; alternatively, a neonate may present in extremis, with hypoxia, hypercapnia and mediastinal shift caused by hyperinflated lung tissue (Figure 30.1). When a child presents acutely, urgent lobectomy is indicated.

### Congenital Cystic Abnormalities of the Lung

There are three main types of congenital cystic abnormalities.

- Congenital cystic adenomatous malformation
- Pulmonary sequestration
- Bronchogenic cysts

In common with congenital lobar emphysema, there is a spectrum of disease. Symptoms can be caused by mass effect or by secondary infection.

### Congenital Cystic Adenomatous Malformation (CCAM)

CCAM results from localised arrest of maturation of fetal lung. A disorganised mass of air and/or blood-filled cysts is present which does not usually communicate with normal lung (Figure 30.2). An antenatal diagnosis is often made, but the

* Many thanks to Dr Simon Haynes, who wrote the first edition of this book chapter, much of the content of which has been used in this revision.

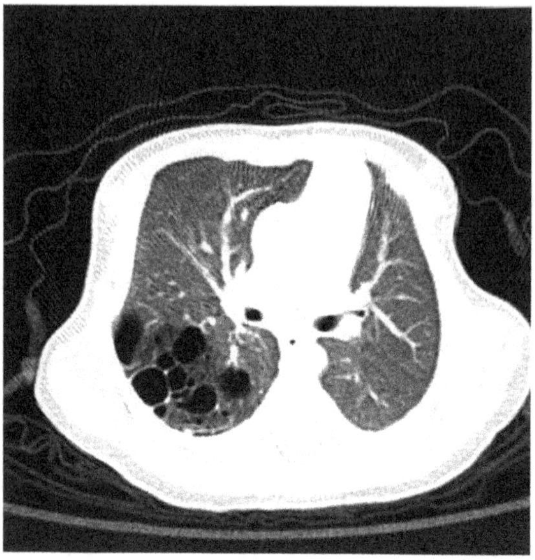

**Figure 30.2** CT scan showing congenital cystic adenomatous malformations in the lung.

immediate course of action depends on the clinical condition of the child once born. Resection of the abnormal mass may be required urgently to relieve compression, although this is not usually as marked as with congenital lobar emphysema. The affected area may be removed electively later in childhood to prevent infection and to remove the abnormal tissue, which has potential to undergo malignant change.

### Pulmonary Sequestration

This is a separate bronchopulmonary mass or cyst which is disconnected from the bronchial tree and has a separate blood supply arising from the aorta. It forms when a supernumerary lung bud arises from the primitive foregut. Other congenital abnormalities are present in 65% of cases. Appropriate preoperative investigation (e.g. contrast CT scan) is required to identify the blood supply.

### Bronchogenic Cysts

These are solitary, unilocular and often mucus filled. They are often an incidental radiographic finding but may become infected.

## Acquired Pathology

### Thoracic Tumours in Children

Primary lung malignancies are rare in children. Extensive intrathoracic tumours such as neuroblastoma may require de-bulking or resection through a thoracotomy. Such tumours are not usually intrapulmonary. Thoracotomy may be required for metastatectomy.

### Anterior Mediastinal Mass

Anterior mediastinal masses are a common presenting feature of haematological malignancy, such as lymphoma, or occasionally primary malignancy. Histological diagnosis of a mediastinal mass is essential to direct therapy. Mediastinal masses can compress the trachea, bronchi or great vessels. Respiratory symptoms are frequently the presenting feature and may be rapidly progressive. Occasionally a child with a mediastinal mass presents in extremis with airway obstruction. Stridor, respiratory difficulty at rest or orthopnea are particularly concerning signs. CT scan images obtained preoperatively are particularly helpful to identify compression of major structures. Preoperative steroids may relieve symptoms to some extent in haematological malignancy but may make the mass shrink quickly and provoke tumour lysis syndrome.

Although most children requiring anaesthesia for biopsy of a mediastinal mass tolerate the procedure without major incident, catastrophic airway and cardiovascular compromise can occur. Alterations in chest wall muscle tone, for example following administration of neuromuscular blocking drugs, or minor postural changes can provoke total airway obstruction or occlude venous return. Such complications must be anticipated following induction of anaesthesia. Splinting the obstruction with a rigid bronchoscope and/or turning the patient prone may rescue the situation. If this does not relieve the obstruction, the only solution may be the emergency provision of cardiopulmonary bypass. For this reason, surgery for mediastinal masses should be performed by paediatric cardiac surgeons in a cardiac surgical unit.

### Pleural Collections

Pleural drainage became incorporated into surgical practice in 1917 to treat empyema associated with the influenza pandemic. Pleural drainage removes air, blood or other fluid from the pleural space, allowing lung re-expansion and eliminating mediastinal shift. Negative intrapleural pressure during spontaneous respiration cannot be achieved if gas or fluid intervenes between the two pleural layers.

## Empyema

Empyema is a complication of bacterial pneumonia (usually pneumococcal) in approximately 5–10% of children. It results in inflammatory debris forming a thick, inelastic covering of the lung, restricting expansion, often accompanied by a purulent pleural effusion. Areas of lung may be necrotic, with the potential for the development of a bronchopleural fistula.

Children with this condition are frequently systemically unwell with fever and bacteraemia and may have been ill for several days or weeks before presenting for surgery. Some children will be septicaemic and haemodynamically compromised; fluid resuscitation may be necessary. Blood should be cross-matched; many of these children have become anaemic during the illness, and blood loss from the inflamed lung surface is occasionally significant. Severely ill children may require a period of optimisation in intensive care before proceeding to surgery and may require postoperative ventilation. Oxygenation is often marginal at presentation and may be compromised further during one-lung ventilation (OLV). Most previously well children improve markedly after decortication.

Video-assisted thoracoscopic surgery (VATS) and decortication is the surgical treatment of choice to break down the fibrin strands and evacuate the pus. In patients with marked pleural thickening and encasement of the lung, thoracotomy and open decortication may be required. The thick inflammatory debris encapsulating the lung is excised, allowing the lung to re-expand, and any necrotic tissue is removed.

## Lung Abscess

This may be associated with primary bacterial infection but may also be precipitated by foreign body inhalation. It may require lung resection. Destruction of lung tissue and erosion into a bronchus with bronchopleural fistula formation may have occurred. Although OLV may not assist with the surgical field, its use may prevent soiling of the non-operative lung and may be necessary at intubation in the presence of a bronchopleural fistula.

## Bronchiectasis

Chronic infection damages the muscular and elastic components of affected bronchi. It is a feature of cystic fibrosis. In children, it is often associated with underlying immune compromise or immune suppression and is a common long-term complication of children receiving organ transplantation in early life. Surgical resection of localised disease is indicated to prevent infection of normal lung tissue. Provision of OLV is indicated during resection to prevent soiling and infection of the healthy lung.

## Chest Wall Deformity

Pectus excavatum is more common than pectus carinatum. Unless extremely severe, the indication for correction is cosmetic, and children undergoing this surgery should be old enough to understand and to consent to surgery themselves. The Ravitch procedure involves a major incision across the chest, detachment of costal cartilages from the sternum and surgical re-modelling of the sternum. This has been replaced by the minimally invasive Nuss procedure. A curved steel bar is inserted under endoscopic guidance under the sternum and then rotated 180° to raise the sternum. Safe insertion of the Nuss bar requires thoracoscopy with $CO_2$ insufflation to create space anterior to the mediastinum for its insertion. Whichever procedure is used, the major issue is the control of postoperative pain. Strategies include thoracic epidural analgesia, paravertebral block (either via single-shot or catheter infusion) and patient-controlled analgesia (e.g. with morphine and ketamine). Each approach has a distinct risk-benefit profile.

## Anaesthesia for Thoracic Surgery: Specific Considerations

The importance of preoperative assessment and continuing communication with the surgical and operating theatre staff cannot be overstated, and use of the WHO Safe Surgery Guidelines to ensure the correct side is operated on is mandatory. If lung isolation is planned, topical local anaesthetic to the larynx and trachea can be used, as repeated manipulation may be required to position the tracheal tube correctly. Nitrous oxide is contraindicated in thoracic anaesthesia as it may diffuse into and expand any gas-filled cavity.

## Vascular Access

Thoracic surgery may involve the mobilisation of large blood vessels, or operating on inflamed, friable tissue. Intra-operative bleeding can be brisk during tumour surgery, and significant plasma losses from either raw tissue surfaces or consequent to lymphatic disruption can occur during the postoperative period. Adequate venous access is essential for fluid replacement, and cross-matched blood should be available. Central venous pressure monitoring can be misleading in the lateral decubitus position, but central venous cannulation is indicated if haemodynamic instability is anticipated or if there is inadequate peripheral venous access. Invasive arterial pressure monitoring is helpful because of the potential for intraoperative haemodynamic instability and for blood gas analysis.

## Hypoxic Pulmonary Vasoconstriction (HPV)

HPV is the mechanism by which the body limits blood flow through unventilated or hypoxic areas of lung. If HPV is inhibited, then the flow of deoxygenated blood increases through non-ventilated areas of lung. Much has been written about the inhibitory effects of inhalational anaesthetic agents on HPV, but in practice it is not a problem unless high concentrations of inspired agent are used.

## Lateral Decubitus Position

Most thoracic procedures require the patient to be in the lateral decubitus position, operative side uppermost. Increased ventilation/perfusion (V/Q) mismatch may result in hypoxaemia as:

- Surgical retraction of the upper (operative) lung or OLV causes collapse of the operative lung.
- The dependent lung may be compressed by the mediastinum and abdominal organs.
- HPV may be impaired by inhalational anaesthetic agents.

The effect of the lateral decubitus position on V/Q mismatch may be more marked in infants than older children. In older children with unilateral lung disease, oxygenation is usually better when the patient is in the lateral decubitus position with the healthy lung 'down'. The hydrostatic pressure difference between upper and lower lungs diverts blood flow away from the upper lung to the healthy lower lung. This pressure gradient is less in infants, making this phenomenon less important. Also, infants have a compliant thoracic wall, which supports the lower lung less effectively; during tidal ventilation, airway closure is more likely to occur because functional residual capacity (FRC) approaches closing volume. Consequently, in infants with unilateral lung disease, oxygenation is improved with the healthy lung 'up', although this is clearly not practical during surgery.

The effect on oxygenation is noticeable during surgery in the lateral decubitus position in infants and young children. A predictable sequence of events occurs:

- FRC increases when moved from supine to the lateral position.
- On opening the pleural space, FRC decreases to 25% below baseline, falling further to 50% of baseline during lung retraction (if OLV is not used).
- FRC then returns to the baseline on completion of surgery.

Oxygenation follows a similar sequence, and provided it is within defined boundaries, modest hypoxaemia is acceptable, and surgery can usually proceed.

## Lung Retraction

Surgical access to the operative lung can be facilitated by ventilating only the dependent lung, allowing the operative lung to collapse. In adults and older children, OLV is achieved relatively easily. In smaller children, this is more challenging, so the surgeon often needs to retract the operative lung for adequate exposure. This necessitates effective dialogue between surgeon and anaesthetist, particularly as there may also be some mediastinal distortion. When lung is retracted, there is decreased lung compliance. This may be accompanied by hypoxaemia; typically, the $SpO^2$ will decrease to 85–90%. If there is no further perturbation in the surgical field, $SpO^2$ will gradually increase as hypoxic pulmonary vasoconstriction lessens the volume of blood passing through the collapsed lung. Lung retraction should be gentle, to avoid both lung contusion and mediastinal compression, which occludes venous return to the heart, which in turn causes haemodynamic compromise. Positive end expiratory pressure

(PEEP) should be used during a thoracotomy. This maintains lung volume in the 'down' lung, both aiding oxygenation and supporting the mediastinum (which then maintains its position in the chest cavity).

## Bronchoscopy

The anaesthetist undertaking paediatric thoracic work should be able to use a flexible bronchoscope to assist with accurate tracheal tube (TT) or bronchus blocker placement, as well as to allow tracheobronchial toilet. Competence in fibreoptic bronchoscopy is also useful in evaluating extrinsic airway compression, subglottic stenosis and tracheomalacia, although these and other laryngotracheal investigations are more commonly undertaken by ENT surgeons.

The smallest flexible fibreoptic bronchoscope with a suction channel has a diameter of 2.8 mm; without a suction channel, it is 2.2 mm. There are two important considerations when choosing the correct-sized bronchoscope: whether it can fit smoothly into the TT, and whether you are able to ventilate around it (Figure 30.3). There are useful formulae to help with this:

- For the bronchoscope to fit smoothly down the TT, the outer diameter of the bronchoscope (ODB) needs to be <90% of the internal diameter (ID) of the TT: ODB/IDTT <0.9.
- For there to be sufficient space around the bronchoscope to allow for some ventilation to occur, it needs to take up <50% of the ID of the TT: ODB/IDTT <0.7.

For example, although a 2.8 mm scope will fit down a 3.5 TT (ODB/IDTT = 2.8/3.5 = 0.8), the ratio is greater than 0.7, so it will not be possible to ventilate whilst the bronchoscope is in place. It is important to note that although some ventilation will occur during bronchoscopy, patients who are critically unwell can decompensate rapidly due to the increase in airway resistance and reduction in ventilation.

Techniques for rigid bronchoscopy in adults cannot simply be transposed to small children. A jet ventilation technique may cause barotrauma in children with normal lungs and cannot be recommended for paediatric practice. When lungs are poorly compliant or there is airway obstruction, air is poorly entrained. In children, ventilation through a rigid bronchoscope is performed by attaching a Mapleson F breathing system to the side arm of a Storz bronchoscope, occluding the main channel by a diaphragm, a window or the operator's thumb. If there is airway obstruction, for example caused by an impacted foreign body, air trapping in the lungs can be problematic; expiration must be unimpeded and of adequate duration. A rigid telescope inserted through a small bronchoscope also causes expiratory embarrassment. A 1.9 mm telescope inside a 3.0 mm internal diameter bronchoscope or a 2.8 mm telescope in a 3.5 mm bronchoscope are the smallest acceptable combinations.

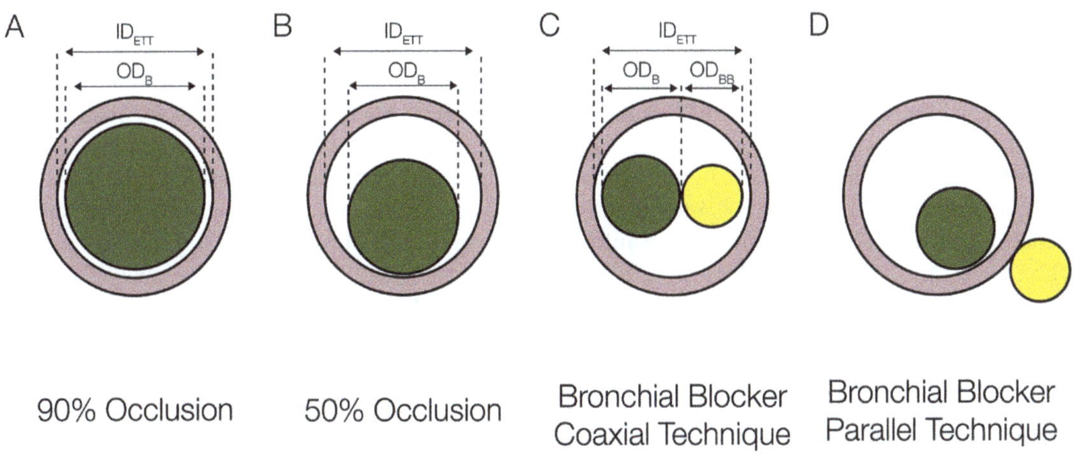


**Figure 30.3** (A) Bronchoscope able to fit into ETT, but no ventilation, $OD_B/ID_{TT} < 0.9$. (B) Allowing for some ventilation, $OD_B/ID_{TT} < 0.7$. (C) Coaxial technique, bronchoscope and bronchial blocker able to fit, $(OD_B + OD_{BB})/ID_{TT} < 0.9$. (D) Parallel technique with bronchial blocker placed outside of the ETT.
*Notes:* Green circle = bronchoscope; yellow circle = bronchial blocker; pink circle = ETT).

Maintenance of anaesthesia during rigid bronchoscopy can be with inhalational or intravenous agents, the latter having the advantages of reduced pollution with anaesthetic gases and a lower carbon footprint.

## One-Lung Ventilation

Lung isolation is standard practice in adult thoracic surgery. The non-operative lung alone is ventilated, allowing the operative lung to deflate. This improves surgical access whilst reducing operating times and lung trauma caused by surgical retraction. Contamination of the non-operative lung and trachea by blood or pus draining from the operative lung may be minimised. In adults, OLV is readily achieved using a double-lumen tube; one lumen lies in a mainstem bronchus, the other in the trachea and the inflatable cuff around the bronchial lumen allowing lung isolation. Double-lumen tubes are not available in small sizes, so OLV in children requires alternative strategies (Figure 30.4). The smaller the child, the harder it is to achieve this, so greater justification for its use is required. Strategies for OLV in children include use of:

- An endobronchially placed single lumen tracheal tube
- Bronchial blockers
- A Univent tube
- A conventional double-lumen tube

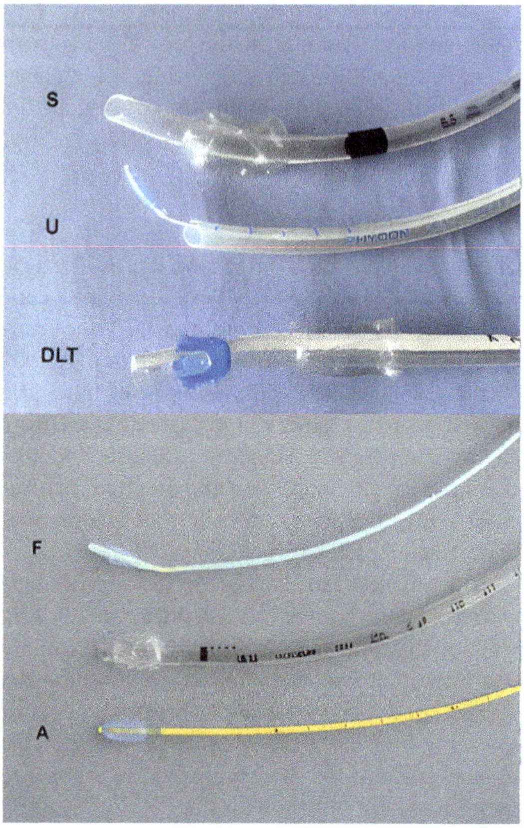


**Figure 30.4** Airway management: Univent-tube (U) (3.5 mm ID) and 26 French DLT (DLT) in relation to a standard ETT (S) (6.5 mm ID). Five French Fuji (F) and Arndt (A)-bronchial blockers next to a 3.5 mm ID ETT.
*Source:* Semmelmann A, Kaltofen H, Loop T. Anesthesia of thoracic surgery in children. *Paediatric Anaesthesia* 2018 April; 28(4):326–31. Reproduced with permission of Wiley.

## Single-Lumen Tube

This is the simplest method in a small child and can usually be achieved in babies from around 3 kg upwards, although the smaller the patient, the more difficulty is encountered. The mainstem bronchus on the non-operative side is intubated with a conventional tube that is 0.5 mm diameter smaller than normal. Placement of a TT into the right main bronchus is easier than the left due to the shallower right bronchial angle. A blind approach for left main bronchus intubation involves rotating the TT through 180° after traversing the glottis, raising the child's right shoulder and turning their head to the right. The tube is then advanced until breath sounds are no longer audible on the right. If a tube is advanced without these manoeuvres, it will usually enter the right main bronchus.

Tube placement assisted by a fibreoptic bronchoscope is the preferred method. The bronchoscope is loaded with the TT, placed into the desired bronchus and, once in position, the tube is advanced off the bronchoscope. In small babies, this is not simple; the bronchoscope is easily dislodged as the tube is advanced. If right bronchial intubation cannot be achieved easily, and a fibreoptic bronchoscope is not available to guide placement, a mirror image technique of that used for left-sided intubation may help.

Tolerances in small children for correct tube position are as little as 2–3 mm, and positioning the tube to ensure that the upper lobe remains ventilated can be awkward. The upper lobe bronchus on either side may originate very close to the carina, and its orifice may be occluded by the tube tip or cuff. Failure to ventilate the upper lobe is suggested by persistently low oxygen saturation

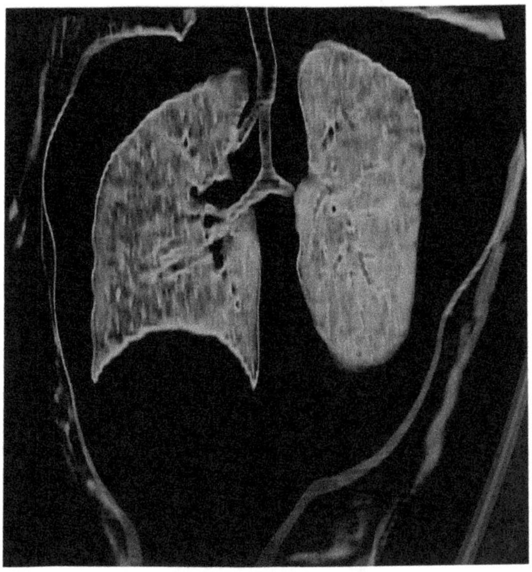

**Figure 30.5** Scan showing aberrant tracheal bronchus.

and is confirmed by failure to hear breath sounds at the lung apex. This is a particular problem on the right side because of the shorter distance between the carina and the origin of the upper-lobe bronchus or when a cuffed tube is used. Difficulty may also occur when selectively intubating the right main bronchus, as the upper lobe bronchus can arise at the carina or directly from the trachea (Figure 30.5). The right upper lobe bronchus arises from the trachea in pigs, and so-called 'pig bronchus' is a normal variant in up to 2% of humans.

Chest auscultation to check tube position is important after positioning for surgery is completed. Moving a child, especially a small infant, frequently disrupts what seemed to be perfect one-lung ventilation due to the tube moving very slightly. Loss of satisfactory OLV can also be due to failure to create an adequate seal in the bronchus with an uncuffed tube, leading to inadequate collapse of the operative lung. An alternative technique is to intubate the trachea with a cuffed tube, position the patient on the operating table and then use the bronchoscope to selectively intubate the appropriate bronchus. However, cuffed tubes are more prone to occluding the upper lobe bronchus and also may slip out of the bronchus. It is very important not to overinflate the cuff once placed in the bronchus, causing inadvertent damage. A disadvantage of selective bronchial intubation with a single lumen is the inability to deliver continuous positive airway pressure (CPAP) or suction down the operative lung.

## Balloon-Tipped Bronchial Blockers

Bronchial blockers can be used from the age of approximately 6 months to 8 years. They feature a balloon at their distal tip, which is passed under bronchoscopic guidance into the bronchus of the operative lung. It is then inflated under direct observation to ensure that an appropriate position and seal has been achieved, using the lowest balloon volume. The bronchial blocker is passed within (coaxial) or alongside (parallel to) a single-lumen TT. For the parallel technique, the bronchial blocker is first passed into the glottis followed by the TT.

Several balloon-tipped catheters have been described including vascular balloon catheters used off license. These include:

- Arndt blockers
- Uniblocker (Fuji systems)
- Vascular balloon catheters
    - Fogarty arterial embolectomy catheters
    - Miller atrioseptostomy catheters

### Arndt Blockers

Arndt bronchial blockers are the smallest commercially available devices and have the advantage of a nylon looped wire that slides over the bronchoscope to aid positioning (Figure 30.6). Once this wire is removed, it cannot be replaced (which may make repositioning more difficult). The Arndt catheter has a central lumen, allowing for CPAP and suctioning of the operative lung. The smallest Arndt catheter is 5 Fr, which has an outer diameter of 1.7 mm; for the bronchial blocker and bronchoscope to fit down the TT coaxially, the smallest TT for a 5 Fr Arndt catheter and a 2.2 bronchoscope would be a 4.5 mm, suitable for a two-year-old child:

$$(OD_{BB} + OD_{B})/ID_{TT} = (2.2 + 1.7)/4.5 = 0.86$$

A parallel insertion technique (alongside the TT) enables the use of bronchial blockers in smaller children. This technique can be used from the age of six months, with a 5 Fr Arndt catheter and a 3.5 microcuff TT.

### Uniblocker (Fuji Systems)

The Fuji Uniblocker is a stiff, polyurethane covered catheter with an angled tip. It is available

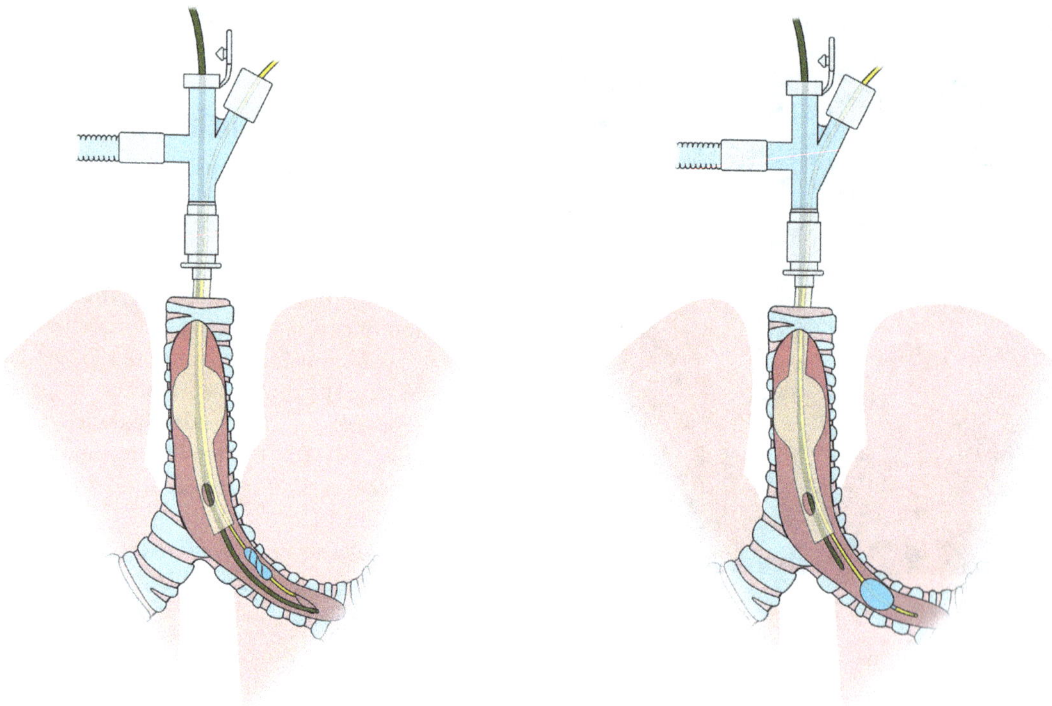

**Figure 30.6** Schematic diagram of coaxial Arndt bronchial blocker placement with multi-port airway adapter. The removable distal wire loop aids placement using a flexible bronchoscope passed down an ETT.

in 5 Fr, which can be used in children up to the age of about eight years. Unlike the Arndt blocker, it does not have a central channel for suctioning or CPAP delivery.

### Vascular Balloons

Although not designed as bronchial blockers, vascular balloon-tipped catheters have been used successfully for one-lung ventilation in paediatric patients. A commonly used catheter is the Fogarty arterial embolectomy catheter, in sizes 2 Fr to 5 Fr. All except the 2 Fr and 3 Fr catheters have a guidewire enabling the tip to be guided endobronchially. An alternative vascular balloon-tipped catheter is the 5 Fr Miller atrioseptostomy catheter, which has a pre-formed angled tip, aiding placement. Neither the Miller or Fogarty catheters have a central port for suction or CPAP.

Bronchial blockers designed for airway use (Arndt and Uniblocker) have high-volume, low-pressure balloons, thus minimising mucosal trauma, and should be used in preference to vascular balloon catheters which have high-pressure balloons. All balloons should be inflated under direct observation to minimise the volume used to produce an adequate bronchial seal.

The parallel technique may be easier when using a stiffer bronchial blocker with an angled tip, such as the Univent tube or vascular balloon catheters.

## Univent Tube

The Univent tube from Fuji Systems Corporation in Tokyo is a conventional tracheal tube with a second lumen dedicated to a bronchial blocker. As the second lumen is an integral part of the tube, displacement of the blocker is unlikely unless the tube itself is dislodged. If double-lung ventilation is required, the bronchial blocker can easily be withdrawn into its lumen. The second lumen reduces the cross-sectional area of the ventilating lumen, thus restricting the size of the bronchoscope that can be used to position the bronchial blocker. For paediatric use, the Univent tube is available in 3.5 and 4.5 mm ID. However, the Univent tube is bulky; the outer diameter of a 3.5 mm ID Univent tube has an external diameter similar to a 5.5–6.0 mm ID uncuffed tube. It is therefore only suitable for use from the age of about six years.

## Double-Lumen Tubes (DLT)

These entail two cuffed tubes of unequal length moulded together; the shorter tube sits in the trachea and the longer in the bronchus. Inflating the bronchial cuff allows diversion of ventilation to either lung, according to whether the bronchial or tracheal lumen is ventilated. The cuff protects each lung from contamination by infected debris or blood from the contralateral side. Insertion is performed via direct laryngoscopy; the DLT is advanced through the larynx, then rotated through 90° to the appropriate side, and the bronchial component is advanced into the corresponding bronchus. Use of a fibreoptic bronchoscope is very helpful in achieving successful placement. A DLT allows suction and the application of CPAP, thus improving oxygenation, to the operative side. Although bulky and rigid, there are few reports of airway trauma associated with their use.

DLTs are available in left- or right-sided tubes, although left-sided tubes are more frequently used to minimise occlusion of the right upper lobe bronchus. DLTs are of limited use in children, as the smallest available size is 26 Fr, which can be used from about the age of eight years. A helpful guide to size the correct DLT is:

$$\text{Size} = (\text{Age} \times 1.5) + 14.$$

Once the patients are fully grown, the correct-sized DLT is based on gender and height (Figure 30.7). Females who are <1.6 m require a 35 Fr DLT, whereas females >1.6 m are more suited to 37 Fr. In males who are <1.7 m, 39 Fr is usually appropriate, whilst males >1.7 m need a 41 Fr DLT.

## Indications for OLV

Single-lung ventilation is difficult to achieve in children and so should be justified in its use.

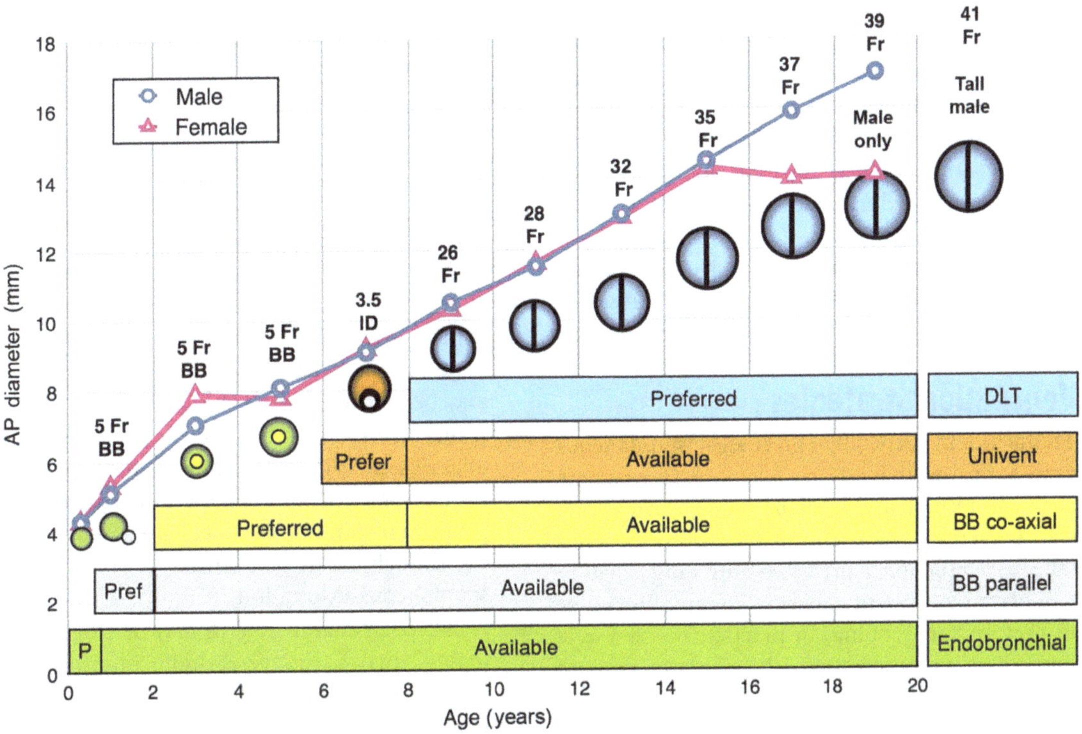


**Figure 30.7** Anteroposterior trachea diameter versus age for male and female paediatric patients. Trachea diameters are from cadaveric and radiologic studies. Male and female airway sizes are similar until 15 years of age, when the female trachea stops growing, but the male trachea continues to grow. Superimposed is the preferred airway device for lung isolation for a given age, placed on the graph at the given diameter of the device. Note that in order to use an airway device for a certain age, the diameter of that device must be smaller than the trachea AP diameter at that age. DLT = double-lumen tracheal tube; Univent = Fuji Univent tracheal tube; BB coaxial = bronchial blocker coaxial technique; BB parallel = bronchial blocker parallel technique; Endobronchial = endobrochial intubation with selective laser trabeculoplasty (SLT).

*Source:* Letal M, Theam M. Paediatric lung isolation. *BJA Education* 2017 February; 17(2):57–62. Reproduced with permission of Elsevier.

- Strong indication for OLV:
  - Major gas trapping in one lung or pleural space, such as bronchopleural fistula and congenital lobar emphysema
  - Lobectomy for bronchiectasis or similar need to prevent airway soiling by blood or infective material
  - Minimally invasive thoracic surgery
- Moderate indication for OLV:
  - Lobectomy or pneumonectomy for cystic malformations or tumour
  - Anterior spinal surgery
  - Oesophageal or aortic surgery
- Contraindication to OLV:
  - Unacceptable hypoxia after institution of OLV
  - Technical inability to isolate one lung safely

## Video-Assisted Thoracoscopic Surgery

As in other surgical specialties, minimally invasive thoracic surgery has gained increasing acceptance. Advantages including reduced pain and faster recovery. Surgical instrument development has enabled VATS even in neonates. Satisfactory surgical exposure requires distancing of the lung from the chest wall; carbon dioxide insufflation into the hemithorax can be used to achieve this, either alone or in combination with OLV. Care by the operator is required to avoid creating excessive intrapleural pressure and compromising venous return; insufflation pressure should be kept between 4 and 6 mbar.

## Ventilation Strategies

Thoracotomy generally precludes spontaneous ventilation, as there is an inability to generate negative intrapleural pressure, and mediastinal shift prevents lung expansion. Occasionally, spontaneous ventilation is preferred until lung isolation is achieved to prevent a tension pneumothorax, or to prevent gas trapping. In practice, this is rarely immediately problematic or life-threatening, and muscle relaxation and positive pressure ventilation are usually safe.

In severe congenital lobar emphysema, novel ventilatory modes may be needed to allow some exhalation. Trial and error may identify the best means of ventilating the child until the chest wall has been opened; in some instances, spontaneous ventilation may be maintained. To allow for adequate oxygenation in neonates with severe disease, extreme hypercapnia may need to be tolerated until the chest wall is opened, using a technique with a very slow respiratory rate and no PEEP. Haemodynamic compromise caused by mediastinal shift resolves instantly; the pleural space is opened and the hyperinflated lobe delivered through the chest wall. OLV may be impossible to achieve safely in cases presenting acutely because of hypoxia and distorted tracheobronchial anatomy. In asymptomatic cases, OLV prevents or, at worst, reduces gas trapping in the emphysematous lobe caused by the instigation of positive pressure ventilation.

During surgery, ventilation is tailored to the individual patient and may require unusual settings. Modified ventilatory strategies to optimise exhalation may be required. The whole surgical team should be aware of the need for either urgent pleural drainage or thoracotomy. A modern ventilator offering spirometry is useful; manual ventilation may be necessary in small infants. Permissive hypercapnia may be prudent. A sudden change in compliance may reflect either surgical manipulation or tube displacement, and dialogue between surgeon and anaesthetist is essential. End-tidal capnography may underestimate $PaCO_2$, particularly if OLV is used.

## Pleural Drainsrains

There are three important components to a pleural drain:

- A tube. This should be large enough. Small drains are adequate for gas, but larger drains may be required for fluid, blood or pus.
- A one-way valve is required (usually an underwater seal). This allows expulsion of air during spontaneous expiration or positive pressure inspiration and prevents re-entry of air through the drain during spontaneous inspiration.
- A collecting chamber. This may be single, or the unit may have several drains in series to prevent increased resistance to drainage as fluid levels increase.

Suction applied to the collecting chamber increases the pressure gradient between pleural space and collecting chamber. Bilateral pleural drains should not be connected to the same suction source lest differential resistance to drainage results in mediastinal shift. Pleural drains should not be clamped or inadvertently occluded, especially in patients receiving positive pressure ventilation – failure to drain pleural air can quickly cause a tension pneumothorax. A drain connected to a suction unit with the suction turned off has the same effect as clamping the drain. Stopping suction on a pleural drain requires disconnection from the suction unit.

## Regional Anaesthesia

Epidural analgesia has traditionally been seen as the gold standard for thoracic surgery due to its role in attenuating the stress response and providing optimal postoperative analgesia. Other regional techniques are increasingly being used (e.g. paravertebral, erector spinae plane blocks) that have fewer limitations and improved safety profiles. Neuraxial block performed under US guidance is becoming more common in children and may improve safe insertion of epidurals. Multiple epidural techniques are used.

### Epidural

Thoracic epidural can be provided either by a catheter inserted at the level of the operation, or, in smaller children, it may be threaded up the epidural space after caudal insertion. The aim is for the catheter tip to lie in close proximity to the spinal segment of the corresponding surgical incision, thus using lower infusion rates of local anaesthetic than a more distant catheter. Epidural analgesia requires careful postoperative supervision.

### Paravertebral Block

Paravertebral blocks (PVBs) are well established in adult thoracic surgery as they provide good intra- and postoperative analgesia and have been shown to be a safe and effective method of pain relief in children. PVBs are performed under ultrasound guidance, unilaterally or bilaterally, using either single-shot or a continuous infusion catheter technique. PVBs cover up to four dermatomal levels, so multilevel injections may be required, particularly to cover for chest drain insertion. For a thoracotomy, needle insertion should be at the level of T6. Under US guidance, the caudad and cephalad spread can be accessed by scanning in a paramedian longitudinal plane. A dose of 0.5 ml $kg^{-1}$ for children usually covers four dermatomes, with an infusion rate of 0.2 ml $kg^{-1}h^{-1}$.

A catheter may be inserted into the paravertebral space for continuous postoperative analgesia, which has been shown to be an effective and safe method of post-thoracotomy pain relief. The catheter can be inserted under either US guidance or by the surgeon under direct vision. Unlike the epidural space, there are no opiate receptors in the paravertebral space, so additives to the local anaesthetic can be used, such as clonidine.

### Erector Spinae Plane Block

Erector spinae plane block (ESPB) is a fascial plane block, where local anesthetic is placed between the erector spinae muscle and transverse process. Although relatively recently described, it has been shown to be safe, effective and easy to perform, with potentially fewer complications of neuraxial injury and pneumothorax than epidural and paravertebral blocks. ESPBs have a larger dermatomal spread than PVBs, with a dose of 0.1ml $kg^{-1}$ required per dermatome. The local anaesthetic spreads anteriorly to the dorsal and ventral rami and may reach the epidural space. Analgesia has been shown to last up to 12 hours, and this can be extended by the placement of an erector spinae catheter.

A further advantage of ESPBs is the possibility of performing the block in anticoagulated patients, as any haematoma formed will be superficial and compressible.

### Serratus Anterior Plane Block

Although serratus anterior plane block (SAPB) provides safe and effective analgesia after thoracic surgery, there is increasing evidence that ESPB provides superior analgesia and longer duration of action.

### Intercostal Nerve Blocks

Intercostal nerve blocks may provide satisfactory intraoperative analgesia, but their use is limited due to a brief analgesic effect. They are easy to perform, with or without ultrasound or under direct vision at the time of surgery.

## Postoperative Management and Analgesia

Children undergoing intrathoracic surgery require admission to a high-dependency unit postoperatively, and adequate provision must be made for pain management, chest physiotherapy and non-invasive CPAP. Full ventilatory support is sometimes necessary, and paediatric intensive care facilities must be available.

Thoracic surgery is extremely painful, so effective pain management is an essential part of the perioperative pathway of these children. Insufficient analgesia prevents coughing, deep breathing and mobilisation, increasing the risk of respiratory complications.

Post-thoracotomy pain is multi-factorial, with nociceptive and neuropathic pain arising from both somatic and visceral afferents. Successful postoperative pain management strategies must therefore be multimodal. Intra- and postoperative analgesia for thoracotomy requires a combination of regional anaesthetic technique with systemic analgesia, both opioid and non-steroidal. The choice of technique is influenced by the age of the child, the underlying pathological process and the preference and experience of the anaesthetist.

## Systemic Analgesia

Opioid infusion, preferably with patient-controlled or nurse-controlled boluses, is essential for the first 48 hours after thoracotomy. This is required in addition to any single-shot regional techniques, due to a mean duration of thoracic blocks of 10–12 hours. Both regular paracetamol and NSAIDs should also be prescribed as their effect is additive. Good analgesia allows early mobilisation and helps to prevent problems with sputum retention.

NMDA-receptor antagonists, such as ketamine and magnesium sulphate, can be used intraoperatively to reduce postoperative opioid consumption. Dexamethasone, 0.15 mg $kg^{-1}$, should also be administered for both its antiemetic and analgesic enhancing properties.

### Key Points

- Surgical access to the operative lung can be facilitated by ventilating only the dependent lung, allowing the operative lung to collapse. In small children, this is hard to achieve, as double-lumen tubes are only available for children over the age of 8–10 years.
- Anaesthetising a child with an anterior mediastinal mass can precipitate total airway collapse. It may be necessary to insert a rigid bronchoscope to maintain an airway.
- In the infant with congenital lobar emphysema, positive pressure ventilation can lead to acute hyperinflation of the affected lobe with severe respiratory and haemodynamic compromise. It may be necessary to try various ventilatory strategies to identify the best means of ventilating the child until the chest wall has been opened.
- Thoracic surgery can be very painful. Regional and local analgesia should be employed wherever possible, supplemented by patient- or nurse-controlled morphine infusion and regular paracetamol and NSAIDs.

## Further Reading


Hammer G. Single-lung ventilation in infants and children. *Paediatric Anaesthesia* 2004; 14:98–102.

Letal M, Theam M. Paediatric lung isolation. *BJA Education.* 2017 February; 17(2):57–62.

Semmelmann A, Kaltofen H, Loop T. Anesthesia of thoracic surgery in children. *Paediatric Anaesthesia* 2018 April; 28 (4):326–31.

Templeton TW, Piccioni F, Chatterjee D. An update on one-lung ventilation in children. *Anesthesia and Analgesia* 2021 May 1; 132(5):1389–99.

Wilmott RW, Bush A, Deterding R et al. *Kendig's Disorders of the Respiratory Tract in Children*, 9th ed. Elsevier. 2019.

Chapter

# 31 Anaesthesia for Cardiac Surgery in Children

Lucy Hepburn and Kyrie Wheeler

## Introduction

Most children presenting for paediatric cardiac surgery have congenital heart disease (CHD), the incidence of which is around eight per 1,000 live births (see Table 31.1). Without surgical intervention, around 50% of children with CHD would die during childhood, but with improvements in care almost all now survive to adulthood. Acquired diseases are rare but include endocarditis, intracardiac masses and cardiomyopathies. Children with cardiomyopathy present an increasing need for anaesthesia, for instance, for insertion of mechanical support devices, pacing or defibrillator devices or cardiac transplantation.

Approximately 3,600 paediatric cardiac surgical procedures are carried out annually in the United Kingdom, 20% of which are undertaken in neonates. Most are performed via sternotomy using cardiopulmonary bypass (CPB). Technological advances and miniaturisation of bypass circuits mean it is now feasible to undertake complex cardiac repairs in infants under 2 kg. A smaller proportion of procedures are carried out without bypass via a thoracotomy approach, such as creation of systemic to pulmonary artery (PA) shunts, ligation of patent ductus arteriosus (PDA) or simple coarctation repair.

**Table 31.1** Congenital cardiac lesions and their frequency

| Lesion | Frequency (%) |
|---|---|
| Ventricular septal defect | 17 |
| Tetralogy of Fallot | 12 |
| Transposition of the great arteries | 11 |
| Coarctation of the aorta | 11 |
| Atrial septal defect | 10 |
| Hypoplastic left-heart syndrome | 5 |
| Atrioventricular septal defect | 3 |
| Pulmonary atresia | 1 |

Paediatric cardiac surgery may aim to be *corrective*, such as ventricular septal defect (VSD) repair, or *palliative*, such as establishment of a stable single-ventricle circulation or valvotomy for valvular stenosis. Staged surgery at different ages is necessary for complex palliative procedures. CPB is also used for non-cardiac surgery, such as complex tracheal repairs or to facilitate removal of tumours adjacent to the heart or major vessels. Owing to greater long-term survival in children with cardiac disorders, there is an increasing need for expertise in the field of adult congenital heart disease (ACHD). This chapter will cover the principles of anaesthesia for cardiac surgery in children.

## Overview of Surgery for Congenital Heart Defects

It is essential that the anaesthetist has a clear understanding of the anatomy and haemodynamic consequences of any cardiac lesion. A useful classification of CHD is shown in Table 31.2. Each condition may vary widely in severity, with substantial differences in the physiological and haemodynamic consequences.

*Children with inadequate pulmonary blood flow* ('right-to-left' shunting) are cyanosed at birth. Tetralogy of Fallot (ToF) is the most common example and may vary widely in severity. Occasionally infants with ToF require a systemic to PA shunt (modified Blalock–Taussig shunt, or mBTS; see Figure 31.1), but more often early complete surgical repair is possible. Conditions such as pulmonary stenosis may be amenable to valvuloplasty by cardiac catheterisation or surgical intervention. In some cases, obstruction to pulmonary flow is so severe that pulmonary blood flow is maintained from the aorta via the arterial duct ('duct-dependent pulmonary circulation'). An infusion of prostaglandin will be required to keep the duct open prior to surgery or catheter intervention.

*Children with increased pulmonary blood flow* ('left-to-right' shunting) suffer from cardiac failure. Cardiac failure is managed with diuretics until the child has grown enough to allow full surgical correction. Left untreated, excessive pulmonary flow will lead to irreversible pulmonary hypertension. If cardiac failure cannot be controlled medically, or early surgical repair is not feasible, PA banding may occasionally be required to reduce pulmonary blood flow. PA banding is usually undertaken via sternotomy, without CPB, and involves placing a band around the main PA to restrict pulmonary flow. The band is adjusted to reduce PA pressure distal to the band to about half systemic pressure. Oxygen saturation will generally fall to around 85%. The PA band is removed when definitive surgery is undertaken.

*Children with abnormal connections and complex shunting* may have a variable combination of cyanosis and heart failure and usually require major surgery involving CPB in the neonatal period. Infants with hypoplastic left-heart syndrome (HLHS) have a single effective ventricle and 'duct-dependent systemic circulation', with blood flow to the distal aorta from the PA via the arterial duct. In transposition of the great arteries (TGA), adequate mixing between systemic and pulmonary circulations may require the duct to be patent. Prostaglandin infusion will be required in both cases prior to surgery or catheter intervention. Infants with total anomalous pulmonary venous drainage (TAPVD) have pulmonary venous return to the right atrium. In 'supracardiac TAPVD', this may be via an abnormal bridging vein in the thorax, and if there is no obstruction to venous return, it may not be

**Table 31.2** Classification of cardiac surgical disorders

| Category | Specific condition |
|---|---|
| Inadequate pulmonary blood flow (right-to-left shunting) | Pulmonary atresia<br>Pulmonary stenosis<br>Tetralogy of Fallot |
| Excessive pulmonary blood flow (left-to-right shunting) | Patent ductus arteriosus<br>Atrial septal defect<br>Ventricular septal defect<br>Atrioventricular septal defect<br>Aortopulmonary window |
| Abnormal connections (complex shunting) | Tricuspid atresia<br>Transposition of the great arteries<br>Hypoplastic left-heart syndrome<br>Truncus arteriosus<br>Total anomalous pulmonary venous connection |
| Left-ventricular outflow tract obstruction | Aortic coarctation<br>Hypertrophic obstructive cardiomyopathy<br>Aortic stenosis<br>Interrupted aortic arch |

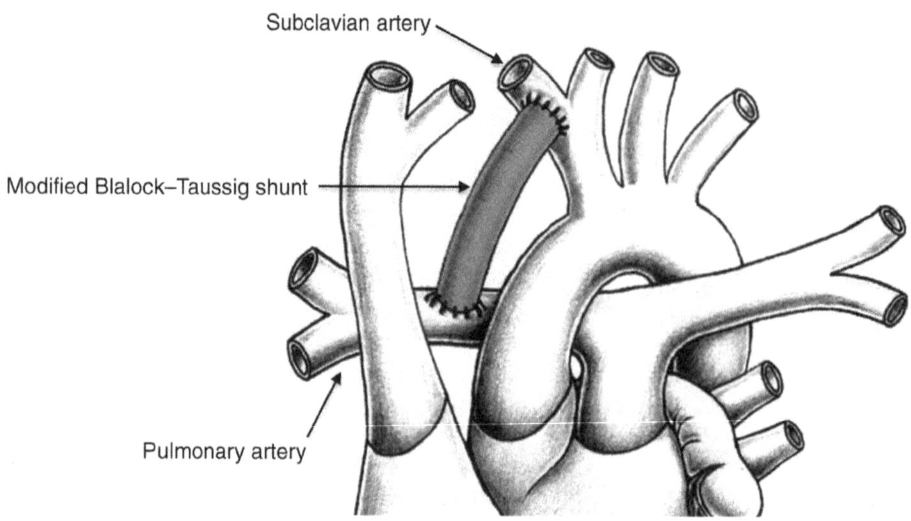


**Figure 31.1** Modified Blalock–Tausig shunt.
*Source:* The PedHeart Resource (www. HeartPassport.com). Courtesy of Scientific Software Solutions, Inc.

detected immediately. In 'infracardiac TAPVD', the pulmonary veins drain into the inferior vena cava (IVC), usually via the hepatic veins. This invariably causes significant pulmonary venous obstruction and requires urgent surgery immediately after birth to maintain oxygenation and cardiac output. The presence of engorged pulmonary veins and profound hypoxaemia may occasionally lead to a misdiagnosis of meconium aspiration syndrome or persistent pulmonary hypertension of the newborn. Obstructed TAPVD may be associated with postoperative pulmonary hypertension.

*Obstructive lesions of the left ventricle* frequently result in left-ventricular hypertrophy and increase in myocardial oxygen demand. Patients are at risk of acute myocardial ischaemia if oxygen demand is further increased by tachycardia or if coronary perfusion pressure falls during anaesthesia. Patients with Williams syndrome and supra-aortic stenosis are particularly challenging and have a high risk of perioperative sudden death. Babies with lesions such as critical aortic stenosis, interrupted aortic arch or severe coarctation may have duct-dependent systemic perfusion and require prostaglandin prior to surgery in the neonatal period.

## Preoperative Assessment and Preparation for Anaesthesia

Successful anaesthesia for CHD surgery requires a meticulous, anticipative approach that starts in the preoperative period. Key features of preoperative assessment include:

- Understanding the anatomy, physiology and haemodynamics of the presenting disorder
- Understanding the proposed surgical procedure, and the consequences of any previous and future surgery
- Determining the clinical condition of the child, particularly cardiac function
- Anticipating the effect of anaesthesia on the circulation

The following considerations are of particular importance:

- *Is the circulation 'duct dependent' or shunt dependent?* For infants with duct-dependent systemic or pulmonary circulation or an mBTs, it is important that the shunt remains patent and that flow through the shunt is 'balanced', meaning that systemic and pulmonary artery blood flow are equal. This balance is determined by systemic vascular resistance (SVR) in relation to pulmonary vascular resistance (PVR). It is important to minimise changes to this balance, including during transport. Oxygen is a potent pulmonary vasodilator, and $FiO_2$ may need to be restricted to room air in some cases.
- *What is the degree of cyanosis?* Children with cyanotic CHD presenting for surgery may be profoundly desaturated, with polycythaemia and coagulopathy. Identification of current anticoagulation therapy, need for perioperative transfusion and expectation of pre- and postoperative haematocrit requirements should be considered.
- *Is myocardial function impaired?* In some lesions, such as cardiomyopathy, there can be severely impaired left-ventricular function. Some patients may already be on inotropic support. The degree of dysfunction is inferred from the ejection fraction (EF) assessed by echocardiography. EF of less than 30% is indicative of poor systolic function. Obstructive lesions may lead to diastolic dysfunction as well as increased metabolic demand.
- *Is there significant pulmonary hypertension?* If so, any hypoxaemia or hypercapnia during induction and intubation will be poorly tolerated. If the right ventricle is significantly hypertrophied or dilated and distorts the left ventricle, systemic hypotension may compromise coronary artery perfusion, rapidly leading to loss of cardiac output. Pulmonary hypertension is a significant cause of anaesthesia-related mortality in children.
- *Is there a septal defect?* If present, it is important to ensure no air bubbles enter the venous system as this can lead to cerebral air emboli, particularly with right-to-left shunting. All infusion lines must be checked meticulously.
- *What is the patient's surgical history?* If there has been a previous sternotomy, there may be fibrous adhesion of the heart to the back of the sternum with the risk of inadvertent injury and significant bleeding during re-sternotomy. This can be a particular problem if there is an

artificial conduit sitting on the front of the heart. During briefing for repeat sternotomy, the anticipated site of emergency cannulation for femoral or jugular bypass should be discussed with the operating surgeon. This has implications for placement of anaesthetic monitoring lines.
- *Is there an existing shunt?* Arterial pressure monitoring can be inaccurate if placed in the same arm as an mBTS.
- *Is there a pacemaker or implantable cardioverter defibrillator (ICD) in place?* It is important to understand the underlying rhythm disturbance. It may be necessary to re-program a pacemaker to fixed pacing mode or disable the ICD before cautery can be used safely.
- *Is intercurrent illness present?* CHD with high pulmonary blood flow can lead to increased susceptibility to chest infections. Undergoing CPB with an acute respiratory tract infection may result in significant postoperative morbidity and increased ICU stay. It can be difficult to differentiate between acute upper-respiratory tract infection and heart failure in some symptomatic children. The decision to proceed with surgery needs to be considered on an individual basis; delay of elective surgery is usually indicated in the presence of fever or an elevated white cell count, but a mild cough or runny nose is generally not a reason to cancel surgery.
- *Medications.* Some children will be dependent on prostaglandin infusion or inotropic support, and it is important these are not interrupted. Others may be on anti-failure medication such as diuretics or captopril. Some children with ToF who suffer from severe hypercyanotic 'tet' spells may be receiving propranolol. A few may be receiving some form of anticoagulant therapy such as warfarin or anti-platelet drugs. It is advisable to continue most medications as close to the time of anaesthesia as possible, particularly anticoagulation in infants who are shunt dependent, or any therapies for pulmonary hypertension.
- *Laboratory investigations.* Chronic cyanosis can result in polycythaemia and coagulopathy. Thrombocytopenia and clotting factor deficiency may be present. Children taking diuretics or in severe cardiac failure may have metabolic derangements such as hypokalaemia.
- *Fasting time* is of particular importance in infants dependent on a small shunt, particularly if polycythaemic. Prolonged starvation leads to dehydration, hyperviscosity and potential shunt thrombosis. Clear fluids should be given until one hour before surgery, ideally continuously via a nasogastric tube, and IV fluids should be started if there is uncertainty about theatre time.

Preparation should begin well in advance of surgery to allow time for understanding of the condition and to answer questions from the family. Discussion should include details of anaesthesia procedures, including induction technique; invasive monitoring (including potential complications); postoperative analgesia; and intensive care pathways. The last should cover duration of postoperative ICU stay and potential cardiorespiratory support, including mechanical circulatory support where relevant. Sedative premedication and topical analgesia should be prescribed as necessary.

## Induction of Anaesthesia

Haemodynamic stability is the goal in the anaesthetic room. Essential monitoring (ECG, audible pulse oximetry and blood pressure) should be started before induction of anaesthesia. In some children, this may be poorly accepted but should be applied at the earliest opportunity. Ideally intravenous access should be obtained before induction; however, this is not always achievable, in which case it should be established as soon as is feasible after loss of consciousness.

Sevoflurane is widely used for inhalational induction and is generally very safe. Uptake of anaesthetic agents from the lungs is slowed in the presence of a large right-to-left shunt, although this is rarely of practical significance. Importantly, any relative overdose of agent will be equally slow to reverse.

For most patients, there is no definite advantage of one intravenous induction agent over another. All anaesthetic agents have haemodynamic effects and should be used with caution. Propofol is suitable if ventricular function is good but should be avoided where a fall in SVR or diastolic pressure must be avoided.

When ventricular function is poor, intravenous induction can be very challenging:

- *Ketamine* is a direct myocardial depressant, but it usually maintains or increases blood pressure, heart rate and cardiac output via sympathomimetic stimulation. It is a commonly used agent particularly when it is important to avoid a fall in SVR. However, in patients who may be surviving on maximal sympathomimetic drive, such as those with significant impairment of myocardial function, ketamine's unopposed depressant action may lead to a profound fall in cardiac output.
- *Fentanyl* is perceived to be a cardiostable agent but may have detrimental cardiac effects in patients whose cardiac output is maintained by sympathomimetic drive as it suppresses the stress response effectively, which can lead to a fall in blood pressure. Fentanyl also reduces heart rate, an important component in maintaining cardiac output in infants, but may be beneficial where tachycardia is detrimental.
- *Etomidate* has negligible effect on myocardial contractility or blood pressure and is a good agent for patients with very limited myocardial reserve, noting concerns about short-term adrenal suppression and pain on injection.

For patients with very poor myocardial function and low cardiac output, such as those presenting for heart transplantation, it is important to remember:

- Circulation times are slowed, so drug effect may be delayed.
- There is preferential blood supply to key organs such as the brain so smaller induction doses are needed.

*The following is the authors' preferred means of induction in high-risk patients:* a small dose of fentanyl (0.5–1.0 mcg $kg^{-1}$ IV) is followed by slow increments of midazolam 50 mcg $kg^{-1}$ IV over 10–15 minutes until the patient is having difficulty keeping their eyes open. At this point, ketamine 0.25–0.5 mg $kg^{-1}$ is administered in boluses followed by the muscle relaxant. Blood pressure should be measured at short intervals throughout induction with close attention to any ECG changes.

Pancuronium is commonly used in cardiac anaesthesia because of its long duration of action. Its modest increase in heart rate is beneficial in opposing the reduced heart rate commonly seen with fentanyl and sevoflurane induction in infants, but it should be avoided where a tachycardia may be detrimental, such as infants with poor cardiac function. Vecuronium and rocuronium are good alternatives, with no impact on heart rate.

When inducing anaesthesia in a child with a shunt or duct-dependent circulation, 'balance' of both pulmonary and systemic circulations must be maintained. In patients with pulmonary-to-systemic shunting, injudicious use of anaesthetic agents may drop SVR, favouring systemic perfusion at the expense of pulmonary blood flow, which may precipitate profound hypoxaemia, bradycardia and cardiac arrest. Conversely, administration of high inspired oxygen concentration or over-ventilation must be avoided in patients with duct- or shunt-dependent systemic perfusion. A fall in PVR will increase pulmonary blood flow at the expense of systemic blood flow. This may lead to poor coronary and end-organ perfusion and could lead to cardiac arrest. Maintaining a higher PVR with low $FiO_2$ will provide adequate flow to the systemic circulation. For many of these patients, oxygen saturation around 80% represents an appropriate balance.

## Maintenance of Anaesthesia

Anaesthesia for CPB surgery is patient-specific but can be institutionally guided. It is acceptable to use a combination of moderate dose opioid, typically fentanyl 15–30 mcg $kg^{-1}$, combined with a volatile agent such as sevoflurane in air or an air/oxygen mix. Nitrous oxide may be used during inhalational induction but should be avoided for maintenance of anaesthesia. In neonates and small infants, volatile agents can cause a profound reduction in blood pressure and cardiac output, and it may be preferable to limit their dose and use higher doses of fentanyl instead. In older children, isoflurane and sevoflurane both cause only a modest fall in SVR and blood pressure at 1–1.5 MAC and are widely used; in these children and those with an anticipated 'fast-track' recovery, excess opioid can and should be avoided. Continuous infusions of propofol or dexmedetomidine are increasingly used and are safe unless cardiac function is very poor.

Regional analgesia in the form of ultrasound-guided paravertebral block (as a single shot or catheter infusion) is opioid-sparing and has gained popularity for its potential in enhanced recovery.

Antibiotic prophylaxis is essential; the choice of antibiotics is guided by institutional protocols and should be administered in the 30-minute period before skin incision.

## Monitoring

ECG, pulse oximetry, capnography and invasive arterial and central venous pressure monitoring are required for all cardiac cases. End-tidal $CO_2$ measurement can be inaccurate in patients with cyanotic CHD and can be up to 2 kPa lower than arterial $pCO_2$ but provides essential confirmation of tracheal tube placement and a useful trend of ventilation. Non-invasive blood pressure monitoring should be used whilst arterial access is being achieved. A urinary catheter should be placed in all patients undergoing CPB.

Invasive arterial and central venous lines must be secure and reliable and should be placed under full aseptic conditions using ultrasound guidance. For CPB cases, it is customary to insert a multi-lumen central venous line in addition to a peripheral line. In most cases, this will be via the internal jugular or femoral vein. Thrombosis of central veins is an unfortunate complication of central venous cannulation in small infants. In neonates with univentricular physiology where cavopulmonary connections will be necessary later, such as those with HLHS, it may be preferable to avoid the internal jugular veins if possible, as SVC thrombosis will compromise subsequent successful repair. An umbilical catheter may be in place in newborn infants. Femoral and iliac thrombosis is a common finding after central venous catheters have been placed for even short periods, and the anaesthetist should be mindful of future surgery and catheter interventions when deciding line insertion sites.

Where central venous access is technically difficult, the external jugular vein can be used for pressure monitoring and to provide access for administration of drugs. Rarely, it may be necessary to start surgery with peripheral access only; a direct transthoracic right-atrial line can be placed by the surgeon once the chest is open, which can be used for drug infusions whilst the atrium is closed.

Arterial access is usually via the radial, femoral or occasionally the axillary artery. The smaller peripheral arteries are sometimes used but may become 'shutdown' and display an artificially low pressure as the patient is cooled. It is best to avoid the ipsilateral upper limb if an mBTS is present or planned, as it is likely to under-read the true pressure. It is important to place the arterial line in the right arm during non-CPB coarctation repair, as the surgeon will clamp the aortic arch proximal to the origin of the left-subclavian artery during repair. Clinicians and families should be aware of the risks of limb ischaemia, and limbs should carefully monitored after a vessel has been cannulated, especially in neonates.

Core (usually nasopharyngeal) and peripheral temperature monitors should be placed in all cases. Core temperature is essential for the conduct of CPB and is also important to ensure mild hypothermia prior to clamping the aorta during coarctation repair.

*Transoesophageal echocardiography (TOE)* offers great advantages perioperatively, allowing confirmation of the diagnosis, detection of a small patent foramen ovale (PFO) not seen on transthoracic echo, detection of air within the heart after cardiotomy and assessment of surgical repair and ventricular function. There are now probes suitable for neonates (3–4 kg), although care must be taken to avoid cardiorespiratory compromise due to compression by the probe. TOE may be undertaken by a suitably trained cardiologist or anaesthetist. It is important that an 'anaesthetic' TOE operator is not also solely responsible for the anaesthesia. If TOE cannot be used, epicardial echocardiography is often employed whilst the chest remains open in the immediate post-CPB period.

*Near-infrared spectroscopy (NIRS)* provides a measure of cerebral and somatic oximetry as a function of regional blood flow. Cerebral NIRS can be useful in monitoring changes in cerebral perfusion related to CPB and to malposition of the CPB cannulae. Use of NIRS has become routine in recent years, although long-term outcome data are not yet available.

## The Pre-bypass Period

For sternotomy, the patient is placed in the supine position with the arms by the sides and a small roll under the shoulders to bring the sternum forward. All lines, monitors and the catheter should be secured, labelled and accessible. Passive cooling is allowed before bypass.

Sternotomy is very stimulating, and adequate opioid, regional and/or volatile anaesthetic is required to blunt a hypertensive response. Following sternotomy, anaesthesia requirements are reduced. Lung compliance usually increases following sternotomy, and ventilatory parameters should be monitored. Haemodynamic instability can occur during mediastinal dissection due to manipulation of the great vessels, impaired venous return, arrhythmias, bleeding or labile pulmonary vascular resistance. Particular vigilance is required if there is a shunt or duct-dependent circulation, as distortion may interfere with pulmonary or systemic perfusion, and it may be necessary to ask the surgeon to pause to allow recovery.

Prior to CPB, heparin is administered (400 IU $kg^{-1}$) to prevent clotting of the extracorporeal circuit, a bolus (dose dependent on circuit size) is also added into the CPB circuit. Heparin should always be administered into a secure line. The adequacy of heparinisation is checked after two to three minutes, usually by the activated clotting time (ACT), which should be above 400 seconds.

## Cardiopulmonary Bypass

It is important for anaesthetists to understand the principles of CPB, although in many centres the responsibility for running bypass during surgery falls to the surgeon and the perfusionist. In some centres, the anaesthetist may also be involved in running the bypass. CPB requires drainage of the systemic venous return from the patient and, following oxygenation, return via a cannula placed in the ascending aorta. The aortic cannula is placed first, and its correct placement within the lumen of the aorta is vital; this is checked by reading the arterial pressure from the CPB whilst testing the line. NIRS may demonstrate a fall in cerebral oxygenation on the rare occasion that the cannula tip is misplaced.

Unlike most adult cardiac cases where a single venous cannula is placed in the right atrium, paediatric CPB usually requires separate venous cannulae in the SVC and IVC to allow intracardiac surgery to be conducted via the right atrium. If there is an additional major source of venous drainage to the heart, such as a left-sided SVC, this may also need to be cannulated. Venous return to the bypass circuit is usually passive and requires appropriately sized cannulae to ensure complete emptying of the heart. CVP should fall to near zero. A vacuum can be added to the CPB if required to facilitate venous drainage. An advantage of measuring CVP in the internal jugular vein is that obstruction to cerebral venous return by the SVC cannula will be apparent. NIRS may also detect a fall in cerebral blood flow.

Once the cannulae are secured, the surgeon instructs the perfusionist to start bypass. Often this may start with just one venous cannula in place. Lung ventilation is continued until both cannulae are in place and the patient is at predicted 'full flow'.

The blood concentration of drugs such as fentanyl will fall substantially on initiation of CPB due to haemodilution and adsorption of the drug to the CPB circuit, so it is usual to give a supplementary bolus of fentanyl immediately before CPB. A volatile agent is administered into the CPB sweep gas by the perfusionist to maintain anaesthesia during CPB. Hypothermia reduces the MAC of volatile agents and metabolism of drugs, so these measures are usually sufficient to maintain adequate anaesthesia. In children in whom CPB is conducted at only mild hypothermia, a hypnotic agent such as midazolam or a propofol infusion may be administered to minimise the risk of awareness.

Blood flow on CPB is non-pulsatile, with flow rates generally around 3 l $min^{-1}m^{-2}$. The perfusionist will use blood gas parameters, venous oxygen saturation levels and NIRS to monitor adequacy of perfusion.

Mean blood pressure on CPB is generally maintained at around 35–60 mmHg. The pressure often falls on institution of CPB due to haemodilution and vasodilation, but this is corrected by the perfusionist within a few minutes. If there is a PDA or an mBTS, this will need to be ligated to prevent flow into the lungs. Other sources of arterial runoff and low pressure, such as aorto-pulmonary collaterals, can be more difficult to manage. If blood pressure remains low, it may be necessary to give a vasoconstrictor such as phenylephrine. NIRS may be useful in monitoring adequacy of cerebral perfusion on CPB. Haematocrit is normally maintained at around 20–25% on CPB; increasing this may also improve blood pressure and cerebral oxygenation.

Many operations are performed with core temperature between 30°C and 34°C to reduce systemic and cerebral metabolic demands, although there is an increasing trend to undertake surgery at near normal temperature. For longer, more complex procedures, the temperature may be reduced to 25–30°C. Some surgery requires hypothermia to 18°C to allow total cessation of bypass. This is known as deep hypothermic circulatory arrest (DHCA) and is discussed in the next subsection.

For many paediatric cardiac procedures, it is necessary to stop the heart by administering a cardioplegia solution into the aortic root. The aorta is cross-clamped to ensure the potassium-containing solution is forced into the coronary arteries. Traditionally this solution was cooled to around 4°C to assist myocardial preservation, but warm blood cardioplegia solutions are increasingly used. Cardioplegia is important for myocardial preservation and is usually repeated every 15–20 minutes. Occasionally, if the procedure is likely to be very short, the heart is fibrillated to prevent ejection and the risk of air embolism whilst repair is undertaken.

## Deep Hypothermic Circulatory Arrest

If surgery is required on the aortic arch or head and neck vessels, and in some other complex repairs, the patient is cooled to 15–18°C and the circulation stopped to allow the aortic cannula to be removed. At least 20 minutes of cooling should occur before the circulation is stopped. Ice packs should be applied to the head to aid brain cooling. It is difficult to quantify the long-term impact of this technique on neurodevelopmental outcome, but DHCA times of greater than 40 minutes are associated with an increased risk of cerebral injury. Because of this risk, some centres use selective cerebral perfusion during DHCA. After the circulation is restarted, an adequate period of re-perfusion and re-warming is required before ending bypass.

## Discontinuing Bypass

Once the surgical repair is completed the patient is rewarmed to 36°C in preparation for coming off CPB. Electrolytes, particularly potassium and calcium, are corrected by the perfusionist. Ultrafiltration may be used to raise the haematocrit above 30%.

The trachea should be suctioned before restarting ventilation and adequacy of ventilation confirmed. Unless there is a physiological contraindication, ventilation is initially with high inspired oxygen and low-dose volatile agent. The volatile can then be increased and inspired oxygen reduced depending upon the haemodynamic and ventilatory parameters after successfully discontinuing CPB.

CPB causes a variable degree of myocardial dysfunction, so it is common to start an inotropic infusion before coming off bypass. Choice of inotrope varies according to local practice and preference and may need to be adjusted post-CPB to address any particular haemodynamic issues. Rhythm disturbances should also be addressed, and it may be necessary to pace the heart to ensure an adequate heart rate, preferably with atrioventricular synchrony. Transoesophageal echocardiography is useful to assess ventricular function and identify any air in the left side of the heart.

If cardiac output or blood pressure is unsatisfactory, it may be necessary to go back on CPB to allow the myocardium time to recover, resolve rhythm disturbances, increase inotropic support or review the surgical repair. Acute rhythm disturbance and ventricular dysfunction are occasionally due to air emboli in the coronary arteries. This is associated with acute ECG changes and usually resolves over a short period. Increasing the blood pressure with an inotropic agent to improve coronary perfusion may be beneficial.

## Modified Ultrafiltration

After successful separation from CPB, some patients will undergo modified ultrafiltration (MUF). This reduces total body water, raises haematocrit and mean arterial pressure and removes inflammatory cytokines. MUF returns warm, 'haemoconcentrated' oxygenated blood into the right side of the heart and can lower pulmonary vascular resistance and attenuate pulmonary hypertension.

## Protamine Administration and Management of Coagulopathy

Protamine is administered to reverse heparinisation once the patient is stable and further bypass runs are unlikely. It is important for the anaesthetist to check that the perfusionist has discontinued the CPB pump suckers before administering protamine, to avoid clotting the circuit. Protamine is infused slowly at a dose of 3–4 mg $kg^{-1}$. Protamine is given slowly, as it can cause increased PVR seen as a temporary reduction in lung compliance and possible hypoxaemia, followed by hypotension.

This is usually short-lived but may require treatment with adrenaline and increased ventilatory support.

Heparin reversal is assessed by checking that the ACT has returned to baseline. Persistent prolongation of the ACT may be caused by residual heparinisation or coagulopathy from any cause (e.g. platelet dysfunction, low fibrinogen). Infusions of platelets, cryoprecipitate or plasma may be required, particularly in neonates. Thromboelastography may be useful in guiding management. Coagulopathy may persist, particularly in neonates, cyanotic patients or those receiving anticoagulant medication.

In patients in whom bleeding is anticipated (complex patients, neonates, patients undergoing repeat sternotomy), antifibrinolytic therapy can be used from the start of the case to reduce bleeding. Tranexamic acid is considered safe and effective in neonates and children, although the optimal dosing regimen remains unclear. The use of aprotinin is controversial given an absence of evidence for superiority over tranexamic acid and following a suggestion of increased complication rates in adults; however, it is still used with ongoing drug surveillance in children, particularly for neonates undergoing complex repairs.

For most patients, we would aim to ensure that haemoglobin is above 100 $gl^{-1}$ in the postoperative period. Haemoglobin should be maintained above 120 $g\ l^{-1}$ in patients with palliated repairs who continue to have oxygen saturations in the 80s.

## Further Management Following CPB

Following satisfactory haemostasis, epicardial pacemaker leads are attached, chest drains are inserted and the chest is closed. Most patients are managed postoperatively on the intensive care unit. Adequate sedation and analgesia are required prior to termination of the volatile agent at the end surgery. A propofol infusion can be useful for transfer. A clear and comprehensive handover to the intensive care team is essential.

In some infants, particularly neonates who have undergone long and complex surgery, sternal closure leads to tamponade of the heart and impaired function. In these infants, the sternum may be stented open and the wound protected with a silicone membrane. The chest is closed after two to three days when cardiac function has improved.

## Pacemakers in Cardiac Surgery

Rhythm disturbances may occur after paediatric cardiac surgery and epicardial pacing wires are routinely placed. Heart block may occur after repairs involving the ventricular septum, and atrial dysrhythmias may occur because of suture lines in the atrium. Patients undergoing tetralogy of Fallot repair are particularly prone to junctional tachycardia. Dysrhythmias are poorly tolerated in lesions such as univentricular repairs and heterotaxy. Some patients will require pacemaker support after bypass.

It is important for the anaesthetist to understand pacemaker codes and which settings to use. The pacemaker code is a series of letters describing the type of pacing. The first letter represents the chamber being paced, the second the chamber being sensed and the third the response to sensing. The chambers are atria (A), ventricle (V) or both/dual (D). Pacing is inhibited (I), triggered (T) or both (D) on sensing; pacing being delivered regardless of sensing is designated by the letter 'O'. Permanent pacemakers are more sophisticated and often have a fourth and fifth letter in the code.

In the presence of AV nodal block, dual chamber pacing is required and DDD mode is selected. The atria are paced using AAI or AOO for bradycardia requiring treatment in the absence of AV nodal block.

## Fast-track Surgery

Increased pressure on health care resources and scrutiny on outcomes has led to renewed interest in enhanced recovery programmes and early extubation, occasionally in theatre, coupled with short-stay intensive care management following certain cardiac procedures. The spectrum of suitable cases is growing beyond atrial septal defect and simple VSD surgeries. All cases should fulfil certain criteria, including adequate haemostasis, normothermia, minimal inotropic support and minimal ventilatory requirement.

For patients in whom early extubation is planned, multimodal analgesia should be started in the operating theatre. This will include intravenous paracetamol, local analgesic infiltration to the sternal wound or regional analgesia and an intravenous morphine infusion, including nurse-controlled (NCA) or patient-controlled (PCA) analgesia. The historical use of high-dose opioid anaesthesia hinders early extubation and fast-tracking. An anaesthetic technique using moderate doses of fentanyl (10–15 mcg $kg^{-1}$) with reversal of short-acting muscle relaxants is more appropriate.

# Specific Conditions

## Blalock–Taussig Shunt

An mBTS is a GoreTex™ tube from the subclavian artery to the pulmonary artery (see Figure 31.1). Surgery may be undertaken via thoracotomy or sternotomy. Where possible, the monitoring arterial line should not be placed in the ipsilateral arm. Heparin 100 IU $kg^{-1}$ IV is given once the subclavian end of the shunt has been completed. On completion of surgery, it is important to maintain an adequate blood pressure to ensure blood flow through the shunt, and on occasion inotropic support may be necessary. Balancing the circulation is critical and is usually determined by the choice of size of the shunt, occasionally by applying a clip to the shunt if the shunt is too large. Oxygen saturation of 70–80% in air should be expected following completion of the shunt. Excessive shunt flow leads to increased pulmonary flow and reduced systemic flow, high oxygen saturation and signs of low systemic cardiac output. If there is very high runoff from the systemic circulation into the shunt, diastolic pressure can be very low, leading to severe myocardial ischaemia. This can also occur postoperatively as PVR falls during the neonatal period and may require shunt revision.

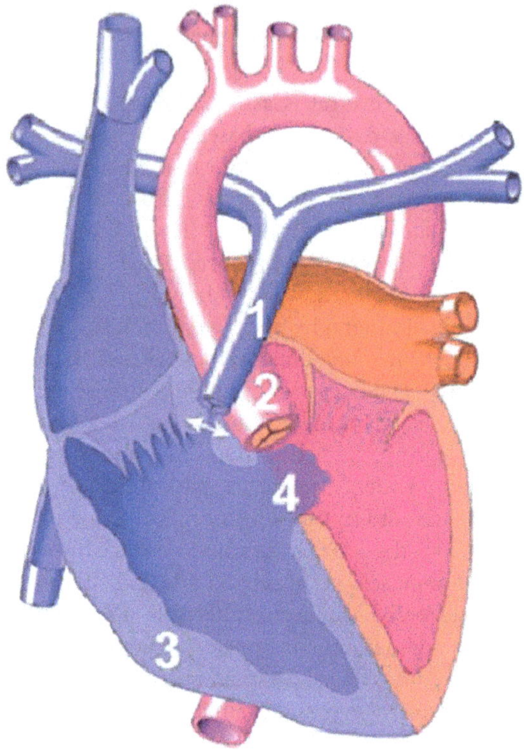


**Figure 31.2** Tetralogy of Fallot. Narrowed pulmonary valve and artery (1) with narrowed right ventricular infundibulum (arrows), with aorta (2) over-riding a ventricular septal defect (4) and hypertophied right ventricle (3).
Source: The PedHeart Resource (www.HeartPassport.com). Courtesy of Scientific Software Solutions, Inc.

## Tetralogy of Fallot

In this condition, there is right-ventricular outflow tract obstruction (RVOTO) with right-ventricular (RV) hypertrophy, a VSD and an aorta that 'over-rides' the VSD (see Figure 31.2). There is a wide spectrum of severity. At one end is the patient with virtually no more than a VSD – the 'pink tetralogy'. At the other end is the very cyanosed patient with total right-ventricular outflow tract obstruction due to pulmonary atresia and right-to-left shunting across the VSD. In some, the main and possibly the branch pulmonary arteries are hypoplastic; it can be very difficult to obtain an acceptable surgical result in these patients. Another variant has an absent pulmonary valve, which results in a hugely dilated pulmonary artery that can cause significant airway compression, particularly of the left main bronchus.

The classic TOF has a variable degree of RVOTO (and therefore cyanosis) due to a narrowed pulmonary valve annulus, combined with thick infundibular (or sub-valvar) muscle bundles which can spasm to further narrow the outflow. These children have intermittent hypercyanotic spells, known as 'tet' spells, in which spasm of the right-ventricular infundibulum occurs, increasing right-to-left shunting through the VSD. The muscular infundibulum is sensitive to the effects of catecholamines, so spells can be brought on by stress and can be ameliorated using beta blockers. Beta agonists such as adrenaline should be avoided in these patients.

Hypercyanotic spells can be triggered by crying, a fall in SVR at induction of anaesthesia and surgical manipulation. The management of a spell includes administering 100% oxygen, giving a fluid bolus, a dose of opioid such as fentanyl and physical measures to increase SVR such as pushing the patient's knees up to the chest. If these measures are unsuccessful, a vasoconstrictor such as noradrenaline by infusion or phenylephrine 1–5 mcg $kg^{-1}$ should be administered. Some experts advocate beta blockade with propranolol 50–100 mcg $kg^{-1}$ if the heart rate is high. Esmolol 500 mcg $kg^{-1}$ over one minute followed by an infusion at 50–200 mcg $kg^{-1}$ $min^{-1}$ is an alternative.

Tetralogy of Fallot is repaired using a patch to close the VSD and excising hypertrophied muscle bundles from the right-ventricular outflow tract. It may be necessary to enlarge the outflow tract or the valve annulus with a patch. Widening the pulmonary valve with a transannular patch will produce pulmonary regurgitation. This can make post-bypass management challenging if the hypertrophied right ventricle is poorly compliant. Adequate cardiac output requires a high filling pressure rather than increased inotropic support with catecholamines such as adrenaline. Tachycardia is unhelpful, but maintaining SVR is useful. A phosphodiesterase inhibitor such as milrinone (inodilator/lusitropic effect) combined with noradrenaline is often used. Surgery carries a risk of heart block postoperatively, as the conduction tissue passes close to the borders of the VSD. Occasionally a sinister dysrhythmia known as junctional ectopic tachycardia (JET) occurs which may lead to very poor cardiac output. This is treated with cooling, amiodarone, electrolyte optimisation and minimising inotropic support.

## Transposition of the Great Arteries (TGA)

In TGA, the aorta arises from the right ventricle and the PA from the left. A VSD may also be present. The condition is incompatible with life unless there is a source of mixing such as an atrial septal defect (ASD), VSD or PDA, without which oxygenated pulmonary venous blood cannot reach the systemic circulation. Patients are usually managed with a prostaglandin infusion preoperatively, and a balloon atrial septostomy is performed if there is inadequate mixing.

The arterial switch operation (ASO) involves disconnecting the great arteries and attaching them to the correct ventricle. The coronary arteries will need to be transposed. Unsatisfactory coronary artery re-anastomosis leading to myocardial ischaemia and poor cardiac output is a major cause of postoperative problems. Following bypass, the left ventricle can be non-compliant, and fluid boluses should be administered cautiously to avoid left-atrial enlargement and coronary distortion. Milrinone and adrenaline are useful in combination following ASO. Measurement of left-atrial pressure (with a line directly placed by the surgeon) can allow early detection of left-ventricular dysfunction and guide fluid and inotrope therapy.

The origin of the coronary arteries lies very close to the PA following repair. Elevation in PA pressure can occlude the coronaries, compromising left-ventricular function, so measures to minimise pulmonary vascular resistance are important.

## Single-Ventricle Circulation

Historically, children with defects where the right ventricle was underdeveloped, for example tricuspid atresia, would be managed with a systemic to pulmonary artery shunt but would die in late childhood or early adulthood due to complications of cyanosis. In the 1960s, Fontan described a palliative operation where pulmonary blood flow was achieved by directly connecting the right atrium to the pulmonary arteries. Although this 'single-ventricle' solution was a major advance, complications such as atrial dysrhythmias were significant, and long-term survival remained poor. The Fontan procedure has undergone several modifications and now involves the staged connection of the SVC and the IVC directly to the pulmonary artery, with improved good-quality long-term survival. The total cavopulmonary connection (TCPC) can be used whichever ventricle is underdeveloped, with the developed ventricle becoming the 'systemic' ventricle.

Creating a single-ventricle circulation usually involves three stages. During the neonatal period, PVR is high, and a systemic shunt (mBTS) is performed. The second stage, a Glenn (superior cavopulmonary) shunt involving the anastomosis of the SVC to the right PA is created at around three to five months of age when the PVR has fallen, and sufficient flow at venous pressure can be achieved through the pulmonary arteries. The mBTS is taken down at this time (see Figure 31.3). The operation creates an end-to-side anastomosis from SVC to the right PA so blood perfuses both lungs; this is the bidirectional Glenn (BDG). Oxygen saturation will usually be in the 80s after

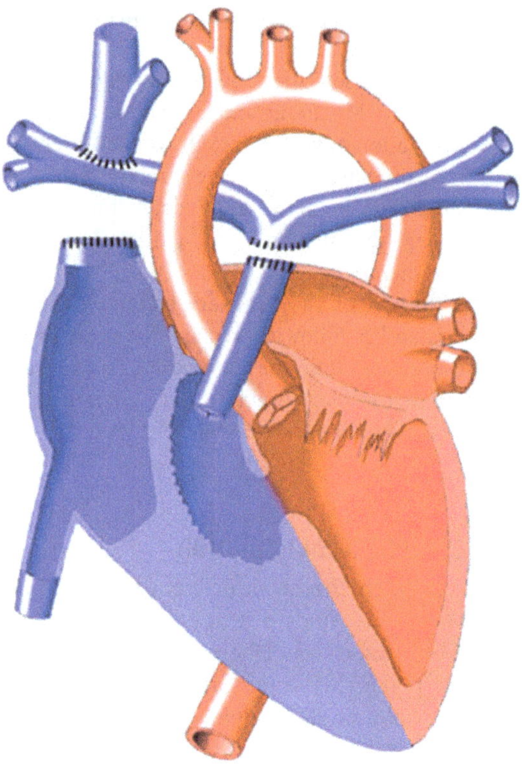

**Figure 31.3** Bidirectional Glenn shunt (BDG) in tricuspid atresia, showing anastomosis of the superior vena cava to the right pulmonary artery.
*Source:* The PedHeart Resource (www.HeartPassport.com). Courtesy of Scientific Software Solutions, Inc.

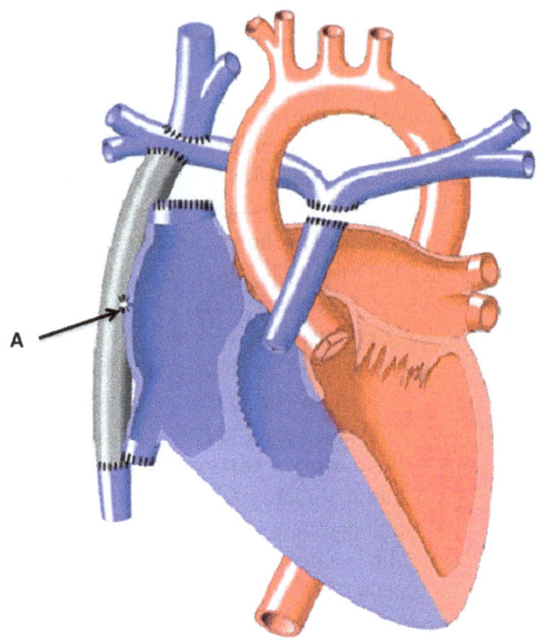


**Figure 31.4** TCPC in tricuspid atresia. Both the superior and inferior vena cavae are connected to the right pulmonary artery. There is a fenestration (A) between the IVC to PA conduit and the atrium.
*Source:* The PedHeart Resource (www.HeartPassport.com). Courtesy of Scientific Software Solutions, Inc.

a BDG. It is important to recognise that pressure measured in the internal jugular vein reflects pulmonary perfusion pressure. This 'venous pressure' must be maintained higher than normal, often 12–15 mmHg, to ensure an adequate transpulmonary pressure gradient. Patients benefit from a low intrathoracic pressure and being in a slightly head-up position after surgery.

The third stage, TCPC completion, in which the IVC is anastomosed to the PA, is usually undertaken between the age of one and five years. This will only be successful if PVR is low. Ideally the transpulmonary gradient, the difference between systemic venous pressure and pressure in the common atrium, should be less than 10 mmHg after the TCPC.

If PVR is high, there will need to be high systemic venous pressure to drive blood across the lungs, and there may be poor filling of the systemic atrium and low cardiac output. Transpulmonary gradient will be high, and there may be poor oxygenation, pleural effusions, ascites and renal dysfunction. In this situation, the surgeon may 'fenestrate' the TCPC by creating a small hole between the GoreTex™ tube and the systemic atrium, allowing systemic venous blood to shunt through this fenestration to the systemic atrium at times of increased pressure (see Figure 31.4). This can improve preload and cardiac output but will be at the expense of lower oxygen saturation. Intrathoracic pressure should be kept low, and these patients benefit from early transition to spontaneous ventilation and extubation. Dysrhythmias are poorly tolerated, and pacing may be necessary.

## Hypoplastic Left-Heart Syndrome

In HLHS, the left ventricle is severely underdeveloped and aortic arch atretic; distal aortic blood flow is initially dependent upon ductal flow from the pulmonary artery. The Norwood operation for HLHS makes use of the right ventricle as the systemic ventricle and creates a neo-aorta using the main pulmonary artery. The branch PAs are disconnected from the main PA and are supplied by either an mBTS or, in the Sano modification, an RV-to-PA conduit.

**Table 31.3** Manipulating PVR and SVR

| Direction of change of vascular | Intervention resistance |
|---|---|
| PVR ↑ | Hypercapnia<br>Hypoxia<br>Acidosis<br>PEEP<br>High airway pressure<br>Atelectasis |
| PVR ↓ | Hypocapnia<br>Alkalosis<br>High $FiO_2$<br>Low haematocrit<br>Nitric oxide<br>Prostacyclin (epoprostenol)<br>Milrinone<br>Low airway pressure |
| SVR ↑ | Vasoconstrictors<br>Hypothermia<br>Raising haematocrit |
| SVR ↓ | Vasodilators<br>Anaesthetic agents<br>Low haematocrit<br>Warming |

As both the pulmonary and systemic circulations are supplied by the same ventricle, it is important to balance SVR and PVR to maintain adequate pulmonary and systemic perfusion (see Table 31.3). This usually necessitates low inspired oxygen and a moderately raised $PaCO_2$ to maintain PVR. When appropriately balanced, arterial oxygen saturation will be around 75–80%. These patients can be very challenging perioperatively as they can rapidly develop very poor systemic output if PVR is allowed to fall. Limiting inspired oxygen concentration to $FiO_2$ 0.21 is crucial in this situation. Progression via a Glenn to a TCPC is as described in the previous section.

## Coarctation Repair

Coarctation may present in the neonatal period or later in childhood. Neonatal coarctation often presents with severe shock when the PDA closes at around four to seven days of age and can be mistaken for sepsis. Immediate management is to attempt re-opening of the duct with prostaglandin infusion to allow perfusion of the distal aorta from the pulmonary artery. There may be severe left-ventricular dysfunction, and ventilatory and inotropic support may be required. Surgery to repair the coarctation is undertaken when cardiovascular and metabolic stability has been restored. Volatile agents are poorly tolerated in these neonatal patients, and a balanced technique with high-dose fentanyl is routinely used.

Surgery is usually via a left thoracotomy, although occasionally in neonates it can be easier to undertake via sternotomy. During the repair, the surgeon will clamp the aorta, usually for a period of around 15–20 minutes, which places spinal cord perfusion at risk. Moderate central cooling should be achieved before the clamp is applied. In older patients, blood pressure (measured in the right arm) may rise significantly during this period, and it may be necessary to increase the volatile agent or occasionally start a vasodilator. It is important to stop these a few minutes before the aortic clamp is removed to avoid a catastrophic fall in blood pressure and to have volume replacement ready. Dialogue with the surgeon is essential.

## Anaesthesia for Ventricular Assist Device Implantation and Cardiac Transplantation

Children requiring a ventricular assist device (VAD) present with poor cardiac function and reserve. Meticulous pre-anaesthetic planning and induction is key. Intravenous, fully monitored induction is preferred, with the theatre team on standby for immediate CPB support. Children presenting for VAD support as a bridge to transplant most commonly have dilated cardiomyopathy but could have restrictive disease or congenital heart disease. They are likely to be supported on inotrope infusions and with poor end-organ perfusion. The important aspects of anaesthesia are as previously described and include a balanced technique with appreciation for slow circulation times and a reduced requirement for most medications. The child may be supported with a left-sided device only or with biventricular support. Once supported by a VAD, the child is anticoagulated to prevent thromboembolic complications. Routine monitoring may be challenging if a non-pulsatile VAD is used, since pulse oximetry and non-invasive BP measurement require pulsatile flow to function. However, once safely supported by a VAD, the child should be more haemodynamically stable. It is important to act on monitoring, filling pressures and the alarm functions of the support system to maintain cardiac output.

Cardiac transplantation includes a multitude of clinical considerations for the anaesthetist and close collaboration with the transplant team. The presence of mechanical support, an implantable defibrillator or pacemaker, anticoagulation management, pulmonary hypertension, previous sternotomies and vascular access should be assessed. Other issues include management of patient and parental anxiety and support for the family after being called in during inconvenient hours or after a long time on a waiting list. Anaesthesia should be administered with care as described previously, in liaison with the transplant coordination team concerning the timing of organ arrival. The perfusionists and surgeons should be on standby in case of instability on induction of anaesthesia. The anaesthetist is required to start the immunosuppression regimen during surgery and to provide meticulous attention to coagulation and infection control. Providing optimal conditions for surgery and ongoing care can make this a challenging yet rewarding anaesthetic to give. It is not uncommon for patients to require a short period of extracorporeal membrane oxygenation (ECMO) post-transplant, usually for a period of 48–72 hours.

### Key Points

- Successful anaesthesia for paediatric cardiac surgery requires a meticulous, anticipative approach that starts in the preoperative period.
- Many infants with congenital heart disease require a 'balanced' circulation in which changes in pulmonary or systemic resistance with anaesthesia can lead to severe adverse haemodynamic disturbances.
- Patients with unrepaired tetralogy of Fallot with severe right-ventricular outflow tract obstruction can develop life-threatening profound hypoxia during induction if systemic resistance falls and may need vasoconstrictor support.
- Children who are very cyanosed and polycythaemic will often have abnormal coagulation.

## Further Reading

Andropoulos DB, Stayer SA, Russell IA, Mossad EB, eds. *Anesthesia for Congenital Heart Disease*, 2nd ed. Wiley-Blackwell. 2010.

UK National Institute for Cardiac Outcomes Research. Available at: www.nicor.org.uk. Accessed 3 April 2024.

Chapter 32

# Anaesthesia for Cardiac Catheterisation and Other Investigative Procedures in Children*

Marc Cohen and Graham Derrick

## Introduction

Since the publication of the previous edition of this chapter, the principles of caring for children in the cardiac catheterisation laboratory (cath lab) remain much the same. Advances in technology and novel devices allow catheter-based interventions in increasingly complex cases of congenital and acquired heart disease, often replacing or postponing the need for a surgical approach. Even extremely preterm infants (some less than 800 g) can now be offered interventional procedures in the catheter lab. Conversely, there is a reduced need for cardiac catheterisation as a purely diagnostic tool, as non-invasive imaging modalities such as cardiac CT and MRI continue to increase in their application and sophistication.

The anaesthetist may find themselves undertaking high-risk, complex cases, with challenges inherent to the cath lab, in a location which may be remote from the main theatre suite. Anaesthetists managing children with complex congenital cardiac disease must understand the pathophysiology of these patients and the effects that anaesthesia and any intervention will have on their underlying physiology. Table 32.1 lists cardiac catheter laboratory procedures.

**Table 32.1** Cardiac catheter laboratory procedures

| | Procedure |
|---|---|
| **Diagnostic** | Diagnostic catheter/ angiography<br>Coronary angiography<br>Endomyocardial biopsy<br>Pulmonary vascular resistance study<br>Transoesophageal echocardiography |
| **Interventional** | Septal defect closure<br>Vessel occlusion<br>Balloon valvotomy<br>Balloon angioplasty<br>Stent placement<br>Balloon atrial septostomy<br>Percutaneous valve implant |
| **Electrophysiological studies (EPS)** | Conduction system mapping<br>Ablation of arrhythmogenic focus<br>Pacemaker insertion<br>Loop recorder insertion<br>Placement of implantable cardioverter defibrillator (ICD)<br>Cardioversion |
| **Miscellaneous** | Drainage of pericardial effusion |

## Risk

Data from the Pediatric Perioperative Cardiac Arrest Registry show that children with congenital heart disease account for nearly a third of perioperative arrests. Paediatric cardiac catheterisation carries a risk of cardiac arrest of around 0.8% and a mortality risk of 0.2%. This is significantly higher than routine paediatric anaesthesia (about 20 times higher). Scoring systems have been developed to help quantify this risk, such as the Catheterisation Risk Score for Pediatrics (CRISP; see 'Further Reading'). Risk factors which increase the likelihood of a life-threatening event during cardiac catheterisation include:

- Age less than one year
- More than two haemodynamic indicators of vulnerability (low mixed venous saturations,

* Many thanks to Ian James and Sally Wilmshurst, who wrote the first edition of this book chapter, much of the content of which has been used in this revision.

elevated systemic ventricle end-diastolic pressure, low systemic arterial oxygen saturation, elevated pulmonary artery pressure)
- Greater procedural complexity (valvuloplasty, pulmonary artery stent placement, ventricular septal defect closure)

Particular attention must be given to children on a single ventricle pathway, those with a cardiomyopathy and children with pulmonary hypertension. These groups have the highest anaesthesia-related mortality in paediatrics.

## Environment

The cath lab environment itself may add to the difficulty managing clinically challenging cases. It is often an isolated suite, away from the operating theatres and the support of anaesthesia personnel and resources, with the additional challenge of limited functional space. There may be reduced access to the patient once the procedure is under way, with imaging equipment hindering airway manoeuvres or additional vascular access, which in an emergency can be troublesome. Long anaesthesia circuits are required to reach the patient, and this should be taken into account when ventilating infants. It is important to identify those cases in which it is prudent to have additional expertise present for the case.

Temperature regulation must be considered. Small babies, particularly premature infants and neonates, lose heat very quickly under anaesthesia. Forced-air warmers, fluid warmers and warming mats should be used to maintain normothermia.

Staff working in the cath lab must keep safe from radiation exposure and wear protective shielding (wraparound lead aprons, thyroid guards and eye shields). Dosimeter badges should be worn to monitor cumulative radiation exposure, and attempts should be made to stay as safe as possible by using mobile lead screens and minimising exposure time.

## World Health Organisation Checks and Briefs

Crucial to a successful cardiac catheter procedure is the preoperative discussion, or brief. There may be a large team of interventionalists, anaesthetists, anaesthetic assistants, scrub nurses, running nurses, physiologists, radiographers and observers. In some cases, a full cardiac theatre team is also present. The brief should include introductions, presentation of the patient's history (led by the operator), the intended procedure, any special requirements, discussion of risk and complication management during the procedure, any additional staff that may need to be called, the need for and location of blood products, potential need for an intensive care bed or other escalations and other factors, including pregnancy test results and infectious alerts. A routine 'sign in' should be performed before induction of anaesthesia. The routine 'time out', which re-confirms the patient identity, consent and preparation for the procedure, should include checks such as the presence of distal limb pulses and pressure area protection, and whether there are new members of the team who were missing from the initial brief. During the procedure, it may be necessary to call out an update, especially if there is a complication or a change of plan, because the events may not be immediately evident to the whole team. An interim check is necessary if additional procedures are planned, such as magnetic resonance scanning, in which case a full metal compatibility check must be completed. After the procedure, with the instrument and swab counts completed, a 'sign out' is performed and recorded before the child is woken up or taken to ICU.

## Diagnostic Cardiac Catheterisation

Diagnostic catheterisation is performed to collect data regarding the child's cardiovascular anatomy, haemodynamics, cardiac function and response to administered medications. Measurement of arterial, mixed venous, pulmonary venous and pulmonary arterial oxygen saturations allows determination of blood flow using the Fick principle. If oxygen consumption is measured, systemic blood flow (Qs), pulmonary blood flow (Qp) and the pulmonary to systemic flow ratio, commonly referred to as Qp:Qs, can be calculated (Box 32.1). In a normal series circulation, cardiac output equates to Qs; in patients without a cardiac shunt, Qp and Qs should be equal. Shunt lesions (septal defects, ducts, surgical shunts, collateral arteries) will alter this ratio. In patients with a parallel circulation, such as single ventricle, cardiac output will equal Qs + Qp.

Measurement of oxygen consumption is difficult and requires a mass spectrometer and a sealed

**Box 32.1** Haemodynamic calculations.

| Haemodynamic variable | Normal values |
|---|---|
| ***Flow*** *(based on the Fick equation)* | |
| Systemic output (Qs) = $VO_2/(C_{ao}O_2 - C_{mv}O_2)$ | **3.5–5 (l $min^{-1}$ $m^{-2}$)** |
| Pulmonary flow (Qp) = $VO_2/(C_{pv}O_2 - C_{pa}O_2)$ | **3.5–5 (l $min^{-1}$ $m^{-2}$)** |
| ***Shunt fraction:*** | |
| Because of the technical difficulties of measuring oxygen content for shunt calculation, in practice shunt fraction is often calculated using saturation measurements from a number of different sites by the following equation: | |
| Pulmonary to systemic (Qp:Qs) = $(S_{ao}O_2 - S_{mv}O_2)/(S_{pv}O_2 - S_{pa}O_2)$ | **1:1–1:1.2** |
| Mixed venous saturation ($S_{mv}O_2$) can be approximated from: | |
| $[3(S_aSVC) + (S_aIVC)]/4$ | **0.65–0.75** |
| ***Resistance:*** | |
| Pulmonary (PVRI) = (PAP – LAP)/Qp | **Newborn 8–10 Woods units $m^2$** |
| (common to substitute PA wedge for LAP) | **Older children 0.6–2 Woods units $m^2$** |
| Systemic (SVRI) = (AoP-RAP)/Qs | **Newborn 10–15 Woods units $m^2$** |
| (note indexed resistance is expressed as Wood units•$m^2$, not Wood units $m^{-2}$. This is because the denominator (Qp or Qs) is already an indexed value, calculated by absolute flow/BSA. | **Older children 15–30 Woods units $m^2$** |

*Notes:* $VO_2$ = oxygen consumption; CO = cardiac output; $CaoO_2$ = aortic arterial oxygen content; $CmvO_2$ = mixed venous oxygen content; $SO_2$ = oxygen saturation; Qp = pulmonary flow; Qs = systemic flow; ao = aorta; mv = mixed venous; pa = pulmonary artery; pv = pulmonary vein; Hb = haemoglobin; PVR = pulmonary vascular resistance, PVRI = indexed pulmonary vascular resistance; PAP = pulmonary artery pressure; SVC = superior vena cava; IVC = inferior vena cava; SVR = systemic vascular resistance; RAP = right-atrial pressure; LAP = left-atrial pressure; AoP = aortic pressure

ventilator system to allow collection of all expired gases. Alternatively, standard assumed values of oxygen consumption are commonly used, though the available nomograms have been shown to be very inaccurate. Thermodilution is an alternative method of determining cardiac output, although this cannot be used in the presence of a cardiac shunt. MRI provides gold standard flow measurements but is only available in specialised centres (see the section 'Cardiac MRI and CT').

Catheterisation data often form the basis for important decisions, for instance whether a patient is suitable for cardiac transplantation or closure of a shunt lesion such as a ventricular septal defect. It is important that the physiological state of the patient remains constant during the procedure; the inspired oxygen fraction, ventilation and depth of anaesthesia should remain stable. If changes to these parameters are made, it is important for the anaesthetist to communicate these to the cardiologist, to determine whether the physiological measurements need to be repeated under constant conditions.

Direct pressure and flow measurements can provide calculation of systemic and pulmonary vascular resistance (Box 32.1). Cardiac output (CO) can be indexed to body surface area (BSA) such that the Cardiac Index (CI) = CO/BSA. Absolute pulmonary vascular resistance (PVR) is referred to in Wood units, but indexed PVR (PVRI) is referred to in Wood units $m^2$ (because PVRI = PVR/CI, or PVRI = PVR/CO/BSA). Indexed PVR would usually be under 2 Wood units $m^2$ in health. Intracardiac and intravascular pressure measurements also provide information about cardiac function and obstructions to flow across valves and vessels and are more accurate than those derived using echocardiography.

Additional diagnostic information is obtained with angiography, which involves the injection of radiographic contrast medium to outline heart structures, great vessels, venous connections and any abnormal vessels such as collaterals or malformations. This can be crucial in establishing the exact anatomical nature of some complex cardiac anomalies. Coronary angiography may be undertaken when echocardiography is unable to answer concerns about coronary anatomy or perfusion. Coronary artery disease is the most common complication of cardiac transplantation, and coronary angiography is part of the routine interval follow-up of these patients. Contrast medium is iodine-based and of varying osmolarity. Hyperosmolar solutions are avoided in children, as they are associated with flushing, hypotension, bradycardia and renal impairment. Adequate hydration is essential in children undergoing angiography, particularly those with pre-existing renal dysfunction, because of the small risk of contrast-induced nephropathy. Anaphylaxis to contrast can occur but is rare. Where contrast allergy exists, an alternative is angiography with carbon dioxide which is rapidly absorbed into solution before embolic phenomena may occur. Intravascular ultrasound (IVUS) uses a fine intracoronary ultrasound catheter to identify early plaque formation within the coronary arteries. It may be utilised in children over 20 kg.

## Interventional Cardiac Catheterisation

Interventional procedures involve the introduction of a variety of devices into the heart or major vessels. These may be:

- Balloons, which are expanded with contrast solution to dilate valves or vessels.
- Stents – balloon-expandable or self-expanding which are implanted to widen a vessel.
- Devices that can be deployed to occlude septal defects, paravalvar leaks, collaterals and other vessels.
- Coils, positioned to occlude vessels such as a patent arterial duct and collateral arteries or veins.
- Artificial valves – transluminal implantation of a valve, such as the Melody Valve® (pulmonary valve) or an aortic valve in adults (transcatheter aortic valve implantation, or TAVI). Off-license use of devices and valves are occasionally considered, for instance the Melody Valve® in the tricuspid position.

## Access to the Heart and Major Vessels

The right side of the heart and pulmonary arteries are accessed via the femoral vein, the jugular vein or occasionally the hepatic vein. The internal jugular vein is preferred for endomyocardial biopsy as it provides easier access to the right ventricle and may be necessary in other cases if the femoral or iliac vessels are blocked. Internal jugular, axillary or subclavian vein access will also be required if it is necessary to measure the pressure in the pulmonary artery after a Glenn anastomosis (in which the SVC is connected to the pulmonary artery).

The left side of the heart and major arterial vessels are usually accessed from the femoral artery or from the right side of the heart via a septal defect or trans-septal puncture. The cardiologist may insert a femoral arterial monitoring line even when left heart catheterisation is not planned. In the absence of an atrial septal approach, it can be difficult and arrhythmogenic to pass a catheter retrogradely across the mitral valve, and so an alternative, indirect method of assessing left-atrial pressure is the pulmonary capillary wedge pressure (more accurately known as the pulmonary *arterial* wedge pressure). This is obtained by wedging a balloon-tipped catheter into a pulmonary artery and measuring the pressure distal to the balloon. This is commonly used for left-atrial pressure for calculation of transpulmonary pressure or pulmonary vascular resistance.

Introducer sheaths are placed using the Seldinger technique under ultrasound guidance. These allow catheters to be inserted without loss of blood or introduction of air. Relatively large sheaths are sometimes required for implantation of larger devices, and the sheath may need to be upsized during the case. Heparin, 50–100μ $kg^{-1}$, is given to prevent thrombosis for most cardiac catheter procedures and particularly when systemic arterial or left-atrial catheters are employed. Monitoring of adequate anticoagulation is performed using activated clotting times (ACT). At the end of the procedure, it is important that satisfactory haemostasis at the puncture site is achieved before anaesthesia is terminated, as it can be very difficult to control bleeding in a restless, wakening child.

## Anaesthesia

Cardiac catheterisation is seldom painful, apart from the infiltration of local anaesthetic and the placement of an introducer sheath in a vessel, which is usually the most stimulating time for a patient. In older children, some diagnostic procedures can be undertaken under local anaesthesia, supplemented with light sedation if necessary. However, in paediatrics, general anaesthesia is necessary for most cath lab procedures, especially if prolonged.

In the majority of cases, the requirement from the anaesthetist is for a still patient with stable haemodynamics, preferably with parameters as near to normal as possible. Inappropriate anaesthesia and ventilation can adversely affect the haemodynamic data being collected, so the anaesthetist must have a thorough knowledge of these potential changes as well as of the procedures being performed. For example, oxygen saturation data for accurate blood flow measurement are best achieved with inspired oxygen as near to 21% as can be tolerated. Normocapnia is particularly important when pulmonary vascular resistance is being assessed. Hypovolaemia and hypotension may lead to inaccurate determination of flows and shunts. Good communication with the cardiologist is essential.

## Induction

Where possible, full anaesthetic monitoring should be applied before induction. Inhalational or intravenous induction is suitable for cardiac catheterisation and will usually depend on the child's age and preferences. Sevoflurane is the ideal agent for inhalational induction. For intravenous induction, propofol is usually suitable unless a fall in SVR is to be avoided, in which case ketamine may be preferred. In patients with limited cardiac output reserve, such as dilated cardiomyopathy, it is important that blood pressure and coronary perfusion do not fall during induction. A combination of fentanyl 1–2 mcg $kg^{-1}$ and propofol 1–2 mg $kg^{-1}$, titrated gently, works well.

As most procedures are conducted through femoral vessels, it is generally preferable to avoid the lower-limb veins for venous access.

## Airway Management

A supraglottic airway device (SGA) may be appropriate for many straightforward diagnostic cases in older infants and children. For small infants, patients who are clinically unstable and those undergoing interventional procedures, a tracheal tube should be employed. Intubation may be preferred for patients in whom internal jugular venous access is required. If the cardiologist needs to collect all expired respiratory gases to measure oxygen consumption, a cuffed tracheal tube should be used. A cuffed tube will also be advantageous when it is necessary to ensure steady carbon dioxide tension during pulmonary vascular resistance studies.

Controlled ventilation is indicated in most cases, as it allows careful control of the blood gases for haemodynamic data collection and facilitates the short periods of apnoea that are occasionally necessary for accurate pressure measurement and high-quality angiographic pictures.

## Maintenance

Maintenance of anaesthesia with inhalational agents is typically with isoflurane or sevoflurane, which are usually well tolerated and are the volatile agents of choice. Total intravenous anaesthesia (TIVA) has become increasingly popular, with an increased focus on delivering an environmentally friendly anaesthetic. Nitrous oxide should be avoided during cardiac catheterisation.

A small dose of fentanyl (1–2 mcg $kg^{-1}$) may be given before inserting a transoesophageal echocardiography (TOE) probe, to blunt the pressor response it induces. Opioid analgesics are otherwise seldom required. Many procedures are undertaken as day cases, so a plan for post-discharge analgesia should be made. Long-acting local anaesthetic infiltration to the puncture site is usually adequate for post-catheter pain relief along with paracetamol, given either intravenously during the procedure or orally afterwards. There is a significant incidence of nausea and vomiting following inhalational anaesthesia for cardiac catheterisation despite avoidance of opioids, and antiemetics should be given.

## Monitoring

Full monitoring should be used for all catheterisation procedures. Multi-lead ECG is generally part of the routine cardiac electrophysiological data displayed, so a separate anaesthetic ECG is not usually required after induction. Distal perfusion can be impaired in the limb used for catheter access; non-invasive blood pressure and pulse oximetry should be applied to the contralateral leg or the upper limbs. End-tidal $CO_2$ can be significantly affected by cyanotic heart disease, owing to venous admixture and impaired pulmonary blood flow, and may underestimate $PaCO_2$ by up to 2 kPa. In general, the greater the degree of cyanosis, the greater the end-tidal to arterial $pCO_2$ gradient. Invasive blood pressure monitoring is seldom required in diagnostic catheterisation but may be indicated in unstable patients or those with severe pulmonary hypertension. Depth of anaesthesia monitoring should be used if neuromuscular blocking agents are administered together with TIVA.

Intravenous fluids are required for all but the shortest procedures, especially if contrast is being used.

## Positioning

For most procedures where biplane X-ray imaging is used, the patient is positioned supine with the arms above the head. Care must be taken that the brachial plexus is not stretched. Exposure is less than during surgical procedures, but temperature monitoring and active warming should be available. Procedures can take many hours and pressure areas must be protected. In some procedures, for instance carotid access procedures, the head-toe position may be reversed, and particular attention must be paid to the placement of the breathing system and intravenous lines. For patients on extracorporeal membrane oxygenation (ECMO), there can be significant challenges in transferring the patient safely on to the X-ray table in such a way as to permit satisfactory fluoroscopy, adequate access for the anaesthetist and interventional cardiologist and very occasionally for the cardiac surgical team.

## Interventional Procedures

When an intervention involves inserting a device, the cardiologist may request that the anaesthetist give antibiotics according to the local guidelines. This will be discussed at the preoperative brief.

- *Device closure:* Device closure of an arterial duct, atrial or ventricular septal defect, are commonly performed interventional procedures. Patients are usually well, and the procedure is generally straightforward. TOE is useful to ensure correct placement of atrial septal defect (ASD) and ventricular septal defect (VSD) devices, less commonly for duct occlusion. Care must be taken to monitor that the TOE probe does not compress the tracheal tube and impair the ventilation of the patient. Rarely, device displacement may occur and complications develop according to the site of displacement. For instance, an atrial septal occluder may displace and impinge on an atrioventricular valve. Mostly, device displacements can be managed by retrieval using endovascular techniques, but occasionally urgent open-heart surgery is necessary for retrieval. Transcatheter closure of a VSD is technically more challenging and is associated with more complications, particularly heart block and valve damage. During any procedure involving stiff catheters and wires crossing the tricuspid valve, transient hypotension can occur.
- *Vascular occlusion*: This is performed for aorto-pulmonary collaterals or veno-venous connections. These patients are usually relatively well, although on occasion there can be a degree of high-output failure. Again, there is always the risk of the occlusion device embolising, necessitating retrieval.
- *Valvotomy:* This may be carried out in the early neonatal period for critical pulmonary valve stenosis or for critical aortic valve stenosis. Both these groups of patients can be seriously ill and may have a duct-dependent circulation, requiring a prostaglandin infusion to maintain ductal patency. In both procedures, a balloon is dilated across the valve for several seconds, resulting in a short period of absent cardiac output.
- *Critical aortic stenosis:* This has a significant risk of cardiac arrest during the procedure, due to catheter- or wire-induced ventricular fibrillation. There is usually a hypertrophied and poorly functioning left ventricle, and inflation of the balloon tends to obstruct coronary perfusion. Volatile agents are poorly tolerated, and it is our practice to use high-dose fentanyl and oxygen. Hypovolaemia is also poorly tolerated, and inotropic support may be necessary. Resuscitation drugs should be close at hand. Balloon dilatation can cause acute aortic regurgitation, which may ultimately need surgery, though this would usually be tolerated acutely. These patients will nearly always need pre- and postoperative intensive care support. Emergency ultrasound-guided transcarotid aortic valvotomy has been performed in patients too unstable to move to the cath lab.

- *Critical pulmonary stenosis:* There will be profound cyanosis as a result of right-to-left shunting across the atrial septum, and acidosis is common. The pressure-loaded right ventricle may be poorly functioning and may be further compromised during occlusion of the pulmonary valve. Pulmonary regurgitation may be produced, though this is better tolerated than aortic insufficiency. The hypertrophic right ventricle may need a high filling pressure after relief of the afterload; vasodilators and aggressive diuresis should be avoided, and occasionally beta blockade is employed.
- *Balloon dilatation:* Such dilation of the aortic and pulmonary valves may be necessary in older children, and the greater the obstruction the greater the likelihood of ventricular hypertrophy and dysfunction.
- *Angioplasty and stent placement*: Re-coarctation of the aorta, pulmonary artery stenosis or narrowing of the superior vena cava may be treated with balloon angioplasty. It may be necessary to place an endovascular stent to maintain adequate vessel patency, although this necessitates a larger introducer sheath, with a higher risk of vascular damage. Acute complications include rupture of the vessel being dilated, which may require management with balloon tamponade, implant of a covered stent or urgent surgery. Most centres will ensure that surgical cover is provided. Although rare, there is the possibility of displacement and embolisation of the stent.
- *Infant right-ventricular outflow tract stent*: This procedure has become more established to protect pulmonary blood flow in patients with tetralogy of Fallot. Access is via the femoral or internal jugular vein. During the procedure, there may be profound cyanotic spells and low cardiac output because of splinting of the tricuspid valve. The procedures can be challenging because the delivery of the stent requires an introducer sheath to be advanced into the pulmonary artery.
- *Neonatal ductal stent*: In patients with duct-dependent systemic or pulmonary blood flow, ductal stenting may be considered. A ductal stent to maintain pulmonary blood flow is intended to be restrictive, to prevent over-circulation of the lungs. A ductal stent to maintain systemic blood flow must be unrestrictive and is usually done as a hybrid procedure, in conjunction with bilateral pulmonary artery banding performed by the surgeons.
- *Neonatal balloon atrial septostomy (BAS):* In transposition of the great arteries (TGA), it is essential that there is adequate mixing of systemic and pulmonary venous blood in the period prior to surgery. Where this is inadequate it will be necessary to create a communication at atrial level. This is performed by passing a balloon-tipped catheter across from the right to left atrium through the foramen ovale, inflating it and then withdrawing it sharply back into the right atrium, tearing the septum in the process. It may be necessary to repeat this a few times to achieve an adequate communication. These neonatal patients may be extremely cyanosed and acidotic, but rapidly improve once the septostomy is performed. In an already ventilated patient, it is most common to undertake these cases at the bedside on the ICU under echocardiographic guidance. Neonates who are not intubated will require an anaesthetic to allow the procedure to take place, usually in the cath lab with ultrasound guidance or even full radiological imaging.
- *Atrial septal puncture and atrial septostomy*: In patients with severe pulmonary hypertension, it may be beneficial for them to have an atrial communication; this allows decompression of the right side of the heat and augmentation of left-sided filling to maintain cardiac output during times of pulmonary hypertensive crisis. Atrial septal puncture may be performed in the cath lab, followed by graded balloon dilatation of the atrial septum. These patients are at high risk for adverse cardiac events under anaesthesia, and the procedure carries additional risk because of the orientation of the atrial septum bowing towards the free wall of the left atrium.
- *Percutaneous valve placement*: The development of a percutaneously implanted pulmonary valve, fashioned from a platinum/iridium alloy stent containing bovine jugular vein valve (the Melody Valve®), has revolutionised the management of right-ventricular outflow tract dysfunction (stenosis or regurgitation) which would otherwise require major open-heart surgery. There is a

risk of device migration and damage to intracardiac structures and vessels. The cardiologist will carefully assess the proximity of the coronary arteries because of the risk of coronary artery distortion as the stent is implanted. If the coronary arteries are deemed too close, the procedure will be abandoned.

## Hazards/Complications

Although most diagnostic procedures are uncomplicated, for some children the nature of the cardiac lesion being investigated is such that induction of anaesthesia may be hazardous. For example, a fall in systemic vascular resistance or blood pressure in children in whom coronary perfusion is borderline can lead to significant haemodynamic compromise and cardiac arrest. Infants with severe pulmonary hypertension and cardiomyopathy are particularly vulnerable.

In addition to the risks of device embolisation already mentioned, there are several potential complications associated with cardiac catheterisation in general:

- *Dysrhythmias:* Atrial and ventricular arrhythmia can be precipitated by the manipulation of catheters within the heart. Repositioning of the catheter may resolve the problem, but occasionally DC cardioversion may be necessary. Heart block can occur as the atrioventricular (AV) junction is navigated, particularly in AV discordant circulations, and will usually settle over a few minutes, though on occasions it can last longer. Pacing facilities must always be available in the cath lab but are usually not needed.
- *Coronary ischaemia:* During coronary angiography, ischaemic changes may rarely be encountered. They are most likely to be related to deep intubation of the coronary artery, or coronary spasm. If these changes do not resolve following repositioning or withdrawal of the catheter, glyceryl trinitrate (GTN) can be administered directly into the coronary artery. During IVUS, intracoronary GTN is given before the guidewire is passed to allow introduction of the IVUS catheter. The small dose, given locally, is unlikely to create a systemic effect.
- *Hypotension:* This can be caused by hypovolaemia, rhythm disturbances or impaired ventricular function exacerbated by volatile anaesthetic agents.
- *Impaired cardiac output*: Balloon dilatation of aortic or pulmonary valve stenosis will totally obstruct flow from the ventricle. This is for a few seconds only and is usually well tolerated. On occasion it can lead to profound decompensation and cardiac arrest.
- *Hypoxaemia:* Passing catheters into vessels that are the only or the main source of pulmonary blood flow can lead to profound desaturation.
- *Perforation of cardiac chambers or major vessels:* Although rare, it is important to consider the possibility of perforation of a cardiac chamber resulting in tamponade, or of a major vessel, if there is an otherwise unexplained fall in blood pressure or signs of reduced cardiac output during or after the procedure. An echo should be obtained urgently to assess this. Retroperitoneal haematoma from a perforation in the abdominal or iliac vessels should also be considered, particularly if there has been difficulty advancing a catheter from the femoral vessels.
- *Vascular injury:* Thrombosis of the artery used for catheterisation is a known complication, despite the use of heparin administered at the time of catheterisation. Regular assessment of the limb pulses and temperature is an important part of routine postoperative management, and there should be a protocol in place for the management of a limb with signs of arterial insufficiency.
- *Haematoma:* This may occur at the site of vascular access at the end of the procedure or several hours later, particularly if heparin has been given.

## Premature Infants

Cardiac catheterisation in premature infants is becoming more common. Transcatheter duct occlusion is now available from three days of age and 700 g weight. Anaesthetic equipment may be less suited for use in babies less than 1 kg, and careful planning between the neonatal service and the anaesthetist is necessary. A neonatal ventilator may be needed (particularly in the presence of premature lung disease), which may affect the way the anaesthetic is planned and delivered. Transport of the infant between the cath lab and neonatal unit needs to be carefully planned. Vascular access can be challenging. Other considerations include temperature control (e.g. warming intravenous fluids, use of heating mats), avoidance of over-hydration and monitoring blood glucose. The cardiologist may also ask for a nasogastric tube or oesophageal temperature probe to be present as a radiographic landmark.

## Hybrid Procedures

Hybrid procedures describe those involving either a cooperative approach by cardiologists and surgeons, or a combined radiological imaging procedure.

Hybrid surgical procedures can be challenging and require coordination between the many members of the different teams at the preoperative brief. Examples of surgical hybrid procedures include the hybrid Norwood operation, which involves direct pulmonary artery branch banding by the surgeon, and the implantation of a ductal stent by the cardiologist, often via direct puncture of the pulmonary artery. Other examples include per-ventricular closure of a ventricular septal defect and direct stent implantation into the pulmonary artery right-ventricular outflow tract. Repair of left pulmonary artery sling in our centre has evolved into a hybrid procedure, involving the cardiology team, to include an exit epicardial echocardiogram and angiogram.

Hybrid imaging procedures may involve catheters being positioned conventionally in the fluoroscopy facility and then moving the patient with catheters in situ into the MRI suite. This allows the combination of pressures and MRI data to be collected simultaneously, such as for the accurate assessment of PVR. A standardised system of checks for safety is necessary, including the exclusion of metallic objects from the field and ensuring the security of fluid-filled monitoring tubes through which significant bleeding could occur should they become disconnected.

## Electrophysiological Studies

Children present for electrophysiological studies (EPS) to identify the source of an arrhythmia and potentially to ablate an abnormal focus or pathway. Most of these patients have normal ventricular function, and many suffer from paroxysmal supraventricular tachycardias. Most commonly these are re-entry or accessory pathway tachycardias such as sinoatrial node re-entrant tachycardia (SARNT), atrioventricular (AV) nodal re-entrant tachycardia (AVRNT) or Wolff–Parkinson–White syndrome and atrioventricular re-entry tachycardia (AVRT).

The procedure involves the insertion of catheters with multiple electrodes along their length into the coronary sinus via the right heart, to stimulate and map the electrical pathways. Access can be from the femoral or subclavian vein. Once the abnormal pathway has been identified, it is ablated by radio-frequency energy delivered by another catheter. The size of the 'burn' necessary to fully ablate the focus varies and the procedure can be prolonged. Where the abnormal focus lies close to the AV node, radiofrequency carries a high risk of heart block; a newer technique involving cryoablation with a super-cooled catheter appears to be safer, though recurrence risk is higher.

Anaesthesia is generally straightforward, as these children are usually otherwise well. Many arrhythmias are provoked by stress and suppressed by deep anaesthesia; the latter should therefore be avoided, as it may make it more difficult to identify the focus. TIVA is a good option, combined with depth of anaesthesia monitoring to avoid excessively deep anaesthesia. Isoflurane at 1–1.5 MAC supplemented with a small dose of fentanyl is an alternative. Isoprenaline is often used to provoke dysrhythmia, and adenosine may be given to help identify an aberrant pathway. Adenosine may induce bronchospasm and should be avoided in children with asthma. Dexamethasone as antiemetic prophylaxis should be avoided in these patients, as its anti-inflammatory effect may ameliorate the 'burn' and compromise the ablation. The procedures can be prolonged; appropriate methods to monitor and maintain temperature should be used.

## Implantation of Pacemakers and Other Devices

Some permanent pacemakers are implanted in the catheter laboratory, usually in the left subclavicular region, with transvenous pacing leads inserted into the subclavian vein. Where the nature of an intermittent dysrhythmia cannot be identified, an indwelling ECG loop recorder may be implanted in the subclavicular or parasternal area. Anaesthesia is generally straightforward and should include intravenous and topical analgesia, together with prophylactic antibiotics.

## Implantable Cardioverter Defibrillator (ICD)

Several disorders are associated with sudden death in childhood due to an arrhythmia which may be prevented by an ICD. These include:

- Hypertrophic obstructive cardiomyopathy (HOCM)
- Catecholaminergic polymorphic ventricular tachycardia (CPVT)
- Arrhythmogenic right-ventricular cardiomyopathy (ARVC)
- Long QT syndrome
- Brugada syndrome

Many of these patients will have experienced a life-threatening arrhythmia or have a family history of sudden cardiac death. The procedure requires the placement of ventricular pacing leads via the subclavian vein and ICD device insertion in the subclavicular or axillary area. The device is designed to detect ventricular tachycardia or fibrillation and deliver an electrical shock to cardiovert. It will also pace where necessary. Once inserted, it is necessary to test that it is working satisfactorily by inducing ventricular fibrillation. Resuscitation drugs should be on hand, and external defibrillation pads should be placed in case the device does not function as intended. Inducing ventricular fibrillation can lead to severe cardiac decompensation in some patients, such as those with severe cardiomyopathy, and invasive arterial pressure monitoring and central venous access should be used.

Induction of anaesthesia can be challenging in patients with severe HOCM, particularly those with significant left-ventricular outflow tract obstruction (LVOTO), exacerbated by systolic anterior motion (SAM) of the mitral valve and with diastolic dysfunction. The LVOTO is dynamic, and it is important to avoid increased sympathetic activity that may increase it. Adequate ventricular filling is essential, so maintaining good hydration preoperatively, for example with intravenous fluids, and avoiding tachycardia are important. These patients will often be on β-blockers, which should not be stopped, and anxiolytic premedication is recommended. For induction a combination of fentanyl 1–2 mcg $kg^{-1}$, slow incremental doses of midazolam 50 mcg $kg^{-1}$ over a few minutes, and a small dose of propofol works well. Sevoflurane can be used where intravenous induction is not appropriate.

## Lead Extraction

The need for pacing or an ICD is usually a lifelong burden. The battery of an implanted device is limited. Battery-depleted pulse generators can be replaced so long as the implanted endovenous leads are working as planned (threshold, capture, etc.). Growth of a child, or simply the passage of time, may cause dysfunction of pacing leads and indicate replacement. Under such circumstances, there may be an indication to extract old pacing leads, to allow space within the vessel for the new leads. These procedures may be difficult when the leads have been in for an extended period because they can become tethered or encased in fibrous or calcified tissue. Various modalities and specialised procedures (telescoping sheaths, laser sheaths, rotational mechanical cutters) may be employed to separate leads from tethering tissue and can be prolonged and dangerous with risk of laceration of the major vein (SVC or brachiocephalic vein). A surgical team must be on standby and be prepared to repair catastrophic injury. Whilst mobilising the surgical team, it may be necessary to tamponade a lacerated vessel by gently inflating a large balloon in the vein. Major haemorrhage protocols must be in place, including rapid infusion equipment. Unusual surgical approaches to access the vessel may be necessary (e.g. division of the clavicle). Another risk of lead extraction is lead fracture and embolisation of fragments of the lead, which may involve more specialised catheter techniques for retrieval.

## Pericardial Effusion Drainage

Insertion of a pericardial needle or drain to relieve a pericardial effusion is usually performed under echocardiographic guidance. General anaesthesia can be challenging as these patients may have a severely compromised circulation from cardiac tamponade, rendering them highly preload dependent. Positive pressure ventilation reduces preload and so is avoided if possible. Ketamine is often advocated as an induction agent as it allows spontaneous ventilation to be maintained whilst maintaining myocardial contractility and SVR.

Profound hypotension can occur when the effusion is drained as the heart becomes acutely underfilled, and it is important that the effusion is drained slowly. Adequate venous access for rapid volume administration is essential. The situation is not helped by the need for the patient to be semi-erect to facilitate the effusion gravitating to the base of the heart. In adolescents, it may be safer to undertake this under local anaesthesia if possible.

## Cardiac MRI and CT

Cardiac MRI and magnetic resonance angiography (MRA) are increasingly used in the diagnosis and assessment of congenital heart disease, particularly for demonstrating 3D anatomical relationships and quantifying blood flows. It has the advantage that there is no radiation, although there is the need for MRI-compatible equipment and a general anaesthetic, as the scans are long. There is generally a need for short periods of apnoea, so controlled ventilation is required.

Many cardiac CT scans are very quick and can often be undertaken with sedation, or in small infants with appropriate swaddling. General anaesthesia may be needed for CT angiography, as a cannula will be needed for the contrast, and a short breath-hold may be required. CT coronary angiography requires a heart rate of around 80 bpm; dexmedetomidine is useful in achieving this.

These investigations are often undertaken to plan further surgical procedures in patients reliant upon a systemic to pulmonary shunt and who may be polycythaemic. It is vitally important to avoid dehydration, and clear oral fluids should be maintained until one hour before the procedure (or two hours if known reflux). Where this is not possible, intravenous fluids should be administered before anaesthesia.

## Further Reading

Hill KD, Du W, Fleming GA et al. Validation and refinement of the catheterization risk score for pediatrics (CRISP score): an analysis from the congenital cardiac interventional study consortium. *Catheterization and Cardiovascular Interventions* 2019 January; 93 (1):97–104.

Lam J, Lin E, Alexy R et al. Anesthesia and the pediatric cardiac catheterization suite: a review. *Pediatric Anesthesia* 2015: 25(2):127–34.

Lasa JJ, Alali A, Minard CG et al. Cardiopulmonary resuscitation in the pediatric cardiac catheterization laboratory: a report from the American Heart Association's Get with the Guidelines–Resuscitation registry. *Pediatric Critical Care Medicine* 2019 November; 20 (11):1040–7.

Latham GJ, Yung D. Educational review: current understanding and perioperative management of pediatric pulmonary hypertension. *Pediatric Anesthesia* 2019; 29(5):441–56.

Levy D, Bigham C, Tomlinson D. Anaesthesia for patients with hereditary arrhythmias; part I: Brugada syndrome, and part II: congenital long QT syndrome and arrhythmogenic right ventricular cardiomyopathy. *BJA Education* 2008; 18(6): 159–65 and 2008; 18(8):246–53.

Qureshi S, Pushparajah K, Taylor D. Anaesthesia for paediatric diagnostic and interventional cardiological procedures. *Continuing Education in Anaesthesia and Critical Care and Pain* 2015; 15(1):1–6.

Chapter

# 33 Anaesthesia for Children with Cardiac Disease Undergoing Non-cardiac Surgery

Ellen Rawlinson

## Introduction

Congenital heart disease (CHD) is one of the most common birth defects, occurring in approximately one in 150 live births. Extracardiac anomalies requiring surgical intervention within the first year of life occur in 30% and are often associated with recognised syndromes (Table 33.1). Advances in surgical strategies and medical care mean that around 90% of affected children will survive to adulthood. These children experience the same childhood illnesses and injuries as those without CHD and may present to their local hospital requiring elective or emergency surgery. Overall, children with CHD undergoing non-cardiac surgery (NCS) are at increased risk of perioperative morbidity and mortality and can present a significant challenge to the anaesthetist. However, this increased risk does not extend to all children with CHD, only to defined higher-risk groups, and it is clear that with appropriate planning and expertise even those with significant disease can tolerate major surgery with few complications.

## Aims and Limitations

This chapter aims to discuss the principles underlying the management of children with CHD: it includes risk stratification to distinguish those who would benefit from specialist care from those who may be safely managed in their local hospital. There are three main limitations. Firstly, few studies consider children with CHD undergoing NCS with much of the available information coming from cardiac catheterisation. The impact of other surgical procedures on risk is not completely characterised. Surgery involving changes in position (prone or Trendelenburg), major fluid shifts or laparoscopic approaches changing intracavity pressures may produce physiological effects that alter these risks. Secondly, most outcome data from which risk stratification systems are derived from large US databases that do not provide perioperative management details, including where the surgery was performed (large versus small hospitals, teaching versus peripheral) or who delivered the care (cardiac or general paediatric anaesthetist). Finally, children with CHD represent an extraordinarily heterogeneous group of patients. Furthermore, in a rapidly advancing field, observed complications may relate to outdated treatment strategies, making application to current practice difficult. As such, it is not possible to describe an anaesthetic technique suitable for all patients. The approach presented here is consequently a general one, based on applied physiology and informed by the available evidence where possible.

## Pathophysiology of Different Circulations

When considering the child with CHD for NCS, a comprehensive understanding of the cardiac lesion is imperative. The likely effects of anaesthesia and surgery can then be anticipated. A simple classification of cardiac disorders is given in Table 33.2, and some common physiological patterns are now discussed.

### Left-to-Right Shunts: 'In Series' Circulations

In some cardiac conditions, the dominant path of blood flow follows that of a structurally normal heart: separate systemic and pulmonary circulations operate in series. This is the situation for most types of repaired CHD. Unrepaired conditions that function 'in series' include atrial septal defects (ASD) ventricular septal defects (VSD) and patent ductus arteriosus (PDA). Blood flows through the defect down a pressure gradient, creating a left-to-right shunt, increased pulmonary blood flow (PBF) and volume overload of the right

**Table 33.1** Congenital syndromes and associated cardiac lesions

| Anomaly & genetic basis | CHD (%) | Typical cardiac lesion | Relevant clinical features |
|---|---|---|---|
| Down syndrome<br>– trisomy 21 | 40-50 | AVSD<br>VSD | Cervical spine instability<br>Prone to pulmonary hypertension<br>Obstructive sleep apnoea |
| DiGeorge / velocardiofacial syndrome<br>– 22q11 deletion | 70-75 | Interrupted aortic arch<br>Tetralogy of Fallot<br>Truncus arteriosus | Immune deficiency from absent thymus<br>- irradiated blood, freq. chest infections<br>Hypocalcaemia<br>Cleft lip and/or palate |
| Turner syndrome – monosomy X | 25-40 | Coarctation of aorta<br>AS / bicuspid Ao valve | Scoliosis<br>Strabismus |
| Williams syndrome – 7q11.3 deletion | 75-80 | Supravalvar AS<br>Pulmonary stenosis | Skeletal/joint abnormalities<br>Dental abnormalities |
| Noonan syndrome | 70-80 | Pulmonary stenosis<br>HOCM | Cervical spine: syringomyelia, Arnold Chiari<br>Pectus carinatum/excavatum |
| VACTERL association | 40-80 | ASD / VSD<br>Tetralogy of Fallot<br>Truncus arteriosus | Tracheoesophageal fistula +/– oesophageal atresia<br>Anal atresia<br>Renal and vertebral anomalies |
| CHARGE association | 75-80 | Tetralogy of Fallot<br>Various others | Choanal atresia<br>Cranial nerve palsy IX/X: swallowing problems<br>Cleft lip and/or palate |
| Goldenhar syndrome | 30-60 | Tetralogy of Fallot<br>ASD / VSD | Hemifacial microsomia: difficult intubation<br>Cleft lip and/or palate |
| Duchenne muscular dystrophy<br>X-linked dystrophin gene | 60-75 | Cardiomyopathy | Respiratory muscle weakness<br>Scoliosis |

*Notes:* AVSD = atrioventricular septal defect; VSD = ventricular septal defect; AS = aortic stenosis; HOCM = hypertrophic cardiomyopathy; ASD = atrial septal defect.

ventricle. Potential consequences include pulmonary hypertension and cardiac failure. Structurally small defects are termed restrictive: the physiological effects are such that treatment can often be deferred. Larger 'unrestrictive' defects can lead to severe cardiac failure in infancy. The degree of shunt can be quantified using the Qp:Qs ratio (where Qp is pulmonary blood flow and Qs is systemic blood flow), estimated from two-dimensional echocardiography (ECHO). Elevation of the normal 1:1 ratio to 2:1 or above is usually associated with symptoms of heart failure.

## Parallel or 'Balanced' Circulations

More significant anatomical defects allow mixing of oxygenated and deoxygenated blood and lead to systemic and pulmonary circulations operating in parallel. Examples include infants with large unrepaired atrioventricular septal defects (AVSD) and truncus arteriosus. Flow to the systemic or pulmonary vascular beds depends on the relative resistances of each circuit, so flow is dependent on the 'balance' between systemic vascular resistance (SVR) and pulmonary vascular resistance (PVR). High flow to one area compromises flow

**Table 33.2** Classification of congenital cardiac lesions

| Type of disorder | Common examples |
|---|---|
| **Acyanotic cardiac lesions** | |
| **Left-to-right shunts – excessive pulmonary blood flow** | |
| 'Restrictive' lesions | Small ASD, VSD, PDA |
| 'Non-restrictive' lesions | Large VSD, PDA<br>AVSD, AP window |
| **Left-ventricular outflow tract obstruction** | |
| | Coarctation of the aorta<br>Interrupted aortic arch<br>Aortic stenosis<br>HOCM |
| **Cyanotic cardiac lesions** | |
| **Right-to-left shunts – inadequate pulmonary blood flow** | |
| | Tetralogy of Fallot<br>Tricuspid atresia<br>Pulmonary stenosis/atresia |
| **Complex shunts with obligatory common mixing** | |
| | Transposition of the great arteries<br>Hypoplastic left heart syndrome<br>Truncus arteriosus<br>TAPVD |

*Notes:* PDA: patent ductus arteriosus, AP: aorto-pulmonary window; TAPVD = total anomalous pulmonary venous drainage.

**Table 33.3** Factors affecting pulmonary blood flow

| Factors reducing PBF | Factors Increasing PBF |
|---|---|
| **Increased PVR** | **Reduced PVR** |
| Hypoxia | High inspired oxygen |
| Hypercarbia | Hypocarbia |
| Acidosis | Alkalosis |
| Hyperinflation | Normal inflation volumes |
| ↑ Haematocrit | ↓ Haematocrit |
| **Decreased SVR** | **Increased SVR** |
| Pyrexia | Hypothermia |
| Anaesthetic agents: | Vasoconstrictors |
| - propofol | Sympathetic stimulation |
| - high dose volatiles | |
| Sympathetic block | |

to the other. Excessive PBF causes pulmonary oedema and poor systemic perfusion and can lead to coronary and splanchnic ischaemia, whereas inadequate PBF causes cyanosis. Anaesthetic interventions can have a significant effect on blood flow in these circumstances. Oxygen is a potent pulmonary vasodilator and will increase PBF at the expense of systemic perfusion. Conversely, large doses of induction agents may reduce SVR sufficiently to reverse a left-to-right shunt and cause profound hypoxia. Factors affecting pulmonary and systemic blood flow are given in Table 33.3.

## Duct-Dependent Circulations

The concept of a balanced circulation is particularly important in patients who are duct dependent. In some complex CHD, neonates rely on flow through the ductus arteriosus to maintain either systemic blood flow, such as hypoplastic left-heart syndrome (HLHS), interrupted aortic arch (IAA) or pulmonary blood flow, such as pulmonary atresia. An infusion of prostaglandin E is required to maintain ductal patency until surgery can occur. A well-balanced circulation produces saturations of 75–85%, with higher saturations indicating excessive PBF. Where systemic perfusion depends on the duct, ventilation in room air with moderate hypercapnia and respiratory acidosis may be required to increase PVR, reduce PBF and prevent systemic hypoperfusion, metabolic acidosis and possible cardiac arrest.

## Single-Ventricle Circulations

Biventricular repair to create a normal 'in series' circulation is not always possible, so some affected children will be palliated with a circulation based on one functional ventricle. The functional single ventricle (SV) is utilised to pump blood around the body whilst pulmonary blood flow is passive down a pressure gradient from the pulmonary artery (PA) to the left atrium (LA). The archetypal SV circulation is HLHS, but there are a large number of cardiac defects that follow this pathway. Most children require a first-stage surgical intervention in the neonatal period, the nature of which is determined by the underlying lesion. For HLHS, this is the Norwood operation, utilising the right ventricle as the systemic SV, with the formation of a 'neo-aorta' from the anatomical hypoplastic aorta and the main

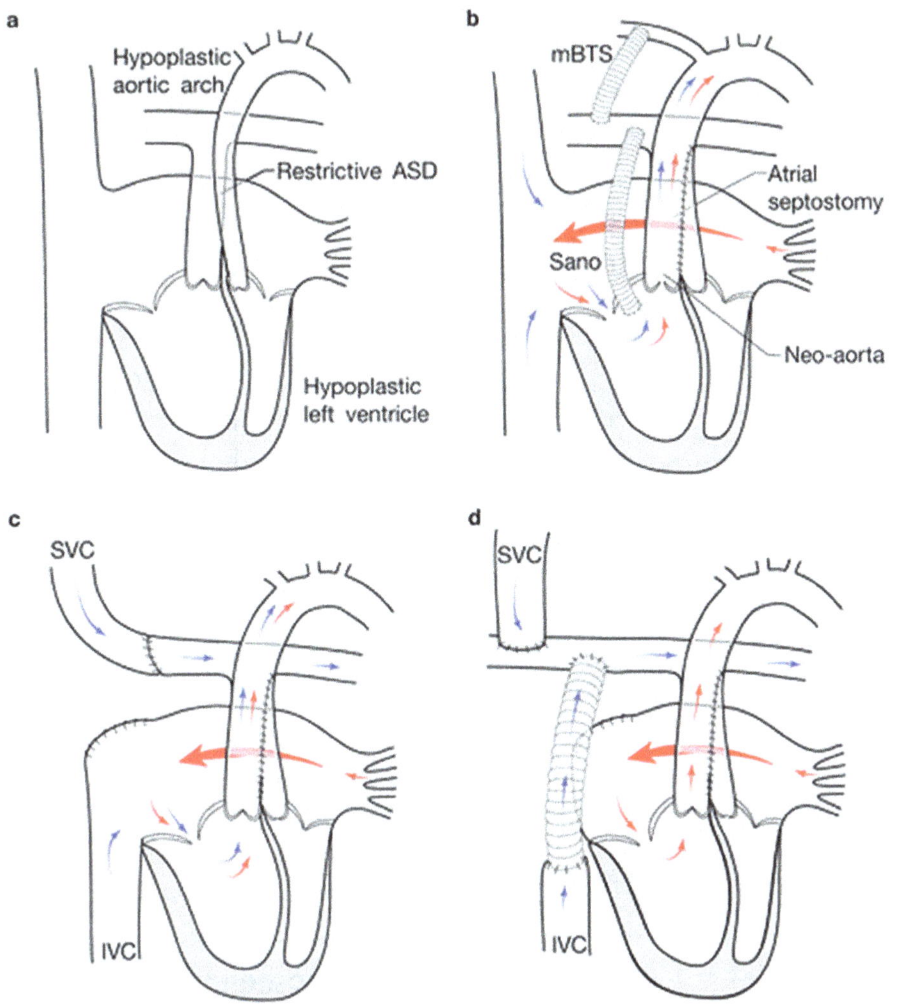


**Figure 33.1** (a) Hypoplastic left-heart syndrome with a small left ventricle, hypoplastic aortic valve and arch and atrial septal defect. (b) Norwood procedure: anastomosis of the aorta to the pulmonary artery and atrial septostomy, ligation of PDA and formation of either a modified Blalock–Taussig (BT) shunt or Sano (right ventricle to pulmonary artery) shunt. (c) Bidirectional Glenn: connection of the superior vena cava (SVC) to the right pulmonary artery (RPA) and ligation of either a BT or Sano shunt. (d) Fontan: inferior vena cava (IVC) also connected to the RPA, shown here using the currently favoured extracardiac conduit.

pulmonary artery, and the creation of a modified Blalock–Taussig (BT) shunt or a Sano shunt to establish pulmonary blood flow (Figure 33.1). For other lesions, pulmonary artery banding or formation of a BT shunt may suffice in the first instance (Figure 33.2).

The second stage is common to all and involves the formation of a Glenn shunt at around three to five months (Figure 33.1c). This involves connecting the superior vena cava (SVC) to the right pulmonary artery (RPA), with the removal of any remaining shunts. Postoperatively, the child remains cyanosed (oxygen saturations 75–85%), and the ventricle remains volume loaded, receiving venous return from both inferior vena cava (IVC) and pulmonary veins. As the child grows, the proportion of venous return from the SVC reduces from the 60% seen in infancy towards adult values of around 35%, and pulmonary blood flow becomes inadequate. The third stage of total cavopulmonary circulation (TCPC) or Fontan procedure is performed between three to five years and involves connecting the IVC to the RPA, such that all systemic venous return now flows passively directly into the pulmonary circulation. A ‘fenestration’ may be created as part of the procedure; this is a surgical connection between the conduit connecting the IVC to the RPA and

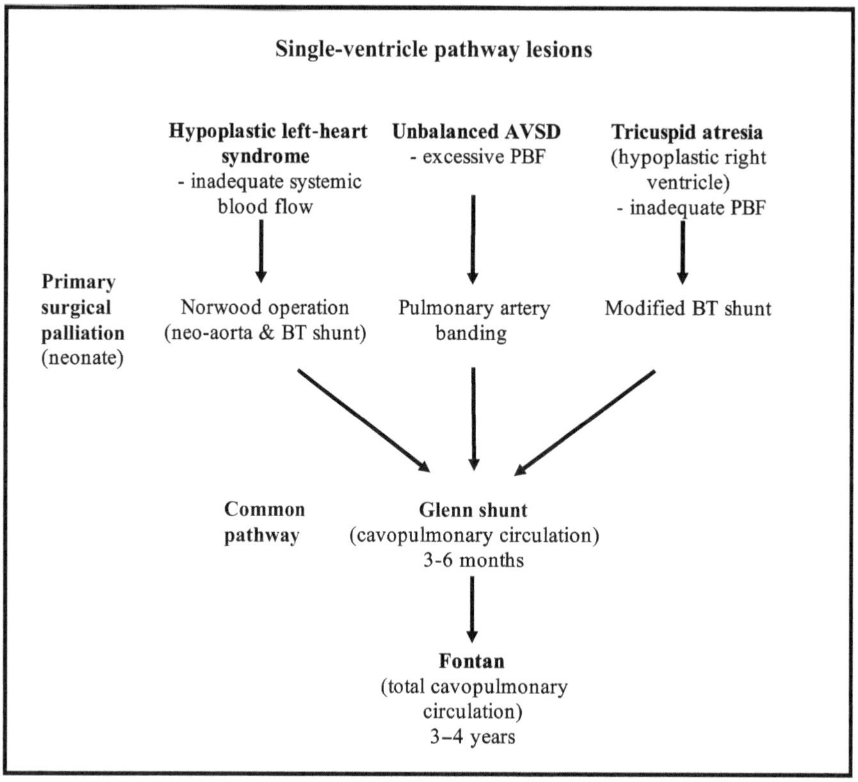


**Figure 33.2** Spectrum of congenital cardiac lesions that are ultimately palliated with a single ventricle surgical strategy. AVSD: atrioventricular septal defect; BT: Blalock–Taussig.
*Source:* Reprinted with permission from Smith S, Walker A. Anaesthetic implications of congenital heart disease for children undergoing non-cardiac surgery. *Anaesthesia and Intensive Care Medicine* 2018; 19(8):414–20. doi: 10.1016/j.mpaic.2018.04.011.

the common atrium and can act as a 'pressure-relief' valve. If PVR is high and PA pressure is elevated, deoxygenated blood can bypass the lungs and enter the heart directly, ensuring that the systemic ventricle remains adequately volume loaded, maintaining cardiac output even in the presence of high PVR, but leading to desaturation. In general, children with an un-fenestrated Fontan should be almost fully saturated, but those with a fenestration may not be.

With single-ventricle physiology (SVP), increases in PVR and intrathoracic pressure associated with intermittent positive pressure ventilation (IPPV) can reduce PBF. The choice of ventilatory strategy represents a compromise. The advantages of spontaneous ventilation, which promotes PBF by generating negative intrathoracic pressure, should be set against the advantages of IPPV with respect to greater control in avoiding hypoxia and hypercapnia. When required, IPPV should be optimised with pressures and inspiratory times minimised to facilitate PBF.

## Physiological Consequences of Heart Disease in Children

### Cardiac Failure

Cardiac failure in children may be a consequence of structural CHD or due to an intrinsic disease of heart muscle (cardiomyopathy). Regardless of aetiology, the common end result of a volume- or pressure-overloaded ventricle is a failing heart that is unable to meet everyday physiological needs. Children with severely limited cardiac reserve function at or near maximal cardiac capacity even when resting and are reliant on sympathetic tone to maintain their cardiac output. Anaesthetic-induced reductions in sympathetic drive or SVR can produce significant haemodynamic compromise. Left-ventricular systolic dysfunction is defined as an ejection fraction (EF) of less than 55%. There are no formal definitions for degrees of dysfunction, but EF less than 40% should be considered moderate and less than 30% severe. A significant degree of impairment may exist without symptoms, but when present symptoms of cardiac failure include tachypnoea, tachycardia, sweating episodes (e.g. when feeding), hepatomegaly and failure to thrive. Anaesthetic induction will be prolonged, whether intravenous or by inhalation, so patience is required to avoid excessive drug administration. These children represent a high-risk group and should be managed in a specialist centre wherever possible.

## Cyanosis

Children with unrepaired or partially palliated CHD will commonly exhibit cyanosis, and oxygen saturations of 70–80% can be well tolerated for several years. Cyanosis is seen in cardiac conditions with right-to-left shunts and obligatory intracardiac mixing such as BT shunts and Glenn circulations. The main aim during anaesthesia is to maintain oxygenation at a level the child is accustomed to. In the presence of a structural shunt, it will not be possible to achieve 'normal' saturations, although it is relatively common to see an intraoperative rise in oxygen saturations with higher fractions of inspired oxygen and a fall in PVR. End-tidal $CO_2$ monitoring is inaccurate in cyanosed patients and reads up to 2 kPa less than arterial $CO_2$; however, the relationship is reasonably reliable, so end-tidal $CO_2$ can still be used as a proxy for ventilatory efficacy. The hypoxic ventilatory response is blunted in children with cyanosis, so the risks of postoperative respiratory depression are increased.

Chronic cyanosis affects most major organ systems, but the haematological effects are most pertinent to anaesthesia. Increased erythropoietin production causes increased haemoglobin, haematocrit and viscosity, maintaining oxygen delivery without elevating cardiac output. The haemoglobin level should not be allowed to fall below 110–120 g $l^{-1}$, with transfusion started early if there is surgical blood loss. However, a haematocrit over 65% can actually reduce oxygen delivery due to increased red cell rigidity. Hyperviscosity is associated with cerebral vein and sinus thrombosis and stroke; the risks are highest in children with fever, dehydration, iron deficiency and those under five years. Preoperative haemoglobin higher than 180 g $l^{-1}$ (haematocrit >60%) should prompt consideration of intravenous fluid therapy to reduce this. Cyanosis is associated with an increased risk of bleeding via multiple effects on the clotting pathway, and this remains true even when preoperative clotting tests are normal. In children taking aspirin to maintain shunt patency, the risk of shunt thrombosis is usually greater than the risk of bleeding, so in most cases aspirin therapy should continue.

## Pulmonary Hypertension

Pulmonary hypertension (PHT) is defined as a mean pulmonary artery pressure (PAP) above 25 mmHg at rest. Whilst over 50% of cases are idiopathic, PHT may develop secondary to a number of cardiac conditions. Children with CHD at risk include those with left-to-right shunts and excess PBF, such as AVSD, or those with prolonged pulmonary venous obstruction or high left-atrial pressure, for example following repair of total anomalous pulmonary venous drainage (TAPVD). Other causes include chronic lung disease, sickle cell disease or syndromic associations such as Down. There is a wide spectrum of severity, but PHT is a clear predictor of increased perioperative morbidity and mortality. Those with suprasystemic PAP are eight times as likely to experience a major complication as those with subsystemic PAP. The key principle of anaesthesia is to avoid a rise in PVR, which in turn may precipitate acute right-ventricular failure. Cardiac arrest in this setting is difficult to recover from. Factors which elevate PVR include acidosis, elevated $PaCO_2$, hypoxia, hypothermia, increased sympathetic stimulation (from inadequate anaesthesia) and increased airway pressure. Appropriate management of all these factors will reduce PVR, improve RV function and minimise any right-to-left shunting.

## Arrhythmias

Children with CHD may be at risk of arrhythmias following surgical intervention, although this risk may not manifest until several years later. Atrial arrhythmias are most common following atrial septal/ sinus venosus defect repairs and atrial switch operations (Mustard and Senning). Conduction defects from damage to the atrioventricular node and bundle of His are commonest following ventriculotomy or right ventricle to pulmonary artery conduit; children with single-ventricle physiology or following tetralogy of Fallot or Ebstein's repairs are at particular risk. In addition to those associated with structural CHD, there is a heterogeneous group of primary malignant arrhythmias, sometimes referred to as cardiac channelopathies, which predispose children to life-threatening perioperative events. This group includes long QT syndrome (LQTS), Brugada syndrome, arrhythmogenic right-ventricular cardiomyopathy (ARVC) and catecholaminergic polymorphic ventricular tachycardia (CPVT).

All children with CHD should have a preoperative ECG. Whilst right bundle branch block (RBBB) is a common and usually benign finding, ventricular ectopics are an ominous sign as 30% of these patients will eventually die suddenly. The optimal anaesthetic strategy is not well defined. In general, it is recommended that factors known to lower the threshold for ventricular ectopics are avoided; these include hypoxia, acidosis, hypercarbia and large doses of local anaesthetic with adrenaline. Prolongation of the QT interval is associated with polymorphic ventricular tachycardia (Torsades de Pointes) particularly in those with long QT syndromes. Both propofol and sevoflurane appear to have little effect on the QTc (QT interval corrected for heart rate), whereas other drugs prolong it and should be avoided, such as ondansetron, ketamine, suxamethonium and most adrenergic agents. Magnesium is the treatment of choice should a polymorphic tachycardia develop, and prophylactic infusion in those at risk has been advocated.

**Table 33.4** Factors associated with increased risk of perioperative morbidity

| |
|---|
| Age: less than 2 years |
| Higher ASA grade |
| Multiple comorbidities |
| Emergency surgery |
| Complex lesions:<br>- Single ventricle physiology, notably: unrepaired; with BT shunt/prior to Glenn formation; failing Fontan<br>- Cardiomyopathy<br>- Left-ventricular outflow tract obstruction, e.g. aortic stenosis |
| Presence of long-term complications:<br>- Cyanosis<br>- Cardiac failure<br>- Arrhythmia |
| Pulmonary hypertension particularly with suprasystemic pressures |

Source: ASA: American Society of Anesthesiologists physical status classification.

## Risk Stratification

Children with CHD presenting for NCS are at significantly increased risk of perioperative morbidity and mortality when compared with those without. Recent analysis of the US Pediatric Health Information System database that includes some 500,000 surgical cases per year demonstrated that overall mortality rates in children with CHD were almost nine times greater than in those without (1.06% vs 0.12% in 2019). However, the outcomes for children with CHD appear to be improving; between 2015 and 2019, the mortality rate in children with CHD decreased significantly from 1.16% to 1.06%, whilst the rate in those without CHD remained unchanged.

Risk is not evenly distributed across this population, and a summary of identified risk factors taken from a heterogeneous group of both single centre and large database studies is given in Table 33.4. The American College of Surgeons (ACS) National Surgical Quality Improvement Program (NSQIP) database categorises CHD according to residual cardiac lesion and functional status into minor, major or severe categories (Table 33.5). The data demonstrate that children with minor CHD are at no greater risk than the general population for overall mortality (1.2% vs 1.7%), cardiac arrest or adverse events. This group of children may be safely managed in their local hospital according to usual protocols, without needing transfer to specialist centres solely on the basis of their CHD.

For children in the major and severe ACS NSQIP categories, the same database has been used to develop the Pediatric Risk Assessment (PRAm) score, designed to prognosticate the perioperative risk of mortality. PRAm identifies eight important factors which are weighted to produce a score of 1–10 (Table 33.6), and validation studies have shown good discrimination for prediction of in-hospital mortality. Scores of $\leq 3$ are associated with a low risk of mortality (OR 1.54, 95% CI: 0.78–3.04), scores 4–6 with a medium risk (OR 4.19, 95% CI: 2.56–6.87) and scores $\geq 7$ with high risk (OR 22.15, 95% CI: 15.06–32.59). This scoring system emphasises the significance of the functional severity of disease as well as markers of

**Table 33.5** ACS NSQIP risk stratification for CHD

| Classification | Definition |
|---|---|
| Minor CHD | Cardiac condition with or without medication and maintenance, e.g. ASD, small to moderate VSD without symptoms<br>Repair of CHD with normal cardiovascular function and no medication |
| Major CHD | Repair of CHD with residual haemodynamic abnormality with or without medications, e.g. tetralogy of Fallot with free pulmonary regurgitation, HLHS including Stage 1 repair |
| Severe CHD | Uncorrected cyanotic CHD<br>Patients with documented pulmonary hypertension<br>Patients with ventricular dysfunction requiring medication<br>Listed for heart transplant |

**Table 33.6** PRAm score: multivariate risk score to predict postoperative mortality

| Variable | OR | 95% CI | Risk score |
|---|---|---|---|
| Emergency procedure | 1.7 | 1.2–2.3 | +1 |
| Severe CHD | 1.7 | 1.2–2.4 | +1 |
| Single ventricle physiology | 1.8 | 1.1–3.0 | +1 |
| Surgery in preceding 30 days | 2.0 | 1.4–2.9 | +1 |
| Inotropic support | 2.1 | 1.4–3.0 | +1 |
| Preoperative CPR | 2.5 | 1.3–4.6 | +2 |
| Acute or chronic kidney injury | 4.4 | 2.0–9.8 | +3 |
| Mechanical ventilation | 7.8 | 5.4–11.2 | +4 |

*Notes:* OR = odds ratio; CI = confidence interval; CPR = cardiopulmonary resuscitation.

critical illness. It also reinforces SV physiology as a major risk factor. Unfortunately, the ACS NSQIP data provides no information about which professionals performed the surgery (general paediatric or cardiac anaesthetist) or what setting the surgery occurred in (large or small, teaching or peripheral hospital). Additionally, some nuance may be lost by the classification of all children with PHT in the severe category. However, PRAm represents the best tool currently available for objective scoring of risk, which may be helpful in determining allocation of resources.

# Anaesthetic Management

## Preoperative Assessment

A comprehensive understanding of the anatomy, physiology and risk factors of the underlying CHD lesion is essential before proceeding with anaesthesia. Consideration of the appropriate location for surgery is also imperative. Children with minor CHD appear to be at no greater risk than their peers without CHD, so they may be managed locally as expertise and facilities allow. Transfers in this population are unnecessary and place additional burdens on families and specialist centres. However, it is clear that children in higher-risk categories experience increased perioperative morbidity and mortality. An evidence-based approach supports transfer and management where full specialist facilities are available, including cardiology, cardiac anaesthesia and paediatric intensive care support. Early communication and cooperation between specialist and local services are essential to ensure that transfers for high-risk children who *may* require surgery are facilitated in a timely manner. In children who are functionally limited by their disease, serious consideration should be given to whether surgery is truly essential, whether the child is in an optimal state to proceed and whether deferral until after further cardiac intervention is possible.

Preoperative assessment includes a routine anaesthetic history and examination, determination of long-term complications and identifying those features associated with high-risk categorisation (discussed in the previous section). In addition, specific attention should be paid to the following elements:

### Echocardiography

A recent ECHO should be acquired and reviewed preoperatively. It provides invaluable information both in confirming the current structural arrangement and providing an assessment of cardiac function. ECHO reports use standard terminology and usually follow a sequential segmental analysis to provide the following information: atrial position and venous drainage; atrioventricular (AV) and

**Table 33.7** Common echocardiography terms

**Cardiac position:**
*Levocardia:* normal position cardiac mass with apex to left
*Dextrocardia:* mirror-image cardiac mass with apex to right and right-ventricle anterior
*Dextroversion:* cardiac mass rotated with apex to right but left-ventricle anterior
*Dextroposition:* cardiac mass displaced to right but apex remains to the left

**Atrial situs – the situation of the atrial chambers:**
*Situs solitus*: normal atria & abdominal organs
*Situs inversus:* mirror image atria & abdominal organs
*Situs ambiguous:* no clear lateralisation
Left-/right-atrial isomerism: two morphological left/right atria

**Atrioventricular connections (AVC):**
Concordant AVC: usual connection of atria to ventricles
Discordant AVC: left atrium connected to right ventricle, right atrium connected to left ventricle
Double inlet left/right ventricle: two ventricle heart but >50% override of atrial to ventricular connection due to malaligned septa
Absent left/right AVC: mitral or tricuspid atresia

**Ventriculo-arterial connections (VAC):**
Concordant VAC: usual connection of ventricles to aorta and pulmonary artery
Discordant VAC: left ventricle connected to pulmonary artery and right ventricle to aorta (TGA)
Single-outlet VAC: aortic or pulmonary atresia
Double-outlet right ventricle: two ventricle heart but >50% override of aorta from right ventricle

**Valve descriptions and sizes:**
The z-score describes the number of standard deviations from the mean of the normal size, e.g. a z score of −3 shows the valve is 3 standard deviations smaller than expected

**Doppler flow & pressure gradients:**
Velocity of flow between chambers may be used to estimate the pressure gradient using the formula:
Pressure (mmHg) = 4 × velocity $(m\ s^{-1})^2$

ventriculo-arterial (VA) connections; abnormal shunts and direction of flow; ventricular dimensions and function; and coronary and arch anatomy. Table 33.7 provides a summary of common terms.

A small amount of tricuspid regurgitation (TR) is considered normal, and the velocity of the regurgitant jet is indicative of the pressure difference between right atrium and ventricle. In PHT, this can give an indication of PAP using the simplified Bernoulli equation $\Delta P = 4V^2$ (P = pressure difference (mmHg), V = peak velocity $(ms^{-2})$): a TR jet of >4 $ms^{-1}$ indicates a high probability of severe pulmonary hypertension.

## Intercurrent Respiratory Tract Infection

Children with increased PBF are more susceptible to respiratory tract infections, and distinguishing infection from cardiac failure can be difficult. In children with PHT or Glenn circulation, infection has a greater than expected effect on PVR. Intercurrent infection should be considered a contraindication to elective surgery, as the perioperative risk of hypoxaemia is increased.

## Medication

In general, cardiac medications should be continued as usual. Cardiac medications are not associated with clinically important preoperative electrolyte disturbances in children presenting for cardiac surgery, so routine testing is unnecessary. Some anaesthetists omit angiotensin converting enzyme (ACE) inhibitors on the morning of surgery to avoid hypotension on induction. Data on this phenomenon in adults are conflicting and in children is non-existent. Aspirin is commonly used to prevent shunt thrombosis and should be continued if possible. Children taking warfarin will need admission for conversion to intravenous heparin therapy and appropriate monitoring. In children taking the newer direct inhibitors of activated factor X, there should be liaison with haematology specialists.

## Endocarditis Prophylaxis

Some children with CHD are generally at increased risk of developing infective endocarditis (IE). However, the evidence that prophylactic antibiotics are effective at preventing perioperative IE is limited, and current NICE guidelines limit their use significantly (see Table 33.8).

## Pacemakers and Defibrillators

The indication for insertion and the features of the device should be ascertained and the current status of the device interrogated by a cardiac physiologist. Remember that in smaller children the box will be implanted in the sub-costal region rather than below the clavicle, and that pacing leads will be epicardial

**Table 33.8** Guideline for infective endocarditis prophylaxis

| |
|---|
| **Conditions at risk for infective endocarditis:** |
| Acquired valve disease with stenosis or regurgitation |
| Previous infective endocarditis |
| Hypertrophic cardiomyopathy |
| Valve replacement |
| Structural congenital heart disease including surgically corrected/palliated lesions but excluding those listed next |
| **Conditions NOT at risk for infective endocarditis:** |
| Isolated atrial septal defect |
| Fully repaired ventricular septal defect |
| Fully repaired patent ductus arteriosus |
| Endothelialised closure devices |
| **Procedures NOT requiring antibiotic prophylaxis even for at risk conditions:** |
| Dental procedures |
| Upper and lower GI tract procedures |
| GU tract, including urology, gynaecology and obstetrics |
| Upper and lower respiratory tract including ENT and bronchoscopy |

rather than endovascular. In general, sensing functionality should be switched off for the duration of the procedure to avoid electromagnetic interference. If the underlying rhythm is insufficient to maintain adequate haemodynamics, then temporary programming to an asynchronous, non-sensing mode may be appropriate. Implantable cardiac defibrillators (ICD) should have their shock delivery capacity disabled and external defibrillator pads applied remote from the ICD site. The response of pacemakers to magnets is not predictable without knowledge of the device, so they should be avoided. However, in a true emergency all commonly available ICDs may have their shock function disabled by taping a medical grade magnet to the skin. Some devices will emit a tone whilst so disabled. The device should revert to its usual settings once the magnet is removed, although a formal check should be performed as soon as possible.

## Perioperative Care

Many different anaesthetic techniques have been described and utilised successfully in children with CHD undergoing NCS, but no single approach can be recommended for all scenarios. In general, prolonged spontaneous ventilation with high-dose volatile agent is potentially hazardous for many: a balanced technique including controlled ventilation and the use of opioids to reduce the dose of volatile agent is usually preferable. Fluid depletion is tolerated poorly in a number of conditions, notably children with shunts and single-ventricle circulations, so preoperative fasting should be kept to a minimum. If fluid replacement is desired but intravenous access is difficult, then preoperative administration of isotonic fluids via nasogastric tube should be considered.

### Premedication

For the majority of children with CHD, the decision to administer premedication may be made according to the anaesthetist's usual assessment of probable compliance. Children with CHD may require multiple procedures under general anaesthesia, so ensuring a calm induction is important from a long-term psychological perspective. Oral midazolam has a long history of successful use, and more recently oral dexmedetomidine has been shown to be equally safe and effective. In some high-risk sub-groups where stress and anxiety can worsen haemodynamics, sedative premedication is strongly recommended. This includes children with dynamic left-ventricular outflow tract obstruction such as hypertrophic cardiomyopathy, where agitation may worsen the degree of obstruction, and those with significant pulmonary hypertension, where agitation may precipitate a pulmonary hypertensive crisis.

### Induction and Maintenance

All the volatile agents are associated with dose-dependent reductions in SVR (and probably PVR) and myocardial contractility. There are variable effects on heart rate and rhythm. Gas induction with sevoflurane is widely utilised, but particular care should be taken in children with trisomy 21 (Down syndrome), who appear susceptible to bradyarrhythmias with this technique. Even when gas induction is planned, preoperative application of topical local anaesthetic to appropriate venous access sites can be helpful. It allows intravenous access to be obtained at lighter planes of anaesthesia and can therefore help reduce the length of time the child is exposed to high concentrations of volatile agent. At maintenance concentrations, isoflurane and sevoflurane have minimal effect on contractility or shunt fraction, although animal studies suggest that myocardial depression with both agents is greater in the presence of a pulmonary artery band. Their use has been widely described in several large case-series of high-risk children for NCS, and the available evidence cannot recommend one agent over the other.

The two most studied intravenous agents for induction in children with CHD are propofol and ketamine. In children undergoing cardiac catheterisation, propofol decreases SVR and mean arterial pressure, whilst PAP and PVR remain unaltered. In the presence of a shunt, propofol leads to a reduction in left-to-right shunt and an increase in right-to-left shunt, thus reducing PBF, which can lead to clinically relevant reductions in oxygen saturations. Judicious use of propofol for induction may be appropriate, but it is best avoided in those with impaired myocardial function and pulmonary hypertension and in patients with right-to-left shunts. Total intravenous anaesthesia (TIVA) with propofol may be considered as an option for maintenance for some surgeries in children with some forms of CHD, but the literature suggests that this approach is not routine. Ketamine has minimal effects on cardiac output, SVR, heart rate and blood pressure. It is a direct myocardial depressant, but haemodynamic stability is maintained by central sympathetic stimulation. It is well tolerated in children with CHD, including those with pulmonary hypertension, and represents the agent of choice in this group and in those where a reduction in SVR is undesirable. However, it should be used with caution in children who are already catecholamine depleted, such as those with severe cardiomyopathy, where the direct myocardial depressant effects may become apparent with significant haemodynamic consequences. Ketamine infusions may be used for maintenance where preserving SVR is important, such as a severe left-ventricular outflow tract obstruction, but should be accompanied by additional sedative medication such as benzodiazepines to avoid unwanted neuropsychiatric side effects, particularly in older children.

### Analgesia

Opioids, including morphine, fentanyl and remifentanil, have minimal direct effects on either myocardial contractility or systemic and pulmonary vascular resistance. Intraoperatively they are effective at blocking responses to noxious stimuli that may precipitate a pulmonary hypertensive crisis in those at risk. In general, they may be used in a routine manner, including as postoperative infusions as the surgery requires. However, in children with cardiac failure whose cardiac output is dependent on sympathetic stimulation, administration of opioids may obtund the stress response and sympathetic drive and should be titrated with great caution. Regional anaesthetic techniques have been described and used effectively, although reports are rare and include only small numbers. Epidurals with general anaesthesia have been reported in neonates with complex, uncorrected cardiac disease with no complications, and there are case reports of spinal anaesthesia being used alone in infants. Care should be taken in those children taking anticoagulants for their cardiac condition.

### Postoperative Monitoring

Identifying the appropriate postoperative location for a child should be part of preoperative planning. The decision will be influenced by many factors, including the nature and severity of the cardiac lesion, the extent of the surgery and the situation of appropriate beds in the operating institution. A cardiology ward in a large teaching hospital with an extensive cardiac surgical practice will be able to support more significant non-cardiac interventions than a general paediatric ward in a district general hospital, where involvement with a high-dependency unit (HDU) or even a paediatric intensive care unit (PICU) may be indicated. Children with some conditions, such as Williams and Brugada syndrome, require prolonged postoperative monitoring even after relatively minor surgery, as the increased risk appears to extend further than usually expected into the postoperative period.

## Further Reading

Faraoni D, Vo D, Nasr VG, DiNardo JA. Development and validation of a risk stratification score for children with congenital heart disease undergoing noncardiac surgery. *Anesthesia Analgesia* 2016; 123 (4):824–30.

Ing RJ, Ames WA, Chambers NA. Paediatric cardiomyopathy and anaesthesia. *British Journal of Anaesthesia* 2012; 108(1): 4–12.

Latham GJ, Yung D. Educational review: current understanding and perioperative management of pediatric pulmonary hypertension. *Pediatric Anesthesia* 2019; 29(5): 441–56.

Levy, D, Bigham, C, Tomlinson, D. Anaesthesia for patients with hereditary arrhythmias; part I: Brugada syndrome, and part II: congenital long QT syndrome and arrhythmogenic right ventricular cardiomyopathy. *BJA Education* 2008; 18(6):159–65 and 2008; 18(8):246–53.

Taylor D, Habre W. Risk associated with anesthesia for noncardiac surgery in children with congenital heart disease. *Pediatric Anesthesia* 2019; 29: 426–34.

Chapter 34

# Anaesthesia for Urological Surgery in Children*

Alice Miskovic and Usman Ali

## Introduction

Paediatric urology theatre lists comprise a range of minor through to major complex cases. The children are often well, but impaired renal function is not uncommon. In addition to routine preoperative assessment, children should have a urine culture to exclude concurrent urinary tract infection (UTI), and coordination with the surgical team will guide antibiotic prophylaxis, which will also be dependent on previous culture results and local protocol. In this chapter, we discuss the anaesthetic management of a sub-specialty that allows for a variety of general and regional anaesthetic techniques to be applied.

## Minor Procedures

Common procedures include:

- Cystoscopy
- Resection of posterior urethral valves
- Circumcision
- Insertion of suprapubic (SP) lines
- Hypospadias repair
- Orchidopexy

## Cystoscopy

Indications for cystoscopy vary from investigation of minor renal tract abnormalities to follow-up after reconstructive or tumour surgery. Antibiotic prophylaxis is required. A supraglottic airway device (SGA) with spontaneous ventilation is standard practice except in neonates where intubation and ventilation are usually required. Cystoscopy is stimulating; fentanyl 1–2 mcg $kg^{-1}$ is needed after induction of anaesthesia with adequate depth of anaesthesia to avoid laryngospasm and provide postoperative analgesia. PRN paracetamol, ibuprofen (>3 months old and providing renal function is normal; or an alternative non-steroidal anti-inflammatory [NSAID]) and oral morphine 100–200 mcg $kg^{-1}$ can be prescribed.

* Many thanks to Dr Angus McEwan, who wrote the first edition of this book chapter, much of the content of which has been used in this revision.

## Resection of Posterior Urethral Valves

Posterior urethral valves (PUV) are the most common cause of urinary tract obstruction and only occur in boys. They are usually a sporadic occurrence, appearing early in fetal development with an incidence of 1:8,000. The severity of obstruction varies widely. Regardless of severity, the effects on the renal tract are lifelong. Those with minimal obstruction may not present until a later age, with recurrent UTI, enuresis or renal impairment. The bladder capacity is typically abnormal with vesico-ureteric reflux and bladder augmentation surgery (see the section 'Bladder Augmentation (Ileocystoplasty) and Mitrofanoff Formation' later in this chapter) may be required to preserve renal function. Monitoring of renal function is needed throughout life. One third of these boys will progress to end-stage renal failure. In children undergoing renal transplantation, 10–15% have a diagnosis of PUV. In the most severe cases, there is oligohydramnios, renal failure and lung hypoplasia requiring neonatal intensive care or possible incompatibility with life. Most commonly, bilateral hydronephrosis without renal impairment is detected antenatally. A cystoscopy is performed in the first few days of life to resect the PUV, with a check cystoscopy repeated one to two months later, occasionally with further resection. A circumcision can be performed at the initial PUV resection to reduce the rate of UTI. Neonatal airways are managed with tracheal intubation; larger infants undergoing a check cystoscopy can be managed with an SGA and spontaneous ventilation. The baby is positioned at the far end of the operating table in a 'natural' lithotomy position, which may necessitate long ventilator tubing. Antibiotic prophylaxis is required. For isolated PUV resection, fentanyl 1–2 mcg $kg^{-1}$ usually provides adequate analgesia, although some colleagues may perform caudal without additives. If circumcision is required, a caudal provides excellent analgesia. Local anaesthetic dose should be halved in neonates (e.g. maximum levobupivicaine 1 mg $kg^{-1}$). Oral paracetamol is prescribed postoperatively, and fluid balance monitored as a large volume of urine may be produced after relief of the bladder outlet obstruction.

## Circumcision

Medical indications include phimosis, paraphimosis, balanitis, balanitis xerotica obliterans and recurrent UTI. Outside of the neonatal group, an SGA with spontaneous ventilation is used. A caudal provides optimal analgesia. Clonidine 1–2 mcg $kg^{-1}$ can be safely used as an additive to prolong analgesia but should be avoided in neonates and ex-premature infants. A penile block can be performed when a caudal is contraindicated. Regular paracetamol, NSAIDs and PRN oral morphine are prescribed postoperatively.

## Insertion of SP Lines

Suprapubic line insertion is the temporary placement of a suprapubic catheter for postprocedure urodynamic testing. It can be carried out with face mask anaesthesia, or an SGA. One mcg $kg^{-1}$ fentanyl is useful, as bladder filling and catheter insertion are stimulating. Prophylactic antibiotics are required. Postoperatively, treatment for bladder spasm may be required with oral oxybutynin 1.25–2.5 mg every 8–12 hours whilst the catheter remains in place.

## Hypospadias Repair

Hypospadias is a congenital malformation of the urethral meatus where the opening is on the ventral surface instead of the tip of the penis. It occurs in 1:250 boys. It may be associated with cryptorchidism, chordee (curvature of the penis) and other urogenital anomalies but is most often an isolated finding with normal renal function. Hypospadias can be defined as anterior (mild displacement of meatus), middle (meatus on ventral surface of penis) or posterior (meatus significantly displaced; scrotal, perineal).

Surgery takes between one and three hours, with the aim to resolve the chordee, extend the length of the urethra to create the meatus at the tip of the penis and perform circumcision. If further tissue is required, a two-stage procedure may be carried out. Posterior auricular tissue or buccal mucosa are used as grafts. For complex hypospadias, a group and screen should be performed.

Anaesthesia with an SGA and spontaneous ventilation is usual unless a buccal mucosal graft is expected. In this case, a south-facing RAE tracheal tube positioned to one side of the mouth is suitable, although some surgeons prefer nasal intubation. A throat pack should be used according to local guidelines. Caudal analgesia with clonidine is ideal for hypospadias repair, and antibiotic prophylaxis should be administered. Postoperative paracetamol, NSAIDs and PRN morphine are prescribed, and oxybutynin may be needed for bladder spasm. Minor hypospadias repair can be performed as a day-case procedure. More complex repairs require an overnight stay. All children return for a dressing change under anaesthesia the following week. There has been concern over an increased risk of urethrocutaneous fistula after hypospadias repair in boys receiving caudal anaesthesia (see 'Further Reading'). The authors' institutional practices have not currently been altered due to the lack of prospective data and local audit data suggesting no association.

## Orchidopexy

Orchidopexy is performed for an undescended testis (cryptorchidism). The aim of surgery is to fix the testis in the scrotum. It is a common congenital anomaly with an incidence of 2–8% and is more common in premature infants as the normal inguino-scrotal testicular descent occurs between 25 and 35 weeks gestation. Spontaneous descent is uncommon after 1 year, and orchidopexy should be performed between 6 and 18 months old, with the aim to improve fertility and reduce the occurrence of testicular cancer (see 'Further Reading'). Examination under anaesthesia will determine if the testis is palpable in the inguinal canal. For a palpable testis, an open procedure is performed with small incisions in the groin and scrotum. For an impalpable testis, laparoscopy is needed to identify its location, which may be 'true' in the path of descent or 'ectopic', such as in the perineal or femoral region. If the testis can be brought down to the scrotum without tension, a single-stage procedure is performed. Many intra-abdominal testes require a two-stage, or 'Fowler–Stephens', operation. This involves division of the testicular vessels, so that the blood supply to the testis is via the vas deferens. The second stage occurs six to nine months later once collateral blood supply is fully developed.

An SGA and spontaneous ventilation with a caudal are appropriate for open orchidopexy. An ilio-inguinal block with infiltration of local anaesthesia to the scrotal incision is an alternative to a caudal. Laparoscopic orchidopexy requires tracheal intubation. Antibiotics are not routinely necessary. A caudal block remains the ideal analgesia, with infiltration of local anaesthetic at the umbilical port site. Paracetamol, NSAIDs and PRN oral morphine provide adequate postoperative analgesia.

## Major Procedures

Laparoscopy is frequently used for many of these procedures, and worldwide, urology has seen the greatest use of robotic surgery within paediatrics. However, only few institutions in the United Kingdom currently offer paediatric robotic surgery. All cases will require antibiotic prophylaxis.

Major urological procedures include:

- Pyeloplasty
- Ureteric re-implantation
- Nephrectomy
- Resection of Wilms' tumour (nephroblastoma)
- Bladder exstrophy and epispadias repair
- Bladder augmentation (ileocystoplasty) and formation of Mitrofanoff
- Renal transplant

## Pyeloplasty

Hydronephrosis caused by pelviureteric junction (PUJ) obstruction resulting in a poorly functioning kidney, recurrent UTI or pain is managed with an open, laparoscopic or robotic-assisted pyeloplasty (RAP). Open procedures are significantly faster and cheaper than laparoscopy and RAP, but RAP has high success rates and children have significantly shorter length of stay. Complication rates do not differ, and techniques continue to vary between institutions. PUJ obstruction is quite rare (1:1,500 children), usually unilateral, and even if the kidney is poorly functioning, renal impairment is uncommon due to a normal contralateral kidney. Persistent dilatation in the postnatal period with poor function on micturating cystourethrogram is an indication for surgery in infants. Whatever the surgical technique, intubation and ventilation are needed. For open procedures in small babies, the incision is small (approximately 3 cm). A group and screen are not required. Analgesia options include local anaesthetic (LA) infiltration, transversus abdominis plane (TAP) block, or quadratrus lumborum (QL) block. A morphine NCA can be prescribed if a block is not performed, although it is not often required for more than 24 hours. Oral morphine 200 mcg $kg^{-1}$ is adequate if the child has had a regional technique, along with simple analgesics, including NSAIDs in the presence of a normal contralateral kidney.

## Ureteric Re-implantation

Ureteric re-implantation is required for significant vesico-ureteric reflux (VUR) or obstruction causing retrograde urinary flow which has not responded to less invasive endoscopic treatment, for example cystoscopy and 'Deflux' bulking injections. Untreated VUR causes recurrent UTI, renal scarring and ultimately chronic renal impairment. Surgery typically involves a small lower abdominal transverse laparotomy, although laparoscopic and robotic-assisted procedures are described. Blood loss is minimal, but a group and screen should be available. Invasive monitoring is not necessary. Surgical time is approximately two hours, and regional anaesthesia is ideal with a caudal block or epidural. Postoperative bladder spasms are treated with oral oxybutynin and diazepam, but a continuous caudal or lumbar epidural infusion manages bladder spasms most effectively unless contraindicated.

## Nephrectomy

Nephrectomy and heminephrectomy are required for a complete or partial non-functioning kidney respectively, severe hydronephrosis or nephroblastoma (which is discussed separately in the next section). Surgery is usually laparoscopic or robotic assisted. A group and screen should be available for a benign laparoscopic nephrectomy. One unit of blood should be cross-matched for open or heminephrectomy and four units for a transplant nephrectomy. Invasive monitoring is not routinely required. Positioning is either prone or lateral, with usual precautions for prone positioning necessary. As with pyeloplasty, LA infiltration, TAP or QL block are useful for laparoscopic or robotic-assisted nephrectomy. If an open nephrectomy is planned or conversion required, an epidural, TAP/QL block or morphine NCA/ PCA can be used.

## Wilms Tumour (Nephroblastoma)

Wilms tumours account for 90% of renal tumours in children and around 5% of all childhood malignancy. Long-term prognosis is good, with >90% five-year survival. However, morbidity is high, with significant chemoradiotherapy-related side effects such as cardiotoxicity, ototoxicity, peripheral neuropathy, scoliosis, infertility and secondary malignancy. Wilms tumour is associated with specific syndromes relating to WT1 gene mutation, including WAGR (Wilms, aniridia, genito-urinary malformation, developmental delay) and Denys–Drash (Wilms, nephrotic syndrome, male pseudohermaphroditism). Multiple other syndromes have been associated with Wilms, including Beckwith–Wiedemann, trisomy 18 and neurofibromatosis-1. Children usually present under the age of five years with an abdominal mass. Late presentation may be with fever and weight loss or abdominal pain and haematuria if the tumour bleeds or extends into the renal pelvis or ureter. Tumour extension into the inferior vena cava (IVC) and right atrium (RA) occurs in 4% and 1% of cases respectively. Metastases occur in the lungs and lymph nodes, less commonly the liver. Paraneoplastic syndrome can result in hypertension (50% cases), hypercalcaemia or acquired von Willebrand disease and coagulopathy. Imaging with ultrasound, CT and MRI aids staging and surgical planning. Chest X-ray and tumour biopsy determine histology and spread. Bilateral nephroblastoma occurs in 5% of cases, more commonly in girls. Neoadjuvant chemotherapy reduces tumour size and vascularity but is not used in all treatment regimens. Cardiopulmonary bypass is required as a joint procedure with cardiothoracic surgeons if the tumour remains in the IVC/RA after chemotherapy. Postoperative chemotherapy is usually needed to treat residual disease, and around 20% of children will require additional radiotherapy. Full blood count, coagulation and renal function should be checked preoperatively. Antihypertensive medication should be continued perioperatively, other than angiotensin converting enzyme (ACE) inhibitors, which should be omitted on the morning of surgery. Hypertension often resolves after nephrectomy. Children who have had preoperative chemotherapy will have central venous access, which can be used for induction of anaesthesia and for invasive monitoring along with an arterial line. If no central access is present, it should be obtained, as well as large-bore peripheral venous access. All lines should be in the upper body, as on occasion the IVC must be clamped during surgery. Compression or kinking of the IVC during tumour resection or, less commonly, major haemorrhage result in haemodynamic instability. One unit of blood should be cross-matched. Large tumours cause atelectasis and reduced functional residual capacity but also delayed gastric emptying, which should be taken into consideration when planning induction of anaesthesia. It should be anticipated that syndromic patients, e.g. Beckwith–Wiedemann or trisomy 18, may have a difficult airway. A cuffed tracheal tube is recommended, as ventilation may be difficult during surgery due to increased intra-abdominal pressure, particularly with very large tumours and surgical retraction. Children with pre-existing hypertension should be expected to have labile blood pressure on induction and intubation and should therefore be well hydrated before anaesthesia. Tumour resection has classically been via a large transverse abdominal incision, with considerable third space and evaporative fluid losses. A low thoracic (T9–10) epidural is ideal for intra- and postoperative analgesia. Temperature maintenance is important, requiring fluid and forced-air warmers. Postoperative intensive care is not routinely necessary. For small tumours, laparoscopic resection of Wilms tumour has similar oncological results and reduces long-term morbidity from adhesion-related complications and scarring. Robotic-assisted laparoscopic resection of Wilms tumours have been reported in small numbers with favourable outcomes, although operative time and cost are a consideration.

## Bladder Exstrophy and Epispadias Repair

This is a rare congenital anomaly (1:40,000) where the skin over the bladder develops abnormally, resulting in exposure of the bladder on the anterior abdominal wall. Midline structures fail to fuse; the pelvis is splayed, and the urethra does not develop normally (epispadias). Epispadias can also occur in isolation. Cryptorchidism is typical in boys with bladder exstrophy. Cloacal exstrophy with rectal exposure and associated exomphalos is rarer. Spinal abnormalities such as myelomeningocele or sacral agenesis with spinal cord tethering may be present in cloacal exstrophy. Repair of a myelomeningocele should take precedence over bladder closure, and babies with cloacal exstrophy will also require colostomy formation. Diagnosis is often antenatal and transfer to a specialist centre should occur as soon as possible after birth. The defect is covered with a thin plastic film to prevent fluid and heat loss and minimise infection risk. Surgical closure should occur within the first 48 hours of life. Delayed closure results in a hyperaemic and oedematous bladder, increasing the risk of infection, and renal damage may occur with ureteric obstruction. The risk of bladder carcinoma in later life is also increased. The surgical approach to repair a bladder exstrophy is either 'complete' or 'staged' and varies between centres. The overall aim of surgery is to achieve continence through bladder closure, pelvic opposition and epispadias repair. Complete repair takes three to four hours, involving considerable blood and fluid loss, and does not preclude the need for further surgery. A staged approach requires simple bladder closure and abdominal wall repair within 48 hours of birth, which takes approximately 90–120 minutes, with minimal blood loss. A hip spica may be applied to oppose the pelvis. A Kelly procedure or bladder neck reconstruction and epispadias repair at one to two years of age creates a sphincter with the aim to allow the bladder to hold urine and increase capacity. Bladder augmentation may be required in later years (see the following section). Renal function should be checked and antibiotic prophylaxis administered. All considerations relevant to neonatal anaesthesia apply. Babies should be intubated and have good IV access ideally in the upper limbs. If adequate peripheral access is not possible, central access which avoids the femoral veins due to surgical proximity may be necessary. Fluids should be warmed, and a unit of blood that is likely to be needed should be cross-matched. For a complete repair, an arterial line should be placed due to the risk of haemodynamic instability and major haemorrhage. For simple bladder closure, analgesia is ideally provided with a lumbar epidural to avoid postoperative ventilation. If a sacral pit is present, it is advisable to exclude spinal abnormalities preoperatively using ultrasound. An epidural is contraindicated in cloacal exstrophy due to the associated spinal anomalies. If an epidural is contraindicated or not possible to site, high-dose opiates and postoperative ventilation are required. Some surgeons prefer babies to remain ventilated for a short period postoperatively to reduce the risk of wound dehiscence.

## Bladder Augmentation (Ileocystoplasty) and Mitrofanoff Formation

The aim of a cystoplasty is to increase bladder capacity, reduce urinary tract infection, achieve continence and preserve renal function. Children with bladder or cloacal exstrophy, posterior urethral valves, spina bifida or anorectal anomalies who have not responded to intermittent catheterisation or bladder neck Botox injections may be offered augmentation. A Mitrofanoff stoma is constructed for lifelong intermittent catheterisation. Those with a neuropathic bladder may also have severe constipation and benefit from an antegrade continence enema (ACE) stoma at the same operation. The surgery involves a segment of ileum being anastomosed to the superior aspect of the bladder to increase capacity (ileocystoplasty), and the appendix is anastomosed between the bladder and abdominal wall, producing a stoma which will not leak urine (Mitrofanoff). Bowel preparation is required preoperatively with 48 hours of clear fluids. Renal function and electrolytes should be checked and one unit of blood cross-matched. This group of children will have had multiple operations and may have perioperative anxiety necessitating premedication or play specialist and psychology input. They are at risk of latex allergy due to long-term intermittent catheterisation. Surgical approach is classically via a laparotomy, although there are case reports and series of children undergoing laparoscopic and robotic-assisted bladder augmentation. Surgery is prolonged, taking four to six hours. Standard anaesthetic considerations for a laparotomy are required with antibiotic prophylaxis and appropriate vascular access for potential blood and fluid replacement. A low thoracic epidural is ideal for open procedures unless contraindicated.

## Chronic Kidney Disease and Renal Transplantation

Aetiology of chronic kidney disease (CKD) in children varies with age. Under the age of six, congenital abnormalities or hereditary conditions predominate, such as obstructive uropathy, renal dysplasia, polycystic kidney disease and Alport syndrome. Acquired conditions (e.g. glomerulonephritis, nephrotic syndrome) are more common over the age of six. The multi-systemic effects of CKD must be taken into consideration for anaesthesia. These include chronic anaemia secondary to reduced erythropoietin production, reduced red cell survival and iron and folate deficiency, with haemoglobin (Hb) concentrations in the region of 60–70 g $l^{-1}$. Coagulation may be deranged due to platelet dysfunction, bone marrow depression causing thrombocytopenia or heparin from dialysis. Electrolyte abnormalities are common and include hyperkalaemia, hypocalcaemia, hyperphosphataemia and hyper-/hyponatraemia depending on the aetiology. Full blood count, electrolytes and coagulation should be checked preoperatively, and knowledge regarding urine output, fluid balance, fluid restriction, baseline blood pressure and dry weight is vital for any child with CKD undergoing anaesthesia. Oliguric children are at risk of cardiac failure and pulmonary oedema due to fluid overload, whilst polyuric children are at risk of hypovolaemia. Hypertension is common but not universal and may result in left-ventricular hypertrophy. Other cardiovascular consequences include arrhythmia and cardiomyopathy. Respiratory reserve may be reduced by the presence of pleural effusion or diaphragmatic splinting from ascites. Echocardiogram, electrocardiogram and chest X-ray should be considered before anaesthesia. Additional complications with implications for anaesthesia are peripheral neuropathy, encephalopathy, seizures, delayed gastric emptying, reduced immunity, polypharmacy and altered pharmacodynamics and pharmacokinetics (see Chapter 2).

Renal transplantation is the treatment of choice for children with end-stage renal failure. Pre-emptive transplantation improves growth, quality of life and survival when compared with dialysis. Approximate graft survival at five years is 90% for a live donor compared to 80% for a deceased donor renal transplant. The principles of anaesthetic management include preoperative optimisation, stable intraoperative haemodynamics, optimal perfusion of the transplanted organ and good postoperative analgesia. If required, haemodialysis usually occurs the day before surgery and should be avoided for four to six hours preoperatively to minimise residual heparinisation. Two units of blood should be cross-matched. The anaesthetist should be familiar with local protocols, including antibiotic prophylaxis, fluid management and administration of aspirin and immunosuppression. Children who are dialysed frequently have labile blood pressure, particularly at induction of anaesthesia; fluid boluses and vasoconstrictors may be required. Large-bore peripheral access is necessary for intra- and postoperative fluid replacement. Isotonic crystalloid, such as compound sodium lactate or Plasma-Lyte 148, are suitable for intraoperative fluid requirements. Arterial blood pressure monitoring is necessary in younger children (<20 kg) where the transplant is anastomosed to the IVC and aorta or in older children with relevant comorbidity (where the organ in anastomosed to iliac vessels). The femoral artery should be avoided in children undergoing iliac vessel transplant due to risk of graft vessel thrombosis, but also in younger children who will inevitably require further iliac transplantation in later life. Peripheral or arterial access and non-invasive blood pressure cuffs should not be placed in limbs with arteriovenous fistulae. Central venous pressure (CVP) monitoring is essential via a size-appropriate triple-lumen central venous catheter or a permacath if already in situ. CVP is kept >10 $cmH_2O$ to optimise renal perfusion. Dopamine can be attached to the CVC and primed for children undergoing anastomosis to the IVC and aorta for use at the time of vascular unclamping. Intraoperatively, the patient should be volume loaded, and transfused with packed red cells with a transfusion threshold of Hb <70 g $l^{-1}$. IVC and aortic anastomoses may require heparin prior to aortic cross-clamping. These cases require large volumes of fluid: up to 200 mls $kg^{-1}$ is not unusual. Communication between the surgeon and anaesthetist is vital for timing of drugs as well as at the point of vascular clamping and reperfusion. Most renal transplant protocols will ask for 1–2 mg $kg^{-1}$ furosemide +/– mannitol to be administered prior to unclamping, and at this point the dopamine may be started at 3–15 mcg $kg^{-1}$ $min^{-1}$, titrated to effect. Hypotension is common as the new kidney fills with blood. Vasoconstrictor boluses such as 0.5–1 mcg $kg^{-1}$ phenylephrine are often required as the systemic vascular resistance drops. Meticulous control of blood pressure is crucial to minimise the risk of graft failure due to thrombosis. Target blood pressure is dependent on donor pathophysiology and anatomy. Close communication with the surgeon as to how the kidney appears and feels at reperfusion is essential. There is a risk of arrhythmia secondary to hyperkalaemia when the kidney preservation fluid enters the circulation at unclamping. At our institution, intravenous salbutamol, bicarbonate and calcium chloride are the preferred treatment for hyperkalaemia. The problems of re-perfusion are exacerbated in small children receiving a large kidney. A TAP block provides good intraoperative analgesia for iliac anastomoses. Postoperative analgesia with a TAP catheter inserted under direct vision by the surgeon minimises opiate requirements. A morphine NCA/PCA is otherwise indicated, and it is the aim to extubate this group of children. Some institutions may use epidurals. For children <20 kg undergoing IVC and aorta transplantation, opioid analgesia is typically used intraoperatively. This group of patients remains ventilated postoperatively, usually for one night in order to stabilise haemodynamics after large fluid shifts, and because transplantation of an adult kidney into a small child can impact on ventilation and wound closure. A transplant ultrasound is performed in theatre or the recovery unit. Postoperative fluid balance is managed by the renal team and involves maintenance fluids and replacement of hourly urinary losses.

**Key Points**

- Paediatric urological surgery is amenable to a variety of regional anaesthesia techniques.
- Antibiotic prophylaxis is required for cystoscopy, major urological and reconstructive procedures.
- Major surgery requires close teamwork with the urologist to identify the complexity of the surgery, positioning needs and appropriate vascular access.
- Wilms nephrectomy can result in major haemorrhage, especially without neoadjuvant chemotherapy or if heminephrectomy is performed.
- Renal transplantation is a major vascular procedure in young children. It involves close teamwork with the surgeons, nephrologists and transplant team.

## Further Reading


Cho A, Thomas J, Perera R et al. Undescended testis. *BMJ* 2019; 364:I926.

Clarke S, Cave J. Paediatric robotic surgery. *Annals* 2018; 100:18–21.

Guruswamy V, Barbour R. Anaesthesia for children with renal disease. *BJA Education* 2015; 15:294–8.

Leslie, SW, Sajjad, H, Murphy, PB. Wilms tumour. StatPearls. 2020. Updated 1 July 2020. Jan_. PMID: 28723033.

Mumford, L, Maxwell, H, Ahmad, N et al. The impact of changing practice on improved outcomes of paediatric renal transplantation in the United Kingdom: a 25 year review. *Transplant International* 2019; 32:751–61.

Taicher, BM, Routh, JC, Eck, JB et al. The association between caudal anesthesia and increased risk of postoperative surgical complications in boys undergoing hypospadias repair. *Pediatric Anesthesia* 2017; 27:688–94.

Chapter 35

# Anaesthesia for Hepatobiliary Surgery, Including Transplantation, in Children

James Bennett and Peter Bromley

## Introduction

Liver disease is rare in children; however, its consequences may be devastating. Care for children with liver disease is usually provided in specialist liver units, but children may present to non-specialist centres, so it is important that all anaesthetists treating children should be aware of the principles of management for this group.

This chapter will consider normal hepatic function, the pathophysiology of liver disease, common conditions that present to the anaesthetist working in a specialist unit and a brief discussion of hepatic transplantation in children.

## Anatomy

The liver is a large abdominal organ, typically 5% of the body weight of a neonate, falling to 2% by adolescence. It lies in the right-upper quadrant and is divided into left and right lobes and smaller caudate and quadrate lobes.

The blood supply to the liver consists of the portal vein and hepatic artery, which together comprise around 25% of the cardiac output. The portal vein provides two thirds of the liver blood flow, but hepatic artery flow can increase to compensate for reduced flow in the portal vein, even in the presence of advanced liver disease. The portal vein drains the intestines and receives flow from the superior mesenteric and splenic veins. Thus, the portal vein carries deoxygenated blood with the products of digestion at relatively low pressure, whereas the hepatic artery carries oxygenated blood at systemic pressure from the aorta via the celiac trunk. The hepatic artery has alpha- and beta-adrenergic receptors, thus arterial flow is in part modified by the autonomic nervous system. The vessels enter inferiorly via the porta hepatis and divide repeatedly within the liver along with the biliary tree; the Couinaud system divides the liver into eight functional segments according to the course of these vessels. The segments are not macroscopically apparent but are important in regional perfusion, and the implications of this arrangement for the venous and biliary drainage of the liver must be carefully considered during and after hepatic surgery.

The venous drainage of the liver is via the left, middle and right hepatic veins. These vessels are short, valveless and empty into the inferior vena cava (IVC). The bile ducts leave the liver at the porta hepatis; the left and right bile ducts join to form the common hepatic duct. The cystic duct from the gallbladder joins the common hepatic duct to form the common bile duct, which ultimately empties into the second part of the duodenum.

Microscopically, the liver is divided into lobules organised around small branches of the portal vein, hepatic artery and the bile ducts in the portal tracts. Blood perfuses the lobules via sinusoidal vessels that ultimately drain into the central hepatic veins.

## Normal Liver Physiology and Pathophysiology of Liver Disease

Knowledge of normal liver physiology is essential for understanding the effects of liver disease. The liver is a complex organ with myriad functions; those that are important to anaesthetists include:

- Synthesis
- Catabolism and excretion
- Intermediary metabolism – carbohydrates, protein, lipid, vitamins and cholesterol
- Immunological functions

### Synthesis

All coagulation factors except factor VIII/vWF (derived from vascular endothelium) are synthesised in the liver. Synthesis of factors II, VII, IX and X is dependent on vitamin K. Bile is necessary for the absorption of the lipid-soluble vitamin K, and impaired bile flow into the small intestine leads to coagulopathy. The half-lives of factors V and VII are only a few hours, so coagulopathy can develop quickly.

Albumin forms the largest fraction of the protein output of liver. Albumin has a long half-life, around 20 days, so levels change slowly in response to changes in liver function. Albumin is an important acid-base buffer, has oncotic effects and is an important determinant of the free fraction of many drugs, but the consequences of low albumin level can be relatively minor. Other plasma proteins, including transport globulins and lipoproteins, are more crucial in maintaining health.

Bile and the bile salts also play an important role in digestion, particularly of lipids.

## Catabolism and Excretion

Bilirubin is the breakdown product of haemoglobin. It is excreted in bile, and the appearance of jaundice can be the first sign of liver problems. Protein catabolism forms amino acids that provide a substrate for gluconeogenesis. Deamination of protein releases toxic ammonia, which is normally safely excreted via conversion to urea by the urea cycle enzymes. The accumulation of ammonia in acute liver failure leads to hepatic encephalopathy, raised intracranial pressure and coma.

Failure of protein catabolism can be very disruptive; for example, if insulin is not removed from the circulation, hypoglycaemia can result. Failure of regulation of other hormones can also be important.

Metabolism and excretion of xenobiotics, including drugs, are also vital. Most of these reactions are phase 1 reactions, carried out by cytochrome P-450 enzymes. Phase 2 reactions are conjugation processes, such as glucuronidation, to create water-soluble compounds that are then excreted in the urine. Some drugs, particularly larger molecules, are excreted in bile.

## Intermediary Metabolism

### Carbohydrates

The liver plays a key role in carbohydrate metabolism and glucose homeostasis. Insulin release after meals promotes hepatic glucose uptake; glucose monomers are phosphorylated to glucose-6-phosphate and then polymerised into glycogen. When energy supplies are low, liver glycogen can be broken down into glucose-6-phosphate and then into glucose that is released into the circulation; the process does not consume any energy as the glucose has already been phosphorylated. Seventy-five per cent of body glycogen is stored in muscle, but this is only for 'local' use; muscle does not contain glucose-6-phosphatase, so glucose cannot be released from muscle glycogen. The liver can store only a limited amount of glycogen, and liver failure rapidly impairs the ability to maintain plasma glucose levels.

### Proteins

The liver is a major site of protein synthesis and catabolism. A wide range of essential proteins are synthesised, including albumin and the clotting factors, as described in the 'Synthesis' section.

Protein catabolism produces amino acids that can be used in energy production via gluconeogenesis or ketone body formation. The handling of dietary protein depends on the liver. End-stage liver disease is commonly associated with marked muscle wasting, and this can be impossible to prevent despite determined nutritional care.

### Lipid and Cholesterol

The liver regulates the distribution of lipid and cholesterol by packaging these substances with apoproteins to form a range of lipoproteins that are essential for health. Lipids can be catabolised and the products directed into gluconeogenesis and the formation of ketone bodies.

## Immunological Functions of the Liver

A sizeable fraction of the cells in the liver (Kupffer cells, pit cells) have immunological functions and are important for the control of pathogens and tumour surveillance.

# FEATURES OF LIVER DISEASE

## Acute Liver Failure

Acute liver failure is a condition resulting from the rapid decline in liver function in patients without evidence of previous liver disease. The presenting features are those of loss of hepatocyte function; there is no associated portal hypertension, and a marked coagulopathy is usual. There is a failure of glucose homeostasis, and intravenous glucose supplementation is usually required, sometimes in large amounts. There is usually a metabolic acidosis with a high serum lactate. The clinical course is variable. Mild disease may recover completely or may progress slowly over some weeks. Conversely, deterioration may be extremely rapid, causing death within a few days if the patient does not undergo urgent liver transplantation. Acute liver failure is associated with high output cardiac failure, and acute renal failure is inevitable if the patient lives long enough. As encephalopathy progresses, it is accompanied by cerebral oedema and raised intracranial pressure. Ascites is generally mild, if present. Bilirubin rarely reaches the high levels seen in some of the chronic cholestatic conditions. Death is usually from cerebral herniation, overwhelming sepsis or circulatory failure.

## Chronic Liver Disease

In chronic liver disease, there are repeated episodes of hepatic damage and regeneration, with fibrosis and eventual cirrhosis. This leads to portal hypertension and cholestasis, as well as loss of liver cell function. Cellular function is often well preserved until end-stage disease; the severity of portal hypertension and cholestasis may vary according to the aetiology of the liver disease and between individuals suffering from the same disease.

## Portal Hypertension

Normal portal vein pressure is 5–10 $cmH_2O$. Increased pressure can lead to the formation of varices and variceal bleeding. There may be ascites and pleural effusions. Hypersplenism may cause thrombocytopenia or pancytopenia. Fluid shifts and other factors may contribute to the hepatopulmonary or hepatorenal syndromes.

## Cholestasis

Obstruction to, or loss of bile ducts as a result of fibrosis will cause jaundice with a conjugated hyperbilirubinemia. Pruritus is common and may severely impair quality of life. Biliary obstruction may lead to cholangitis and systemic sepsis. The lack of bile flow into the gastrointestinal tract can cause malabsorption and steatorrhea, leading to depletion of lipid-soluble vitamins A, D, E and K; coagulopathy due to loss of vitamin K-dependent clotting factors; and accumulation of drugs that are eliminated in bile.

## Hepatocellular Dysfunction

An early indicator of hepatocellular dysfunction is coagulopathy that is not fully corrected by vitamin K. Low albumin levels aggravate ascites, and peripheral oedema may develop. Drug volume of distribution and plasma protein binding may be altered. Drug metabolism may be impaired by the disturbance of either phase 1 or phase 2 conjugation processes. There may be loss of peripheral vascular resistance, causing a high-output low-pressure circulation. Encephalopathy is associated with raised ammonia levels, and there may be enhanced gamma-aminobutyric acid (GABA)-receptor effect and neuroinflammatory processes. Impaired immunity increases the likelihood and severity of sepsis.

## Neonatal Jaundice

Establishing a diagnosis in a baby with jaundice is important as some conditions, such as biliary atresia, have a good prognosis if the baby receives early surgical treatment.

Physiological jaundice is common in neonates; it is worse in the breast-fed baby, but usually disappears by two weeks. Persistent or worsening jaundice requires investigation. Haemolytic disease of the newborn is rare in the developed world since the introduction of anti-D immunoglobulin.

The differential diagnosis of neonatal jaundice includes:

- Physiological jaundice
- Haemolytic disease
- Biliary atresia (or possible choledochal cyst, although this is often asymptomatic, at least initially)
- Neonatal hepatitis and other infections, such as TORCH
- Metabolic disorders (alpha-1-antitrypsin deficiency, galactosaemia, Crigler–Najjar syndrome, etc.)
- Drug reactions

Pale stools suggest bile is not entering the gut normally. Conjugated hyperbilirubinaemia, which causes dark urine, suggests biliary obstruction, whilst unconjugated hyperbilirubinaemia suggests physiological jaundice or haemolytic disease.

## Liver Function Tests

The most important blood tests for assessment of liver function are the coagulation parameters and albumin levels, both indicators of synthetic function. Excretory function can be assessed by the serum bilirubin level; a high proportion of conjugated versus unconjugated fraction implies biliary obstruction; a high unconjugated fraction implies hepatic dysfunction, or that the conjugating capacity has been overwhelmed by haemolysis. The liver enzymes help to indicate the origin and nature of hepatocyte damage: aspartate transaminase (AST) is partially microsomal, whereas alanine transaminase (ALT) is exclusively cytosolic; a high AST/ALT ratio implies cell death (e.g. cirrhosis or tumour secondaries), whereas ALT will rise more in conditions where the cell membrane becomes 'leaky' (e.g. viral hepatitis). Alkaline phosphate (ALP) and gamma glutamyl-transferase (GGT) are both membrane bound and do not 'leak' out. GGT is a marker of enzyme induction, and both ALP and GGT rise when there is biliary obstruction.

## Special Investigations and Imaging

The liver is effectively imaged by ultrasound, and structural abnormalities of liver parenchyma, biliary tree and vasculature can be readily identified. CT with or without contrast may be indicated to define the size of lesions and their relation to major vessels or to guide specific therapeutic options. MRI may provide greater resolution of subtle tissue differences.

Oesophagogastroendoscopy may be indicated to identify varices and thus portal hypertension. Percutaneous liver biopsy can be a valuable investigation, yielding diagnostic histology not available from liver function tests. It is a painful procedure and requires general anaesthesia in most children and carries a significant risk of bleeding. Transjugular liver biopsy maybe indicated in the presence of coagulopathy in acute liver failure. Endoscopic retrograde cholangiopancreatography (ERCP) may be required to diagnose biliary or pancreatic pathology. It usually requires general anaesthesia. Its therapeutic uses include stone extraction from the biliary tree, sphincterotomy of the sphincter of Oddi as well as dilatation or stenting of biliary strictures.

## Anaesthesia for Children with Liver Disease

Some of the common conditions in children with liver disease are described in the following sections. The necessary procedures may be categorised as minor, intermediate and major. In general, a child with liver disease requires a higher intensity of care than a healthy child; even minor or moderate surgery may require invasive monitoring, active warming, fluid therapy and an intensity of perioperative care that might be provided for a major procedure in a normal child. Surgery is high risk in this population, and the child should be offered the best chance of a favourable outcome. If a child presents to a non-specialist unit, advice should be sought and transfer to a specialist unit considered.

## Hepatobiliary Procedures

Hepatobiliary surgery can be divided into procedures for conditions of the biliary tree and for those of the liver itself, although there are obviously some features common to both.

### Biliary Atresia

Biliary atresia is a rare condition of unknown aetiology affecting roughly 1:14,000 live births in the United Kingdom. Around 25% of cases are associated with other anomalies, typically abdominal situs inversus, polysplenia and atrial septal defect. Absence of extrahepatic and (to a variable degree) intrahepatic bile ducts leads to cholestasis, progressive fibrosis and cirrhosis.

The affected neonate is usually born at term. Jaundice and pale stools soon become apparent, and the infant fails to thrive. The presence of hepatomegaly suggests hepatic fibrosis. Investigation reveals a raised conjugated bilirubin, alkaline phosphatase and AST. Serum albumin and prothrombin times are usually normal in the early stages. Abdominal ultrasound reveals contracted or absent gallbladder, and a Tc trimethylbromoiminodiacetic acid (TEBIDA) scan demonstrates failure to excrete radioisotope from the liver into bowel. Liver biopsy demonstrates cholestasis and bile duct proliferation and plugging.

Definitive diagnosis is with an operative cholangiogram which fails to demonstrate bile ducts. Following confirmation of the diagnosis, the surgical team will proceed to the Kasai portoenterostomy procedure. This involves excision of the fibrotic portion of the biliary tree and formation of a Roux-en-Y portoenterostomy to allow bile drainage. The Kasai procedure usually achieves biliary clearance in greater than 50% of infants, and over 40% avoid liver transplantation until at least 10 years of age. The outcomes are worse when performed in infants older than eight weeks of age or with advanced fibrosis or established cirrhosis.

## Anaesthesia for the Kasai Procedure

A systematic approach to preoperative assessment is necessary for infants undergoing this operation. The full blood count may reveal anaemia, but the platelet count is usually normal, as portal hypertension is unusual at this stage. The prothrombin time is generally normal provided the child has received supplementary vitamin K. Standard starvation guidelines can be followed, but the risk of hypoglycaemia should be remembered, and intravenous glucose may be required.

Induction of anaesthesia may proceed according to the anaesthetist's preference. A non-depolarising muscle relaxant is administered, oral tracheal intubation is performed and a nasogastric tube is placed. Anaesthesia is maintained with a volatile agent in a mixture of oxygen and air.

Epidural analgesia has much merit as it offers good postoperative analgesia, promotes early feeding and avoids the risk of opioid accumulation; however, there are concerns about sepsis in the epidural space because of systemic sepsis secondary to ascending cholangitis. Epidural analgesia should be avoided in the presence of coagulopathy or thrombocytopenia.

A safer alternative may be local anaesthetic infiltration and continuous infusion via a subcutaneous catheter sited by the surgical team, in addition to intravenous opioid, using a nurse-controlled analgesia (NCA) pump.

When forming the anastomosis between the Roux-en-Y and the porta hepatis, the liver is retracted, potentially reducing venous return from the IVC. Thus, adequate venous access in the upper limbs is necessary; a central venous catheter may be useful for access, both intra- and postoperatively, and measurement of central venous pressure. Arterial cannulation is generally unnecessary in the absence of associated cardiac anomalies or haemodynamic instability.

As these patients are usually less than eight weeks of age, they are prone to hypothermia; this may be avoided using warmed intravenous fluids and external warming devices.

Extubation at the end of surgery and return to a high-dependency unit is usual. Antibiotic prophylaxis should be continued for five days to prevent postoperative cholangitis. Recurrent cholangitis, cirrhosis and portal hypertension may all occur despite adequate biliary drainage. Rotating courses of antibiotics are often necessary as prophylaxis for cholangitis and nutritional support is useful to help with growth, which may be impaired secondary to a degree of malabsorption.

In the United Kingdom, this surgery is performed in three designated centres, allowing monitoring and timely assessment for liver transplantation, should this become necessary.

# Choledochal Malformations

Choledochal malformations are localised dilatations of the biliary tree. The aetiology is unknown, and the incidence is around 1:100,000 live births. Presentation in infancy is usually with obstructive jaundice, although it may have been detected as a chance finding on antenatal ultrasound. In older children, recurrent abdominal pain is the main feature, potentially with acute pancreatitis.

Choledochal malformations can lead to severe cholangitis, hepatic fibrosis and cirrhosis; there is a risk of malignancy later in life if left untreated. Surgical treatment is by excision of the malformation and formation of a Roux-en-Y anastomosis. Anaesthetic management is similar to that for infants with biliary atresia, but patients with choledochal malformations are generally older and more robust, and prognosis and recovery are usually very good.

# Gallstone Disease

Although considered a disease of adult life, gallstones can affect children with haemoglobinopathies, where haemolysis leads to deposition of pigment stones, children with disorders of cholesterol metabolism and, increasingly, obese teenagers. It rarely affects infants. Presentation is most commonly with right-upper quadrant pain, intermittent jaundice and pancreatitis. Surgical treatment is cholecystectomy, often with intraoperative cholangiography to exclude biliary obstruction due to residual stones in the bile duct. Laparoscopic cholecystectomy is popular because of reduced postoperative pain and shorter recovery time. This approach necessitates a significant pneumoperitoneum and often steep head-up tilt, which may cause some degree of haemodynamic compromise. Good venous access is required. Routine anaesthesia is used, avoiding nitrous oxide owing to its potential to diffuse into gas-filled cavities. Analgesia is usually with intravenous paracetamol, a non-steroidal anti-inflammatory agent, and morphine. Local anaesthetic infiltration to the sites of the laparoscope ports may be useful. Shoulder tip pain secondary to diaphragmatic irritation can be severe but is usually short lasting.

Laparoscopic cholecystectomy may be technically difficult and require conversion to an open procedure. Postoperative pain should be managed with opioid patient-controlled analgesia (PCA) and local anaesthetic infusion to the wound or transversus abdominis plane (TAP) block, or with epidural analgesia. The postoperative course may be complicated by pain, fluid shifts and ileus.

## Hepatic Tumours

Hepatoblastoma is the most common liver tumour encountered in the paediatric population, with an incidence of around 0.77 per million. It is more common in boys. Hepatoblastoma is commonest in children under the age of four years and is associated with conditions such as Beckwith–Wiedemann syndrome and hemihypertrophy. It usually presents as an abdominal mass, which may have become quite large before it is discovered. Full blood count may reveal anaemia, but liver function tests are often normal. α-Fetoprotein (AFP) is a useful diagnostic test and monitor of treatment response. Abdominal ultrasound helps to differentiate hepatoblastoma from other abdominal tumours. CT and MRI scanning provide information about metastatic spread and the relationship of the tumour to vascular structures and thus staging and surgical resectability. Treatment is with chemotherapy (cisplatin and doxorubicin) and surgical resection as guided by the International Society of Paediatric Oncology (SIOPEL) regimen. Children with unresectable hepatoblastoma may be suitable for liver transplantation. Doxorubicin toxicity may lead to cardiomyopathy, and all children should be assessed by echocardiography.

Anaesthesia for liver resection shares many similarities with that for liver transplantation (described in the next section), particularly the risks of severe and rapid blood loss. Issues specific to hepatic resection are the risks of air embolus and hepatic insufficiency. In order to achieve clearance and reduce bleeding, surgical resection is usually by hemihepatectomy or segmentectomy using an ultrasonic scalpel or similar device to divide the liver parenchyma along the planes of the functional anatomical segments. Occasionally very peripheral tumours may be suitable for extra-anatomical resection. Entrainment of air into veins held open in the liver parenchyma can lead to air embolus; this may be minimised by meticulous surgical technique and adequate fluid loading. However, excessive administration of fluid leads to engorgement of the liver and increased bleeding. Fluid administration is therefore usually restricted until after the parenchymal resection is completed. A lower central venous pressure has been shown to reduce bleeding and reduce blood product transfusion. Systemic arterial blood pressure should be maintained with appropriate inotropes and vasopressors to preserve liver perfusion and postoperative liver function. Clamping the portal vein and hepatic artery or vascular exclusion with clamping of the vena cava may reduce bleeding. This has the advantage of increased speed of surgery and reduced blood loss but risks ischaemic damage to the remaining liver and postoperative hepatic dysfunction.

There is always the potential for massive blood loss in these children. Intra-arterial and central venous pressure monitoring and urinary output measurement are mandatory. A wide bore intravenous catheter, in addition to a multiple-lumen central venous catheter, will facilitate rapid infusion of intravenous fluid and blood products. The majority of these patients will have an existing Hickman catheter, which is not adequate for rapid transfusion.

Perioperative hepatic dysfunction is suggested by a progressive base deficit and lactic acidosis. Adequate cardiac output must be maintained. Clotting factors are sometimes needed to support coagulation. There is little evidence to support the use of N-acetylcysteine to aid residual liver recovery. Children with hepatic dysfunction are best managed in the intensive care unit.

For uncomplicated liver resection, epidural analgesia is effective and allows early extubation and return to the high-dependency unit. Epidural analgesia may be high risk in the presence of coagulopathy due to postoperative hepatic dysfunction, so careful consideration should be given to the size of the tumour and expected difficulty of the resection. The infusion of local anaesthetic agents via tunnelled infiltration catheters in the surgical wound is an alternative technique which can provide good analgesia when combined with a morphine NCA.

## Liver Transplantation

Liver transplantation may be a very effective treatment for children with acute or chronic liver disease. The first successful liver transplant was performed on a child with hepatoblastoma in 1967. However, it was not until the introduction of cyclosporin immunosuppression in the 1980s that the procedure became an established therapy for end-stage liver disease.

Children with chronic liver disease can expect a one-year survival of over 90% after liver transplantation. The outcomes for acute liver disease are generally not quite as good. Developments in anaesthesia and critical care, surgery and immunosuppression have greatly contributed to this success; however, the impact of improved nutrition, microbiology and nursing care should not be forgotten.

The variety of conditions causing paediatric liver disease, and their influence on symptoms, is remarkable. Table 35.1 lists some common indications for liver transplantation.

**Table 35.1** Some commoner indications for liver transplantation at various ages

| Disease | Typical age |
|---|---|
| Gestational alloimmune liver disease (GALD)/ neonatal haemochromatosis | Neonatal period |
| Biliary atresia | Infancy and onwards |
| Unresectable hepatoblastoma | Typically <3 years |
| Alagille syndrome | >4 years |
| Progressive familial intrahepatic cholestasis | >4 years |
| A-1-antitrypsin hepatitis | >6 years |
| Glycogen storage diseases | >6 years |
| Autoimmune hepatitis | >10 years |
| Wilson disease, tyrosinaemia | >10 years |
| Cystic fibrosis | Adolescence |

## Acute Liver Failure in Children

About 10% of liver transplants are performed in patients with acute liver disease. The features of acute liver failure are quite different from chronic disease, requiring urgent effective multidisciplinary treatment.

Acute liver failure is a complex illness which evolves following a severe insult to the liver. The aetiology and progression of acute liver failure vary with age. In the newborn, infection and gestational alloimmune liver disease (GALD), previously known as neonatal haemochromatosis, are frequent diagnoses; in older children, viral hepatitis, drugs and toxins are more likely, but often no cause is found.

Acute liver failure is an emergency with a high mortality, requiring rapid diagnosis and management. Early transfer to a specialist unit with transplantation facilities is essential. Children with moderate or severe encephalopathy should be admitted to the intensive care unit for ventilation and invasive monitoring. The high mortality rate in acute liver failure is mainly from circulatory collapse, neurological deterioration and sepsis; it is essential that close attention be paid to haemodynamics and neurology. Hypotension is common and must be treated aggressively due to impaired cerebral autoregulation.

Intravascular volume must be maintained to ensure adequate organ perfusion in the face of high cardiac output and low systemic vascular resistance. Inotropic support, usually noradrenaline, is often required to maintain adequate perfusion pressure. Acute renal failure is common, necessitating renal replacement therapy.

Survival in acute liver failure requires rapid diagnosis, coordinated management and timely liver transplantation if recovery is unlikely; the decision whether to transplant or wait for possible recovery may be extremely difficult. Actual or impending loss of cerebral perfusion, progressive circulatory failure unresponsive to inotropic support and multi-organ failure suggest a low likelihood of recovery, with or without transplantation.

## Assessment of Children for Liver Transplantation

Most liver transplants in the United Kingdom are performed with grafts from cadaveric donors, thus the time available for review and optimisation is limited. In most liver units, potential transplant candidates are fully assessed by a multidisciplinary team before listing. The anaesthetist has an important role as a part of this team assessing all aspects of preparation for liver transplantation. Particularly important features are the severity of the liver disease itself and the effects on other systems, with special regard to the cardiovascular, respiratory, renal and neurological systems.

Irrespective of aetiology and severity, some features of chronic end-stage liver disease and portal hypertension are commonly seen. Patients are often malnourished and display poor growth, reduced muscle mass and thin subcutaneous tissue. The abdomen may be distended due to ascites and hepatosplenomegaly. The skin may demonstrate jaundice, scratch marks from severe pruritis, bruising and dilated veins, particularly around the umbilicus.

## Assessment of Cardiovascular Function

In end-stage liver disease, cardiac output is typically increased and systemic vascular resistance reduced. Fluid retention and peripheral oedema are common despite diuretic treatment. Electrocardiogram (ECG) and transthoracic echocardiography should be reviewed to exclude cardiac abnormalities such as pericardial effusion, cardiomyopathy and congenital cardiac anomalies. Moderate ventricular hypertrophy is reasonably common. Discovery of associated cardiac anomalies allows risk stratification, which includes the danger of paradoxical air embolus during surgery in cases where there is the potential for right-to-left intracardiac shunting. The decision to treat cardiac anomalies either surgically or by interventional cardiological techniques must be balanced by the extra risk of the procedure in a patient with liver disease; it may be difficult to decide which problem to treat first.

## Respiratory Function

Moderate hypoxia and respiratory impairment are common and often secondary to ascites and hepatosplenomegaly, causing basal atelectasis. Pleural effusions are also common, as are lower respiratory tract infections.

The hepatopulmonary syndrome (HPS) is a condition characterised by abnormal blood oxygenation associated with intrapulmonary vascular dilatation in the presence of cirrhotic liver disease. The incidence is variable, and the condition is often insidious and not necessarily related to the severity of the liver disease. The children may demonstrate clubbing and marked hypoxia, particularly on standing. Investigation with contrast echocardiography or a Tc99 radiolabelled microalbumin scan may quantify the degree of shunting. Significant levels of shunting maybe discovered and supplemental oxygen therapy indicated. The outcome with liver transplantation for children with HPS is similar to those without the condition; however, the hypoxia may worsen acutely, necessitating higher inspired oxygen levels and prolonged postoperative ventilation. HPS usually resolves completely in the weeks and months following liver transplant.

## Renal Function

Renal impairment is common in advanced liver disease as a consequence of sepsis, diuretic therapy and hypovolaemia. It may be most accurately assessed by measurement of serum cystatin C, the level of which is unaffected by muscle mass. The hepatorenal syndrome (HRS) is unusual in children.

## Neurological Assessment

Hepatic encephalopathy is not always apparent or recognised but is a worrying sign and difficult to treat. The cause remains elusive, but raised serum ammonia, neurotoxins and neuro-inflammatory processes are implicated. Cirrhotic liver disease may result in portosystemic shunting, allowing potentially neurotoxic intestinal metabolites, normally removed by healthy hepatocytes, to be found in the circulation. There is a significant risk of hepatic encephalopathy following placement of transjugular intrahepatic portosystemic shunts to treat portal hypertension. There may be other causes of impaired consciousness in chronic liver disease, including hyponatraemia, hypoglycaemia, sepsis and impaired metabolism of sedative drugs. Table 35.2 describes the grading of hepatic encephalopathy.

## Anaesthetic Management of Liver Transplantation

Start times for liver transplantation are difficult to predict, but preoperative fasting protocols should

**Table 35.2** Grading of hepatic encephalopathy

| | |
|---|---|
| Grade 0 | Normal |
| Grade I | Minimal drowsiness but oriented; some impairment of cognitive functions or reversal of day/night sleep pattern |
| Grade II | Drowsy, confused, mood swings |
| Grade III | Very drowsy, unresponsive to speech |
| Grade IV | Comatose |

allow most children to drink clear sugar containing fluids up to one hour before induction of anaesthesia. If hypoglycaemia is problematic, a glucose-containing infusion should be commenced.

Sedative premedication, typically oral midazolam, may be given to minimise anxiety, but delayed start times, impaired drug metabolism and fragile clinical state demand pragmatism and sound clinical judgement.

Coagulopathy should be corrected, or partially corrected, with fresh frozen plasma and platelet transfusion, but fluid overload should be avoided. Hyponatremia is common because of fluid retention and diuretics and is associated with increased mortality in those awaiting transplantation. A serum sodium of less than 126 mmol $l^{-1}$ is concerning; lower values than this risk central pontine myelinolysis and should be treated.

After induction of anaesthesia, a higher than usual dose of non-depolarising neuromuscular blocking drug may be required, owing to increased volume of distribution in advanced liver disease and binding to acute phase proteins. Nasal intubation is avoided due to the risks of bleeding. The abdominal distension from ascites and hepatosplenomegaly often makes positive pressure ventilation difficult initially; positive end expiratory pressure (PEEP), high inflation pressures and high inspired oxygen levels may be needed. Ventilation usually improves following opening of the peritoneum and drainage of ascites, although surgical retractors may impede diaphragmatic excursion and make ventilation difficult.

Anaesthesia is maintained with isoflurane in a mixture of oxygen and air, supplemented with an opioid infusion. Neuromuscular blockade is usually maintained with an atracurium infusion.

Manipulation and clamping of the IVC may drastically reduce venous return, so IV cannulae and central catheters are sited in the upper body. Similarly, the infrarenal aorta may be clamped when forming an arterial conduit to the graft, so radial artery cannulation is preferred. Generally, one or two peripheral cannulae and a multiple-lumen central venous line for pressure monitoring and infusion of inotropes and other drugs is required. High risk cases warrant placement of a wide-bore catheter in a central vein to facilitate rapid fluid infusion. Coagulopathy and thrombocytopenia increase the risk of central venous cannulation, and ultrasound guidance is recommended.

Intraoperative hypothermia is common due to the small size of the patient, malnourished state and peripheral vasodilation, which may be exacerbated by rapid transfusion, loss of ascites and implantation of a cold liver graft. The ambient temperature should be raised, and a warming mattress and waterproof drapes used to reduce convection and prevent pooling of fluids and subsequent cooling. IV fluids and surgical wash should be warmed, and inspired gases humidified. Core and peripheral temperature should be monitored.

The major fluid shifts and alterations in cardiac output that occur during liver transplantation have profound haemodynamic effects, making cardiac output measurement useful. Pulmonary artery catheters are rarely used in small children. Transoesophageal echocardiography (TOE) offers a dynamic assessment of ventricular filling, stroke volume and ejection fraction, and it can be used even in small children, although there are concerns about the passage of such a device in the presence of oesophageal varices. Continuous cardiac output measurement by pulse contour analysis is increasingly popular in paediatric anaesthesia and critical care and may be useful during liver transplantation.

Fluid management is initially with crystalloids such as compound sodium lactate solution (Hartmann's or Ringer's solution) at maintenance rates; glucose infusion may be added if hypoglycaemia develops. Ascitic losses, bleeding and alterations in venous return may necessitate infusion of further crystalloid, colloid, and blood products. There is continued debate concerning the risks of hyperchloraemic acidosis and acute kidney injury (AKI) with 0.9% NaCl compared with more balanced solutions. Regular blood gas, glucose, electrolyte and haematocrit measurements can direct the type of infused fluid or other physiological and therapeutic manoeuvres. Changes in coagulation occur as a result of transfusion, dilutional coagulopathy and loss of liver function. Transfusion of coagulation factors and platelets is guided by prothrombin time (PT), activated partial thromboplastin time (APTT) and point of care viscoelastic testing. These parameters change very quickly during transplantation and analysers should be situated in or very close to the theatre, to minimise delays in obtaining data to guide treatment.

Thromboelastography (TEG) is a point of care viscoelastic test used to measure coagulation. It measures the transmitted force from a rotating sample of warmed blood to a wire inserted into the sample. A computer displays these forces in real time as clot forms. Standardised values are produced: reaction time (R), maximum amplitude (MA), α angle and LY30. These results are interpreted to provide an assessment of rate of clot formation, clot strength and fibrinolysis. Thromboelastometry (ROTEM) is a refinement of the technique which employs additional assays to identify specific information about blood coagulation, particularly hyperfibrinolysis.

The liver transplant procedure is classically divided into three phases: dissection, anhepatic and reperfusion. The dissection phase is from skin incision to occlusion of the hepatic artery and portal vein, which is the start of the anhepatic phase. The anhepatic phase ends when blood first reperfuses the transplanted liver.

## Dissection phase

Division of adhesions, venous collaterals and varices may result in considerable bleeding, and large volumes may also be lost as ascites. Transfusion should be guided by filling pressures, haematocrit and coagulation studies. Despite intensive preventive measures, hypothermia and coagulopathy are common. Manipulation of the liver may cause reduced flow in the IVC, reducing venous return and cardiac output. Hypocalcaemia may be aggravated by the citrate load secondary to fresh frozen plasma (FFP) transfusion and should be treated with an infusion of calcium ions; this should be done cautiously to avoid hypercalcaemia.

Intraoperative cell salvage and autologous blood transfusion reduces the requirement for allogenic blood, so reducing risks of donor blood transfusion and cost. There is growing confidence that its use is safe in liver transplantation for malignancy.

## Anhepatic Phase

The anhepatic phase is characterised by sustained reduction of venous return and absence of liver function. Although surgical techniques vary, the IVC and portal vein are often clamped, which leads to reduced cardiac output and hypotension, often accompanied by a compensatory tachycardia. Treatment is with inotropic support and cautious fluid administration to avoid excessive right-sided filling pressures at reperfusion. Clamping the portal vein may lead to congestion of the intestines and can be associated with intestinal perforation and bacterial translocation.

Absent hepatic function leads to profound metabolic changes. Implantation of the ice-cold liver graft reduces core temperature, requiring adjustment of warming devices. Hypoglycaemia is common and often profound, necessitating adjustment of the glucose infusion. A progressive metabolic acidosis develops. Sodium bicarbonate or other acid-buffering solutions should be withheld unless the acidosis becomes so severe that it causes inotrope-resistant hypotension, hyperkalaemia or other dangerous effects. Severe hyperkalaemia at reperfusion carries a risk of cardiac arrhythmias; buffers, calcium, furosemide and dextrose/insulin may be needed.

Towards the end of the anhepatic phase, the liver graft is flushed to wash out potassium, preservation medium, heparin, metabolites, inflammatory mediators, cell debris and air. Crystalloid, colloid or the patient's blood may be used. Before reperfusion, careful attention should be paid to the serum potassium, calcium and acidosis, and fluid and inotrope infusions should be prepared.

## Reperfusion Phase

Unclamping of the IVC leads to a sudden increase in venous return to the heart, so the portal vein is unclamped slowly. The characteristic features of reperfusion are systemic hypotension, increased cardiac output, pulmonary vasoconstriction and hyperfibrinolysis. The definition and characterisation of the post-reperfusion syndrome (PRS) have evolved over the years, and because of this its incidence varies in the literature. It can have a major effect on morbidity and mortality of liver transplantation. Risk factors include increased donor age and prolonged cold ischaemia time for the graft. The pathogenesis of post-reperfusion syndrome is unclear, but endogenous mediators are implicated. Post-reperfusion syndrome is usually transient but may be profound and prolonged, requiring fluid and inotropic support, usually noradrenaline or adrenaline. Often the simplest and most successful strategy is to use the minimum therapy required to support viable circulation until the reperfusion phenomena start to wear off, which may be no more than a few minutes.

Reperfusion coagulopathy is common; thrombelastography (TEG)/rotational thrombelastography (ROTEM) often reveals hyperfibrinolysis, requiring treatment with clotting factors and tranexamic acid or aprotinin. Over-transfusion should be avoided to prevent congestion of the graft, excessive volume loading of the heart and worsening of bleeding. Additionally, there may be significant bleeding from the cut surface of a reduced or split liver graft. This situation can be challenging in the presence of abnormal coagulation.

The surgical team then commences arterialisation of the graft, which requires good systemic arterial blood pressure. In infants undergoing a split liver transplant, an aortic conduit is often required, necessitating temporary aortic clamping.

Following completion of the arterial anastomosis, the biliary anastomosis is performed (usually with a Roux-en-Y) and the abdomen closed. If primary abdominal closure is difficult due to a large donor liver graft, then delayed or staged closure may be required.

Following liver transplantation, the patient returns to the intensive care unit. During the early postoperative phase, vigilance is required; the patient is closely observed for any haemodynamic or respiratory changes, which are promptly acted upon. Abdominal drain losses, temperature and urine output are all monitored closely, along with assessment of graft function. Transabdominal doppler scanning is utilised to assess liver graft perfusion.

## Types of Liver Grafts

The imbalance between the number of children awaiting liver transplantation and the availability of size-matched donor livers has led to innovative surgical techniques to provide more liver grafts and reduce waiting list times and mortality. Smaller grafts and split liver grafts allow adult cadaveric livers to be used even for small infants. Living related grafts have the advantage of allowing scheduling of the liver transplant operation and provision of a high-quality graft, but the risk of morbidity and mortality to the donor is a powerful disincentive.

## Outcomes and Complications after Liver Transplantation

Liver transplantation is one of the most physiologically challenging procedures performed in children, and given the fact the children undergoing transplantation can be extremely sick, it is perhaps surprising that after an uncomplicated procedure, most children can be discharged from the intensive care within 24 hours and from the ward in 7–10 days or even fewer. However, disastrous complications can occur resulting in perioperative mortality. Five-year survival rates of 80–90% are achievable for chronic liver disease but nearer 60–70% for acute liver failure. With meticulous surgical technique and close attention to the treatment of coagulopathy, early returns to theatre for bleeding are rare. Complete normalisation of clotting parameters is not necessary and may even be undesirable; prothrombin time or internationa normalised ratio (INR) less than twice normal is generally acceptable.

- Early graft failure is rare and may necessitate urgent re-transplantation, often within 48 hours.
- Early graft loss (within the first few days or weeks) is usually due to vascular problems (hepatic artery or portal vein thrombosis).
- Graft perfusion may be compromised if abdominal closure is too tight (abdominal compartment syndrome), if the patient becomes hypovolaemic or if there is excessive use of vasoconstrictors.
- Grafts may be lost, or the patient may die, in the first month or two due to infective complications.
- Later complications include problems with immunosuppressive therapy leading to graft rejection or malignancy, particularly post-transplant lympho-proliferative disorder (PTLD). Problems with biliary or venous drainage may require further surgery or radiological intervention.

Overall a re-transplantation rate of about 10% can be expected. Re-grafts take longer, bleed more and suffer worse outcomes from both mortality and morbidity, but success is still achievable, so they are definitely worth trying in most circumstances. Good communication and collaboration and an experienced multidisciplinary team can help achieve the best results. The rewards can also be great, as transplantation provides a realistic hope of near-normal growth and development for children who are desperately ill with end-stage liver disease.

## Key Points

- Jaundice is relatively common in the neonatal period and is usually benign, but warrants investigation to detect serious but treatable conditions
- Chronic liver disease is characterised by portal hypertension, jaundice and relatively preserved synthetic function until end-stage
- Acute liver disease is characterised by hypoglycaemia, coagulopathy, acidosis, raised intracranial pressure and high-output, low-resistance circulatory failure
- Liver transplantation provides the hope of cure from the symptoms of liver disease with excellent survival for many indications.
- Significant liver disease is best treated in specialist units, and so prompt referral is recommended.

Chapter 36

# Anaesthesia for Radiology and Interventional Radiology in Children

Jane Herod

Radiology is a rapidly expanding service in paediatrics, often requiring general anaesthesia. Paediatric interventional radiology is a new speciality, and radiologists can perform an increasing number of procedures to facilitate treatment for some of the sickest patients in the hospital. Examples include tumour biopsy, embolisation of arteriovenous malformations, delivery of intra-arterial chemotherapy and insertion of tunnelled central lines for chemotherapy or long-term inotropic support for cardiac failure patients. The radiology suite is an 'unfriendly' environment for the anaesthetist, with access to the patient often limited by long distances and bulky X-ray equipment, and procedures may occasionally be performed with dimmed lights. Scrupulous attention must be paid to patient positioning, security of lines and tubes and maintenance of normothermia during long procedures. Constant vigilance with respect to both the patient's needs and the demands of the radiologist is required. Good communication and teamwork between the radiology team and anaesthetist are essential to ensure patient safety in this challenging but rewarding area of work. This chapter will describe anaesthesia for interventional radiology, including neuroradiology, computerised tomography (CT) and magnetic resonance imaging (MRI).

## Vascular Access

### Long-Term Vascular Access

This is one of the mainstays of the interventional radiologist. Children require long-term vascular access for the administration of chemotherapy, parenteral nutrition, inotropes or chemotherapy, or short-term access for courses of antibiotics or anti-viral or anti-fungal medication. A cuffed Hickman line or Portacath is inserted, depending on the treatment required and patient or parental preference. Lines are required for the duration of treatment and may remain in place for years unless they become infected.

It is important to assess children carefully preoperatively, as candidates for central access are rarely fit and healthy. Children with cardiomyopathy or severe pulmonary hypertension (right-ventricular pressure approaching systemic pressure) are at particular risk of cardiac arrest under anaesthesia. The risks and benefits of the procedure should be carefully considered, and a backup plan formulated in case of complications.

### Anterior Mediastinal Mass

Children presenting with a haematological malignancy, neuroblastoma or intrathoracic germ cell tumour may have an anterior mediastinal mass (seen in up to 50% of children with non-Hodgkin's lymphoma). This may cause airway compression, superior vena cava (SVC) obstruction or vascular compression, which may result in cardiovascular collapse on induction of anaesthesia. Worrying symptoms and signs include stridor, wheeze, orthopnoea, facial swelling and history of cardiovascular collapse. Review of the preoperative chest X-ray and CT scan is essential to look for a widened mediastinum, compression of the great vessels, tracheal or mainstem bronchus or pericardial or pleural effusion (see Figures 36.1 and 36.2).

It may be preferable to start treatment and delay line insertion for a few days in children with a new diagnosis of lymphoma and severe respiratory symptoms to reduce the risk of anaesthesia. This requires close liaison with the oncologist, as treatment will shrink lymph nodes rapidly and may make diagnosis impossible.

For induction of anaesthesia, children with an anterior mediastinal mass should be placed in a position of comfort (often on the side), and spontaneous respiration should be maintained if possible. If a neuromuscular blocking drug is given and thoracic tone reduced, be prepared for distal airway obstruction; this should be managed by application of continuous positive airway pressure (CPAP), repositioning or intubation with a long tracheal tube; some advocate the use of a rigid bronchoscope to regain airway patency. Vascular access should be placed in the lower limbs if the SVC is obstructed, and intravenous fluids and resuscitation drugs should be available in case of vascular compromise when the child is anaesthetised.

## Tumour Lysis Syndrome

Children with lymphoma or high-count acute lymphocytic leukaemia (ALL) are at risk of tumour lysis syndrome 12–72 hours after starting chemotherapy due to massive release of intracellular metabolites. These children require hyperhydration and treatment with allopurinol or rasburicase to preserve renal function and prevent deposits of uric acid or calcium phosphate in renal tubules. The main chemotherapy drug used for lymphoma is dexamethasone, so children with a new diagnosis of lymphoma or leukaemia should not receive dexamethasone as an antiemetic, as this may inadvertently precipitate tumour lysis syndrome.

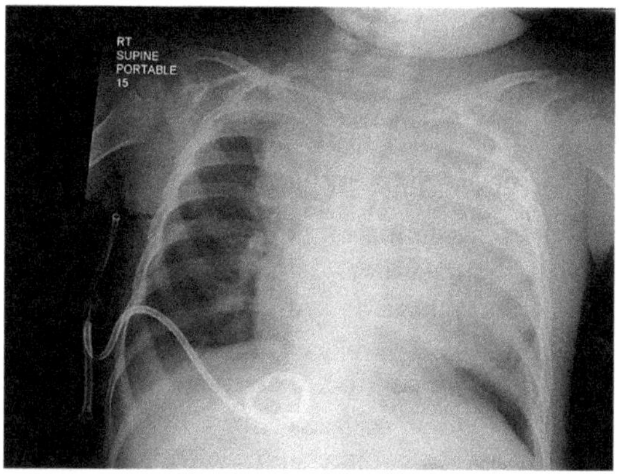


**Figure 36.1** Chest X-ray of child with non-Hodgkin's lymphoma associated with a large anterior mediastinal mass.

For children requiring intermediate duration vascular access (six weeks to six months), a non-cuffed line such as a peripherally inserted central catheter (PICC) is inserted, usually via an antecubital fossa vein, or in infants and small children tunnelled over the chest wall and inserted into the internal jugular vein.

The other types of vascular access lines inserted in the radiology suite are dialysis catheters, either temporary (Vascath®) or long term (Permacath®). These are large-bore catheters, which are 'locked' with heparin 1,000 IU $ml^{-1}$ to prevent line thrombosis and occlusion. The dead space of the line is always printed on the line, and this volume must be aspirated and discarded prior to use to prevent unintentional heparinisation of the patient.

Positive pressure ventilation is usually required in all tunnelled line insertions to decrease the risk of venous air embolism during central vein puncture. If a PICC line is required in older children, a spontaneous ventilation technique may be acceptable, as the line insertion utilises an arm vein only.

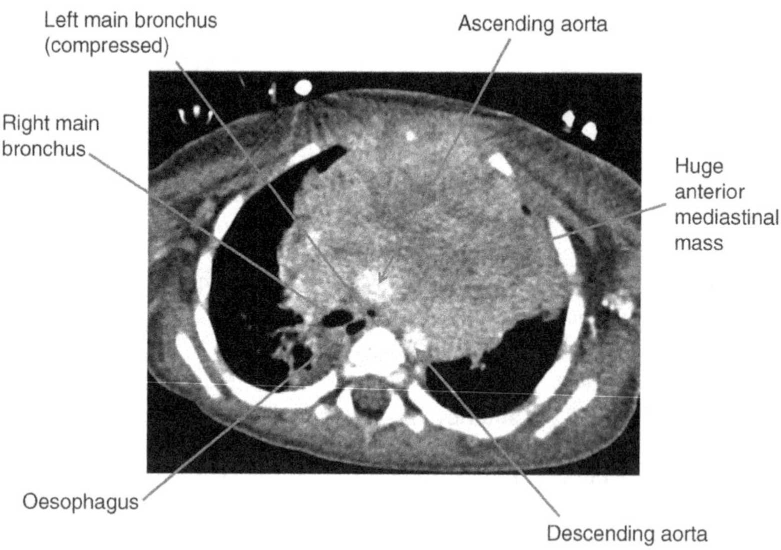


**Figure 36.2** CT scan of child with non-Hodgkin's lymphoma associated with a large anterior mediastinal mass.

A platelet count above $50 \times 10^9\ l^{-1}$ and normal coagulation are required; children with a coagulopathy may require blood products to cover line insertion.

Portacaths and cuffed lines are removed under general anaesthesia, but non-cuffed lines may be removed on the ward. Children with acute myeloid leukaemia (AML), non-Hodgkin's lymphoma, Wilm's, neuroblastoma or bone tumours may have received intensive chemotherapy with anthracyclines (doxorubicin, daunorubicin or epirubicin). They are at risk for anthracycline-induced cardiomyopathy, which may be subclinical. These children require thorough preoperative assessment, and a recent echocardiogram should be reviewed.

## Biopsy of Solid Organs or Tissues

### Liver Biopsy

Diagnostic liver biopsy may be required to determine the nature of acute or chronic liver disease. A Tru-Cut biopsy needle is inserted into the liver under ultrasound guidance, and several core samples are taken using the same tract. The following precautions are taken to reduce the risk of bleeding:

- Platelet count must be at least $100 \times 10^9\ l^{-1}$.
- Coagulation must be normal.
- A collagen gel foam plug is inserted in the biopsy tract at the time of the procedure.

The patient is usually positioned on their side with a bolster placed underneath them to open the gap between the lower end of the rib cage and the iliac crest. Spontaneous ventilation with a supraglottic airway device (SAD) is acceptable. Patients should be observed carefully over the next six hours for signs of ongoing blood loss (pain, tachycardia, hypotension). If the clotting is grossly deranged and the risk of bleeding from the biopsy site is deemed to be great, then a biopsy may be taken via a catheter inserted into the internal jugular vein and passed into the liver via the hepatic vein. If bleeding from the liver does occur, it is contained within the venous circulation.

### Renal Biopsy

Renal biopsy of a native kidney may be required to establish a diagnosis or monitor disease progression, or post-transplant to help confirm or rule out rejection. In order to biopsy a native kidney, the patient is positioned on their side with a bolster placed underneath them, as for liver biopsy. For renal transplants, the kidney is in the iliac fossa, so the patient can remain supine.

### Tumour Biopsies

The same principles apply for liver and renal biopsies. The site of the tumour determines the anaesthetic technique and positioning. Biopsies may be either ultrasound or CT guided. The latter can be quite a logistical feat, as the patient may need to be positioned prone in the CT scanner for the radiologist to locate and biopsy the tumour. All patients must be closely observed after the biopsy for signs of ongoing blood loss.

## Gastrostomy

Percutaneous gastrostomy insertion is another procedure that is being performed more commonly in the radiology suite (see Figure 36.3). The major advantage of fluoroscopic control over the traditional endoscopic method is that the patient can be given a barium meal the day before to outline the colon, which reduces the risk of inadvertent colonic perforation.

A nasogastric tube is inserted under fluoroscopic control, and the stomach is inflated with air to aid distension and ease of percutaneous puncture. A dose of glucagon (40 mcg $kg^{-1}$ IV) is given to cause gastric paresis. Once the stomach has been punctured, a catheter over a wire is passed retrograde up the oesophagus and out of the mouth. A thread is then passed via the catheter, and the gastrostomy tube is attached to this thread. The thread is used to pull the gastrostomy back down through the mouth and oesophagus so that the flange is in the stomach

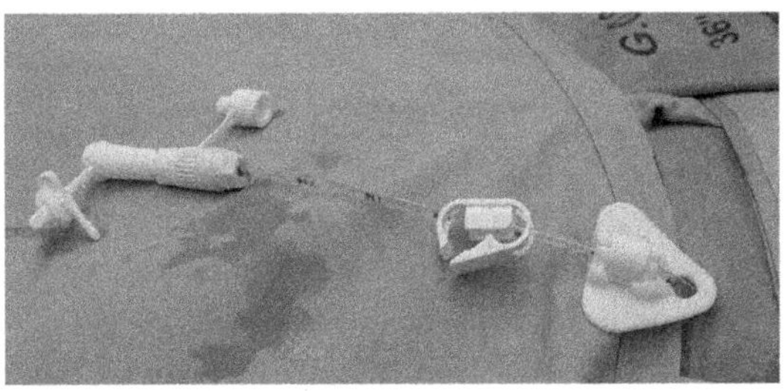

**Figure 36.3** Percutaneous endoscopic gastrostomy tube (PEG). A Freka® PEG feeding tube is shown.

and the tube protrudes from the abdominal wall. The position is confirmed fluoroscopically.

As with any percutaneous gastrostomy, there is a risk of contamination of the abdominal cavity with gastric contents, so prophylactic antibiotics (co-amoxiclav or metronidazole) are given before the start of the procedure. The stomach is usually rested for 6–24 hours after gastrostomy insertion, so postoperative IV maintenance fluids are required.

## Oesophageal Dilatation

There are two main groups of children who present to the radiology suite for oesophageal dilatation: those with a stricture following surgical repair of oesophageal atresia or tracheo-oesophageal fistula (TOF); and those with a stricture secondary to other scarring processes, such as dystrophic epidermolysis bullosa (DEB) or, less commonly, ingestion of caustic soda.

DEB is a hereditary skin disease that is characterised by painful blistering when skin or other stratified squamous epithelial membranes are exposed to shearing forces. Direct pressure does not cause new bullae to form, only shearing forces. Swallowing food boluses results in chronic bullae in the oropharynx and oesophagus, with subsequent scarring and stenosis.

Oesophageal dilatation involves passing a wire, usually via the mouth, across the stricture under fluoroscopic control, followed by balloon inflation. Patients with the most severe form of DEB may have limited mouth opening due to oral strictures, and intubation may be very difficult. These patients usually have a gastrostomy in situ, and a retrograde technique may be used.

Anaesthesia for patients with DEB can be very challenging, and the following precautions should be taken:

- Intravenous access is often difficult due to multiple dressings. Access should be secured with a non-adhesive silicone dressing such as Mepitel®.
- Electrocardiogram (ECG) electrodes should not be stuck to the patient. Placing the electrodes onto pieces of defibrillator pad on the skin makes good electrical contact.
- An adhesive pulse oximeter should be placed on a digit over a covering of plastic food wrap and not straight onto skin.
- The blood pressure cuff should be padded.
- If the patient is intubated, the tracheal tube should be tied using plastic food wrap rather than taped in place.
- The face mask should be lined with paraffin gauze. Gloves should be worn, and it is sensible to protect pressure points on the chin and jaw with paraffin gauze.
- The eyes should be covered with gel pads, and artificial tears may be used to protect the cornea.
- A well-lubricated SAD may be used if a retrograde technique is used, but the mouth opening is often too limited for SAD insertion.
- Great care is needed in transferring the patient onto the X-ray table, using a straight lift rather than a slide.

Even when the utmost care has been taken, anaesthesia is often associated with new bullae formation, and it is sensible to warn the family that this may occur.

## Airway Procedures

### Bronchoscopy, Bronchogram, Tracheal Dilatation or Insertion of Airway Stents

Patients may come to the radiology suite for bronchoscopic, radiographic and intrauminal ultrasound assessment of the airway as part of the management for both congenital and acquired tracheal stenosis or tracheomalacia (see Figure 36.4). Direct bronchoscopy is useful to document the nature and extent of tracheal disease and the presence of abnormal complete tracheal rings. A dynamic contrast bronchogram is required to delineate distal tracheobronchomalacia and define the level of CPAP required to keep the airway patent. Bronchoscopy and bronchogram are both vital parts of the surgical work-up and postoperative follow-up for patients with tracheobronchial abnormalities. Balloon dilatation or insertion of intraluminal stents may be required at suture lines or in the presence of residual stenosis. Granulation tissue may also be managed with stenting (see Figures 36.5 and 36.6).

Patients with congenital tracheal stenosis may have an underlying cardiac abnormality, and an echocardiogram is required as part of their preoperative work-up.

Our preferred anaesthetic technique for bronchoscopy is spontaneous ventilation via a

SAD so that dynamic assessment of the airway can be made during the respiratory cycle, particularly if tracheobronchomalacia is suspected. A pressure manometer inserted into the Ayres T-piece circuit will give an indication of opening pressures required to overcome inspiratory collapse due to tracheobronchomalacia. This method using a SAD may not always be possible, for instance in neonates or those already ventilated, in which case a bronchoscope of appropriate size may be passed via a tracheal tube (see Table 36.1).

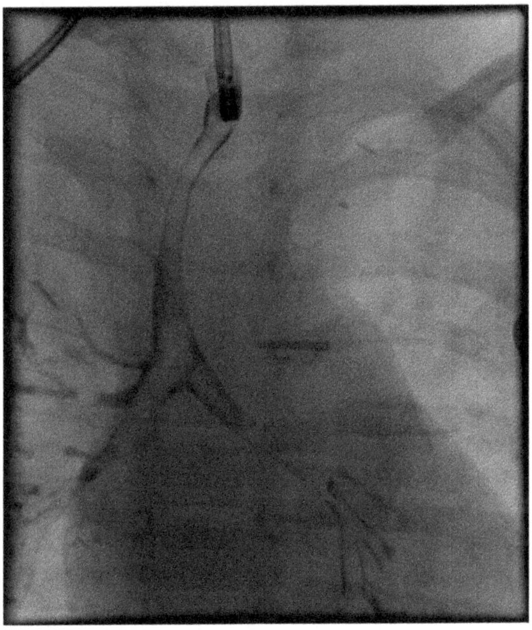

**Figure 36.4** Bronchogram to demonstrate congenital tracheal stenosis.

An angle piece with a self-sealing valve is used to minimise leakage of anaesthetic gases when the bronchoscope is passed down the SAD. Atropine 20 mcg $kg^{-1}$ IV may be given to dry secretions. Topical lidocaine (3 mg $kg^{-1}$) to the larynx and between the cords before endoscopy reduces coughing, although this has the disadvantage of preventing the child from eating or drinking for two hours post-procedure. Passing the bronchoscope through the vocal cords rarely causes coughing/spasm in patients if the child is relatively deep (end-tidal sevoflurane concentration of around 4%). The child may cough if the bronchoscope 'tickles' the carina, and a bolus of 1–2 mg $kg^{-1}$ of propofol is usually enough to prevent or treat this. Transient apnoea associated with the propofol bolus can be overcome by assisting ventilation until spontaneous respiration returns.

A dynamic assessment of the airway is made with the child breathing spontaneously prior to airway stent insertion or balloon dilatation. A bolus of propofol is administered just before the balloon is inflated so that the child is apnoeic and does not cough. This technique allows spontaneous ventilation to return rapidly after the procedure so that the dynamic assessment of the airway can be repeated.

(a) (b)

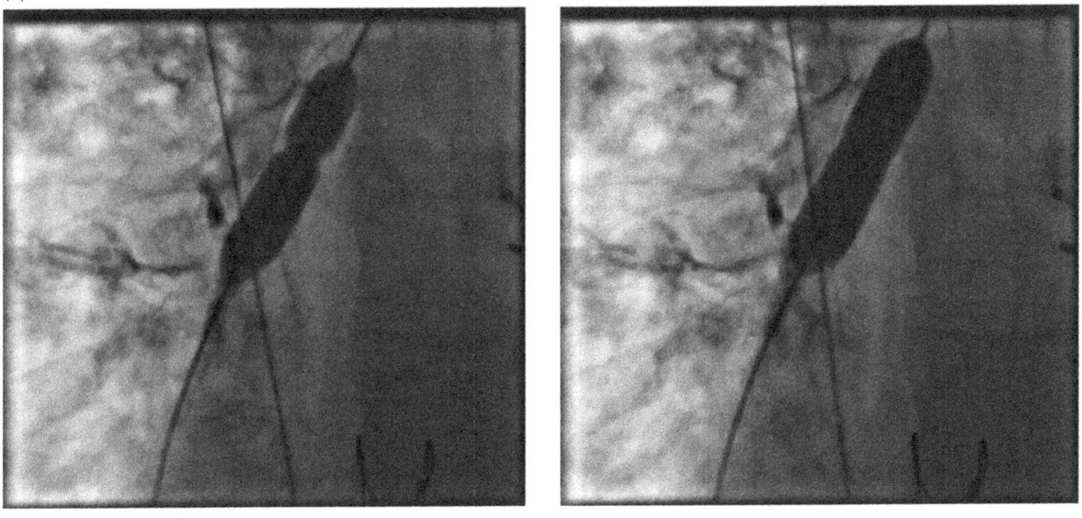

**Figure 36.5** Balloon dilation of residual stricture after repair of congenital tracheal stenosis. (A) Bronchial waist on balloon. (B) Bronchial waist abolished after dilation.

**Table 36.1** Sizing guide for fibreoptic bronchoscopes

| Scope diameter | Minimum internal diameter of tracheal tube (mm) |
|---|---|
| Olympus 2.2 (no suction channel) | 2.5 |
| Storz 2.8 | 3 (tight)<br>3.5 acceptable |
| Olympus 3.8<br>Storz 3.7 | 4 (tight)<br>4.5 acceptable |

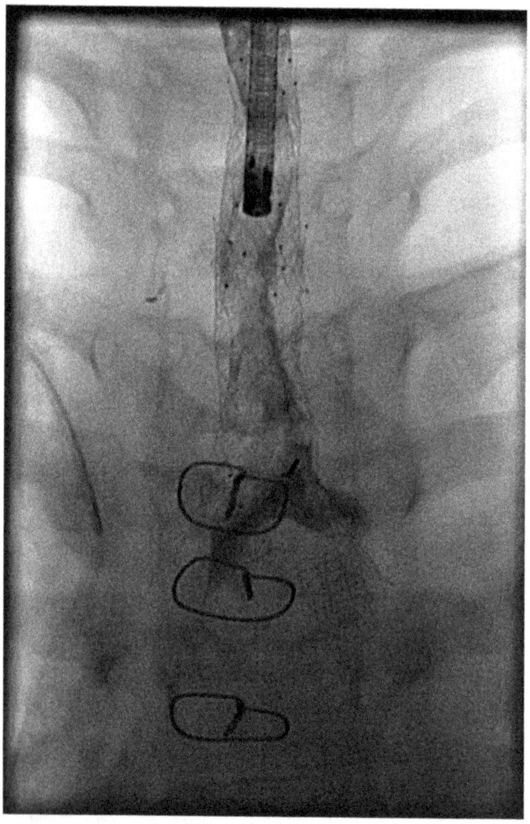

**Figure 36.6** Tracheal stent in situ for residual stricture in severe congenital tracheal stenosis.

## Visceral Angiography

Access for most angiographic procedures is via a femoral artery. It is often best to paralyse and ventilate the patient, as repeated periods of apnoea may be required after injection of contrast, and small movements, even those associated with respiration, cause significant artefacts.

Conventional X-ray contrast (Omnipaque® 240 mg I $ml^{-1}$) is used. As with all contrast media, there is a small risk of prior sensitisation, and a full allergy history should be taken during preoperative assessment in case an alternative is required. A cumulative dose of 5 ml $kg^{-1}$ is the usual maximum, although up to 7 ml $kg^{-1}$ may be given safely. Radiographic contrast media are usually osmotic diuretics, and intravenous fluids should be given during the procedure. 'In-out' catheterisation may be required at the end of the procedure if the bladder is distended. Occasionally, carbon dioxide gas (1 ml $kg^{-1}$ to the nearest 5 ml aliquot) is used as a contrast medium to keep the dose of iodinated contrast medium to a minimum. Hyoscine butylbromide (0.3 mg $kg^{-1}$ IV) is useful to counteract spasm of the gastrointestinal tract before enteric angiography.

The arterial sheaths used for angiography are relatively large, and it is helpful if the child does not cough vigorously during emergence, as this will lead to hematoma formation. For this reason, some advocate topical lidocaine to the cords prior to intubation and plan for deep extubation at the end of the procedure.

## Renal Vein Sampling and Angioplasty

Approximately 10% of children with secondary hypertension have renovascular disease that results from one or more lesions that impair renal blood flow. This is usually secondary to fibromuscular dysplasia of the renal vessels, which is often bilateral. Patients may be taking multiple antihypertensive agents and may have evidence of left-ventricular hypertrophy or even hypertensive cardiomyopathy on preoperative echocardiogram or ECG. There is a common association between renal artery stenosis and disease in other vascular beds, and 20–25% of these patients have cerebral vascular involvement. Cerebral angiography is often performed at the same time as renal imaging.

Children who have severe hypertension resistant to treatment may benefit from either angioplasty or from surgical resection or stenting of a stenosed renal artery. Selective renal vein angiography and sampling allows measurement of local renin secretion to identify those who may benefit from this intervention. It may also be of diagnostic value and helps differentiate these children from those with hypertension due to nephropathy or vesicoureteric reflux.

Angiographic treatment alone (stenting or balloon dilatation) results in improvement in blood pressure control in approximately half of these patients, although re-stenosis may require further treatment. This is especially true when a stent is inserted. Those with severe disease involving the aorta require surgical repair with a Gore-Tex® graft, but they may develop stenosis at the graft site, which will also benefit from angiographic dilatation.

Good control of blood pressure preoperatively is difficult in these children, despite the use of combination therapy. Treatment may be compromised by poor compliance or limitation of dose due to adverse drug side effects.

As with all angiographic procedures, the patient must be completely still during the procedure, and multiple episodes of breath-holding are required. The child should therefore be intubated and ventilated. A loading dose of heparin (75–100 IU $kg^{-1}$) is given prior to balloon inflation if angioplasty is undertaken.

The major complication of any angioplasty is vessel rupture, and vascular surgeons should always be readily available before this procedure is undertaken.

## Pancreatic Venous Sampling

The most frequent cause of prolonged severe hypoglycaemia in infancy is congenital hyperinsulinism, usually secondary to one or more insulin-secreting lesions within the pancreas. This is treated by surgical resection and partial pancreatectomy after localisation of the tumour by pancreatic arterial stimulation and venous sampling.

Pancreatic venous sampling of insulin is usually performed under general anaesthesia in children but may be performed under sedation in the adult population. Both venous and arterial catheters are inserted, and timed samples are taken from the right hepatic vein after injection of calcium gluconate into pancreatic arteries that supply different parts of the pancreas. Diagnosis requires at least doubling of the insulin level sampled from the hepatic vein.

High levels of endogenous catecholamine released due to stress such as intubation may cause a rise in blood glucose concentrations, which in turn can interfere with the interpretation of test results. Deep anaesthesia is therefore ideal. Theoretically, using high concentrations of volatile agents may also interfere with test results, as volatile agents block calcium channels, which in turn reduces insulin release. A balanced anaesthetic to maintain heart rate and BP to within 20% of baseline may be achieved using remifentanil (0.5–1.5 mcg $kg^{-1}$ $min^{-1}$ IV) and volatile anaesthesia with end tidal concentration of 0.5 MAC.

These infants usually require a glucose infusion to prevent profound and dangerous hypoglycaemia due to their insulinoma. The amount of glucose required may be quite substantial, and they commonly require a tunnelled PICC or Hickman line so that glucose 20% or more can be given to maintain normoglycaemia. Regular blood sugar measurement should be taken throughout any intervention and the glucose infusion rate altered accordingly.

## Extracranial Sclerotherapy

This is used to treat cutaneous or peripheral lymphangiomas, either simple or macrocystic-type (cystic hygromas) or vascular arteriovenous malformations (AVM). A sclerosing agent is injected under ultrasound or fluoroscopic guidance into the malformation. The choice of sclerosant depends upon the type of malformation and preference of the radiologist. For microcystic (solid) lymphatic malformations, either doxycycline or bleomycin is used; for macrocystic lesions, either doxycycline or STS 3% (sodium tetradecyl sulphate) is used. Bleomycin injection requires specific anaesthetic considerations. To minimise the risk of lung fibrosis, additional inspired oxygen should be kept to a minimum, with inspired air being ideal. Also, removal of adhesives applied to the skin can cause significant, permanent skin discolouration. Therefore, all adhesives should be avoided. A non-adhesive dressing such as Mepitel® can be used to secure venous access, and ECG dots stuck onto a gel-type defibrillator pad on the chest avoids sticking these dots directly onto the patient's skin.

A course sclerotherapy of sessions is usually required. This may be as a prelude to surgical excision if required. In head and neck lymphangiomas, approximately 90% show improvement after sclerotherapy, and 40% of lesions show complete regression. The anaesthetic technique will be dependent on the site of the lesion. Spontaneous ventilation is usually adequate for extracranial lesions.

Patients with malformations on the face or oral area require a single dose of prophylactic antibiotics (co-amoxiclav or teicoplanin and an aminoglycoside for penicillin allergic patients). A single dose of dexamethasone 0.25 mg $kg^{-1}$ IV up to 8 mg should be given to reduce inflammation in patients with facial or oral lesions.

Sclerotherapy may be quite painful postoperatively and patients may require opioid analgesics such as oral morphine in addition to regular paracetamol and NSAIDs such as ibuprofen or diclofenac.

There is a small risk of hypoglycaemia after sclerotherapy, and so blood glucose level should be monitored twice hourly for the first six hours after the procedure and oral intake encouraged.

## Neuroradiological Interventions

### Cerebral Angiography

Children may require cerebral angiography and/or embolisation of intracranial congenital AV malformations and shunts. These are often first diagnosed after an intracranial bleed. The initial visit to the angiographic suite may be during the acute phase whilst intubated and ventilated in the intensive care unit, possibly whilst requiring inotropic support to maintain cerebral blood flow.

There are three methods of embolising cerebral AVMs: coils, micro-particles or glue. In children, the use of coils is uncommon, as most large, rapidly shunting AVMs are thin walled and may rupture when coiled. Most malformations, shunts and tumours are embolised using either micro-particles or glue. Micro-particles are usually employed in tumours and glue in the embolisation of AVMs, although some operators may wish to use micro-particles for AVMs that have a small shunt component. Where there is a large atrioventricular (AV) shunt, such as vein of Galen aneurysmal malformation, glue is always used. Glue used for embolisation starts to polymerise when the glue comes into contact blood.

The extent of glue dispersion depends upon three variables: the concentration of glue, the speed of injection and the flow velocity within the AV shunt. This last factor is affected by the nature of the lesion and where, in relation to the lesion, the neuroradiologist can place the micro-catheter. The process of glue polymerisation is exothermic, so dexamethasone (0.2–0.25 mg $kg^{-1}$ IV) should be given to reduce inflammation and reduce the risk of 'peri-glue' oedema.

Cerebral angiography carries a small risk of stroke and blindness, which is increased when a lesion is embolised. The neuroradiologist looks specifically for signs of retinal 'blush' during angiography, as embolisation near the origin of the ophthalmic artery would cause permanent visual loss.

There are three possible major intracerebral complications if glue has been used:

- The micro-catheter tip may be retained within the glue.
- Proximal spread of glue due to invagination of the 'glueoma' when the embolisation catheter is removed.
- A vessel is torn when the catheter is removed. This may occur if the catheter has become lodged within the glue ball stuck to the vessel wall and may result in cerebral haemorrhage.

The second two complications are fortunately very rare but contribute to the risk of stroke during the procedure. Cerebral haemorrhage may require further embolisation or surgery such as ventricular drain insertion. Retention of the micro-catheter tip within the glue mass does not usually cause a problem, as the catheter becomes epithelialised with time.

The main systemic risk of cerebral embolisation is that of migration of the embolising material into the extracranial venous circulation and the pulmonary bed. The anaesthetist should look for signs of systemic spread such as a fall in end-tidal $CO_2$ or oxygen saturation. Fortunately, these pulmonary emboli are very small, and the effect is not usually long-lasting.

### Vein of Galen Aneurysmal Malformation (VGAM)

Large AV shunts often present with signs of high-output right-heart failure rather than an intracranial bleed. This is due to the rapid recirculation of blood from the arterial circulation through the AV shunt back to the right heart without passing through the systemic vascular bed. The vein of Galen aneurysmal malformation is a rare but important cause of high-output cardiac failure presenting in neonates (see Figure 36.7).

The vein of Galen aneurysmal malformation (VGAM) is a heterogenous collection of rare midline intracranial choroid arteriovenous (AV) vascular malformations. A VGAM consists of

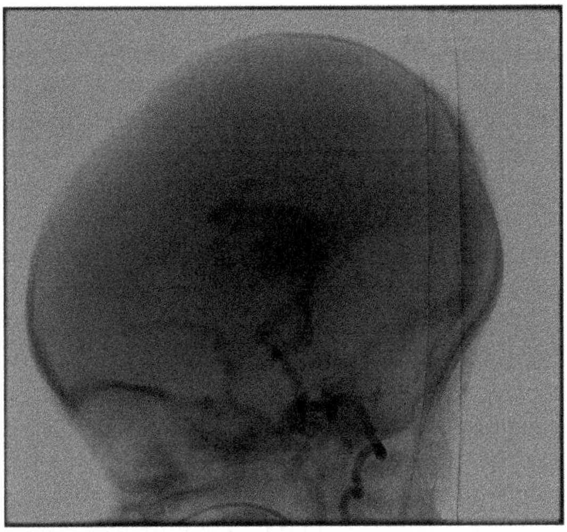

**Figure 36.7** Vein of Galen aneurysmal malformation.

multiple AV shunts draining into a dilated median prosencephalic vein of Markowski, a persistent embryonic vein that is normally absent in adults. The normal vein of Galen is formed by the junction of the internal cerebral veins and passes between the corpus callosum and pineal gland to form the straight sinus as it joins with the inferior saggital sinus. A VGAM is anatomically different from an AV malformation, where the venous drainage is into a dilated, but already formed, vein of Galen.

Without treatment, VGAMs are invariably fatal. Advances in cerebral angiography with early embolisation have improved outcomes significantly, so that in some series, 74% of those who are treated are neurologically normal at follow-up.

Babies presenting with VGAMs have a massive intracranial AV shunt. They usually present in the neonatal period with signs of poor systemic perfusion, pulmonary hypertension and right-heart failure. The systemic vascular resistance is higher than AV shunt resistance; thus blood leaving the left side of the heart goes preferentially to the carotid arteries, through the AV shunt and back to the right heart to cause volume overload and subsequent right-heart failure. Increased pulmonary blood flow may result in pulmonary hypertension (PHT), particularly in the newborn period, and right-ventricular pressure may approach or exceed systemic values.

Diagnosis is made by demonstration of the AVM on cranial ultrasound. A loud bruit may also be heard over the anterior fontanelle. Occasionally a VGAM can be diagnosed antenatally if a third trimester scan is done.

Babies presenting in the first few days of life with poor systemic perfusion and cardiac failure require pre-intervention ventilation and inotropic support in the neonatal intensive care unit (NICU). Milder cases of cardiac failure presenting in the first few weeks of life usually respond to diuretics.

Close cooperation with the neuroradiologist is essential. If the arterial pressure is high during an embolisation run, the glue may spread further than intended, thus unintentionally embolising other areas of the brain. The neuroradiologist will usually ask for a drop in systemic blood pressure (BP) to about two thirds of awake values. Fentanyl 1–2 mcg $kg^{-1}$ and sevoflurane 2–3 MAC is usually sufficient if the patient is fully paralysed. The diastolic BP is often very low and starts to normalise once the AV shunt is embolised. Tachycardia often becomes less pronounced as systemic blood flow increases, though this may not be as obvious in the anaesthetised patient.

All neonates are kept sedated, intubated and ventilated in NICU after VGAM embolisation. Closure of the AV shunt will cause a sudden increase in cerebral (rather than shunt) perfusion, as well as increased systemic perfusion. These factors may result in reperfusion injury, and there is a risk of post-embolisation cerebral bleed. Although right-sided heart failure may start to improve after embolisation, an element of left-sided heart failure often develops, as the left ventricular afterload is now increased.

Blood pressure must be carefully controlled post-embolisation, and an agent such as glyceryl trinitrate (GTN) or sodium nitroprusside (SNP) may be required if simple sedation is not sufficient. Some neuroradiologists heparinise patients after embolisation to prevent retrograde blood clots resulting in ischemic stroke. Heparin should only be started if there has been no bleeding during or after the embolisation procedure. A CT scan is routinely performed at the end of the procedure to determine if this is a safe course of action.

As there are potentially huge changes in both cerebral blood flow and physiology, the AV shunt is usually closed in stages in the first two to three months of life. Children for repeat embolisation are not usually as sick and may no longer require anti-failure medication. Post-embolisation management of these patients, including admission to NICU for ventilation after the procedure, depends on the residual AV shunt and operator preference.

## Intra-ophthalmic Artery Chemotherapy

Selective catheterisation of the ophthalmic artery for intra-orbital chemotherapy is a relatively new but expanding area of interventional neuroradiology.

This is currently reserved as second-line treatment for children with retinoblastoma who have relapsed during or after conventional systemic chemotherapy and cryotherapy. It avoids the need for radiotherapy during a critical time of brain development with the attendant risks of secondary malignancy and developmental delay. Initial results are encouraging, and with more experience this treatment option may become more widely available for other patients.

Access is via the femoral artery as per standard cerebral angiography. A micro-catheter is placed directly into the ophthalmic artery and the chemotherapy agent (e.g. melphalan, topotecan) is slowly infused into the orbit over a period of at least 20 minutes. Response to treatment is assessed two to three weeks later by formal examination under anaesthesia, and if responding, the child will receive further two treatments four to six weeks apart.

Standard cerebral angiography is performed, but there are some additional special considerations:

- The eye is at risk from arterial thrombosis, so a loading dose of heparin (75 IU $kg^{-1}$) is given after femoral access has been obtained.
- Dexamethasone (0.25 mg $kg^{-1}$) is given to reduce orbital and peri-catheter oedema.
- Chemotherapy is very emetogenic, so a dose of ondansetron (150 mcg $kg^{-1}$) is given.

The procedure may also stimulate an unusual oculocardiac reflex. The reaction is unpredictable and can be quite extreme. The first sign is sudden reduction in lung compliance and fall in tidal volume. The end-tidal $CO_2$ trace is like that seen in a patient with bronchospasm, although this is not heard on auscultation and is probably due to acute pulmonary venous congestion. The reaction is accompanied by a fall in oxygen saturation and hypotension, which may be profound. Screening with fluoroscopy shows the heart appears to be poorly contracting ('myocardial stunning'), although the heart rate does not usually fall initially. Bradycardia may occur a few minutes later. The child should be treated with atropine (5–10 mcg $kg^{-1}$ IV), and a bolus of IV isotonic fluid (10 ml $kg^{-1}$) may be required. Resistant hypotension should be treated with IV adrenaline (1–2 mcg $kg^{-1}$).

This reaction is seen when the micro-catheter is flushed, prior to chemotherapy injection. It typically occurs on repeat administration of intra-arterial chemotherapy but has been known to occur on the first treatment. The exact mechanism is unclear but is thought to be due to sensitisation of the ciliary ganglion, the parasympathetic ganglion located in the posterior orbit. Thermal or mechanical stimulation during a repeat procedure results in this unusual phenomenon. Prophylactic IV atropine and slow injection of intra-ophthalmic contrast seems to reduce the severity of the reaction.

## Anaesthesia for CT

CT is used as a diagnostic modality and to monitor treatment in children. It is particularly useful to delineate bony or vascular anatomy with 3D reconstruction to image the lungs or identify intracranial bleeding. High-quality scans require the child to remain still to reduce motion artefact, with breath-holds required for cardiac CT. CT scans are quick (although the dose of radiation is high), and most children do not require anaesthesia. Babies may be managed with 'feed and wrap', and older children will lie still in the scanner, but sedation is generally used for younger children (see Chapter 16). Anaesthesia is required for CT-guided biopsy, cardiac CT (frequent breath-holds) and those children unsuitable for sedation. Particular issues relate to anaesthesia in remote locations, with the added challenge of limited space in the scanner and limited access during the scan. Monitors must be visible from the control room, although the anaesthetist may stay in the scanner if wearing appropriate radiation protection.

## Anaesthesia for MRI

MRI is particularly useful for providing high-quality images of soft tissue and is the technique of choice in neurological, cardiovascular, oncology and musculoskeletal imaging. MRI imaging is based on the physical behaviour of protons in hydrogen atoms in water and phosphorus in ATP when placed in externally applied magnetic fields. Magnetic resonance (MR) scanners therefore contain very strong magnets, between 0.2 and 3 Tesla, and specific safety precautions are required to prevent ferrous objects from being sucked into the scanner. The presence of ferromagnetic implants, including pacemakers, are an absolute contraindication to MRI scanning. The scanners generate weak signals, and it is important to shield external radio-frequency sources such as from monitors.

MR scans are often long, between 30 minutes to 2 hours, depending on the area of interest, and the child must remain still during acquisition of images. The child is relatively inaccessible during the scan, and additional precautions need to be taken because of the magnet. Many older children will be able to manage by watching videos; however, younger, well children may be suitable for non-anaesthetist delivered sedation (e.g. via dexmedetomidine infusion; see Chapter 16). Younger patients who are unsuitable for nurse-led sedation or who require breath-holds during the scan will need general anaesthesia.

Induction of anaesthesia should take place in an anaesthetic room adjacent to the MR room after metal checks have been completed. A spontaneously breathing technique with SAD is suitable for most scans, although small infants should be intubated, as access is limited. Children undergoing cardiac MR require frequent breath-holds and should also be intubated and ventilated. Specific MR-compatible ECG electrodes, cables, saturation and blood pressure cuffs should be used. In an emergency, the child should be taken out of the scanner back to the anaesthetic room, as metal objects such as laryngoscopes and stethoscopes cannot be taken into the scanning room. Ward infusion pumps may malfunction close to the magnet, will need to be transferred to MR-compatible machines, which must be kept outside the immediate vicinity of the magnet (the 50 gauss line). Unstable patients requiring inotropic support may not be suitable for MR scanning for this reason.

### Key Points

- Interventional radiology is a rapidly expanding area in paediatric anaesthesia, with a range of complex procedures now being possible for some of the sickest patients in the hospital.
- Limited access due to X-ray equipment and dimmed lighting requires constant vigilance.
- Scrupulous attention to detail is required, including choice of anaesthetic technique, patient positioning and monitoring.
- Good communication and teamwork are essential to ensure patient safety during radiological procedures. Although both technically and logistically challenging, overcoming these obstacles makes this a very rewarding area in paediatric anaesthesia.
- Special precautions are required for safe anaesthesia in MRI.

## Further Reading


Acevedo J et al. Nonsurgical therapies for lymphangiomas: a systematic review. *Otolaryngology: Head and Neck Surgery* 2008; 138: 418–24.

Cucchiaro G et al. Blood glucose control during selective arterial stimulation and venous sampling for localization of focal hyperinsulinism lesions in anesthetized children. *Anesthesia and Analgesia* 2004; 99: 1044–8.

Dillon MJ et al. Angioplasty for renovascular hypertension in children: 20-year experience. *Pediatrics* 2006; 118:268–75.

Herod J et al. Epidermolysis bullosa in children: pathophysiology, anaesthesia and pain management. *Pediatric Anesthesia* 2002; 12:388–97.

King D et al. Pulmonary function is compromised in children with mediastinal lymphoma. *Journal of Pediatric Surgery* 1997; 32(2):294–300.

Lasjaunias P et al. The management of vein of Galen aneurysmal malformations. *Neurosurgery* 2006; 59(5):S3-184–S3-194.

Phillips TJ et al. Autonomic cardio-respiratory reflex reactions and superselective ophthalmic arterial chemotherapy for retinoblastoma. *Pediatric Anesthesia* 2013; 10:940–5.

Stuart G. Understanding Magnetic Resonance Imaging. Anaesthesia Tutorial of the Week no 177. Available online: https://resources.wfsahq.org/atotw/understanding-magnetic-resonance-imaging/. Accessed 18 April 2024.

Chapter 37

# Anaesthesia for Oncology and Other Medical Procedures in Children

Ioannis Ioannou

## Introduction

There are an increasing number of diagnostic and therapeutic interventions performed outside the theatre environment, and anaesthesia in remote locations is now a routine part of paediatric practice. Anaesthesia is required for painless procedures such as radiological scans where the child must remain immobile, or minor procedures that are uncomfortable or painful, such as lumbar puncture (LP), bone marrow aspirate (BMA) and endoscopy.

Anaesthetists have a key role to play in ensuring that these procedures are undertaken safely and efficiently, whilst minimising pain or distress for the child. The quality of the experience may influence the child's future attitude towards medical care. This chapter will consider the general principles for provision of remote anaesthesia, and specific requirements for oncology patients, muscle biopsy and joint injections. The development of safe sedation services and endoscopy for children is described in Chapter 16, and anaesthesia for radiology is covered in Chapter 36.

## General Principles: Anaesthesia in Remote Locations

Children undergoing minor medical procedures are frequently admitted as day cases. Procedures may be undertaken in the main operating theatre on an ad hoc basis, but it is probably more efficient, and more pleasant for the child and family, to base their care in a dedicated day unit or day-case list. A stand-alone medical procedure unit is ideal for high-volume, rapid turnover services such as oncology or gastroenterology. It is important that in all these situations, the same standards of care are provided as in the main operating suite:

- There should be a clinical lead for anaesthesia in the non-theatre environment, responsible for developing the service, training and revalidation of staff and ensuring safety standards and audit are appropriate.
- The service should ideally be consultant delivered with appropriate supervision of trainees.
- There should be clear policies covering patient selection and preparation, and a forum to discuss high-risk patients at a multidisciplinary team meeting. Children with an abnormal airway, pulmonary hypertension, cardiomyopathy, congenital heart disease or mucopolysaccharidosis or children with unstable disease, ASA III or above, should be discussed as to their suitability for treatment in a remote location. Additional support and planning will be required for high-risk patients.
- There should be appropriately trained theatre and recovery staff, including a trained anaesthetic assistant, and a fully equipped recovery room. Emergency drills should be practised regularly.
- Procedure rooms should be large enough to accommodate equipment and personnel and include full resuscitation facilities, piped medical gases, suction, air exchange and a means of providing ventilation.
- Full anaesthesia monitoring should be available, according to national guidelines.
- There should be full access to appropriate anaesthetic equipment, disposables and anaesthetic drugs. Service contracts for equipment and pharmacy support should be the same as for the main operating theatre.
- There should be regular audit of patient outcomes, training of staff and feedback from parents about the quality of the service.

## Paediatric Oncology

Cancer affects around 1:500 children under the age of 14 years in the United Kingdom, with around

1,900 new cases diagnosed each year (2015–2017). It is the most common cause of death in children aged 1–14 years in the United Kingdom. Since the early 1990s, incidence rates have increased by around a seventh (15%) in the United Kingdom, most likely related to improved cancer diagnosis and registration. Outcomes have improved markedly over the same period of time, owing to more intense treatment regimens with improved support and rescue therapies. The corollary of this is that there are more children surviving with long-term side effects from cancer treatments.

Cancer is more common in boys than girls (54% vs 46 %, respectively, 2015–2017), with most tumours presenting in children less than five years of age. The most common diagnoses are leukaemia, central nervous system (CNS) tumours and lymphomas; the overall five-year survival rate is 82%, but survival varies greatly according to diagnosis (see Table 37.1). Brain and CNS tumours account for most deaths, and retinoblastoma has the best survival rate (99% cure).

Diagnosis in children is often delayed, as childhood cancer is rare and slow to be considered. The child may have non-specific symptoms such as weight loss and listlessness, and then develop signs such as:

- Bruising and petechial haemorrhage, lymphadenopathy or bone pain (haematological malignancy)
- Abdominal distension or pain (Wilms' tumour, (nephroblastoma or neuroblastoma)
- Headache with ataxia (posterior fossa tumour)

Spread to distant sites and bone marrow is common at presentation. The parents are often devastated when the diagnosis is made, and the child frightened, upset and unwell. One of the major achievements of paediatric cancer treatment, and one of the factors that has led to improvements in outcome, has been the centralisation of care and the development of international research registries. The UK Children's Cancer and Leukaemia Group (CCLG) is the national association for the treatment of cancer in children and young people. More than 70% of children with cancer in the United Kingdom are registered as part of a national or international clinical trial. The CCLG is also a registered charity and provides support and information for children and their families. There are currently 19 specialist centres with multidisciplinary teams undertaking the treatment of cancer in children in the United Kingdom, with 'shared care' with non-specialist centres. Treatment is continued over several months or years, and shared care allows children to stay as close to home as possible.

**Table 37.1** UK children's cancer incidence and five-year survival rates

| | Incidence children <14 years (% all cases) | Five-year survival (%) |
|---|---|---|
| Leukaemia | 30 | |
| Acute lymphoblastic leukaemia | | 90 |
| Acute myeloid leukaemia | | 65 |
| CNS tumours | 26 | |
| Astrocytoma | | 95 |
| Ependymoma and choroid plexus tumours | | 60 |
| Embryonal CNS tumours | | 60 |
| Other gliomas | | 44 |
| Lymphoma | 11 | |
| Hodgkin's lymphoma | | 95 |
| Non-Hodgkin's lymphoma | | 90 |
| Soft tissue tumours Rhabdomyosarcoma | 6 | 70 |
| Neuroblastoma | 6 | 67 |
| Nephroblastoma | 5 | 92 |
| Retinoblastoma | 3 | 99 |
| Bone tumours | 4 | |
| Ewing sarcoma of bone | | 66 |
| Osteosarcoma | | 65 |
| Germ cell tumours | 4 | 93 |
| Melanoma/ epithelioma | 4 | |
| Hepatic tumours | 1 | |

*Source:* Cancer Research UK Childhood Cancer – Great Britain and UK and Children with Cancer UK

Anaesthesia may be required at many stages in the care of children with malignancy, for instance BMA, LP or biopsy for diagnosis or staging, routine scans, line insertion or definitive surgery. The anaesthetist must be aware of how the condition affects the child, the effects of treatment and whether the child has undergone surgery, radiotherapy, chemotherapy or a combination of these. Children with cancer require repeated anaesthetics – some children may be relatively well, receiving long-term maintenance chemotherapy, but others may be acutely unwell as a result of their treatment or a complication of treatment.

## Treatment of Specific Conditions

Current approaches to cancer treatment depend on clinical features and biological characteristics of the tumour, response to treatment and extent of residual disease (see Table 37.2).

Chemotherapy is given in cycles to increase efficacy and allow time for recovery. It is given either orally (PO) or IV, with intrathecal chemotherapy given to treat overt or potential CNS disease.

## Standard-Risk Acute Lymphoblastic Leukaemia (ALL)

Treatment of standard-risk childhood acute lymphoblastic leukaemia has a relatively good prognosis, so the aim is to limit exposure to drugs associated with late toxic effects. Children receive induction therapy over four to six weeks to induce remission in blood and bone marrow (steroids, vincristine and daunorubicin), with treatment of CNS disease (intrathecal methotrexate), possible intensification blocks to remove residual cells (methotrexate or asparaginase), a maintenance phase of daily 6-mercaptopurine (6-MP) PO with weekly methotrexate PO and six-weekly intrathecal methotrexate to prevent CNS recurrence. This treatment continues for two to three years.

## High-Risk ALL

High-risk ALL includes presentation <1 year of age, those presenting with high white cell count or CNS disease at diagnosis, those with chromosomal abnormalities such as the Philadelphia chromosome or those with poor response to induction treatment with increased minimal residual disease (MRD) in bone marrow. These children are treated with more intensive chemotherapy regimens associated with increased short- and long-term side effects, as for acute myeloid leukaemia (see the next section). Target drug therapy such as tyrosine kinase inhibitors is used to reduce cell proliferation, and immunotherapy including monoclonal antibodies and CAR T-cell therapy is employed in high-risk patients. Stem cell transplantation may be offered when the child is in first remission or presents with recurrent disease. Radiotherapy may be used for children presenting with CNS or testicular disease.

**Table 37.2** Treatment for children's cancers

| Cancer | Treatment |
|---|---|
| Acute lymphoblastic leukaemia | Steroids, chemotherapy, radiotherapy, target cancer drug, immunotherapy, stem cell or bone marrow transplant |
| Acute myeloid leukaemia | Chemotherapy, radiotherapy, target cancer drugs, immunotherapy, stem cell or bone marrow transplant |
| Hodgkin's lymphoma | Surgery (stage 1 disease), chemotherapy, radiotherapy |
| Non-Hodgkin's lymphoma | Chemotherapy, radiotherapy, donor stem cell or bone marrow transplant if relapse |
| Brain and CNS tumours | Surgery, chemotherapy, radiotherapy for children >3 years and proton beam therapy |
| Neuroblastoma | Surgery, chemotherapy, stem cell transplant, immunotherapy |
| Retinoblastoma | Surgery, laser, cryotherapy, systemic chemotherapy, radiotherapy, selective ophthalmic artery chemosurgery (SOAC) |
| Nephroblastoma | Surgery, chemotherapy, radiotherapy |
| Osteosarcoma | Surgery, chemotherapy, radiotherapy |
| Rhabdomyosarcoma | Surgery, chemotherapy, radiotherapy |

## Acute Myeloid Leukaemia

Acute myeloid leukaemia (AML) has a lower cure rate; treatment involves high-dose induction and intensification chemotherapy that may induce prolonged marrow suppression requiring in-patient stay with associated episodes of febrile neutropenia or mucositis. Stem cell transplantation is often used for children with high-risk disease.

## Solid Tumours

For solid tumours such as Wilms' or neuroblastoma, tumour staging is carried out at diagnosis with CT/MRI, bone marrow and tumour biopsy. Current UK practice is to reduce tumour size and vascularity with several courses of chemotherapy prior to definitive surgery, followed by further courses of chemotherapy or radiotherapy.

## Tumours Associated with Anterior Mediastinal Mass

Children presenting with T-cell ALL, lymphomas, neuroblastoma or intrathoracic germ cell tumour may present with a mass in the anterior mediastinum. This may result in airway compression, superior vena cava (SVC) obstruction or cardiorespiratory collapse in severe cases.

Anaesthesia is required for tumour staging and line insertion. Induction of anaesthesia is particularly high risk for children with an anterior mediastinal mass (see Chapters 30 and 36).

Timing of procedures such as diagnostic BMA, LP and line insertion should be made after discussion with the oncology team. A possible option is to start chemotherapy and monitor symptoms. Biopsies need to be undertaken within five days of starting treatment if an accurate tissue diagnosis is to be obtained.

## Bone Marrow Transplantation

Bone marrow transplantation is used to treat high-risk malignant disease such as relapsed ALL or AML, or non-malignant disease such as aplastic anaemia, severe combined immune deficiency, sickle cell anaemia or inborn errors of metabolism. Stem cells may be obtained from the patient (autologous transplant) or from a matched related or unrelated donor (allogeneic transplant). Autologous transplant is used as 'rescue' after high-dose chemotherapy, and allogeneic transplant is used for treatment of malignant or non-malignant disease.

Autologous stem cells may be obtained from bone marrow harvest or peripheral blood stem cell (PBSC). PBSCs are harvested by apheresis after granulocyte colony stimulating factor (G-CSF) is given to increase the stem cell count in peripheral blood. Allogeneic stem cells may be obtained from bone marrow, peripheral blood or cord blood. Children donating bone marrow to a sibling require general anaesthesia. The child is placed in the prone position and a volume of approximately 10 ml $kg^{-1}$ marrow is collected under aseptic conditions. Intravenous fluids and multimodal analgesia are required. The relative risks and benefits of the procedure to the healthy donor should be considered.

The recipient receives 'conditioning' chemotherapy and/or total body irradiation before transplant, followed by reinfusion of harvested stem cells. Conditioning may result in complete ablation of the recipient bone marrow to remove residual cancer cells, but less aggressive regimens associated with fewer complications are currently being investigated, particularly for non-malignant conditions. The child will require intensive supportive therapy after conditioning and until engraftment occurs and will be extremely vulnerable to infection. Full barrier precautions should be used when treating these patients.

## Graft-versus-Host Disease

Graft-versus-host disease (GvHD) is the term given to the immunological reaction of donor cells introduced to an immunocompromised host. It is usual after allogeneic bone marrow transplantation, and is an indication that engraftment is taking place. It may be useful to clear residual cancer cells. GvHD may also be seen after transfusion of non-irradiated blood to an immunocompromised patient (transfusion-related GvHD).

Acute GvHD occurs within 100 days of transplant and is associated with generalised skin rash, hepatitis and diarrhoea. Severe GvHD has a high mortality. Chronic GvHD occurs later with a more indolent course with characteristics of a chronic autoimmune disease affecting multiple organ systems, including skin, liver and gastro-intestinal tract. Severe GvHD should ideally be prevented, for instance by improved matching of donor and recipient, by less severe recipient conditioning regimens and ensuring the use of irradiated blood in vulnerable patients. Treatment is supportive, including immunosuppression (e.g. steroids, tacrolimus, ciclosporin, mycophenolate [MMF]) or immunotherapy. Children with severe GvHD usually require admission to a paediatric intensive care unit (PICU).

## Side Effects of Chemotherapy Treatment

Cytotoxic agents commonly induce bone marrow suppression, hair loss, nausea and vomiting. Other drug-specific side effects are described in Table 37.3. Children with bone marrow suppression require support with platelet and red cell transfusions, and they may require broad-spectrum antibiotics and removal of a central venous line during a period of febrile neutropenia. G-CSF may be given to aid recovery from neutropenia and allows more intensive chemotherapy to be given in high-risk disease. Some specific complications of treatment relevant to the anaesthetist are described in the next section.

## Steroids and Tumour Lysis Syndrome

Steroids are a mainstay of treatment in ALL, but they are given in short courses, so adrenal suppression is rarely a problem.

Tumour lysis syndrome results from the massive release of intracellular metabolites. It is seen in the first 12–72 hours of the start of treatment in children with high tumour load or high proliferative rate, or those where tumours are very chemosensitive. Anaesthetists should be aware that tumour lysis syndrome may be triggered by dexamethasone given as an antiemetic to a child in an at-risk category; dexamethasone must be avoided in this situation.

**Table 37.3** Commonly used agents and side effects of treatment

| Drug | Conditions treated | Common side effects of drug |
|---|---|---|
| Vincristine | ALL | Myelosuppression, syndrome of inappropriate antidiuretic hormone (SIADH), peripheral neuropathy, mucositis |
| Anthracyclines (daunorubicin,doxorubicin, epirubicin) | Acute leukaemia, sarcoma, Wilms tumour, neuroblastoma, Hodgkin's disease | Myelosuppression, cardiomyopathy, arrhythmias |
| Cyclophosphamide | Non-Hodgkin's lymphoma, neuroblastoma, sarcoma, conditioning prior to bone marrow transplant | Myelosuppression, cardiomyopathy, arrhythmias, haemorrhagic cystitis |
| Ifosfamide | Non-Hodgkin's lymphoma, sarcoma, bone tumours | Myelosuppression, Fanconi's syndrome, renal failure |
| Cisplatin | Neuroblastoma, germ cell tumour | Seizures, hypomagnesaemia, renal failure |
| L-Asparaginase | ALL | Coagulopathy, allergic reaction, pancreatitis |
| Nitrosoureas | | Pneumonitis, renal failure |
| Bleomycin | Hodgkin's disease, germ cell tumours | Allergic reactions, pulmonary fibrosis, Reynaud's |
| Methotrexate | ALL | Myelosuppression, mucositis, pneumonitis, renal failure |
| Actinomycin D | Wilms tumour, sarcoma | Coagulopathy, liver failure, acute respiratory distress syndrome |
| Busulfan | Conditioning prior to bone marrow transplant | Hepatic veno-occlusive disease, seizures |

Children at risk of tumour lysis syndrome include those with:

- High count ALL
- AML
- Hodgkin's lymphoma, non-Hodgkin's lymphoma, Burkitt's lymphoma

Tumour lysis results in hyperuricaemia, hyperkalaemia, hyperphosphataemia, hypocalcaemia and uraemia and is associated with deposits of uric acid or calcium phosphate in the renal tubules. Children present with nausea and vomiting, muscle cramps, renal impairment, seizures or arrhythmias. Children who are at risk should be closely monitored and treated with hydration and rasburicase, which promotes the metabolism of uric acid to soluble metabolites, or allopurinol, which reduces the formation of uric acid.

## Mucositis

Mucositis is painful inflammation and ulceration of all mucous membranes, seen in all children receiving high-dose chemotherapy, 50% of children receiving head and neck radiotherapy, and 5–10% of children receiving standard chemotherapy. Severe mucositis may limit therapy. Treatment is symptomatic with intravenous fluids and total parenteral nutrition (TPN) if required. Abdominal pain should be treated with IV morphine patient- or nurse-controlled analgesia (PCA/NCA), with added ketamine if required.

## Vincristine

Vincristine is neurotoxic; children are monitored for possible sensory or motor neuropathy, and doses adjusted accordingly.

Vincristine and other vinca alkaloids such as vinblastine and vindesine are universally fatal if given intrathecally. There have been more than 50 deaths reported internationally involving accidental intrathecal administration of vinca alkaloids, often due to systems errors and human factors identified as the root cause. Administration of chemotherapy in the United Kingdom is now tightly regulated and can only be given by registered individuals with appropriate training, in designated areas, and following specified checks. Intrathecal and intravenous agents are given on different days, and vincristine is often prepared in intravenous mini-bags to prevent accidental intrathecal administration. Non-Luer spinal needles that are incompatible with intravenous Luer connections have been introduced to prevent such accidents in future.

## Anthracyclines and Other Agents Associated with Cardiac Toxicity

Anthracyclines (doxorubicin, daunorubicin, epirubicin) are commonly used in children with the following conditions:

- AML
- Non-Hodgkin's lymphoma (NHL)
- Wilms tumour
- Neuroblastoma
- Bone tumours

Anthracyclines are cardiotoxic, particularly when given in high doses. Risk factors for anthracycline cardiotoxicity include treatment for relapsed disease, high cumulative dose (>300 mg $m^{-2}$), associated radiotherapy and if there have been signs of early cardiac toxicity. All children are monitored with regular echocardiograms during treatment and long-term follow-up. Mortality associated with overt cardiomyopathy is high (50%), so many of these children will be candidates for cardiac transplantation. Subclinical cardiomyopathy is common (a degree of cardiac impairment has been reported in up to 65% of such children) and may be un-masked at times of increased demand, such as puberty, pregnancy or intercurrent illness, and possibly during anaesthesia and surgery. A high index of suspicion should be maintained when anaesthetising these children, and a recent echo should be available.

Cyclophosphamide is associated with cardiomyopathy or cardiac arrhythmias when used in high doses to induce bone marrow ablation (conditioning) before bone marrow transplant. Fluorouracil is occasionally associated with cardiac toxicity.

## Bleomycin

Bleomycin is used in the treatment of children with Hodgkin's lymphoma and germ cell tumours. It is associated with an inflammatory pneumonitis and progressive pulmonary fibrosis, particularly when given in high doses. Risk factors for bleomycin toxicity include increasing age (toxicity rarely seen in children), increasing dose, radiotherapy and renal impairment.

Bleomycin is used to induce fibrosis in animal models of pulmonary fibrosis and is deactivated in the lungs by pulmonary hydroxylases. The role of oxygen in promoting bleomycin toxicity is controversial, with evidence mainly from case reviews. Hyperoxia should be avoided after recent exposure to bleomycin and if there is evidence of pre-existing pulmonary disease. It is sensible to use the lowest possible inspired oxygen during anaesthesia.

## Anaesthesia for LP and BMA

In our institution, oncology procedures are undertaken on dedicated lists, usually in the dedicated procedure unit, with a senior nurse acting as a list coordinator to book patients, coordinate review by the oncologists and prepare children with up-to-date blood counts. It is our preference to provide general anaesthesia for these short, painful procedures rather than deep sedation or local anaesthesia alone.

From an anaesthesia perspective, the child requires careful assessment, particularly if newly diagnosed, receiving high-dose chemotherapy or suffering from acute GvHD. Active sepsis should be excluded. Children receiving long-term maintenance chemotherapy are generally well and often develop their own 'routine', which is helpful for the anaesthetist to follow.

Commonly accepted minimum platelet counts for procedures are shown in Table 37.4.

BMA and LP are quick procedures and ideally suited to total intravenous anaesthesia (TIVA) with propofol, with assisted/spontaneous ventilation with a face mask. This technique facilitates early discharge home (see Table 37.5 for the suggested protocol). Supplementary local anaesthesia and IV paracetamol are indicated if bone marrow trephine is performed.

Children usually have an in-dwelling central line, which may be used for anaesthesia provided full aseptic precautions are taken when accessing the line. *It is the responsibility of the anaesthetist to ensure that the line is flushed after use to remove residual anaesthesia drugs.*

## Anaesthesia for Radiotherapy

Targeted radiotherapy is used as a primary therapy or to clear microscopic disease in children with CNS tumours, Hodgkin's lymphoma, Wilms tumour, neuroblastoma and sarcoma of bone and soft tissue. Radiotherapy is delivered in fractionated daily doses over six weeks; side effects are localised to the area of treatment and may include redness and blistering of the skin, mucositis, neurocognitive impairment and pituitary damage. Damage to normal tissue is minimised by use of three-dimensional targeted beams (3D conformational radiotherapy, or 3D CRT), and modulating the intensity of the beams (intensity-modulated radiotherapy, or IMRT). Proton beam radiotherapy enables treatment to be targeted at a precise depth, ideal for cranial irradiation in children Radiotherapy units are usually based in adult hospitals, and special arrangements may need to be made for paediatric patients.

Each treatment typically takes 10–45 minutes. The child must remain by themselves in the treatment room and is required to wear an immobilisation device. With careful preparation and play therapy, treatment can often be performed without sedation in children >8 years (and some younger children). When required, a propofol-based anaesthetic is ideal with a SAD for airway control. As for any anaesthesia service for children, trained staff and full monitoring are required. The anaesthetist cannot stay with the child during treatment, and output from the monitors must be relayed to the control room.

**Table 37.4** Minimum platelet count for oncology procedures

| Procedure | Platelet count ($\times 10^9$ $^{-1}$) |
|---|---|
| Line insertion | 100 |
| LP | 50 |
| Trephine | 20 |
| BMA | No minimum count Specified |

**Table 37.5** Alternative anaesthesia protocols for short oncology procedures such as BMA, LP or trephine

| |
|---|
| Propofol 3–5 mg kg$^{-1}$ IV + remifentanil 1 mcg kg$^{-1}$ IV bolus<br>Repeat propofol 1–2 mg kg$^{-1}$ IV if required |
| Propofol 3–5 mg kg$^{-1}$ IV + alfentanil 5 mcg kg$^{-1}$ IV bolus Repeat propofol 1–2 mg kg$^{-1}$ IV if required |

## Anaesthesia for Selective Ophthalmic Artery Chemosurgery (SOAC)

Advanced retinoblastoma that does not respond to conventional treatment or those who develop recurrent disease may require selective ophthalmic artery chemosurgery (SOAC). A microcatheter is inserted into the ophthalmic artery for chemotherapy to be delivered selectively to the affected eye. Typically, three treatment cycles are required with post-treatment examination under anaesthesia (EUA) being performed after each cycle. During catheter placement, profound but transient cardiorespiratory collapse of unknown aetiology has been observed, typically (but not always) during the second cycle. A reduction in tidal volume, a slow rising non-plateauing $ETCO_2$ with difficulty maintaining adequate ventilation is seen, which is followed by a rapid progressive fall in $ETCO_2$ and arterial desaturation. This is accompanied with marked haemodynamic instability with hypotension and bradycardia. Patients should receive prophylactic atropine at induction, and the anaesthetist should have appropriate resuscitation drugs such as adrenaline and fluid boluses prepared to treat such a response.

## Rare 'Non-malignant' Medical Conditions

### Haemophagocytic Lymphocytic Histiocytosis

Haemophagocytic lymphocytic histiocytosis (HLH) is a rare disease presenting in infancy associated with high mortality. It is caused by activation of normal macrophages and T-lymphocytes, which results in an overwhelming inflammatory response with release of cytokines and phagocytosis of normal cells by activated macrophages. It is inherited as an autosomal recessive condition, but secondary HLH may occur in older children after systemic infection, immune deficiency or associated with underlying malignancy. Typical presentation is with fever, skin rash, hepatosplenomegaly and pancytopenia. CNS involvement including seizures is common. Skin, lymph node, liver and bone marrow biopsy confirm diagnosis. Treatment is with supportive therapy followed by bone marrow transplantation.

## Langerhans Cell Histiocytosis

Langerhans cell histiocytosis (LCH) is a rare condition, previously known as histiocytosis X. It is a proliferative disorder of epidermal Langerhans cells, typically associated with lytic lesions in bone, with skin involvement in many cases. Controversy exists as to whether LCH is an inflammatory or malignant condition, but recent evidence suggests that it is a distinct myeloid neoplasm. There is a spectrum of disease, with three typical presentations:

- Eosinophilic granuloma. One or more bone lesions, classically in the skull but may affect other sites, including vertebra or femur. Recurrent mastoiditis and otitis media may occur because of destruction of the mastoid bone. Diabetes insipidus may occur because of destruction of the sella turcica.
- Hand–Schüller–Christian disease. Multifocal disease with classical triad of bony defects of the skull, exophthalmos and diabetes insipidus. Mucocutaneous and systemic involvement may occur.
- Letterer–Siwe disease. Fulminant disorder associated with generalised skin rash, fever, hepatosplenomegaly, lymphadenopathy, bone lesions and marrow infiltration.

Diagnosis is by imaging, skin or bone marrow biopsy. Isolated LCH of bone may be treated by surgical curettage and local injection of steroid. Mild systemic LCH is treated by chemotherapy, particularly where LCH involves vulnerable sites such as the skull or there is a risk of fracture; multi-system disease is treated by chemotherapy but may be associated with up to 20% mortality. Children with diabetes insipidus should continue desmopressin (DDAVP) in the perioperative period.

## Severe Combined Immune Deficiency

Severe combined immune deficiency (SCID) is associated with life-threatening infection, dermatitis, diarrhoea and failure to thrive. SCID results from one of a range of gene defects causing impairment of T-cell, B-cell and NK-cell function. It is inherited as an autosomal recessive condition, X-linked or may be sporadic. A subgroup of children with immune deficiency and DiGeorge syndrome have a hypoplasia of the thymus with absent T-cells (associated with chromosome 22q11 deletion).

Children with SCID present with severe opportunistic infection in the first three months of life, which may be bacterial, viral or fungal, for example *Candida* or *Aspergillus*. Without treatment, SCID is usually fatal by two years of age. Allogeneic bone marrow transplantation is ideally performed before the age of six months to avoid the effects of repeated infections. Children with SCID or other conditions associated with immune deficiency must not receive live vaccines. They must only receive irradiated blood products to prevent GvHD from immunocompetent lymphocytes in donor blood or blood products.

## Neuromuscular Disorders and Myopathy

Muscle biopsy may be required as a diagnostic procedure in children with suspected neuromuscular disorders or in children with mitochondrial myopathy. Muscle is taken from the anterolateral aspect of the thigh, either as a needle biopsy or excised as a small strip. It is a short, painful procedure, usually requiring general anaesthesia, although it can be performed under regional block in older children.

The choice of anaesthesia for muscle biopsy may be difficult. Volatile agents may cause anaesthesia-induced rhabdomyolysis (AIR) in patients with one of the muscular dystrophies or may trigger malignant hyperthermia (MH) in susceptible patients. Conversely, TIVA using propofol may cause propofol-related infusion syndrome (PRIS), particularly if the child has a mitochondrial disorder. PRIS is associated with metabolic acidosis, lipidaemia, bradycardia, rhabdomyolysis and heart failure.

Suxamethonium must not be used in any patient with abnormal muscle, as fasciculations may cause hyperkalaemic cardiac arrest. Non-depolarising muscle relaxants should be avoided or used in reduced dose in a child who has a myopathy.

Children presenting for muscle biopsy usually fall into four main categories:

- *The child presents for investigation as a 'floppy baby'.* It is best to use a volatile anaesthetic rather than use TIVA, which may not be a familiar technique in this age group and may induce significant hypotension.
- *An older child is being investigated for MH or suspected central core disease.* A trigger-free anaesthetic must be given. Central core disease is associated with a mutation of the RyR1 gene and an abnormality of the intracellular ryanodine receptor. It is inherited as an autosomal-dominant disease, but sporadic cases occur. Children present with hypotonia from birth, with truncal weakness, delayed motor milestones, muscle cramps, mild facial weakness, contractures and scoliosis. The disease is slowly progressive, but children generally walk. There is a characteristic appearance on biopsy, and a genetic test from a blood sample is also available.
- *A boy with raised creatine kinase (CK) is being investigated for failure to walk, aged three to four years.* The likely diagnosis is Duchenne muscular dystrophy (DMD). TIVA with propofol should probably be given, as volatile agents may trigger AIR and hyperkalaemic cardiac arrest, usually in recovery when the child starts to move again. There is usually a family history in a boy with DMD, with characteristic hypertrophic calves and global hypotonia. A raised CK should act as a 'red flag' for the anaesthetist. Volatile agents have been used uneventfully in this group but are best avoided, particularly in young DMD patients when they still have significant muscle mass. If it is not possible to obtain venous access in these patients, it is acceptable to use a volatile agent for induction, then switch to TIVA.
- *The child is suspected to have a mitochondrial myopathy.* Prolonged high-dose propofol infusion should be avoided. Mitochondrial myopathies are associated with abnormalities of the electron transfer chain or oxidative phosphorylation. Mitochondrial disorders may be associated with myopathy, encephalopathy, epilepsy, lactic acidosis or gastrointestinal disorders. Mitochondrial myopathies are not associated with MH, and volatile agents are safe. The child should also be given dextrose-containing intravenous fluids to avoid lactic acidosis.

A careful history should be taken and the case discussed with the referring team with respect to the most likely differential diagnosis, so that the risks and benefits of each technique can be assessed. It may be logical to use TIVA as the default technique for all patients (except babies); it avoids the risk of MH or rhabdomyolysis, and since muscle biopsy takes less than 15 minutes, the exposure to propofol will not be long enough to develop PRIS in children with mitochondrial myopathies.

Anaesthesia may be given by intermittent bolus injection, and the airway maintained with a SAD – mix propofol 200 mg with alfentanil 1 mg in a 20 ml syringe and give propofol 3–5 mg $kg^{-1}$ for induction, with increments as required.

## Juvenile Arthritis

Juvenile idiopathic arthritis (JIA) is an autoimmune condition associated with painful swollen joints that may affect children from around six months of age. There are several types of JIA, including:

- Systemic JIA. Associated with fevers, rash, lymphadenopathy and splenomegaly. Inflammation and stiffness may affect any joint.
- Oligoarthritis. Pain, stiffness and swelling affecting the wrist and knees.
- Polyarticular arthritis. Affects small joints of the hands, weight-bearing joints and the neck; more common in girls than boys. Fifteen per cent of children are rheumatoid factor positive and may develop joint damage and erosions.
- Psoriatic arthritis. Associated with psoriatic rash and/or family history of psoriasis.

The treatment of JIA is analgesia (NSAIDs), physiotherapy and exercise. Children who do not respond may be treated with oral methotrexate. Injections of steroids help to reduce pain and disability associated with an acute exacerbation. These procedures are usually undertaken as day cases. Joints to be injected should be clearly marked, and an image intensifier should be available. For large joints, the steroid may be combined with local anaesthetic to reduce post-procedural pain. Injections into multiple small joints are more painful, and morphine may be required.

**Key Points**

- The demand for anaesthesia services outside the main theatre is rising; the same standard of care should be available in all areas.
- Children receiving chemotherapy may be unwell if newly diagnosed, receiving high-dose chemotherapy or suffering from sepsis, or they may be in good health if receiving long-term maintenance treatment. High-dose anthracyclines may cause cardiomyopathy.
- The choice of anaesthetic for undiagnosed muscle biopsy is difficult. TIVA is preferred in older children to prevent anaesthesia-induced rhabdomyolysis and reduce the risk of MH. PRIS is unlikely after a short procedure.
- Children undergoing joint injections are managed as day cases; adequate analgesia is required.

## Further Reading

Culshaw V, Yule M, Lawson R. Considerations for anaesthesia in children with haematological malignancy undergoing short procedures. *Paediatric Anaesthesia* 2003; 13: 375–83.

Kinder RA. Muscular dystrophy versus mitochondrial myopathy: the dilemma of the undiagnosed child. *Paediatric Anaesthesia* 2007; 17:1–6.

McFadyen JG, Pelly N, Orr RJ. Sedation and anesthesia for the pediatric patient undergoing radiation therapy. *Current Opinion in Anesthesiology* 2011; 24:433–8.

Mcleod M, Dobbie M. Anterior mediastinal masses in children. *BJA Education*, 2019; 19:21–6.

Oduro-Dominah L, Brennan LJ. Anaesthetic management of the child with haematological malignancy. *Continuing Education in Anaesthesia Critical Care and Pain* 2013; 13 (5):158–64.

Chapter 38

# Principles of Paediatric Resuscitation

Sophie Skellet

Paediatric basic and advanced life support skills are essential for all anaesthetists. They may be needed occasionally in the operating room or more commonly when anaesthetists are members of clinical emergency/cardiac arrest teams. Data from the National Cardiac Arrest Audit in the United Kingdom (which collects data from in-hospital cardiac arrests [IHCA] attended by emergency teams) indicates that approximately 250 IHCA occur per year in children and infants in contrast to approximately 16,000 adult IHCA each year.

As cardiac arrest occurs less frequently in children than in adults, regular training is essential. Good teamwork is an important element of successful resuscitation, so an emphasis on this should be placed in simulation training and practice. The ideal interval for re-training is unknown, but it is likely that frequent top-ups, several times a year, are most effective.

## Epidemiology

When resuscitating children and infants, the following definitions are used:

- A newborn is an infant just after birth.
- An infant is under the age of 1 year.
- A child is between 1 year and 18 years of age.

The differences between adult and paediatric resuscitation are largely based on differing aetiology. If paediatric guidelines are used in error in a young adult, little harm will ensue, as studies have shown that the paediatric causes of arrest continue into early adulthood.

Adults most commonly have primary cardiac arrests caused by a cardiac arrhythmia reflecting intrinsic heart disease; this is a sudden acute event. Arrest rhythms are commonly ventricular fibrillation (VF) and pulseless ventricular tachycardia (pVT), and they are managed with prompt defibrillation. Children and infants rarely present with primary cardiac arrest, although it can occur with congenital or acquired heart disease or inherited arrhythmia syndromes.

In children, most cardiac arrests are secondary and are caused by hypoxia associated with decompensated respiratory and/or circulatory failure, reflecting the limit of the body's ability to compensate for the effects of underlying illness or injury. Severe tissue hypoxia causes myocardial dysfunction, resulting in profound bradycardia, which typically deteriorates to asystole or pulseless electrical activity (PEA); hence cardiac arrest in children is more often referred to as cardiorespiratory arrest.

In the operating theatre, cardiac arrest in children is rare, most commonly due to respiratory causes, such as loss of airway, or cardiovascular causes such as hypovolaemia due to blood loss or hyperkalaemia associated with rapid blood transfusion. Children with pulmonary hypertension are also a high-risk group of patients. A combination of many factors can often be identified in perioperative cardiac arrest, including poor preoperative condition, inadequate assessment, inappropriate anaesthesia technique or human factors.

A secondary cardiorespiratory arrest in a ward setting is rarely a sudden event but follows a progressive deterioration. The body initially activates adaptive physiological responses compensating for the effects of the deterioration in vital organs (compensated respiratory or circulatory failure). These compensatory responses result in important signs and symptoms that can be recognised, thereby providing an opportunity to intervene before further deterioration. This pattern of deterioration can most easily be recognised and managed using the structured ABCDE (airway, breathing, circulation, disability, exposure) approach which is taught in resuscitation courses. Early intervention in the deteriorating child is crucial, as the outcome from secondary cardiorespiratory arrest is relatively poor in a ward setting.

Even if return of spontaneous circulation (ROSC) is achieved, morbidity and mortality after cardiorespiratory arrest remain high. Data from the Warwick University Out-of-Hospital Cardiac Arrest Outcomes (OHCAO) audit in the United Kingdom between 2014 and 2018 indicate approximately 570 out-of-hospital cardiac arrests (OHCA) per year in children with 9% survival to hospital discharge. Rates of ROSC and survival to hospital discharge after IHCA have improved over the past two decades, with 70% achieving ROSC and 54% of children surviving to hospital discharge. Cardiac arrest outcomes in theatre are better as children are closely monitored. However, many children continue to succumb to severe organ injury (e.g. brain, kidney) or multi-system organ failure 48–72 hours post-arrest.

## Basic Life Support (BLS)

In the management of the collapsed child, several factors are important in maximising the chances of a good outcome. The most important is early recognition and appropriate intervention in children who exhibit signs of respiratory and/or circulatory compromise. Whilst this is essential, there will always be some children in whom respiratory and/or circulatory collapse cannot be prevented. For these children, early BLS, rapid activation of the in-hospital clinical emergency team and prompt, effective advanced life support is crucial in improving mortality and morbidity. The sequence is as shown in the algorithm (Figure 38.1).

BLS is the combination of manoeuvres and skills that provides recognition and management of a person in cardiac or respiratory arrest (without the use of technical adjuncts) and which 'buys time' until the child can receive more advanced treatment. The aim is to achieve sufficient oxygenation and perfusion to 'protect' the brain and other vital organs.

The sequence of actions in BLS is known as cardiopulmonary resuscitation (CPR). For optimum outcome, CPR should start as soon as possible by the first person on the scene. Although ventilation remains a particularly important component of CPR in children, rescuers who are unable or unwilling to provide breaths should be encouraged to perform at least compression-only CPR. A child is far more likely to be harmed if the rescuer does nothing.

Before starting BLS, it is important to remember the 3 S's:

- *Safety*

  Assess the situation and ensure the safety of the rescuer(s) and then the child. There may be a variety of hazards which the rescuer should be alert to whether the situation occurs within or outside the health care environment.

  All bodily fluids should be treated as potentially infectious; put on gloves as soon as practicable and use barrier devices for ventilation (e.g. pocket mask, bag mask ventilation [BMV]) if possible. Most airway procedures are considered aerosol generating and thus require proper (risk-adjusted) personal protection equipment (PPE) in cases of presumed transmittable diseases.

- *Stimulate*

  Establish the responsiveness of the unconscious child by tactile and verbal stimulation but never shake a child vigorously. If the child or infant is unresponsive, further assistance will be required.

- *Shout for assistance*

  Call for help or press the emergency buzzer and summon the clinical emergency team. In the United Kingdom and Europe, the cardiac arrest call number is 2222.

The following subsections describe the elements of the structured ABCDE approach.

## A – Airway

Turn the child or infant supine. In the unconscious child, the tongue is likely to occlude their airway at least partly. This can usually be overcome by using a head-tilt and chin-lift manoeuvre or, if necessary, by performing a jaw thrust.

Head tilt and chin lift: place one hand on the forehead and gently tilt their head back. In infants, the head should be placed in a neutral position. For the child, a 'sniffing' position that causes some extension of the head on the neck will be required. The chin lift is performed by placing the fingertips of the rescuer's other hand on the bony part of the child's lower jaw and lifting the chin upwards. Take care not to compress the soft tissues under the child's jaw as this will occlude the airway.

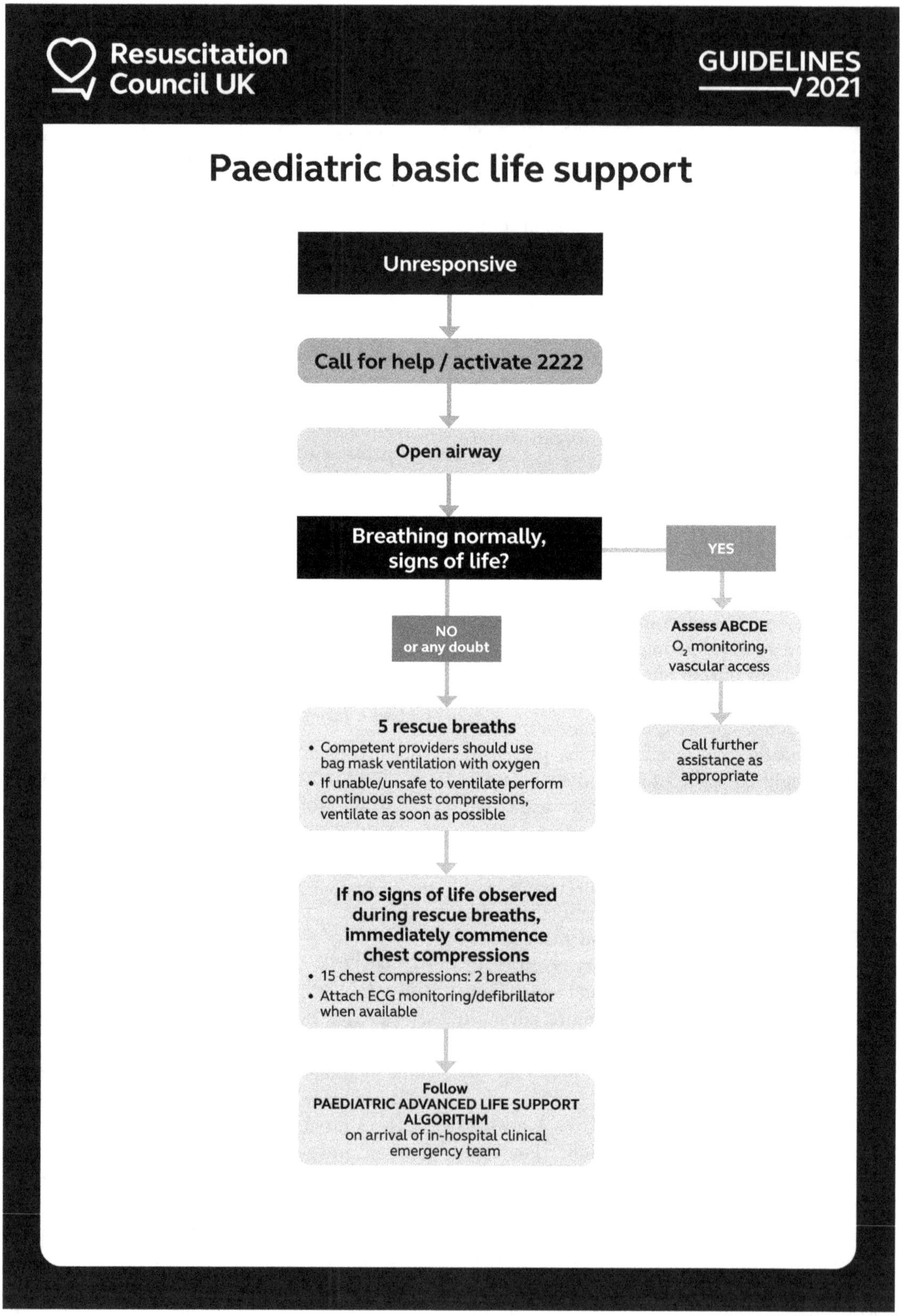


**Figure 38.1** The BLS algorithm.

Jaw thrust: this is the preferred airway opening manoeuvre when cervical spine immobilisation is required. Place hands on either side of the child's head with two or three fingertips of both hands under both angles of the child's lower jaw. With thumbs resting gently on the child's cheeks, lift the jaw upwards. If neck injury is suspected, try to open the airway using jaw thrust alone. If this is unsuccessful, add head tilt gradually until the airway is open. Establishing an open airway takes priority over concerns about the cervical spine.

After airway opening, check in the child's mouth to ensure there is no obvious foreign body present. If one is seen and the rescuer is confident that they can remove it safely, this can be attempted; however, blind finger sweeps should never be performed.

## B – Breathing

After opening the airway, the rescuer needs to assess the child for effective, normal breathing (see Table 38.1).

Keeping the airway open, look, listen and feel for normal breathing by putting your face close to the child's face and looking along the chest whilst simultaneously looking for signs of life (see Table 38.2). Studies have shown that feeling for a pulse is unreliable in determining the presence or absence of a circulation even for trained paediatric health care workers. The evaluation of circulation is now performed by looking for signs of life during the breathing assessment and during delivery of rescue breaths. If a health care worker wishes to also check for a pulse, this should be done simultaneously with the breathing assessment.

**Table 38.1** Assessment of breathing during BLS

| | |
|---|---|
| LOOK | For chest and abdominal movements |
| LISTEN | For airflow at the mouth and nose (+/–additional noises) |
| FEEL | For airflow at the mouth and nose |

**Table 38.2** Signs of life

| Signs of life |
|---|
| Swallowing |
| Spontaneous movements |
| Vocalising |
| Coughing |
| Normal (not agonal) breathing |

Look, listen and feel for no more than 10 seconds before deciding; if you have any doubts about whether the breathing is normal, act as if it is not normal.

If the child's breathing is *not* normal or absent:

- *Give five initial rescue breaths*: While performing the rescue breaths, note any gag or cough response to your action. These responses, or their absence, will form part of your ongoing assessment of signs of life.
- *Give rescue breaths for an infant*: Maintaining an open airway, cover the mouth and nose of the infant with your mouth, ensuring a good seal. Blow steadily into the infant's mouth and nose over one second, sufficient to make the chest rise. Take your mouth away and watch for the chest to fall as air comes out. Repeat this sequence four more times ensuring chest rise and fall.
- *Give rescue breaths for a child older than one year*: Maintaining an open airway, pinch the soft part of the nose closed with the index finger and thumb of your hand on their forehead. Open the mouth a little, but maintain a chin lift. Take a breath and place your lips around the mouth, ensuring a good seal. Blow steadily into their mouth over one second, sufficient to make the chest rise visibly. Take your mouth away and watch for the chest to fall as air comes out. Repeat this sequence four more times ensuring chest rise and fall.
- *Where equipment is immediately, accessible provide ventilation by BMV, using 100% oxygen as soon as this is available*: To provide an adequate seal to the mask, a two-person technique is advocated.
- *If a rescue breath is ineffective, consider airway obstruction or inadequate airway opening*: Try repositioning the head to open the airway or the addition of jaw thrust. Take up to five attempts to achieve an effective breath. If still unsuccessful, move on to chest compressions.

If there are signs of life after the rescue breaths, continue ventilations (12–30 breaths per minute) until the child starts breathing effectively on their own. Unconscious children and infants who are not in cardiac arrest and have normal breathing can have their airway kept open by either continued head tilt and chin lift or jaw thrust. If there is a perceived risk of vomiting, position the unconscious child in a recovery position and check for continued normal breathing once every minute.

## C – Circulation

Following the rescue breaths, if there are no signs of life or you are unsure, immediately start high-quality chest compressions. Chest compressions are serial, rhythmic compressions of the anterior chest wall, intended to cause blood to flow to vital organ tissues.

To perform high-quality chest compressions (CC):

- CC rate: 100–120 per minute for both infants and children.
- Locate the xiphisternum and compress the sternum one finger's breadth above this.
- CC depth: depress the lower half of the sternum by at least one third of the anterior-posterior dimension of the chest (approximately 4 cm for an infant and 5 cm for a child), not deeper than 6 cm (adult).
- Release all pressure on the chest between compressions to allow for complete chest recoil; this optimises venous return and hence cardiac output generated by CC.
- Minimise pauses in CC so that 80% or more of the CPR cycle consists of CC. ROSC is linked to the generation of a coronary perfusion pressure of more than 15 mmHg during CPR.

Coronary perfusion pressure rises when the aortic end diastolic pressure generated by effective chest compressions rises. It takes six to eight compressions to build up sufficient aortic end diastolic pressure, and this will be lost immediately if the compressions stop.

After 15 chest compressions, tilt the head, lift the chin and give two rescue breaths. Continue CC and breaths in a ratio of 15:2. Perform compressions on a firm surface.

The best method for compressions varies slightly between infants and children:

- Infants:
  - Two-finger technique: Recommended for the lone rescuer. Place two fingers of one hand in the correct position on the sternum and depress it by at least one third of the depth of the infant's chest, approximately 4 cm.
  - Two-thumb encircling technique: Recommended for two rescuers and in-hospital resuscitation. There is evidence that this method delivers greater cardiac output than the two-finger technique. Place both thumbs flat, side-by-side, on the lower half of the sternum, with the tips pointing towards the infant's head. Spread the rest of both hands, with the fingers together, to encircle the lower part of the infant's rib cage with tips of the fingers supporting the infant's back. Press down on the lower sternum with your two thumbs to depress it at least one third of the depth of the infant's chest, approximately 4 cm. For small infants, you may need to overlap your thumbs to provide effective compressions.
- Chest compression in children aged over one year:
  - Place the heel of one hand over the lower half of the sternum. Lift the fingers to ensure that pressure is not applied over the child's ribs. Position yourself vertically above the child's chest and, with your arm straight, compress the sternum by at least one third of the depth of the chest, approximately 5 cm. In larger children, or for small rescuers, this may be achieved by using both hands with fingers interlocked.

Do not interrupt CPR at any moment unless there are clear signs of life (e.g. normal breathing, coughing). Two or more rescuers should alternate who is performing chest compressions frequently and/or switch hands to avoid fatigue.

Continue with this sequence, attaching electrocardiogram (ECG) monitoring/defibrillator when available, until the arrival of the clinical emergency team or until the child starts to show signs of life.

# Advanced Life Support

Resuscitation is a continuous process from BLS to advanced life support (ALS). High-quality BLS is the essential foundation of resuscitation and must be continued even when experienced help arrives and appropriate equipment can be used to facilitate the delivery of advanced techniques. The anaesthetist is often a member of the clinical emergency team because of their advanced airway management skills. Good teamworking skills and excellent communication are required to achieve all the simultaneous interventions that are required to optimise outcomes. The sequence is shown in the ALS algorithm (Figure 38.2).

Whilst monitoring is attached, the team leader should confirm cardiac arrest with a short simultaneous check for breathing and signs of life, then immediately direct the team to recommence high-quality CPR.

## Airway and Breathing

The team member tasked with airway and breathing, most often the anaesthetist, should ensure a patent airway by using an airway manoeuvre and provide ventilation, initially by BMV, using 100% oxygen. The concentration of inspired oxygen ($FiO_2$) should not be titrated during CPR. To provide an adequate seal of the mask, a two-person technique is advocated. If BMV can be successfully performed, then continue with this mode of ventilation.

The trachea should only be intubated by experienced personnel (anaesthetists, intensivists) if this can be performed with minimal interruption to chest compressions. Consider intubation if BMV is unsuccessful or becoming more difficult as the resuscitation progresses. A cuffed tracheal tube (TT) should be used, and placement must be confirmed by end-tidal carbon dioxide ($ETCO_2$) monitoring. Once positive pressure ventilation via a TT is being delivered, ventilations can be asynchronous and chest compressions continuous (only pausing every two minutes for rhythm check). In this case, ventilations should approximate to the lower limit of normal rate for age:

- Infants: 25 breaths per minute
- Children 1–8 years old: 20 breaths per minute
- Children 8–12 years old: 15 breaths per minute
- Children >12 years old: 10–12 breaths per minute

In the out-of-hospital setting, studies have suggested that ventilation with BMV rather than attempting tracheal intubation or use of a supraglottic airway (SGA) in the management of paediatric cardiac arrest is associated with better outcomes. In the in-hospital setting, there is insufficient evidence to make a definitive recommendation. Competent personnel may choose to insert an SGA as an alternative to intubation when BMV is unsuccessful; $ETCO_2$ monitoring should be used with an SGA.

For children or infants already on a mechanical ventilator, either disconnect the ventilator and ventilate by means of a self-inflating bag or continue to ventilate with the mechanical ventilator. In the latter case, ensure that the ventilator is in a volume-controlled mode; that triggers and limits are disabled; and ventilation rate, tidal volume and $FiO_2$ are appropriate for CPR. There is no evidence to support any specific level of positive end expiratory pressure (PEEP) during CPR. Ventilator dysfunction can itself be a cause of cardiac arrest.

## Circulation

Once cardiorespiratory arrest is confirmed and CPR recommenced, attach an ECG monitor to allow cardiac rhythm assessment to decide whether the child has a shockable or non-shockable cardiac arrest rhythm (done with no interruption to CPR).

Manual defibrillators can provide ECG monitoring via electrodes or via self-adhesive defibrillation pads. If using pads, place one on the chest wall just below the right clavicle, and one in the mid-axillary line (anterolateral [AL] position). In infants and small children, it may be best to apply the pads to the front (mid-chest immediately left of the sternum) and back (middle of the back between the scapulae) of the chest (antero-posterior [AP] position) if they cannot be adequately separated in the standard positions. There is no evidence to recommend the superiority of one pad position over the other, but the heart must be bracketed between the two pads. Use the largest size pads that fit the chest without touching each other. Pads for children should be 8–12 cm in size and 4.5 cm for infants. Avoid contact between the pads, as this will create charge arcing if defibrillation is needed. Some defibrillators have pads fitted with feedback devices which will help monitor the quality of CPR delivered; these may require AP pad placement. The devices store the data from resuscitation efforts and can be used to debrief teams after resuscitation episodes. There is evidence that guideline-compliant CPR and event debriefs can improve resuscitation outcomes.

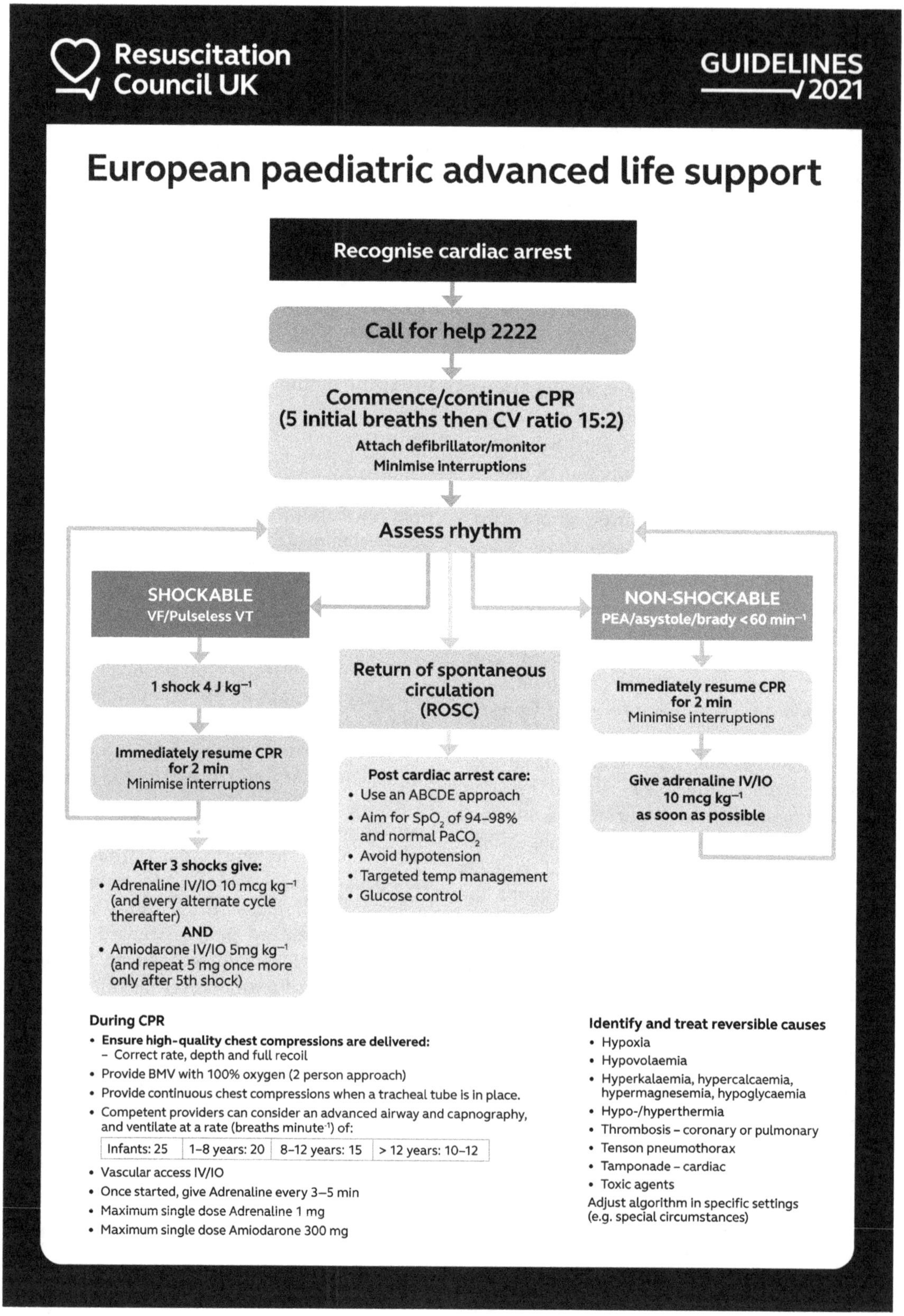


**Figure 38.2** The ALS algorithm.

## Rhythm Assessment

The majority of children and infants (>80%) will have a non-shockable rhythm:

- *Asystole* – no electrical activity of the heart, the ECG is a flat line.
- *PEA* – normal electrical complexes are present on the ECG, but there are no signs of life nor a palpable pulse.
- *Bradycardia <60/minute* – CPR should be started in children and infants who become bradycardic with signs of inadequate perfusion despite adequate respiratory support. Hence providers should rather assess signs of life and not lose time by checking for a pulse.

A few children and infants will have a shockable rhythm:

- VF
- pVT

## Non-shockable (Asystole, PEA, Bradycardia)

- Pause chest compressions briefly to assess the cardiac rhythm on the monitor.
- If a non-shockable rhythm is diagnosed, immediately continue high-quality CPR.
- Obtain intravenous (IV) or intraosseous (IO) access and give 10 mcg $kg^{-1}$ adrenaline (0.1 ml $kg^{-1}$ of 1 in 10,000 solution) as soon as possible after a non-shockable rhythm is identified, preferably within three minutes of identification of cardiac arrest. The same dose of adrenaline should be repeated every three to five minutes (every other cycle) until ROSC is obtained or the rhythm changes and/or CPR is stopped.
- Continue CPR, only pausing briefly every two minutes to check for rhythm change.
  If organised electrical activity is seen, check for signs of life and a pulse. If there is ROSC, continue post-resuscitation care.
- Feeling for a pulse:
  - In a child aged over one year, feel for the carotid pulse in the neck.
  - In an infant, feel for the brachial pulse on the inner aspect of the upper arm.
  - For both infants and children, the femoral pulse in the groin (mid-way between the anterior superior iliac spine and the symphysis pubis) can also be used.
- Consider any reversible causes of cardiorespiratory arrest (4H's and 4T's), and correct as found (see Table 38.3).
- If the patient is intubated, chest compressions can be continuous if this does not interfere with satisfactory ventilation. The ventilation rates during continuous chest compressions differ according to age, as noted in the 'Airway and Breathing' section.
- When performing chest compressions, choose a team member who will be able to deliver them most effectively. Use a rigid surface/back board so that chest compressions are more effective.
- Change the person performing chest compressions at least every two minutes. Watch for fatigue and/or suboptimal compressions and switch rescuers earlier if necessary.
- Once there is ROSC, the ventilation rate should be a normal physiological age-dependent respiratory rate which may then be adjusted to meet the goals of post-resuscitation care. Continue to measure $ETCO_2$ to monitor ventilation and confirm correct TT placement.

## Shockable (VF/pVT)

- As soon as a shockable rhythm is identified, defibrillation should immediately be attempted (regardless of the ECG amplitude). If in doubt, consider the rhythm to be shockable.
- Continue CPR until a defibrillator is available; good team planning before each action will minimise hands-off time and improve the quality of CPR.
- Apply self-adhesive defibrillation pads in the anterolateral or anteroposterior position.
- Charge the defibrillator while another rescuer continues chest compressions.
- Once the defibrillator is charged, pause the chest compressions, ensure all rescuers are clear of the patient and deliver the shock. Minimise the delay between stopping CC and shock delivery (<5 seconds).
- Give one shock of 4 J $kg^{-1}$ if using a manual defibrillator (do not exceed the adult starting dose, 150 J).
- Without reassessing the rhythm or feeling for a pulse, resume CC immediately. Even if the heart is cardioverted to a potential perfusing

**Table 38.3** Identification and treatment of the reversible causes of cardiorespiratory arrest in children and infants (the 4Hs and 4Ts)

| Cause | Consider | Identification | Treatment |
|---|---|---|---|
| H | Hypoxia | History/clinical exam +/– oxygen saturation (if trace picked up) | Ventilation and 100% FiO2 |
| H | Hypovolaemia | History +/– POCUS* | Fluid bolus 10 mls/kg balanced isotonic crystalloid; blood products (major haemorrhage) |
| H | Hyper/ hypokalaemia | History + blood gas analysis: | Correction/reduction of metabolic derangement |
| H | Hypothermia/ hyperthermia | History + core temperature: | External (e.g. blanket), internal (e.g. cold/ warm fluids, extracorporeal circuit) techniques |
| T | Thromboembolism | History +/– POCUS* (e.g. dilated right ventricle) | IV thrombolysis |
| T | Tension pneumothorax | Examine symmetrical air entry +/– POCUS* | Needle thoracocentesis/thoracostomy (trauma) |
| T | Tamponade (cardiac) | History +/– POCUS* (e.g. pericardial fluid collection) | Needle pericardiocentesis/thoracotomy (trauma) |
| T | Toxic/therapeutic disturbance | History/ECG | Specific toxic treatment (e.g. sodium bicarbonate for tri-cyclic drug poisoning) |

*Note*: *POCUS = point of care ultrasound.

rhythm, the myocardium will be 'stunned' and the right ventricle distended with blood. By restarting CC immediately, coronary perfusion pressure will be maintained and help ventricular emptying.

- Consider and correct reversible causes (4Hs and 4Ts, Table 38.3).
- Continue CPR for two minutes, then pause briefly to check the monitor: if still VF/pVT, give a second shock with same energy level, 4J $kg^{-1}$, and strategy for delivery as the first shock.
- Continue to repeat the cycle of shocks at 4J $kg^{-1}$ followed by two minutes of CPR and a brief pause to assess the rhythm for as long as the child or infant remains in a shockable rhythm.
- Immediately after the third shock, whilst chest compressions are ongoing, give adrenaline 10 mcg $kg^{-1}$ IV/IO (0.1 ml $kg^{-1}$ of 1 in 10,000 solution) and 5 mg $kg^{-1}$ amiodarone IV/IO (lidocaine 1 mg $kg^{-1}$ may be used an alternative to amiodarone).
- The same adrenaline dose, 10 mcg $kg^{-1}$ IV/IO, should then be given after every other shock (third, fifth, seventh, etc.) until ROSC. Amiodarone 5 mg $kg^{-1}$ can be repeated once more after the fifth shock.
- Consider escalating the energy dose for the sixth shock in refractory VF/pVT. The 2021 guidelines suggest escalating to 8J $kg^{-1}$ but without exceeding the maximum adult dose (360 J). In refractory VF/pVT, it is also suggested to try alternative pad placement (i.e. change AL to AP position).
- Change the person performing chest compressions at least every two minutes; watch for fatigue and/or suboptimal compressions and switch rescuers earlier if necessary. Team choreography is important.
- CPR should be continued unless:
    - An organised, perfusing rhythm is recognised and confirmed by a clinical assessment indicating signs of life (ROSC).
    - There are criteria for withdrawing resuscitation.
- After the event, debriefing of the team should be conducted, to support the team whilst reflecting on their clinical practice.

## Automated External Defibrillators (AEDs)

AEDs are increasingly available in public places (supermarkets, swimming pools, cinemas, schools), and a national programme is under way in the United Kingdom to map AED locations so that the ambulance dispatcher (when 999 is called) can direct a rescuer to the nearest one available.

Trained providers should limit the no-flow time when using an AED by performing CPR up to the point of analysis (but not during, or the rhythm will not be correctly identified) and immediately after the shock delivery or no shock decision; pads should be applied with minimal or no interruption in CPR. If possible, use an AED with a paediatric attenuator in infants and children younger than eight years (e.g. energy reduced to 50–75 J). If this is not available, use a standard AED for all ages. There have been continuing reports of safe and successful use of AEDs in children less than eight years, demonstrating that AEDs can identify arrhythmias accurately in children and are extremely unlikely to advise a shock inappropriately.

## Capnography

This is mandatory for all intubated patients, including children. Monitoring $ETCO_2$ with waveform capnography reliably confirms TT placement in a child or infant weighing more than 2 kg with a perfusing rhythm. The waveform will appear after four ventilated breaths and indicates that the TT is in the tracheobronchial tree, both in the presence of a perfusing rhythm and during CPR. It does not rule out intubation of a bronchus.

If there is no $ETCO_2$ trace during CPR, then TT placement must be checked. Assume 'No trace, wrong place'.

The $ETCO_2$ value reflects pulmonary blood flow, which in turn reflects cardiac output, so an attenuated $ETCO_2$ waveform or $ETCO_2$ value less than 2 kPa during CPR should direct the team to check the quality of CPR, particularly that of chest compressions, being delivered. A sudden rise in $ETCO_2$ can be an early indication of ROSC. Current evidence does not support the use of a threshold $ETCO_2$ value as an indicator for stopping the resuscitation attempt. Capnography may also be useful for monitoring ventilation when using an SGA or during BMV.

## Physiological CPR

Several recent studies have looked at monitoring of certain physiological responses during CPR, in the critical care or highly monitored setting, that may be used to direct further resuscitative efforts. Parameters studied include invasively measured diastolic blood pressure, $ETCO_2$ and cerebral near-infrared spectroscopy (NIRS). There is some evidence that generation of diastolic blood pressures of $\geq$25 mmHg in infants and $\geq$30 mmHg in children during CPR may improve the chances of ROSC. Whilst this shows promise for the future, evidence is currently insufficient to recommend routine use.

## Point of Care Tests

- Bedside ultrasound (US) may be used by those trained in its use to identify certain reversible causes of cardiac arrest (e.g. cardiac tamponade, pneumothorax), but evidence of benefit on outcome is limited. Most importantly, the use of US should not increase hands-off time or impact the quality of CPR; image acquisition is best done during pauses for rhythm check and/or for ventilations.
- Blood gas analysis may be used to identify reversible causes of cardiac arrest and help direct additional treatments in certain conditions (e.g. hyperkalaemia).

## Transcutaneous Pacing

Pacing is not effective for the management of children and infants in asystole. Nor is it helpful in children or infants with bradycardia secondary to post–cardiac arrest hypoxic/ischaemic myocardial insult or in bradycardia secondary to respiratory failure. Pacing is useful in selected cases of bradycardia caused by complete heart block or abnormal function of the sinus node, and in these situations emergency transthoracic pacing may be life-saving.

## Extracorporeal Life Support (ECLS)

For some children and infants with decompensated cardiorespiratory failure (e.g. severe refractory septic shock or cardiomyopathy or myocarditis with refractory low cardiac output), pre-arrest use of ECLS can be beneficial to provide end-organ support and prevent cardiac arrest. IHCA shortly prior to or during cannulation should not preclude ECLS initiation. Any child or infant who is considered to have any chance of a favourable outcome should ideally be transported as soon as possible to a paediatric centre with ECLS capacity.

Extracorporeal cardiopulmonary resuscitation (E-CPR) is the implementation of veno-arterial extracorporeal membrane oxygenation (VA-ECMO) in a patient with refractory cardiac arrest. E-CPR should be considered early for children and infants with IHCA and a presumed reversible cause when conventional ALS does not promptly lead to ROSC. E-CPR has also been used in the management of children with OHCA in cases of hypothermic cardiac arrest or when cannulation can be done pre-hospitally by a highly trained team, within a dedicated health care system. Whilst this is not yet widely available in the United Kingdom, practice is increasing.

## Management of Cardiac Arrest in Specific Disease States

**Trauma:** Start standard CPR with particular attention to external haemorrhage control, including the use of tourniquets in exsanguinating injury to the extremities; potential need for bilateral thoracostomies (or needle thoracocentesis); and IO/IV access and fluid resuscitation (if possible, with blood or blood products), as well as the use of the pelvic binder in blunt trauma. CC are performed simultaneously with these interventions depending on the available personnel and procedures. Effective CPR must be prioritised over cervical spine immobilisation.

**Hypothermic arrest**: Start standard BLS and assess the heart rhythm. Muscle rigidity in hypothermia will make CC and ventilations more difficult to perform. Hypothermia reduces the effectiveness of defibrillation and resuscitation drugs. If the rhythm is shockable, attempt defibrillation, but if this is unsuccessful continue CC until core temperature >30°C when drugs and defibrillation are more likely to be effective. Drugs given when the core temperature is <30°C may accumulate with resultant toxicity when re-warmed. Never stop resuscitation and diagnose death until the patient has been re-warmed to at least 32°C or cannot be re-warmed despite active measures. In some cases, hypothermia can exert a protective effect on the brain and vital organs, and intact neurological recovery can occur even after prolonged cardiac arrest if deep hypothermia develops before asphyxia. Consider E-CPR where facilities are available to support this.

**Septic shock**: There is no evidence to suggest alterations to standard CPR are of benefit.

**Single-ventricle circulation**: There is no evidence to suggest alterations to standard CPR are of benefit for children and infants with single-ventricle anatomy after stage 1 repair. Prior to repair, infants with shock due to elevated pulmonary to systemic flow ratio may benefit from inducing mild hypercarbia.

**Hemi-Fontan/Fontan circulation**: There is no evidence to suggest alterations to standard CPR are of benefit. For the seriously ill child or infant, hypercarbia achieved by hypoventilation may be beneficial to increase oxygenation and cardiac output. Hypovolaemia is poorly tolerated, and intravenous fluid administration may be necessary. Negative pressure ventilation, if available, may be beneficial for hemi-Fontan, bidirectional Glenn or Fontan circulations by increasing cardiac output. It is reasonable to consider E-CPR early in situations of refractory CA.

**Pulmonary hypertension (PHT)**: If a child or infant with PHT suffers a cardiac arrest, then standard CPR should be performed; it may be beneficial to attempt to correct hypercarbia. Additionally, consider the use of inhaled nitric oxide or aerosolised prostacyclin (PGI2). For children and infants with PHT receiving postoperative care, respiratory management and monitoring should be directed towards avoiding hypoxia and acidosis.

## Prognostic and Family Considerations

There is little evidence to suggest a fixed length of time for CPR after which ongoing efforts are futile, but if there has been no ROSC after 30 minutes of unsuccessful CPR, the team leader should consider stopping the resuscitation. This decision should be made on an individual basis for each child or infant and should consider various factors.

Poor prognostic factors include:

- Unwitnessed arrest
- Prolonged interval from collapse to initiation of CPR
- Asystole as the first arrest rhythm
- Blunt trauma

Good prognostic factors include:

- Witnessed arrest with prompt bystander CPR
- Short periods of CPR
- A shockable rhythm
- Arrest with hypothermia or immersion in cold water

Many parents want to be present during a resuscitation attempt so they can see that everything possible is being done for their child or infant. Studies indicate that being with their child is comforting to the parents and helps them to gain a realistic view of attempted resuscitation and death. Additionally, bereaved families who have been present at the event show less anxiety and depression several months after the death. A dedicated staff member should always stay with the parents to explain the process in an empathetic and sympathetic manner. They can also ensure that the parents do not interfere with the resuscitation process or distract the resuscitation team. When appropriate, physical contact with the child or infant should be allowed.

## Post-resuscitation Care

A child or infant who is successfully resuscitated may suffer from post–cardiac arrest syndrome. This is comprised of multiple organ failure (resulting from hypoxia and ischaemia during cardiac arrest), the effects of the subsequent reperfusion injury and effects from precipitating pathology. It is seen most often in children who remain comatose post-ROSC. Each patient may be affected differently depending on pre-arrest comorbidities, duration of the ischaemic insult and cause of the cardiorespiratory arrest.

A significant percentage of resuscitated children may ultimately die or survive with serious neurological sequelae. Therefore, the main goal of post-resuscitation care is to maintain oxygenation and perfusion to vital organs to prevent secondary organ injury (e.g. hypoxic-ischaemic brain injury, ischaemic myocardial damage, hypoxic pulmonary damage [acute lung injury], acute kidney injury, coagulopathy). For children and infants who have had a cardiorespiratory arrest, the initial step is ROSC, but this is only the first step in the continuous process of resuscitation management.

The ABCDE approach must be followed, and ongoing care of the child who remains comatose post-ROSC is best delivered in a paediatric intensive care unit (PICU). This may require specialist transport. Children who have suffered perioperative cardiac arrest should not be extubated at the end of surgery and should be transferred to the PICU for continuing care.

**Airway and breathing**: In children and infants who do not regain consciousness within 10 minutes of ROSC and for some other clinical indications (e.g. transfer to PICU, CT scan), intubation may be required, if not already undertaken. This will also allow subsequent control of ventilation: hypoxia, hypercarbia and hypocarbia should all be avoided to prevent the deleterious effects on the brain.

If a child wakes but does not return to a fully alert state, analgesia, sedation and muscle relaxants will be required; these will reduce oxygen consumption, facilitate ventilation and help to prevent complications. Neuromuscular blockade may also be needed to facilitate ventilation and prevent shivering during targeted temperature management (discussed later in this section).

A cuffed TT should be used and the cuff pressure monitored. In the non-theatre setting, tracheal intubation should be performed by competent and experienced personnel (usually anaesthetists) following well-defined protocols, having all necessary equipment and drugs at hand, anticipating problems and having a plan B if intubation fails. Capnography is mandatory for all intubated children, and a chest X-ray should be performed to confirm correct placement of TT (between T2 and T3).

Once intubated, children and infants will require gastric decompression with a gastric tube; this is usually via the nasogastric route unless there is a history of head injury when an orogastric tube should be used in case of basal skull fracture. Once there is sustained ROSC, titrate the $FiO_2$ to an $SpO_2$ of 94–98%.

**Circulation:** Continuous re-assessment to ensure haemodynamic stability and prevent further organ failure is important. A stunned myocardium will not tolerate fluid overload, so judicious use of fluid is indicated. Each bolus should be 10 ml $kg^{-1}$ of balanced isotonic fluid, given when there are signs of circulatory failure; 0.9% saline is an acceptable alternative. Clinical assessment of the child's circulation (heart rate, blood pressure, capillary refill time, peripheral temperature, core temperature and urine output) is important and will aid in the evaluation of any treatment response. Re-assessment should look for signs of effectiveness of fluid administration and for signs of fluid overload, which include basal lung crepitations, an expanding liver edge and in older children a raised jugular venous pressure. Use of vasoactive medications (adrenaline and noradrenaline) should be used when fluid-resistant shock exists or the child develops signs of fluid overload. Noradrenaline and adrenaline may be started as peripheral IV infusions (or given IO) but are best given via a central vein if access can be achieved. An arterial line is optimal, as it will allow monitoring of blood gases and continuous blood pressure. An early echocardiogram is helpful in assessing heart function. Serial lactate measurements may also indicate the effectiveness of circulatory interventions. The ideal goal for blood pressure (BP) post-ROSC is unknown, but BP should not be allowed to fall below the fifth centile for age at any point; aim for a mean or systolic blood pressure between the fifth and 50th centile for age. Urine output is a marker of end-organ perfusion, so it reflects circulatory status and should be monitored (>1 ml $kg^{-1}$ $h^{-1}$ in children and >2 ml $kg^{-1}$ $h^{-1}$ in infants).

**Disability:** An assessment of neurological status should be performed early to obtain a post-resuscitation baseline, help identify neurological deficits and aid in predicting prognosis. The conscious level should be assessed with either the AVPU or Glasgow Coma Scale scoring systems. Pupil reactivity, posturing and focal signs should also be noted and regularly recorded. Most children who die after ROSC do so from neurological injury, so efforts need to be directed at protecting the brain from secondary injury. Secondary brain injury can be minimised by:

- Avoiding hypoxia, hypocapnia and hypercapnia; providing adequate oxygen and ventilation, keeping $PaCO_2$ between 4.5 kPa and 6.0 kPa.
- Avoiding and treating hypotension with fluids and vasoactive medications; keeping BP between the fifth and 50th centile for age.
- Recognising and promptly treating seizures, as these are associated with a worse outcome; begin continuous EEG monitoring as soon as possible and check blood glucose.
- Correcting glucose and electrolyte abnormalities.
- Monitoring and promptly treating signs of raised ICP (using 3% saline or mannitol).
- Targeted temperature management (TTM): after ROSC, TTM involves strict control of temperature to avoid hyperthermia (>37.5°C) and severe hypothermia (<32°C) and is mandatory. Hyperthermia post-ROSC is common within the first 48 hours and worsens brain injury. Fever should be treated aggressively with anti-pyretics and active cooling. Two large paediatric randomised controlled trials (Therapeutic Hypothermia after Pediatric Cardiac Arrest [THAPCA] trials) compared mild therapeutic hypothermia (TH, 32–34°C) with therapeutic normothermia (TN, 36.8°C, controlled to prevent temperatures above 37.5°C) following in-hospital and out-of-hospital cardiorespiratory arrest. In both the out-of-hospital and in-hospital groups, there was no significant difference in survival or one-year functional outcome between the two different temperature groups (TH and TN). It may be that the avoidance of fever confers a better outcome and is the important goal in TTM for patients following cardiorespiratory arrest. The optimal duration of TTM is unknown, and different centres use 24, 48 or 72 hours.

**Exposure:** The child or infant will need to be (at least briefly) fully exposed to facilitate a full examination. This may aid in diagnosis and inform specific management (e.g. the purpuric rash of meningococcaemia may prompt treatment with broad-spectrum antibiotics if not already given).

## Resuscitation of the Acutely Unwell Child

The transition from a compensatory state to decompensation may occur unpredictably in children. Therefore, any acutely unwell child should be monitored in the right setting to enable early recognition and appropriate intervention to correct any deterioration in their physiology. Health care systems should implement strategies for early recognition and management of deteriorating children and infants in their institutions, including context-specific guidance, for example children with septic shock.

### Assessment and Management of Respiratory and Circulatory Failure Follows the ABCDE Approach

Assess the respiratory status by evaluating:

- The child's level of responsiveness: hypoxia causes agitation and eventually loss of consciousness.

- Respiratory rate (RR) adjusted for age and in context: pain, fever and anxiety will all increase RR, so trends are more informative than single values.
- $SpO_2$.
- Work of breathing: subcostal and intercostal recession, tracheal tug, head bobbing, chest excursion.
- Air entry on auscultation of the chest.
- The presence of additional noises: stridor, wheeze.

Assess the child's circulatory status by evaluating:

- The pulse rate: trends are more informative than single readings.
- Pulse volume.
- Peripheral and end-organ circulation: capillary refill time (CRT), urinary output, level of consciousness.
- Preload evaluation: jugular veins, liver span, lung crepitations.
- Blood pressure.
- Serial lactate measurements.

It is important to remember that no single finding can reliably identify the severity of the circulatory failure and/or be used as a goal for treatment. Attach an ECG monitor to assess cardiac rhythm in acutely unwell children.

All children need to be reassessed frequently and at least after every intervention.

Most drugs and fluids are administered to children based on their weight. In the emergency department, if the weight of the child is not yet known, the weight of the child should be obtained, in order of preference, by:

- Asking the caregiver for a recent weight
- Using a body length tape with pre-calculated drug doses (Sandell, Broselow)
- Using a paediatric emergency drug chart, such as provided on the European Paediatric Advanced Life Support course
- Using an age-based weight calculation formula:
  - For the age group between 1 and 10 years, the following formula provides an approximation of weight:
    weight (kg) = (age in years + 4) × 2.
  - This formula will underestimate the weight of overweight children, but for most resuscitation drugs, dosage is based on lean body mass (care must be taken to avoid exceeding adult drug doses).
  - An infant weighs approximately 3 kg at birth and 10 kg at one year of age.

## Airway

- Open the airway and keep it patent using head-tilt/chin-lift or jaw-thrust manoeuvres and perform careful suctioning of any secretions.
- Awake children will usually assume their own optimal position; do not try and lie them down or agitate them, as this will make them cry, causing turbulent airflows resulting in increased airway resistance, worsening hypoxia.
- Consider an oropharyngeal airway (Guedel) in the unconscious child, in whom there is no gag reflex, to optimise the airway. Use the appropriate size, measured from the central incisors to the angle of the mandible, and avoid pushing the tongue backwards during insertion.
- Consider a nasopharyngeal airway in the semi-conscious child for airway optimisation (unless the child has a coagulopathy or basal skull fracture). The correct insertion depth should be sized from the nostrils to the tragus of the ear.
- In children and infants with a tracheostomy, respiratory distress may be caused by obstruction of the tracheostomy tube, leading to ineffective ventilation. Check the patency of the tube by suctioning. If a suction catheter cannot be passed, the tracheostomy tube should be removed immediately and replaced. If a clean tube is not available, ventilation via BMV should be given at the tracheostomy stoma site until the tube is cleaned and replaced. If the child's upper airway is patent, it may be possible to provide BMV via the mouth and nose using a conventional bag and mask whilst the tracheal stoma site is occluded. Rarely tracheal intubation via the tracheostomy with a classical endotracheal tube may be needed. It is important that each child/infant with a tracheostomy has an emergency box which includes spare tubes and a pre-defined emergency plan for airway re-establishment.
- Needle cricothyroidotomy is an emergency technique indicated in cases of upper-airway obstruction (e.g. laryngeal obstruction by

oedema, foreign body or major facial trauma) when an emergency surgical airway is not available. It should only be undertaken when ventilation by BMV or a supraglottic airway device and TT intubation have failed. (See Chapter 22.)

As there is virtually no $CO_2$ removal, this technique only provides temporary oxygenation until a definitive airway can be provided, that is, tracheal intubation or a tracheostomy. Expert help must be sought as soon as possible.

## Breathing

- Start oxygen therapy if $SpO_2$ <94%.
- For infants or children with chronic conditions, use a threshold of $SpO_2$ 3% below known baseline.
- Maintain $SpO_2$ 94–98 % with as little supplemental oxygen as possible.
- Avoid sustained $SpO_2$ readings of 100% except when it is known to be beneficial, such as for carbon monoxide poisoning or pulmonary hypertension. There is no benefit to giving oxygen if $SpO_2$ is within range.
- If $SpO_2$ cannot be monitored, use 100% oxygen for children and infants with signs and symptoms of respiratory and/or circulatory failure and titrate the oxygen as soon as possible.
- Consider either high-flow humidified nasal cannula oxygen or non-invasive ventilation (NIV) for children with respiratory failure and hypoxaemia not responding to low-flow oxygen.
- For high-flow humidified nasal cannula oxygen, flows of 2 l $kg^{-1}$ $min^{-1}$ are commonly used for children up to 12 kg, plus 0.5 l $kg^{-1}$ $min^{-1}$ for each kilogram thereafter to a maximum of 50 l $min^{-1}$.
- BMV is the recommended first line method to support ventilation. It is important to use an appropriately sized bag for age to support the tidal volume delivered whilst avoiding hyperinflation.
- If BMV is ineffective or ventilation will be prolonged, progress to tracheal intubation. An SGA will not be well tolerated in child with intact pharyngeal reflexes.
- Tracheal intubation provides a secure airway, and this together with subsequent mechanical ventilation enables secure delivery of both oxygen and positive end expiratory pressure (which will help improve oxygenation). Personnel experienced in airway management should intubate children and infants. Cuffed TTs should be used (except in small infants) with monitoring of cuff inflation pressures.
- All equipment and drugs should be pre-prepared, and the use of a checklist is advised.
- Plans for failure of intubation also need to be reviewed before the procedure.
- Confirm the TT position is correct by clinical assessment, auscultation of the lung with air entry in all areas, capnography and chest X-ray.
- When initiating mechanical ventilation, use a tidal volume appropriate for the size and weight of the child (5–7 ml $kg^{-1}$) and adjust respiratory rate and expiratory time according to age and pathology. Look for normal chest rise. Avoid hyperinflation as well as hypoventilation.
- Only use $ETCO_2$ as a surrogate for arterial $PaCO_2$ when correlation has been demonstrated.
- If the condition of a child being ventilated via mask, SGA or TT suddenly deteriorates, consider the following causes, best recalled using the acronym DOPES:
  - D stands for displacement of airway device.
  - O for obstruction (TT, airway circuit, airway, head position).
  - P for pneumothorax.
  - E for equipment problem (oxygen, tubing, connections, valves).
  - S for stomach (distention can alter diaphragm mechanics).

## Circulation

- Peripheral IV lines are the first choice for vascular access in children who remain responsive to pain. In an emergency, limit the time for placement to five minutes (two attempts).
- For infants and children, the primary rescue alternative is IO access. Health care workers who may encounter an acutely unwell child should be competent in IO placement and have regular retraining in the different devices and

puncture sites used in their workplace. IO infusion is painful, so appropriate intraosseous analgesia will be required before giving the first fluid bolus in every child and infant, unless comatose. Confirm placement clinically and monitor for extravasation, which can lead to compartment syndrome.

- Children and infants with a febrile illness and no signs of shock should not receive fluid bolus therapy.
- Recommendations for fluid administration in shock for children and infants in the UK health care system with intensive care availability are 10 ml $kg^{-1}$ bolus, repeated up to 40–60 ml $kg^{-1}$ in the first hour, titrated to patient response with repeated reassessment and discontinued if signs of fluid overload develop. Signs of fluid overload include hepatomegaly, bilateral basal lung crackles and jugular venous distention.
- Use balanced isotonic crystalloids as first choice of fluid bolus (Hartmann's, Ringer's, Plasmalyte, Normosol); if these are not available, 0.9% saline is an acceptable alternative.
- Consensus opinion suggests that in the setting of fluid- and inotrope-resistant septic shock intubation is indicated even in the absence of respiratory failure.
- In suspected septic shock, start broad-spectrum antibiotics as soon as possible after initial ABCDE assessment, ideally within the first hour of treatment, and obtain blood cultures before starting, if this can be done without delaying therapy.
- In haemorrhagic shock, keep crystalloid boluses to a minimum (maximum 20 ml $kg^{-1}$), and give blood products early to children with severe trauma and circulatory failure (use a strategy that focuses on improving coagulation). Avoid fluid overload, but try to provide adequate tissue perfusion whilst awaiting definitive damage control and/or spontaneous thrombosis.
- Give tranexamic acid 15 mg $kg^{-1}$ loading dose (maximum 1 g) over 10 minutes followed by 2 mg $kg^{-1}$ per hour to all children and infants requiring blood transfusion after severe trauma and/or significant haemorrhage, as soon as possible (within three hours).
- In children and infants with persistent decompensated circulatory failure after multiple fluid boluses, vasoactive drugs should be started early as a continuous infusion via either a central or peripheral line. Use either noradrenaline or adrenaline as first-line vasoactive drugs (dopamine is no longer recommended but can be used if adrenaline and noradrenaline are not available).
- **Unstable bradycardia**: Only consider atropine in children where bradycardia is caused by increased vagal tone.
- **Unstable tachycardia**: In children and infants with decompensated circulatory failure due to either supraventricular (SVT) or ventricular tachycardia (VT), the first choice for treatment is immediate cardioversion at a starting energy of 1 J $kg^{-1}$ body weight. Double the energy to 2 J $kg^{-1}$ if the initial electric cardioversion is unsuccessful. Consider up to 4 J $kg^{-1}$, guided by expert help. If the child or infant is still conscious, use adequate analgesia and sedation (e.g. intranasal or intramuscular ketamine) with airway management. If an IV line can be rapidly sited, IV analgesia and sedation (e.g. ketamine) can be used, but IV access attempts must not delay cardioversion. In children and infants with presumed SVT with good compensation, vagal manoeuvres (ice immersion, Valsalva techniques) can be tried. If this has no immediate effect, proceed with IV or IO adenosine. The dose depends on age; for a child 1–11 years, for example, the dose is 100 mg $kg^{-1}$, increased in steps of 50–100 mg $kg^{-1}$ every one to two minutes if required, the dose to be repeated until tachycardia terminated or maximum single dose of 500 micrograms $kg^{-1}$ (maximum 12 mg) given. An initial dose of 150 micrograms $kg^{-1}$ is used in infants. In children over 12 years, the initial dose is 3 mg, increasing to 6 mg, then 12 mg. Each dose of adenosine should be given intravenously by rapid bolus followed by immediate saline flush in a large vein as close to the heart as possible (the heart is the site of action).

Ensure an ECG rhythm strip is recording to evaluate response and for later expert evaluation (exercise caution with adenosine if there is known sinus node disease, pre-excited atrial arrhythmias, heart transplant or severe asthma). Even in stable patients, electrical cardioversion should always be considered.

In case of Torsade de pointes VT, magnesium IV 25–50 mg $kg^{-1}$ (maximum 2 g) should be given over 10–15 minutes; the dose may be repeated once if necessary (check local protocols).

## Foreign Body Airway Obstruction (FBAO)

A child will react immediately to a foreign body in the airway by coughing to try to expel it. If the child can still cough effectively, this must be encouraged, as a spontaneous cough is not only safer but probably more effective than any manoeuvre. If coughing is absent or becoming ineffective, the child's airway is at risk of complete obstruction, and immediate intervention is required.

Most choking events occur during play or feeding and are therefore frequently witnessed. If unwitnessed, FBAO should be suspected when the onset of respiratory symptoms (coughing, gagging, stridor, distress) is very sudden and there are no other signs of illness; a history of eating or playing with small items immediately before the onset of symptoms will alert the rescuer. The management is shown in the algorithm (Figure 38.3).

If the child is coughing effectively (fully responsive, loud cough, taking a breath before coughing, still crying or speaking), no manoeuvre is necessary. Encourage the child to cough and continue monitoring the child's condition.

If the child's coughing is or becomes ineffective (decreasing consciousness, quiet cough, inability to breathe or vocalise, cyanosis), ask for help and determine the child's conscious level.

If the child or infant is still conscious but has ineffective coughing, give five back blows. Back blows are intended to loosen the object for the child to be able to then expel it. If back blows do not relieve the airway obstruction and the child is still conscious, then chest thrusts or abdominal thrusts should be given; five chest thrusts for infants and five abdominal thrusts for children. Thrusts increase the intrathoracic pressure, which will facilitate the expulsion of the foreign body. Following chest or abdominal thrusts, reassess the infant or child.

If the foreign body has still not been expelled and the child/infant remains conscious, continue the sequence of five back blows and five chest (for infant) or five abdominal (for children) thrusts. The aim is to relieve the obstruction with each thrust rather than to complete the sequence. Do not use abdominal thrusts (Heimlich manoeuvre) for infants.

If the object is expelled successfully, assess the child's clinical condition. It is possible that part of the object may remain in the respiratory tract and cause complications. If there is any doubt or if the victim was treated with abdominal thrusts, the child needs further medical review in hospital.

If the infant/child with foreign body airway obstruction is, or becomes, unconscious, move to treatment with the paediatric BLS algorithm.

Back blows for an infant:

- Support the infant in a head-downwards, prone position to enable gravity to assist. A seated or kneeling rescuer should be able to support the infant across their lap.
- Support the infant's head by placing the thumb of one hand at the angle of the lower jaw and one or two fingers from the same hand at the same point on the other side of the jaw. Do not compress the soft tissues under the infant's jaw, as this will exacerbate the airway obstruction.
- Deliver up to five sharp back blows with the heel of one hand in the middle of the back between the shoulder blades.

Back blows for a child over one year:

- Back blows are more effective if the child is positioned head-down. A small child may be placed across the rescuer's lap as with an infant. If this is not possible, support the child in a forward-leaning position and deliver the back blows from behind.
- Deliver up to five sharp back blows with the heel of one hand in the middle of the back between the shoulder blades.

Chest thrusts for infants:

- Turn the infant into a head-downwards supine position. Place your free arm along the infant's back and encircle the occiput with your hand. This will be easiest whilst the rescuer is sitting and their arm supporting the infant's back can rest on their thigh.
- Identify the landmark for chest compression (the lower sternum approximately a finger's breadth above the xiphisternum).

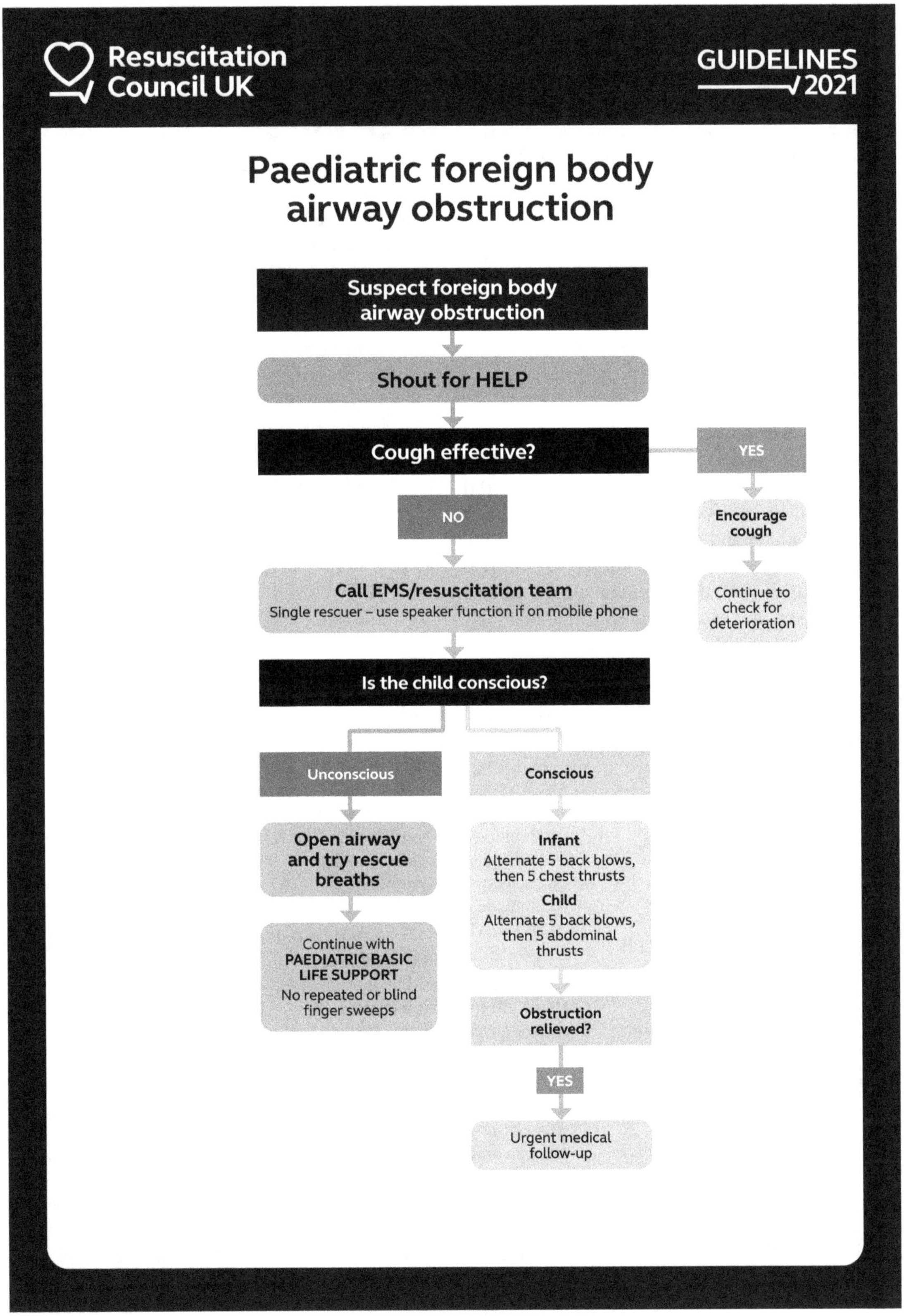


**Figure 38.3** The FBAO algorithm.

- Deliver up to five chest thrusts, comparable to chest compressions but sharper in nature and delivered at a slower rate.

Abdominal thrusts for children over one year:

- Stand or kneel behind the child. Place your arms under the child's arms and encircle their torso.
- Clench your fist and place it between the umbilicus and xiphisternum.
- Grasp your fist with the other hand and pull sharply inwards and upwards.
- Repeat up to four more times. Ensure that pressure is not applied to the xiphoid process or the lower rib cage, as this may cause abdominal trauma.

In recent years, several anti-choking devices have become available on the market. A recent systematic review (with broad study inclusion criteria) looking at these devices identified only a small case series of manikin and cadaver studies, which were limited to a single device type. No reports of harm were identified, but their limited use in clinical practice means it is too early to conclude that their use is harm-free. The review recommended the need for further research before device use can be supported in practice.

**Key Points**

- Children and infants most often have a secondary cardiorespiratory arrest.
- Evaluation of the acutely unwell child with a systematic ABCDE approach will allow early intervention and help prevent deterioration to cardiorespiratory arrest.
- Teamwork is essential to good outcomes; regular training and simulation practice are recommended.
- High-quality CPR is essential to maximise chances of ROSC.
- In cardiorespiratory arrest, signs of life are used to evaluate circulation, as pulse detection is poor even in trained health care workers.
- Good post-ROSC care is important. Avoid hyperoxia and hypo- and hyperventilation, employ TTM and avoid fever (>37.5°C).

## Further Reading

Berg RA, Sutton RM, Reeder RW et al. Association between diastolic blood pressure during pediatric in-hospital cardiopulmonary resuscitation and survival. *Circulation* 2018;137(17):1784–95.

Couper K, Hassan A, Ohri V, Patterson E, Tang H, Bingham R, Olasveengen T, Perkins G. Removal of foreign body airway obstruction: a systematic review of interventions. On behalf of the International Liaison Committee on Resuscitation Basic and Paediatric Life Support Task Force Collaborators. *Resuscitation* 2020; 156:174–81.

Lavonas EJ, Ohshimo S, Nation K et al. International Liaison Committee on Resuscitation (ILCOR) Pediatric Life Support Task Force. Advanced airway interventions for paediatric cardiac arrest: a systematic review and meta-analysis. *Resuscitation* 2019; 138:114–28.

Maconochie IK, Aickin R, Hazinski MF et al. Pediatric life support: 2020 international consensus on cardiopulmonary resuscitation and emergency cardiovascular care science with treatment recommendations. *Resuscitation* 2020; 156:A120–A155.

Moler FW, Silverstein FS, Holubkov R et al. Therapeutic hypothermia after in-hospital cardiac arrest in children. *New England Journal of Medicine* 2017; 376(4):318–29.

Moler FW, Silverstein FS, Holubkov R et al. Therapeutic hypothermia after out-of-hospital cardiac arrest in children. *New England Journal of Medicine* 2015; 372 (20):1898–908.

Naim MY, Burke RV et al. Association of bystander cardiopulmonary resuscitation with overall and neurologically favorable survival after pediatric out-of-hospital cardiac arrest in the united states: a report from the CARES surveillance registry. *JAMA Pediatrics* 2017; 171 (2):133–41.

National Cardiac Arrest Audit, UK. Available at: https://ncaa.icnarc.org/Home. Accessed 24 April 2024.

Resuscitation Council UK. 2021 Guidelines. 2021. Available online: www.resus.org.uk/library/2021-resuscitation-guidelines. Accessed 10 April 2024.

Skellett S, Orzechowska I, Thomas K, Fortune PM. The landscape of paediatric in-hospital cardiac arrest in the United Kingdom National Cardiac Arrest Audit. *Resuscitation* 2020; 155:165–71.

Sutton R, Reeder RW, Landis WP et al. Ventilation rates and pediatric in-hospital cardiac arrest survival outcomes. *Critical Care Medicine* 2019; 47:1627–36.

Tibballs J, Weeranatna C. The influence of time on the accuracy of healthcare personnel to diagnose paediatric cardiac arrest by pulse palpation. *Resuscitation* 2010; 81:671–5.

University of Warwick, UK. Out of Hospital Cardiac Arrest Outcomes Audit. Available online: https://warwick.ac.uk/fac/sci/med/research/ctu/trials/ohcao. Accessed 10 April 2024.

Van de Voorde P et al. European Resuscitation Council Guidelines 2021: Paediatric Life Support. *Resuscitation* 2021; 161:327–87.

Chapter 39

# Trauma in Children

Hannah Lewis, Naomi Edmonds and Breda O'Neill

## Introduction

Trauma is the leading cause of death in children worldwide. The causes of trauma and pattern of injury vary with age, with peaks in infancy and adolescence. Males are affected more frequently than females across all age groups except in infancy, where there is a 50:50 split. Blunt injury is responsible for >80% of fatalities. Falls from less than two metres and road traffic collisions (RTCs) are the most common mechanisms of injury in most age groups. Non-accidental injury (NAI) is the most frequent mechanism of injury in infants. There has been a substantial increase in penetrating trauma due to knife and gunshot injury in adolescents in recent years in the United Kingdom, particularly in urban areas. Currently, 10–20% of adolescent trauma is due to penetrating injury and responsible for 10–20% of paediatric trauma call activations in many major trauma centres (MTCs). Penetrating injuries have a high injury severity score (ISS) at presentation, increased activation of major haemorrhage protocols and a significant mortality of around 25%. The highest mortality (>50%) is seen with gunshot injuries to the head and injuries to the neck and thorax.

The incidence of major trauma in childhood increases in summer months, related to increased daylight hours and outdoor activities. Trauma calls are most common at the weekend and after school. Limb injuries are the most common and in isolation are not associated with high mortality. Traumatic brain injury (TBI) is the leading cause of disability and mortality, with the highest mortality seen in children with TBI combined with thoracic or abdominal trauma.

## Provision of Trauma Services

Management of paediatric trauma in the United Kingdom has been transformed with centralisation of services and the creation of regional networks. This followed recommendations from several bodies, including the 2007 UK National Confidential Enquiry into Patient Outcome and Death (NCEPOD) report 'Trauma: Who Cares?', which found that care could be improved in more than 50% of cases.

Regional networks consist of a major trauma centre (MTC), which provides care to severely injured patients 24 hours a day, and linked local trauma units (TUs) that manage patients with less severe injuries. The ISS is used to describe trauma severity, with the highest score of 75 defining the most critically injured. Moderate injury is defined as an ISS of score of 9–15, and severe injury an ISS of >15. The ISS cannot be calculated at the scene at the time of injury. Pre-hospital triage is used to identify moderate and severe injuries to determine which cases should go directly to an MTC (see Table 39.1). If transfer times are long, cases may be taken to a local TU for rapid stabilisation prior to transfer. However, 30–50% of children bypass the pre-hospital triage system and are brought directly to hospital by parents or guardians. Care must be standardised and skills maintained across the whole paediatric network, especially the provision of life-saving interventions in local hospitals.

In the United Kingdom, there are currently 33 MTCs: 27 in England, four in Scotland, one in Wales and one in Northern Ireland. Twenty-one have paediatric services and are either paediatric only or co-located with adult services. Hospitals providing trauma care for children (MTCs and TUs) have dedicated standard operating procedures (SOPs) and up-to-date local guidelines. All units contribute data to the Trauma Audit and Research Network (TARN), which is a national UK audit that collects data on all children injured who are admitted to hospital for >3 days or admitted to intensive care and/or any mortality. Since the reconfiguration of services, practice between institutions has become more

**Table 39.1** Paediatric injuries triaged to major trauma centres

| |
|---|
| Haemodynamic instability not explained by anxiety or pain |
| Traumatic amputation |
| Signs of bruising to chest or abdomen |
| Glasgow coma score (GCS) <13 |
| Penetrating injury |
| Open long bone/multiple long bone fractures |
| Pelvic fracture |
| Spinal injury with abnormal neurology |
| Skull fracture |
| Burn surface area >20 % if <12 years old or >30 % if >12 years old. Facial burns or circumferential burns |
| High-risk mechanism of injury – death of a same vehicle occupant, ejected from a vehicle, under a train, fall >2 floors (>20 feet), amputation above wrist or ankle or trapped under a vehicle (not a motorcycle) |

standardised, and outcomes have improved, with a higher proportion of severely injured children surviving to hospital discharge.

## The Role of the Anaesthetist

The anaesthetist is an integral member of the trauma team and may be involved throughout the patient pathway, including in pre-hospital care. Trauma care in hospital begins with resuscitation and stabilisation in the emergency department (ED), potentially combined with transfer to radiology for diagnostic imaging, surgical interventions, procedures in interventional radiology (IR), provision of analgesia and postoperative care in the paediatric intensive care unit (PICU). Regional anaesthesia is increasingly important, particularly for complex polytrauma patients in the perioperative period.

## Trauma Calls, Primary Survey and Imaging

When there is a trauma call, there should be a team brief before the patient arrives, led by the trauma team leader (TTL). Everyone is identified by name, role and the available patient information shared:

- Patient age and mechanism of injury
- Observations, including conscious level
- Obvious life-threatening injuries (including airway problems and uncontrolled haemorrhage)

Trauma calls can be stratified by level of injury (mild, moderate or severe). Advanced trauma calls are for the most seriously injured, for example suspected or confirmed major haemorrhage, cardiac arrest at scene, serious head injury or polytrauma. Additional senior support should be available for these cases, including specific teams such as neurosurgery where there is a suspected serious head injury. An advanced trauma call should alert the theatre team that surgical intervention may be required, triggering a pause in theatre to allow the theatre coordinator to liaise with the trauma team to plan theatre allocation. The anaesthetic consultant should be called early if their presence is anticipated. Anaesthetic drugs should be prepared and airway equipment made ready. Once the patient arrives in hospital, there should be a structured handover from the pre-hospital team to the trauma team.

The primary survey is performed to identify and treat any life-threatening injuries. The anaesthetist simultaneously assesses the airway, adequacy of ventilation and conscious level.

In adult trauma, early whole-body CT within 60 minutes of arrival has been shown to improve survival. Children are sensitive to ionising radiation, and there are concerns that repeated exposure to X-ray may increase the lifetime risk of malignancy. It is recommended that only children suffering severe polytrauma should undergo whole body CT, with a more tailored approach for other cases.

Comprehensive guidelines are available from the National Institute for Health and Care Excellence (NICE) for head and neck imaging in TBI (see the section 'Traumatic Brain Injury'), and the Royal College of Radiologists provide additional recommendations for imaging in chest, abdomen or pelvic injuries (see Figure 39.1). If an isolated cervical spine (C-spine) injury is suspected, cervical X-rays are normally sufficient to exclude bony injury. Chest X-ray (CXR) is a relatively sensitive screening tool and is performed as part of the primary survey in major trauma.

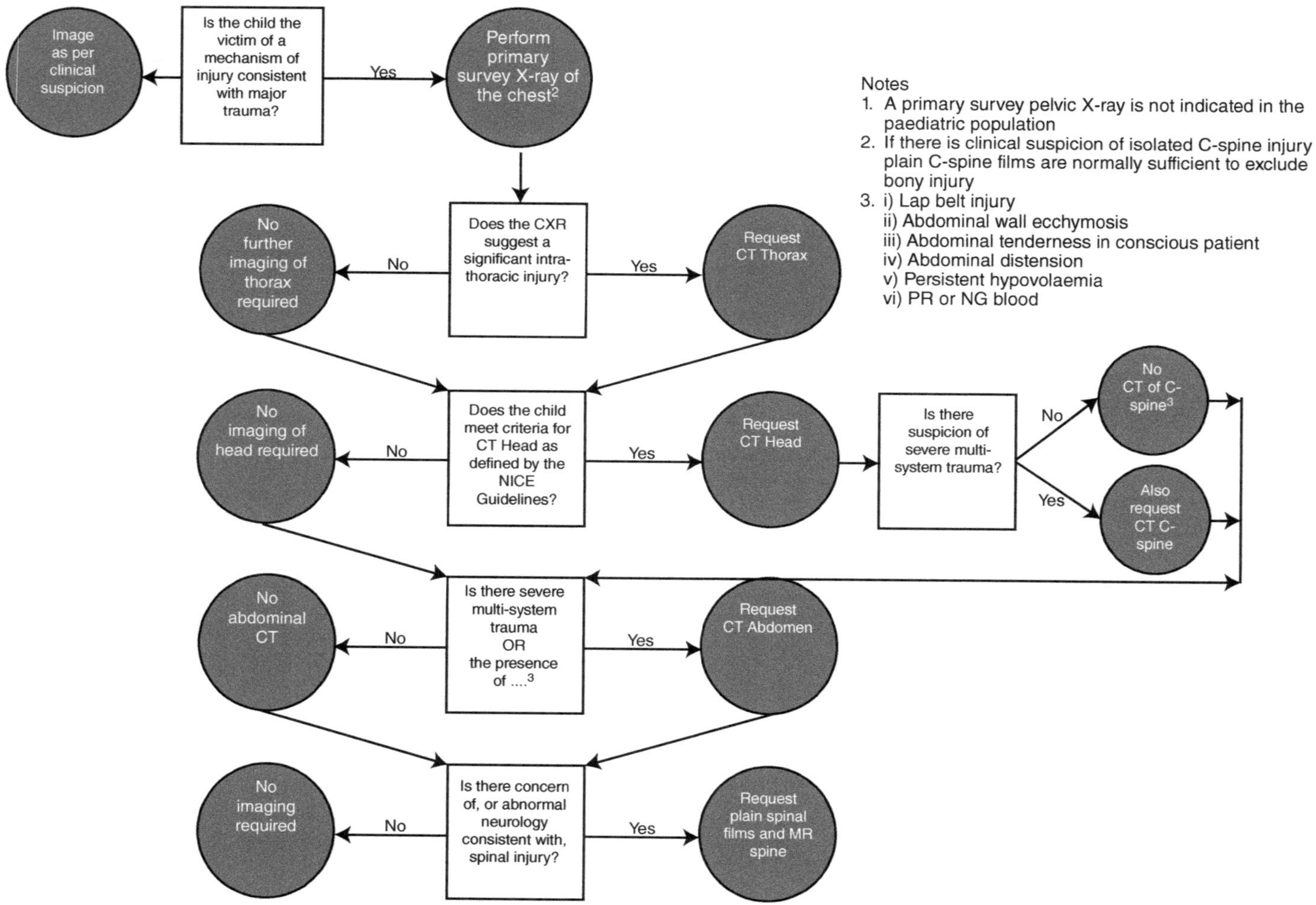


**Figure 39.1** Paediatric emergency department major trauma imaging decision tool.

Children with an abnormal CXR or severe mechanism of injury should undergo a computed tomography (CT) chest examination. Pelvic X-ray and focused assessment with sonography in trauma (FAST) scans have low sensitivity and are no longer recommended as part of the primary survey. The Royal College of Radiologists Paediatric Trauma Protocols recommend CT abdomen in major trauma or if there is suspicion of abdominal injury, for instance tenderness, ecchymosis, distension, a lap belt injury and/or blood per rectum or in the nasogastric (NG) tube.

Intravenous access should be obtained and standard blood tests taken: full blood count, group and cross-match, clotting, urea and electrolytes, liver function tests including lipase, blood gas and point of care coagulation testing in major trauma, if available.

The child may be awake, distressed and frightened, and it is essential to maintain good verbal and non-verbal communication at all times. Play therapists can provide useful distraction for procedures and increase cooperation, especially if parents are not present. Analgesia is sometimes necessary during the primary survey. Small boluses of opioid (fentanyl 0.5 mcg $kg^{-1}$ or morphine 25–50 mcg $kg^{-1}$) or ketamine (0.5 mg $kg^{-1}$) are suitable. The ED should have a sedation and pain relief protocol for children. Intranasal opioids such as fentanyl (2 mcg $kg^{-1}$) or diamorphine (100 mcg $kg^{-1}$) can be given whilst intravenous access is obtained. Even low doses can impair ventilation and cause hypotension, so opioids must be used carefully and titrated to effect.

## Airway Management

Airway patency must be checked as soon as the patient arrives in the ED. C-spine protection must be maintained if there is any suspicion of injury. Collars are often poorly fitting and not well tolerated in younger children. Manual in-line stabilisation or collar and blocks are used in preference if there is a suspicion of cervical spine injury. The anaesthetist should lead patient transfers or log-roll procedures carried out during the secondary survey.

The child should be monitored with continuous pulse oximetry, non-invasive blood pressure, electrocardiogram (ECG) monitoring and capnography (if intubated). Oxygen saturations can be unreliable if the child is cold, and blood pressure readings may be inaccurate at extreme highs and lows (mean arterial pressure is more reliable). Initial steps in airway management involve the application of high-flow oxygen delivered via a non-rebreather mask and, if there is airway obstruction, basic airway manoeuvres to open the airway and restore patency:

- Apply gentle suction to clear the upper airway of blood, secretions and vomit. It is important not to cause further trauma or reflex vomiting.
- Open the airway with a jaw thrust to maintain C-spine immobilisation. Consider an oropharyngeal airway if there is a reduced conscious level.
- Decompress the stomach with a wide-bore orogastric or NG tube (ensure there are no concerns about base of skull fracture before NG placement).
- If the patient has already been intubated by the pre-hospital team, ensure correct tracheal tube position with capnography monitoring and auscultate the chest to ensure bilateral air entry. Document the grade of intubation, size and position of the tube. Tube position should be confirmed on imaging.
- Report any obvious scalp lacerations to the TTL. These can be a significant source of blood loss, especially in small children and infants.

The main indications for intubation are airway obstruction, respiratory inadequacy or a reduced conscious level (see Table 39.2).

The decision to intubate should be made at a senior level, by the anaesthetist and the TTL, with agreement from the rest of the trauma team. A simple neurological assessment should be carried out before intubation to document the Glasgow Coma Score (GCS), any focal neurological signs and pupillary responses.

## Induction of Anaesthesia

Induction of anaesthesia can obtund compensatory vasoconstriction and lead to significant haemodynamic instability in a child who is hypovolaemic. In TBI, this can cause a detrimental reduction in cerebral perfusion pressure (CPP). Choice and dose of induction agent should take into account the haemodynamics and neurology of the child. Ketamine is a sympathomimetic and maintains cardiovascular stability to a greater extent than other agents. It also has analgesic

**Table 39.2** Indications for intubation in paediatric trauma

| |
|---|
| Airway obstruction |
| Severe TBI with reduced conscious level; causing loss of pharyngeal tone and airway protection |
| Vomit or blood or secretions in the airway |
| Penetrating neck trauma, expanding haematoma causing airway compression |
| Direct airway trauma |
| Maxillofacial trauma |
| **Inadequate ventilation** |
| Severe TBI; causing loss of ventilatory drive |
| Intoxication |
| **Respiratory failure (type 1 or 2)** |
| Lung contusions |
| Pneumothorax |
| Haemothorax |
| **Polytrauma** |
| **Major haemorrhage** |
| **Transfer to tertiary major trauma centre** |

properties and is the preferred induction agent in severe trauma. Propofol and thiopentone reduce myocardial contractility and vascular tone. This can cause cardiovascular collapse in a shocked patient. Opioids are used to obtund the response to laryngoscopy and reduce the amount of induction agent required. Short-acting opioids such as fentanyl cause less cardiovascular instability and histamine release compared to longer-acting drugs such as morphine. Large boluses of fentanyl can still cause haemodynamic compromise, and use should be titrated to effect. Rocuronium has largely replaced suxamethonium for muscle relaxation. It has a quick onset of action, avoids detrimental side effects of suxamethonium (raised intracranial pressure [ICP] and intraocular pressure [IOP]) and can be readily reversed with sugammadex. A frequently used induction technique is ketamine 1–2 mg $kg^{-1}$, fentanyl 1–2 mcg $kg^{-1}$ and rocuronium 1–1.5 mg $kg^{-1}$. Anaesthetic agents, common doses and side effects are shown in Table 39.3.

Gastric emptying is reduced from the time of injury, and children are at risk of aspiration following trauma. A modified rapid sequence induction (RSI) should be considered, with the child in a head-up position. Children are prone to desaturation at induction, which may be exacerbated by chest injuries and/or pain, causing shallow breathing. The child should ideally be pre-oxygenated, although compliance may be a problem with younger or frightened children. Cricoid pressure can distort the anatomy and make the view difficult at laryngoscopy. There is limited evidence of benefit of cricoid pressure in children, and it should be removed if it interferes with the view of the glottis.

Intubation may be difficult in trauma due to C-spine immobilisation, facial and neck injuries and ongoing oropharyngeal bleeding. Video laryngoscopy should be considered in experienced hands, as it causes less C-spine movement, although the view may be obscured by bleeding. Intubation may be helped by removal of the cervical collar and blocks, and C-spine protection is maintained with manual in-line stabilisation (MILS). Suction should be on and ready to remove any debris obscuring the view at laryngoscopy. In severe maxillofacial or neck trauma, a potential difficult airway should be declared. Intubation should be performed by the most senior member of the anaesthetic team with an ENT surgeon in attendance. A supraglottic airway should be available as a rescue device to maintain oxygenation in failed intubation. Front of neck access is required in a 'can't intubate, can't ventilate' situation. Fortunately, this is rare in paediatrics, but formal tracheostomy is the technique of choice in this situation.

Correct position of the tracheal tube should be confirmed by capnography and auscultation, checking for bilateral air entry. High airway pressure, low tidal volume and reduced oxygen saturation may indicate ventilatory problems, potentially due to insufficient muscle relaxant, endobronchial intubation or light anaesthesia. Pulmonary causes need to be excluded, such as secretions plugging the airway or aspiration of blood or gastric contents. The former can usually be addressed with gentle suction with saline down the tracheal tube. In addition, there may be pulmonary injury with contusion or pneumothorax, in which case positive pressure ventilation may convert a simple pneumothorax to a tension pneumothorax. This is suggested by reduced breath sounds on the side of the pneumothorax, high airway pressures and potentially cardiovascular collapse. Needle decompression or thoracostomy is required followed by chest drain insertion.

Injury to the airway may be indicated by surgical emphysema following the start of positive

**Table 39.3** Anaesthetic agents used in trauma patients

| Anaesthetic agent | Dose | Effects |
|---|---|---|
| Ketamine | 1–2 mg $kg^{-1}$ (induction dose)<br>10–45 mcg $kg^{-1}$ (maintenance of sedation/anaesthesia) | Analgesia, sedation and anaesthesia. Preserves cardiovascular stability and CPP better than other induction agents. |
| Fentanyl | 1–2 mcg $kg^{-1}$ | Sympatholytic and analgesic. Obtunds response to laryngoscopy. Can cause hypotension with bolus doses. Titrate to effect. |
| Propofol | 1–2 mg $kg^{-1}$ | Anaesthesia and sedation. Causes haemodynamic instability in hypovolaemic shock. Not recommended in severe trauma. |
| Thiopentone | 2–5 mg $kg^{-1}$ | Anaesthesia and sedation. Causes haemodynamic instability in hypovolaemic shock. Not recommended in severe trauma. |
| Alfentanil | 10–20 mcg $kg^{-1}$ | Sympatholytic and analgesic. Obtunds response to laryngoscopy. Can cause hypotension with bolus doses. Titrate to effect |
| Morphine | 0.1–0.2 mg $kg^{-1}$ (bolus dose)<br>10–40 mcg $kg^{-1}hour^{-1}$ (maintenance of sedation/ anaesthesia) | Analgesic. Can cause histamine release and hypotension. Used for sedation and maintenance of anaesthesia. |
| Rocuronium | 1–1.5 mg $kg^{-1}$ (RSI dose)<br>0.5–1 mg $kg^{-1}$ (subsequent bolus doses) | Rapid onset within 60 seconds. Reversed with sugammadex.<br>Has largely replaced suxamethonium. |
| Atracurium | 0.5 mg $kg^{-1}$ | Slower onset of action. Can cause histamine release and hypotension.<br>Not suitable for RSI. |
| Suxamethonium | 1–2 mg $kg^{-1}$ | Rapid onset of action.<br>Causes increased ICP and IOP.<br>Largely replaced by rocuronium. |
| Volatile agents: sevoflurane/ isoflurane | Titrate to effect and MAC | Used in theatre for maintenance of anaesthesia.<br>Cause vasodilation and hypotension. |
| Nitrous oxide | - | Not used in severe trauma. Causes cerebral vasodilation and increased ICP. Diffuses into and increases air-filled spaces rapidly. Can convert a simple pneumothorax to a tension. |

pressure ventilation. Bronchoscopy will be needed to identify where the injury is and guide surgical planning. Instituting positive pressure ventilation may cause cardiovascular collapse in major haemorrhage. Blood transfusion should be ongoing if this is predicted.

Penetrating injuries have increased in the adolescent population in recent years. Penetrating neck trauma (injury extending below the platysma muscle) can be life threatening and cause significant airway compromise. An expanding neck haematoma quickly obstructs the airway, necessitating definitive airway management in ED. Intubation may become increasingly difficult as oedema and swelling distort the laryngeal anatomy. If the patient is unstable (surgical emphysema, airway compromise, hemiparesis or a rapidly expanding pulsatile neck haematoma), they should be taken directly to theatre for airway management and surgery. If the patient is stable, a

**Table 39.4** Physiological values in children: normal values and values in severe trauma

| Age (years) | Respiratory Rate (breaths per minute) | Heart rate (beats per minute) | | Systolic BP (50th centile) (mmHg) | |
|---|---|---|---|---|---|
| | | Normal | Suspect >40% blood loss | Normal | Suspect >40% blood loss |
| <1 | 30–40 | 110–160 | >160 | 80–90 | <70 |
| 1–2 | 25–35 | 100–150 | >150 | 85–95 | <80 |
| 2–5 | 25–30 | 95–140 | >140 | 85–100 | <80 |
| 5–12 | 20–25 | 80–120 | >120 | 90–110 | <90 |
| <12 | 15–20 | 60–100 | >100 | 100–120 | <90 |

CT neck is often obtained to plan further management. Good decision-making at senior level is critical.

## Major Haemorrhage

The increase in penetrating trauma in adolescents has resulted in a rise in major haemorrhage trauma calls. Major haemorrhage occurs in 3–4% of paediatric trauma calls, with more than 50% of deaths occurring in the first 24 hours. Major haemorrhage is a cause of preventable death in trauma.

Haemorrhage can be concealed or obvious. Hospital definition of paediatric major haemorrhage is transfusion of 1–1.5 times the total blood volume (TBV) acutely or over a 24-hour period or ongoing losses of >2ml $kg^{-1}$ $min^{-1}$. These definitions work well in elective surgical settings, although less well in trauma. Pre-hospital definitions are important to allow teams time for preparation. In this situation, major haemorrhage is declared in the presence of confirmed or suspected haemorrhage, cardiac arrest at the scene and/or heart rate or blood pressure >20% above or below normal for the age of the child. The emphasis is on the importance of ongoing clinical assessment and reassessment, particularly in a rapidly changing resuscitation situation.

Major haemorrhage is often 'under-called' in paediatric trauma. The reasons for this are multifactorial. Children have excellent compensatory mechanisms and can lose 25–40% of TBV before a reduction in systolic blood pressure is seen. Hypotension is often a late pre-terminal sign. A prolonged capillary refill time and narrow pulse pressure are more reliable signs of early shock. The definition of major haemorrhage paediatric trauma is not clear-cut, with the definition of haemodynamic instability depending on the age of the child. This and the fact that up to 50% of trauma presentations are self-referrals by parents or guardians, bypassing pre-hospital triage systems, can make paediatric major haemorrhage management more complex. Normal values for cardiorespiratory variables by age are shown in Table 39.4.

## Intravenous Access

Adequate intravenous access must be obtained on arrival (with formal laboratory blood tests as described in the section 'Trauma Calls, Primary Survey and Imaging'). Access can be difficult in younger children or those in shock with cold peripheries. Excessive time should not be spent attempting IV access, and intraosseous (IO) access should be performed after two failed IV attempts. The tibial tuberosity is the most common site used. Other sites are the anterolateral surface of the femur and the tibia proximal to the medial malleolus. Limbs with fractures should be avoided. Flow rates are limited through an IO needle, and they can become dislodged easily. Intraosseous access is therefore only a temporary measure until more reliable access is obtained.

Blood products must be warmed before administration. Rapid infuser devices are used to simultaneously warm and deliver products quickly via the IV route. A rate of >100 ml $min^{-1}$ is achieved by devices using a countercurrent exchange method and magnetic induction. It is important to set pressure alarms when using devices that are not exclusively paediatric. The cannula site should be checked regularly to ensure it is working. Maximum flow rates are limited by

**Table 39.5** Rates of flow and IV/IO access

| IV/IO cannula/ needle | Rates of flow (with gravity) (ml min$^{-1}$) | Rates of flow (with pressure) (ml min$^{-1}$) |
|---|---|---|
| 14G cannula | 236.1 | 384.3 |
| 16G cannula | 154.7 | 334.4 |
| 18G cannula | 98.1 | 153.1 |
| 20G cannula | 64.4 | 105.1 |
| 22G cannula | 35.7 | 71.4 |
| 25G IO needle | 68.2 | 204.6 |

the size of the cannula (see Table 39.5). Rates of flow of >100 ml min$^{-1}$ are not possible through smaller gauge cannula (22G and 24G).

## Invasive Monitoring

Wide-bore cannulae are used for rapid resuscitation. If expertise allows, ultrasound-guided central venous access can be established for further monitoring and access. The site (femoral, internal jugular or subclavian) depends on access and preference of the practitioner. The presence of a pelvic binder and cervical collar limit femoral and internal jugular access respectively. The subclavian vein is associated with increased complications, including pneumothorax and inadvertent arterial puncture. The risk of pneumothorax is mitigated if there are thoracostomies. The size of central line depends on the age of the child (see Table 39.6).

Arterial access should be established early in major haemorrhage, but placement should not interfere or delay resuscitation. Arterial lines are used for gas sampling and point-of-care tests. The waveform provides information about blood pressure and vascular filling. A narrow waveform and wide variation in systolic pressure with respiration imply ongoing hypovolaemia.

## Damage Control Resuscitation

Coagulopathy begins at the time of injury. Tissue damage releases tissue factor and activates the clotting cascade. This leads to consumption of

**Table 39.6** Paediatric central line sizes

| Age | Weight (kg) | Size |
|---|---|---|
| 0–6 months | >10 | 4 Fr |
| 6 months–4 years | 10–20 | 4.5 Fr–5 Fr |
| 4–12 years | 20–40 | 5 Fr |
| >12 years | >40 | 7 Fr |

clotting factors. Ongoing bleeding causes systemic hypoperfusion and tissue hypoxia. The resulting endothelial damage causes fibrinolysis and clot breakdown. The combination of this endogenous multi-factorial process is called acute traumatic coagulopathy (ATC). It can present on admission to hospital prior to transfusion. ATC is particularly pronounced where there is a high injury burden. Hypothermia, metabolic acidosis, haemodilution and hypocalcaemia are all modifiable factors that worsen ATC.

Acute traumatic coagulopathy and the modifiable factors create a vicious cycle called trauma-induced coagulopathy (TIC). The principles of damage control resuscitation are to reduce TIC:

- *Haemostatic resuscitation.* Replacing ongoing blood losses with blood products, guided by major transfusion protocols and point-of-care testing (see the following section). This reduces haemodilution and coagulopathy. Crystalloid and colloid are avoided. They increase transfusion requirements, coagulopathy, multi-organ failure and mortality.
- *Temperature control.* Correction of hypothermia. Measure core temperature and minimise exposure. Active warming with fluid warmers and warming blankets. Increase environmental temperature.
- *Permissive hypotensive resuscitation.* There is little evidence for this strategy in children; however, targeting a mean arterial pressure (MAP) at the lower end of normal for the age of the child is common practice. A higher MAP may be necessary in coexisting TBI.
- *Wound management and damage control surgery.* Apply direct pressure to the wound. Pelvic binders and tourniquets reduce bleeding. Damage control surgery (DCS) is aimed at wound decontamination and control of bleeding, with definitive surgery after a period of stability in PICU.

**Table 39.7** Biochemical electrolyte correction

| Electrolyte abnormality | Management |
|---|---|
| Hypocalcaemia ($Ca^{2+}$ > 1.0 mmol $l^{-1}$) | Calcium gluconate (or chloride) 10% 0.5 ml $kg^{-1}$ up to 20 ml maximum. Give over 15 minutes. Aim for ionised calcium > 1.0 mmol $l^{-1}$. Repeat as necessary. |
| Hyperkalaemia $K^+$ 6.0–7.0 mmol $l^{-1}$ or ECG changes are present (tented T waves, wide QRS, prolonged PR interval or absent/small P waves). | **For cardiac protection** Calcium gluconate (or chloride) 10% 0.5 ml $kg^{-1}$ up to 20 ml maximum. Give over 15 minutes. **To reduce serum potassium** Insulin infusion 0.05–0.1 units kg hour $^{-1}$. Monitor blood glucose levels. Nebulised salbutamol 2.5 mg (<25 kg) or 5 mg (>25 kg) Repeat as necessary Continue cardiac monitoring Consider 8.4% sodium bicarbonate 1–2 ml $kg^{-1}$ in severe metabolic acidosis Consider dialysis for refractory hyperkalaemia |

- *Electrolyte correction.* Calcium is integral to the clotting pathway. Ionised calcium should be kept greater than 1.0 mmol $l^{-1}$. Potassium levels increase with metabolic acidosis and transfusion and should be corrected if >7.0 mmol $l^{-1}$ or with ECG changes (see Table 39.7).

## Haemostatic Resuscitation

Red blood cells (RBC) and fresh frozen plasma (FFP) are given initially in a 1:1 ratio with additional platelets and cryoprecipitate guided by major haemorrhage protocols and point-of-care testing. An initial bolus of 10–20 ml $kg^{-1}$ of RBC (in 5 ml $kg^{-1}$ aliquots) should be given in major haemorrhage. O-negative blood is given in the emergency setting whilst waiting for cross-matched blood. Group specific blood is preferred; this takes approximately 15 minutes to obtain, whilst a full cross-match takes 40–45 minutes. The volume of FFP/octaplas is matched for every 10–20 ml $kg^{-1}$ of RBC given.

Tranexamic acid 15 mg $kg^{-1}$ over 10 minutes (maximum 1 g) should be given within three hours of injury. Adult practice is to give a larger dose of 2 g of tranexamic acid, and paediatric practice may change to reflect this. The CRASH-2 (Clinical Randomisation of an Antifibrinolytic in Significant Haemorrhage) trial found this higher dose reduced death from haemorrhage but was less likely to be effective given more than three hours after injury and may increase the relative risk of death. If bleeding persists platelets (15 ml $kg^{-1}$) and cryoprecipitate (10 ml $kg^{-1}$) should be given. As a guide, platelets should be given after every 30 ml $kg^{-1}$ of RBC or if indicated by laboratory results (platelet value $<100 \times 10^9\ l^{-1}$) or point of care coagulation testing. Cryoprecipitate should be given if fibrinogen is <1.5 g $l^{-1}$ or if indicated by point-of-care testing. Consider using adult major haemorrhage protocols in children >50 kg.

Point-of-care testing is used to guide ongoing transfusion requirements and is performed at the bedside. Thromboelastometry (ROTEM®) and thromboelastography (TEG®) are examples of point-of-care tests that help to identify factors leading to ongoing bleeding and allow specific tailored resuscitation. They measure the viscoelastic properties of whole blood from initiation of coagulation to fibrinolysis. The median and reference range for normal values vary depending on the age of the child. Local protocols should be used to interpret ROTEM® and TEG® values. An example ROTEM® algorithm for a child >50 kg is as follows:

- Clotting time, extrinsic assay (EXTEM CT) >80 s – give four units of FFP
- Fibrinogen assay at 5 minutes (FIBTEM A5) <10 mm – give two pools of cryoprecipitate

- Clot amplitude at 5 minutes (EXTEM A5) < 40 mm and FIBTEM A5 ≥ 10 mm – give one pool of platelets
- Maximum lysis, extrinsic assay (EXTEM ML) >15% – give 1 g of tranexamic acid and four units of FFP

## Theatre Conduct in Damage Control Surgery

Leadership and theatre preparation are important in DCS:

- The theatre team leader should be identified and roles allocated. A runner should be identified to take samples to the laboratory and collect blood products, and a scribe be appointed to document events.
- The ED team leader should conduct a formal handover to the theatre team.
- The operating table should be arranged in a crucifix layout (+/– extended arm boards depending on age of child) for ease of access to the patient.
- Blood bank must be informed that the patient is now in theatre.
- The airway and resuscitation trolley should be moved into theatre.
- Equipment including chest drain, thoracotomy kit, invasive lines, ultrasound, rapid infuser devices and fluid warmer should be in theatre.
- Theatre temperature should be increased.
- The World Health Organisation (WHO) trauma checklist should be performed.

## Transfusion Endpoints in DCS

This varies depending on local protocols. Common targets used are as follows:

- Haemoglobin 80–100 g $l^{-1}$ or haematocrit >0.3.
- Fibrinogen >1.5 g $l^{-1}$.
- Ionised calcium >1.0 mmol $l^{-1}$.
- PT <1.5 (less sensitive in the context of major haemorrhage).
- Platelets >75–100 × $10^9$ $l^{-1}$.
- Blood gas – improving lactate and metabolic acidosis.
- Clinical endpoints – normal heart rate/blood pressure/capillary refill time/warm peripheries. Values at the higher end of normal should be used in patients with coexisting TBI.

## Other Causes of Shock in Trauma

Haemorrhage is the most common cause of shock in trauma patients. It is important to consider other causes that may be coexistent:

- Neurogenic
- Spinal trauma, massive TBI
- Obstructive shock
- Tension pneumothorax
- Cardiac tamponade

## Vasopressors and Inotropes

The evidence for the use of vasopressors in haemorrhagic shock in children is limited. There may be a role for short-term use in refractory hypotension, in failure to respond to fluid resuscitation and in spinal injury. Inotropes are often needed in conjunction with vasopressors, titrated to effect. Supranormal blood pressures will exacerbate bleeding and disrupt clot formation.

## Traumatic Brain Injury

Traumatic brain injury is the leading cause of mortality and morbidity in paediatric trauma. Non-accidental injury should always be considered in children <2 years. The severity of TBI is classified using the GCS, with a modified GCS for use in younger pre-verbal children (see Table 39.8). A GCS score of 3–15 is allocated depending on the child's best eye, verbal and motor responses at the time of injury. TBI is classified as mild (GCS 13–15), moderate (GCS 9–12) or severe (GCS ≤ 8). Initial motor score correlates with prognosis.

Neurological status can be assessed in awake children by assessment of conscious level, pupillary responses and presence of localising signs. Children with a GCS ≤ 8 or who are agitated require intubation and ventilation for airway and neuroprotection. Intracranial pressure (ICP) monitoring is recommended in children with severe TBI and GCS < 8 and/or who are intubated and ventilated.

The NICE 2014 guidance (updated in 2019) recommends a CT head is performed within one hour in children if there is any of the following: suspicion of NAI; depressed, basal or 'open' skull fracture; GCS < 14 (or < 15 in infants); focal neurological signs; post-traumatic seizure in the absence of epilepsy history; or any bruise or swelling >5 cm in an infant. A CT head is also

**Table 39.8** Paediatric Glasgow coma scale

| GCS | Score | Infants | Older children |
|---|---|---|---|
| 4 | Eye opening | Spontaneously | Spontaneously |
| 3 | | Verbal | Verbal |
| 2 | | Pain | Pain |
| 1 | | No response | No response |
| 5 | Speech | Babbles and coos normally | Orientated |
| 4 | | Spontaneous irritable cries | Confused |
| 3 | | Cries to pain | Inappropriate words |
| 2 | | Moans to pain | Incomprehensible sounds |
| 1 | | No response | No response |
| 6 | Best motor response | Normal spontaneous movement | Follows commands |
| 5 | | Withdraws to touch | Localises pain |
| 4 | | Withdraws to pain | Withdraws from pain |
| 3 | | Abnormal flexion to pain | Abnormal flexion from pain |
| 2 | | Extension to pain | Extension to pain |
| 1 | | No response | No response |

indicated in the presence of more than one of the following: amnesia for >5 minutes, loss of consciousness for >5 minutes, a severe mechanism of injury, three or more discrete episodes of vomiting and/or persistent drowsiness. A C-spine CT is performed with the CT head in the context of major polytrauma. Radiological clearance of the C-spine allows removal of a collar. This can reduce venous engorgement and help with ICP management.

The outcome after TBI depends on the extent of the initial intracranial insult (the primary injury) and development of any secondary injury. Secondary injury is exacerbated by hypotension, hypoxia and cerebral oedema. Careful management is required to provide neuroprotection and reduce secondary injury.

Neuroprotection involves control of factors that increase ICP or reduce cerebral perfusion pressure (CPP) (CPP = MAP – ICP). CPP should be maintained at a minimum of 40 mmHg; infants >40–50 mmHg, children >50–60 mmHg and adolescents >60 mmHg (as per adult guidelines). Vasopressor infusions should be used to achieve adequate CPP, with noradrenaline, ideally given centrally, as the first line. Temperature should be controlled to ensure normothermia and the ventilation set to achieve arterial carbon dioxide ($PaCO_2$) of 4.5–5.5 kPa. Arterial sampling is recommended to validate the end-tidal carbon dioxide ($ETCO_2$) readings, as there can be a discrepancy between $ETCO_2$ and $PaCO_2$, particularly in smaller children. Hyperthermia and high $PaCO_2$ cause cerebral vasodilation and increase ICP. Hyperventilation and a low $PaCO_2$ cause cerebral vasoconstriction, which can lead to ischaemia and infarction. Simple measures to reduce ICP involve nursing the patient in a head-up position and ensuring tracheal tube is secured appropriately with tapes, avoiding compression of neck veins.

Intracranial lesions causing a mass effect (acute subdural or extradural haematoma) require urgent neurosurgery and should be operated on ideally within four hours of injury. This is a time-critical emergency, and urgent transfer is required if the child is not at a neurosurgical centre; potentially by the local team, rather than waiting for the retrieval team. A refractory ICP >20 mmHg despite maximum medical therapy and signs of impending herniation are indications for decompressive craniectomy.

Anaesthesia for emergency neurosurgery should aim to maintain neuroprotection. Blood loss can be significant and require transfusion, particularly in smaller children and infants with open cranial sutures. Blood should be available in theatre, and adequate IV access available (ideally two wide-bore cannulas). Invasive lines should not delay surgery and can be sited intraoperatively if required. Cardiovascular instability may occur following the first burr hole or incision of the dura. It is possible to extubate children with isolated uncomplicated head injury at the end of surgery, which also aids neurological assessment. Children with more severe head injuries or polytrauma will usually require postoperative PICU care. Cerebral oedema often increases in the first 24–48 hours postoperatively.

Maintaining ICP <20 mmHg improves outcomes. Hypertonic saline (3%) is recommended in preference to mannitol to control ICP if required. A bolus of 3–5 ml $kg^{-1}$ is given over 10–20 minutes to treat sustained ICP >20 mmHg or if there are signs of impending herniation. Sedation and analgesia can be used to treat raised ICP. Boluses of sedative drugs risk hypotension and cerebral hypoperfusion and should be used with caution. Propofol is not recommended for prolonged sedation or treatment of raised ICP in children.

Refractory ICP >20 mmHg can be managed with high-dose barbiturate therapy. Prophylactic seizure treatment is recommended to reduce the occurrence of early post-traumatic seizures (PTS) within seven days, with either phenytoin or levetiracetam. Steroids and hypothermia are no longer recommended to reduce ICP or improve outcome in TBI.

The CRASH-3 trial published in 2019 demonstrated a reduction in head injury–related mortality in adults with mild and moderate TBI who received tranexamic acid within three hours of injury, but there have been no publications relating to children yet.

## Chest Trauma

Thoracic injuries account for less than 10% of paediatric injuries but have a high mortality. Eighty-five per cent are blunt trauma, mainly caused by road traffic accidents. Penetrating chest injuries are more likely to cause traumatic cardiac arrest. NAI must be considered in younger children with rib fractures.

A small body surface area and increased compliance of the chest wall make children more vulnerable to thoracic injury. The ribs have not undergone complete ossification, and large amounts of energy from impact are transmitted readily, with risk of serious injury to underlying intrathoracic structures. The presence of rib fractures suggests severe injury, particularly in young children. Small mediastinal shifts can cause significant ventilatory and cardiovascular compromise.

Pulmonary contusions are the most common form of thoracic injury. This may cause varying degrees of hypoxia and respiratory distress, depending on severity. Life-threatening major thoracic injuries include tension pneumothorax, cardiac tamponade, massive haemothorax, airway injury and aortic rupture. These should be identified and treated rapidly during the primary survey. A CXR in ED is a good screening tool. Anterior pneumothoraces are often not seen on CXR. A CT chest is not performed routinely in children but is indicated following a serious mechanism of injury or where the initial CXR is abnormal.

Positive pressure ventilation can convert a simple pneumothorax to a tension pneumothorax, and a chest drain should be sited if this is anticipated. Ketamine or short-acting opioids can be used for sedation for chest drain insertion. Low chest wall penetrating injuries can rupture the diaphragm, resulting in intraperitoneal injury.

The majority of simple chest injuries can be managed conservatively with early effective analgesia, high-flow oxygen and chest physiotherapy. A chest drain is often the only intervention needed. Severe injuries require surgical intervention in theatre and management on PICU postoperatively. Deterioration post-induction of anaesthesia should be anticipated if haemostatic resuscitation is ongoing. Major haemorrhage should be managed as detailed in the section 'Major Haemorrhage'.

Emergency thoracotomy is performed to control massive haemorrhage usually associated with penetrating injury. The surgeon can cannulate the right atrium for rapid volume replacement if other access has not been possible. If the patient is too unstable for transfer to theatre or has a traumatic cardiac arrest, a resuscitative thoracotomy can be performed in ED. Transfer to theatre to achieve definitive vascular control should occur as soon as return of spontaneous circulation (ROSC) is achieved.

## Traumatic Cardiac Arrest and Resuscitative Thoracotomy

The Paediatric Emergency Research in the United Kingdom and Ireland (PERUKI) Consensus Statement on management of paediatric traumatic cardiac arrest states 'good airway management with a supraglottic airway device (SAD) or tracheal tube (TT) to maintain oxygenation and ventilation, rapid volume replacement with warmed blood products and a resuscitative thoracotomy in penetrating trauma, improve survival'. The PERUKI group suggests the following life-saving interventions are used initially in paediatric traumatic arrest, in preference to chest compressions and defibrillation:

- External haemorrhage control
- Oxygenation and ventilation
- Bilateral thoracostomies
- Haemostatic resuscitation with warmed blood products
- Use of a pelvic binder

These interventions are not recommended in traumatic arrest secondary to hypoxia (drowning or asphyxiation). There is no consensus regarding the role of adrenaline in a paediatric traumatic cardiac arrest, and the normal Advanced Paediatric Life Support algorithm should be followed. Cautious use of adrenaline to avoid hypertension and exacerbation of bleeding is advised following ROSC.

Resuscitative thoracotomy is well established in the adult trauma algorithm and improves survival. Most evidence for resuscitative thoracotomy in paediatrics is in adolescents with penetrating chest injury. Evidence for benefit is less clear in blunt injuries. Indications are a penetrating chest injury causing traumatic cardiac arrest or peri-arrest in ED or five minutes prior to arrival. The aim is to control massive haemorrhage (and to clamp the aorta when needed) to provide internal cardiac massage and to relieve any underlying cardiac tamponade. Aggressive haemostatic resuscitation should begin whilst preparations for thoracotomy are made.

Decisions regarding when to stop resuscitation are guided by duration of cardiac arrest and response to the aforementioned interventions.

## Rarer Thoracic Injuries

### Aortic Rupture

This is very rare and due to rapid deceleration injuries. Death at the scene is common due to massive haemorrhage into the left side of the chest. Children who survive present in shock and require massive transfusion. A widened mediastinum is seen on CXR. A transoesophageal echo (TOE) is useful to define the injury. Emergency cardiothoracic surgery is needed to repair or replace the damaged aorta.

### Tracheobronchial Injury

This occurs in $< 3\%$ of thoracic injuries. Children present with subcutaneous emphysema, airway obstruction and hypoxia. A classic sign is an air leak and persistent pneumothorax despite chest drain. Lung isolation reduces the air leak and improves ventilation and oxygenation. This is achieved with placement of the tracheal tube beyond the level of injury, a bronchial blocker or double-lumen tube (DLT), although DLTs are only available for children $>10$ years old. Airway placement should be confirmed with flexible bronchoscopy, although any significant airway bleeding will preclude use. Definitive management is with thoracic surgery to repair the fistula.

### Diaphragmatic Rupture

This rare injury occurs more frequently on the left side of the chest. Abdominal viscera can herniate into the thoracic cavity, causing respiratory distress and mediastinal movement. An NG tube should be sited to decompress the gastrointestinal (GI) tract. Surgical correction may be required.

## Intra-abdominal and Pelvic Trauma

Children are vulnerable to abdominal injuries. The liver and spleen are relatively unprotected, as they are larger and extend below the thoracic cage. The anterior-posterior diameter of the abdomen is smaller, and energy forces can be widely dissipated within the intra-abdominal structures. Injuries to the abdomen can involve the solid organs (liver, spleen and pancreas) or hollow viscera (bowel and bladder) or be vascular in nature. The spleen is the most common solid organ injured.

Management strategy is guided by the haemodynamic status and the American Association for the Surgery of Trauma Organ Injury Scale (OIS), which describes and grades the severity of traumatic organ injuries based on initial CT imaging. Classification grades for the liver, kidney and spleen are most frequently used. Between 80–95%

of abdominal injuries can be managed conservatively, especially blunt injuries. This has the advantage of avoiding morbidity associated with high-risk surgery and preserves organ function. This is particularly important in splenic injury to preserve immune function and avoid post-splenectomy sepsis. Risk factors for failure of conservative management are a high ISS at presentation, a high organ injury grade and multiple organ injuries. Early identification of failure of conservative management is key.

## Trauma Laparotomy

Indications for a trauma laparotomy are haemodynamic instability, abnormal findings on CT (free air or fluid), peritonitis and/or evisceration or omental herniation. Massive traumatic haemorrhage should be anticipated and managed as detailed in the section 'Major Haemorrhage'. The surgeon should be scrubbed in the operating theatre prior to induction of anaesthesia. Fentanyl or ketamine can be used for induction as outlined previously. The tamponade effect of retroperitoneal or intra-abdominal bleeding is lost on surgical opening; in extreme cases, this can cause hypovolaemic cardiac arrest.

Complex abdominal injuries require initial DCS to control bleeding, decontaminate the area (in cases of intestinal perforation) and stabilise the child. Definitive surgery should be planned after a period of stability in PICU. There is a risk of abdominal compartment syndrome following abdominal injuries. Clinical signs include increased ventilation pressures, hypotension, reduced urine output and a rising lactate. Intra-abdominal pressures should be measured in PICU to aid early identification.

## Interventional Radiology

IR is a well-established component of the adult trauma algorithm. Advances in endovascular techniques and equipment and increasing experience of interventional radiologists with smaller children have made interventional procedures an important option in paediatric trauma. Most reports are in adolescents, with increasing case reports in younger children.

IR procedures, mainly embolisation, may be performed as a primary procedure or when conservative management fails. Indications include extravasation of contrast on CT and/or ongoing bleeding. This is suggested by a persistent tachycardia (despite sufficient analgesia) and a falling haemoglobin with ongoing requirement for blood transfusion. Main techniques for embolisation are with a coil or a gelfoam slurry. Complications include failure to control bleeding and conversion to an open technique, infarction distal to the embolisation site, infection and post-procedure re-bleeding. Anaesthesia for IR can be challenging in a remote site. Monitoring and IV lines require careful positioning for accessibility during the procedure. Extensions to IV lines are often needed. The theatre team must be ready if conversion to an open technique is required. This is invariably due to massive haemorrhage.

## Pelvic Injury

Pelvic injury is rare in children, the management is mainly conservative and there is a good prognosis. Pelvic fractures in adolescents can cause a massive retroperitoneal haemorrhage. A pelvic binder is used to tamponade the bleeding and prevent further fracture movement until definitive intervention. The binder may remain in place for up to 24 hours. Movement should be by limited log-rolls restricted to 15–30° only to preserve clot stability. Active arterial bleeding will benefit from embolisation of pelvic or iliac vessels in IR. Removal of the binder in IR to allow for cannulation of femoral vessels can cause further haemorrhage and haemodynamic instability. The binder should be released slowly with blood products available for transfusion. Retroperitoneal packing can be used to manage venous bleeding in centres where IR is not immediately available. Perineal, rectal and urinary tract injuries should be anticipated when there is a pelvic fracture.

## Penetrating Abdominal Trauma

Penetrating abdominal trauma is increasingly common in children and adolescents. The principles of management are similar to those for blunt trauma, although surgery is required more often. A CT scan can be performed if the child is haemodynamically stable, with the anaesthetist present in case of deterioration. Patients with stab injuries and a normal CT scan can undergo a period of close observation, but patients with gunshot injuries often require immediate surgery. The patient must be examined for an exit wound in gunshot injuries, and diaphragmatic, cardiac or thoracic injury considered in all penetrating injuries. Diaphragmatic injury on CT is not obvious, and exclusion with laparoscopic surgery is sometimes required, although it should be avoided if there is haemodynamic instability.

## Limb Trauma

Mortality associated with isolated limb trauma is uncommon. Stabilisation of long bone fractures reduces blood loss and provides analgesia. This is achieved with external fixation devices or application of a cast to more distal fractures. Occasionally emergency surgery is needed when there is compromise to the limb. Displaced supracondylar fractures can cause damage to the brachial artery or nerve injury (median or radial). Concerning neurovascular signs are increased pallor, changes in sensation, muscle weakness and reduced or absent peripheral pulses. Neurovascular compromise must not be missed in the context of a polytrauma patient with other distracting significant injuries. Open fractures should be closed as an emergency to reduce the risk of infection.

## Anaesthesia for Minor Trauma

Most minor trauma cases can be managed semi-electively. The exception is where there is neurovascular compromise to the affected limb or an infection risk from an open fracture (see the previous section). Common minor injuries include facial lacerations, nailbed injuries and limb fractures or dislocations. Immobilisation combined with oral paracetamol and ibuprofen often provides sufficient analgesia, and in most cases children can go home and have the surgery the next day as a day-case procedure under general anaesthesia.

The anaesthetist is occasionally asked to provide IV procedural sedation in the emergency department at the time the child presents. This is usually to facilitate sutures for a laceration, relocation of a dislocated limb (for example, shoulder or elbow) or removal of a foreign body (commonly from the ear or nose in young children). The anaesthetist will be responsible for providing the sedation, managing the patient's airway and monitoring the child whilst the sedation wears off. Intravenous ketamine 1–2 mg $kg^{-1}$ (titrated to effect) is most often used. Intravenous ketamine provides 10–20 minutes of 'surgical' sedation with complete recovery around 40 minutes after administration. This has the advantage of treating the problem in one hospital visit and avoids the need for a general anaesthetic and day-case surgery. The child should be discharged home with appropriate verbal and written advice following the sedation.

## Violence Reduction Strategies

The rise in interpersonal violence in adolescents makes violence reduction strategies increasingly important. Adolescents who suffer penetrating trauma are a vulnerable group, often young males from deprived backgrounds. Up to 40% of cases will re-present with a more severe injury. Usual safeguarding measures aimed at younger children may not be sufficient to provide the protection needed, and specialist violence reduction teams should be involved.

Risk factors should be identified whilst the patient is in hospital. The following should trigger referral to a violence reduction team:

- The history is not consistent with the injury.
- The patient has presented to hospital before with a similar injury pattern.
- The patient and/or their family are concerned for their safety on discharge.

An independent caseworker should be assigned through the local authority before discharge home. Examples of teams in London are the St Giles SOS project, Oasis Youth Support and Redthread. Caseworkers, who have an insight into the nature of how and why these children get injured, have an important role in building rapport and trust with individuals. The aim is to implement suitable safeguarding measures to prevent subsequent violence.

## Further Reading

Blain S, Paterson N. Paediatric massive transfusion, *BJA Education* 2016; 16:269–75.

Jones S, Tyson S, Young M et al. Patterns of moderate and severe injury in children after the introduction of major trauma networks. *Archives of Disease in Childhood* 2019; 104:366–71.

Kochanek PM, Tasker R, Carney N et al. Guidelines for the management of pediatric severe traumatic brain injury, 3rd ed.: update of the brain trauma foundation guidelines. *Pediatric Critical Care Medicine* 2019; 20: S1–S82.

London Major Trauma System. Management of Paediatric

Trauma Guidelines. 2020. 1–36. Available online: www.c4ts.qmul.ac.uk/downloads/pan-london-paediatric-trauma-guidelines-summaryrelease-compressed.pdf. Accessed 7 October 2020.

National Confidential Enquiry into Patient Outcome and Death (NCEPOD). Trauma: Who Cares? 2007. 1–26. Available online: www.ncepod.org.uk/2007report2/Downloads/SIP_summary.pdf. Accessed 7 October 2020.

National Institute for Health and Care Excellence. Head Injury: Assessment and Early Management. 2014 (last updated 2019). 1–60. Available online: www.nice.org.uk/guidance/cg176/resources/head-injury-assessment-and-early-management-pdf-35109755595493. Accessed 7 October 2020.

Chapter 40

# Burns in Children

Bruce Emerson and Joseph Hussey

## Introduction

Burns are a common injury throughout the world and are mostly preventable. A moment of inattention by a guardian, or an older child playing with fire, can lead to a lifetime of burn care. Children have a higher incidence of burns than adults, although most burns are small. Burns over 10% require formal fluid resuscitation to mitigate the effects of systemic oedema and burn shock. Definitive treatment involves non-operative techniques, such as application of dressings or, for larger or deeper injuries, operations to debride the wound and apply skin grafts. Each burn generates background, breakthrough and procedural pain that must be managed effectively. Small burns may be complicated by infection, larger burns by multiple organ failure. The outcomes are generally good, and children can survive and thrive even after very large injuries. Anaesthetists are involved in all aspects of burn care once a child reaches hospital, and they are an essential part of the multidisciplinary burn care team. The aim of this team is to deliver faster healing and better pain control and to prevent complications. This chapter will describe current burn care for children in the United Kingdom.

## Definition and Epidemiology

A 'burn' is defined as an area of coagulative necrosis of tissue. Burns involve the destruction of one or more layers of the skin and/or subdermal structures. Burns are a very common injury in all age groups; fortunately, large burns requiring hospital admission are not. In 2019, 7,061 children with burns presented to specialist burn services in the United Kingdom, according to the Children's Burns Trust, UK.

As with many victims of trauma, patients with significant burn injury are over-represented in areas of deprivation, and there are often coexisting social and psychological factors at play. This is particularly important in children, where it is estimated around 10% of admissions have safeguarding concerns.

## Classification and Aetiology

Burns are classified in terms of size (percentage of body surface area), depth and aetiology.

Accurate estimation of burn size is important to guide fluid resuscitation and prognosis. Children are particularly difficult to assess due to their changing body surface area proportions as they grow. Useful tools include the Lund and Browder chart for estimating larger burns (Figure 40.1) or the 'rule of one' for smaller burns. This uses the patient's palm area, which stays relatively constant at 1% of total body surface area (TBSA) throughout life. Novel smartphone apps are available for this use, some being validated for research. Burn erythema is *not* included in size estimations.

Depth estimation is used to guide clinical treatment and prognosis. This is a 'dynamic' process. Superficial burns may convert to deeper ones later, particularly if resuscitation is inadequate or wound infection happens. The degree of burn depth injury is a function of thickness of skin (infants have thin skin) and the 'dose' of energy imparted by the burn incident. The dose of energy is in turn a function of temperature and time exposed. An adult would need their skin exposed to a temperature of 70°C for only one second to sustain a deep burn. The energy dose resulting in a deep burn in an infant would be significantly less than this. Since 2010, all areas of the United Kingdom are required to limit bathing outlet temperatures in new homes to 48°C, following a successful campaign by the British Burn Association and Children's Burns Trust.

Burn depth is generally estimated according to the wound appearance (Figure 40.2). Laser

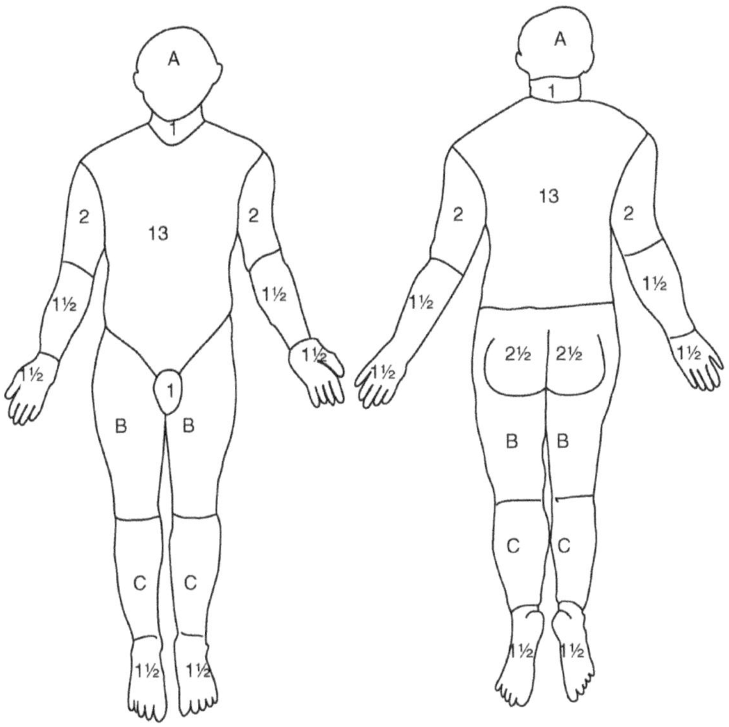


**Figure 40.1** Lund and Browder chart for estimating the size of burn. The numbers on the figure represent percentage of total body surface area. The letters reflect age-specific areas (see the associated table). The Depth of Burn table allows differentiation between superficial and deep burns.

| Area | Age | | | | | |
|---|---|---|---|---|---|---|
| | <1 | 1 | 5 | 10 | 15 | Adult |
| A - ½ of head | 9½ | 8½ | 6½ | 5½ | 4½ | 3½ |
| B - ½ of one thigh | 2¾ | 3¼ | 4 | 4½ | 4½ | 9¾ |
| C - ½ of one leg | 2½ | 2½ | 2¾ | 3 | 3¼ | 3½ |

| | Depth of burn | |
|---|---|---|
| | Superficial | Deep |
| | *Shade on figure* | *Diagonal lines on figure* |
| **Region** | % | % |
| Head | | |
| Neck | | |
| Anterior trunk | | |
| Posterior trunk | | |
| Right arm | | |
| Left arm | | |
| Buttocks | | |
| Genitalia | | |
| Right leg | | |
| Left leg | | |
| **Total** | | |

doppler technology, which measures dermal blood flow, can also be used if visual estimation of burn depth is equivocal. Generally, the deeper the burn, the longer the healing time and the higher the morbidity.

In the United Kingdom, the aetiology of most paediatric burns are thermal scald injuries. A common presentation to a specialist burns service is the '10% scald in a 10-month, 10 kg toddler' resulting from spilt hot drinks. Scalds from unprotected cooking liquids at ground level are common in the developing world.

The six most common causes of burns or skin loss presenting to specialist secondary burn services are:

- Thermal (scald, flame, contact, cold)
- Electrical injury
- Chemical (acid/alkali) injury
- Radiation
- Friction
- Medical skin loss (toxic epidermal necrolysis, staphylococcal scalded skin syndrome)

These all have differences in terms of clinical course and treatment.

Depth of burn

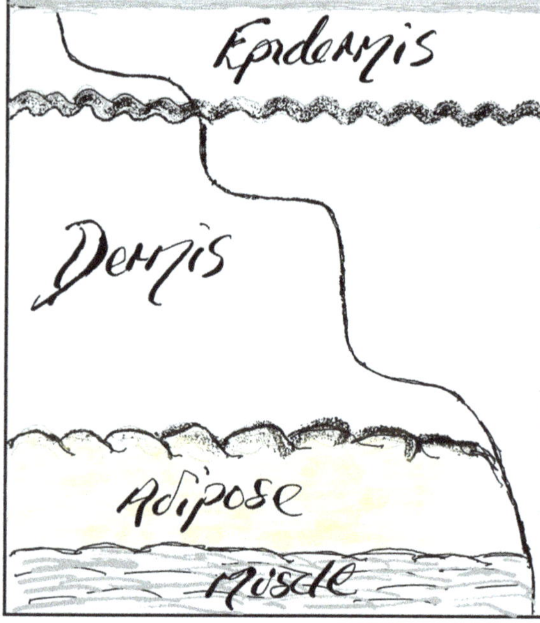


| Appearance, signs & symptoms | Expected recovery time with no intervention |
|---|---|
| **Superficial**<br>Erythema – blanches to touch.<br>Dry & non-blistering.<br>Painful. | Not included in burn size calculation.<br><br>3–4 days. |
| **Superficial Dermal**<br>Pink – blanches to touch & brisk capillary refill.<br>Wet & blistering.<br>Very Painful. | Heals in around 7–14 days with dressings. Scarring unlikely. |
| **Deep Dermal**<br>Darker red – mixed capillary staining.<br>Sluggish blanching to touch (if any) and sluggish capillary refill.<br>Painful but less than more superficial wounds. | Heals > 21 days. Scarring likely. Often requires excision and skin graft. |
| **Full Thickness**<br>Tough white/grey eschar.<br>No blanching to touch.<br>Anaesthetic but 'dull' pain can still be present. | Will not heal without surgical intervention. |
| **Subdermal**<br>Involving muscles & bone.<br>As per full thickness wound.<br>Evidence of myoglobinuria. | Will not heal without surgical intervention. |

**Figure 40.2** Depth of burn – diagnostic features and clinical course of healing.

## Depth of Burn-Diagnostic Features and Clinical Course of Healing: Pathophysiology of Burn Injury

The skin is the largest organ system in the human body and is involved in the protective and immunological response to infection as well as many other physiological processes. Damage from burn results in the release of pro-inflammatory molecules (cytokines, chemokines, etc.), causing a local inflammatory response and, in the case of larger burns, a systemic inflammatory response involving non-burned tissues. The degree of the systemic response tends to be proportional to burn size and depth; however, there is notable interindividual variation. In larger burns, there is a widespread marked increase in microvascular permeability, leading to oedema and intravascular volume depletion. Careful fluid replacement is required to maintain vital organ perfusion and minimise burn depth conversion whilst minimising oedema. The acute systemic response tends to be at its peak around four hours after the burn and tails off 36–48 hours after injury. Hypovolaemia and hypotension are *not* generally a feature immediately following an isolated burn injury – other possible causes should be investigated.

A compensatory anti-inflammatory response and hypermetabolic syndrome often occurs 48–72 hours post-injury, resulting in an immune dysfunction, raised basal metabolic rate and hyperdynamic circulation for some 18 months after large burns.

## Inhalation Injury

Smoke inhalation is common when exposed to fires occurring in enclosed spaces, such as in housefires, and is the leading cause of mortality in these situations. Smoke is composed of soot particles and chemicals, both inorganic and organic, which cause direct damage to the airways. In addition, systemic toxins such as carbon monoxide and hydrogen cyanide are produced from the burning of materials in a relatively hypoxic atmosphere. The fractional inspired oxygen ($FiO_2$) in housefires is estimated to be around 0.12.

Smoke inhalation tends to cause thermal injury above the glottis, leading to oedema and threatening the patency of the airway. This swelling often gets worse with time and after formal fluid resuscitation has started. Below the glottis, chemicals can cause airway inflammation, bronchospasm, epithelial damage, pulmonary oedema and acute pulmonary hypertension, leading to an acute respiratory distress syndrome.

The carbon monoxide molecule has a very high affinity for haemoglobin and myoglobin. It causes a 'left shift' in the haemoglobin oxygen dissociation curve leading to tissue hypoxia. Systemic effects are experienced at haemoglobin carbon monoxide (HbCO) saturation levels over 15%. Over 50%, there is a very high mortality risk. Specific treatment involves the administration of supplemental oxygen therapy at high concentration until the HbCO is under 10%. At the time of writing, routine use of hyperbaric oxygen therapy is not recommended for acute carbon monoxide poisoning. Standard pulse oximeters do not specifically detect carboxyhaemoglobin, and significant poisoning can occur with normal oxygen saturation ($SpO_2$) readings. If poisoning is suspected, an arterial blood gas sample should be obtained to confirm this.

Hydrogen cyanide is released from burning synthetic materials often contained in furniture. It is a potent mitochondrial toxin that interferes with aerobic metabolism and leads to a profound lactic acidaemia and dysfunction of organ systems with high oxygen requirements. The brain and heart are often affected, presenting as unconsciousness and an early shock state respectively. In addition to supportive measures, specific antidotes should be given as early as possible (preferably pre-hospital), particularly if any of the aforementioned features are present. A commonly used antidote in the United Kingdom is high-dose intravenous hydroxocobalamin, such as Cyanokit®, at 70 mg $kg^{-1}$ (a maximum of 5 g) over 15 minutes. A second dose can be given depending on severity of poisoning and stability.

## Referral Criteria

Children, particularly infants, can become unwell, even following small burns. There are nationally and locally agreed guidelines governing the referral of patients to specialist burns services.

The UK national burn care referral guidance of 2012 has the following minimum thresholds for referral to specialist burns services:

- *All* burns over 2% TBSA.
- *All* full thickness burns.
- *All* circumferential burns.
- Any burn not healed in two weeks.
- Any burn with a suspicion of non-accidental injury should be referred to a burn unit/centre for expert assessment within 24 hours.

In addition, the following factors should prompt a discussion with a consultant in a specialised burn care service and consideration given to referral:

- All burns to hands, feet, face, perineum or genitalia.
- Any chemical, electrical or friction burn.
- Any cold injury.
- Any unwell/febrile child with a burn.
- Any concerns regarding burn injuries and comorbidities that may affect treatment or healing of the burn.
- If there is any suspicion of toxic shock syndrome (TSS), then refer early.

## Management of Burn Injury in Children

The management of burn injury in children can conveniently be classified into:

- Emergency burn care and resuscitation
- Acute burn care (including critical care, surgery and rehabilitation)
- Post-burn reconstruction

Anaesthetists are integral to all aspects of management as part of the wider multidisciplinary team.

## Emergency Burn Care and Resuscitation

Pre-hospital first aid and extraction should involve a 'safe approach', particularly at house fires or if an electrical injury is suspected. The burning process should be stopped as soon as possible (the stop-drop-roll campaign describes actions to take if clothes catch fire).

The benefits from cooling a burn wound with clean cool water are described up to three hours following injury by arresting damaging enzymatic processes. Cooling should be carried out using water under 20°C for at least 20 minutes following removal of clothing (unless these have melted on to the wound). Care needs to be taken to avoid hypothermia with large burns.

Emergency care and initial assessment of large burns are best carried out in an emergency department or major trauma centre prior to transfer to the burn service. Burns are a classic 'distracting' injury. To avoid missing coexisting injuries, a careful systematic assessment of the patient should be carried out according to established trauma principles described in previous chapters.

The history should be carefully tailored to alert personnel to the possibility of coexisting injury (e.g. housefire, road traffic accident, blast, electrical injury, fall/jump). However, most burn injuries presenting to hospital are isolated.

## Burn-Related Aspects to the Primary Survey

### Airway and Cervical Spine Control

- History: fire in an enclosed space, trapped casualties, extricated unconscious, presence of explosion, other fatalities involved.
- Signs: intra-oral burns and soot present, deep peri-oral or neck burns, facial/neck oedema
- Symptoms: voice changes, stridor, dysphagia, tachypnoea or respiratory distress

If any of these features is present, there should be a low index of suspicion for significant inhalation injury and an ensuing threatened airway. Consideration should be given to securing the airway *early* with a cuffed and uncut tracheal tube.

> Note: it is very unusual for a child with a facial- or upper-body scald injury to require intubation to secure the airway. In the rare cases when this is required, there is often evidence of boiling fluid ingestion (intra-oral scalding) or deep burn to the front of the neck resulting in direct transmission of heat, damaging the glottic structures underneath.

If there is a history of a significant exposure to smoke, particularly in an enclosed environment and evidence of tissue hypoxia (high lactate) or early organ dysfunction (e.g. shock, unconsciousness), then consideration should be given to the possibility of systemic poisoning with carbon monoxide and/or hydrogen cyanide. Specific treatment should be given as previously described. There is no rapid turnover blood test to diagnose cyanide poisoning, and therefore clinical and biochemical surrogates are used to make the diagnosis.

## Breathing and Ventilation

Extensive full thickness burns to the anterior trunk may form a restrictive eschar (tight coagulated dermis) impeding ventilation. Releasing escharotomies can improve matters; however, these need to be adequate and carefully done under anaesthetic to avoid damage to underlying structures. Cutting diathermy should always be used, as catastrophic bleeding can occur.

## Circulation and Haemorrhage Control

### Shock Due to a Cutaneous Burn Does Not Occur Immediately

If a child has evidence of shock early in presentation, then alternative causes such as haemorrhage or poisoning should be investigated and treated.

Reliable intravenous access should be placed for any burn over 10%. This can be difficult if burns are extensive. Intraosseous access can be life-saving in this situation.

## Disability and Neurological Status

### A Reduced Conscious State Is Not Associated with Cutaneous Burns

If a child has a reduced state of consciousness, then alternative causes such as head injury and poisoning should be investigated and treated.

## Exposure and Environmental Control

Clothing should be removed unless it has melted. Burn size and depth should be estimated and documented as described earlier. Burns should be covered with a loose, non-adherent covering such as paraffin gauze or clingfilm. Children with extensive burns lose temperature rapidly, and active warming should be instituted to prevent this.

## Intravenous Fluids

Resuscitation fluids should be given according to established paediatric trauma guidelines if shock is present. Large cutaneous burns result in a systemic inflammatory response and temporary microvascular capillary leak syndrome that can eventually lead to severe hypovolaemia and 'cold' shock. The capillary leak tends to be at its peak around four hours after burn and tails off 36–48 hours after injury. Different fluid resuscitation formulae based on burn size have been described to compensate for the first 24 hours of capillary leak. The most commonly used worldwide is the Parkland formula using Hartmann's solution, Ringer's lactate or other 'balanced' salt solution (2–4 ml $kg^{-1}$ % $burn^{-1}$ over 24 hours).

All formulae are estimates and make no allowance for different burn depth or interindividual variation in systemic response. Under-resuscitation and over-resuscitation can both lead to morbidity and mortality, therefore infusion rates should be titrated according to response using markers such as urine output.

Young children have a large basal fluid requirement. It is easy to under-resuscitate if this is not taken into account or over-resuscitate if this is added to the full Parkland volume. In our institution, we recommend the following:

Start formal burn fluid resuscitation in burns over 10% TBSA (not including erythema) using Hartmann's solution, calculated from the time of burn.

For children <30 kg:

- 1 ml $kg^{-1}$ % $burn^{-1}$ given as a constant infusion in the first eight hours post-burn
- 1 ml $kg^{-1}$ % $burn^{-1}$ given as a constant infusion in the following 16 hours
- Plus maintenance fluid given according to Holliday–Segar formula (this may require a balanced glucose-containing solution if very young)

For children >30 kg:

- 2 ml $kg^{-1}$ % $burn^{-1}$ given as a constant infusion in the first eight hours post-burn
- 2 ml $kg^{-1}$ % $burn^{-1}$ given as a constant infusion in the following 16 hours
- No maintenance fluid

Urine output aim is 0.5–1 ml $kg^{-1}$ $h^{-1}$ or up to 2 ml $kg^{-1}$ $h^{-1}$ if there is evidence of myoglobinuria. Infusion rate should be titrated accordingly. Low urine output should not be aggressively 'chased' with fluid boluses if the child is otherwise well. A urinary catheter is recommended for burns over 20% TBSA.

## Analgesia

Burns are extremely painful including, contrary to popular belief, full thickness burns. Strong analgesia using intravenous opioids is often required. Diamorphine or fentanyl are effective alternatives that can be given intranasally for rapid but short-action analgesia. Ketamine is a valuable analgesic but should only be administered by practitioners skilled in its use. Non-steroidal anti-inflammatory drugs (NSAIDs) are effective but are associated with gastrointestinal bleeding and acute kidney injury; they should not be used in children with 'resuscitation-sized' burns. One of the most effective analgesic interventions is the application of wound coverage, which should be done following inspection.

## Burn-Related Aspects to the Secondary Survey

A 'head-to-toe' examination should take place with special focus on the limbs and presence of circumferential eschar causing compartment syndrome. Releasing limb escharotomies may be required. As with chest escharotomies, these should be carried out under anaesthesia by an experienced clinician using a cutting diathermy.

Burns are tetanus-prone injuries. Immunisation status should be ascertained. Booster vaccine and human tetanus immunoglobulin may be indicated. Prophylactic antimicrobial therapy is not usually indicated unless surgical procedures such as escharotomy take place.

Transfer to a specialist burn service is not often time critical and should only take place once the patient is comfortable and stable. A paediatric critical care transport service will often transfer children with large burn injuries.

## Electrical Injury

Children of all ages are at risk of electrical injury due to accidents at home or misadventure. High-voltage electrical injuries are associated with large burns and extensive tissue damage (rhabdomyolysis and compartment syndrome). Domestic supplies are associated with direct myocardial injury and arrythmias. If there is a history of loss of consciousness or electrocardiogram (ECG) changes (the most common arrythmia being atrial fibrillation), the child should be monitored for 24 hours post-injury even if tissue injury is not apparent.

## Chemical Burns

Chemical burns are often associated with the workplace or an assault. As such, they are rare in children. Accidental ingestion of a corrosive substance does occasionally happen; these cases should be referred urgently to a paediatric general surgeon, as internal aero-digestive complications can be fatal despite minimal cutaneous burn.

If cutaneous chemical burns do occur, they should be liberally irrigated with saline or water until the measured pH is within physiological limits. If available, amphoteric aqueous washing solutions such as Diphoterine® are highly effective against corrosive and irritant chemicals and can be used on both skin and eyes.

## Acute Burn Care (Including Critical Care, Surgery and Rehabilitation)

Burn care is a surgical specialty involving both operative and non-operative interventions, supported by a large multidisciplinary team. Anaesthetists are key members of this team, providing specialist knowledge and skills in the areas of anaesthesia, sedation, critical care and pain management throughout the child's journey.

The broad surgical aims are:

- Accurate assessment of burn size and depth and development of a treatment plan. Immediate surgery (e.g. escharotomy) should be performed as soon as possible. Planned treatment may be operative or non-operative (dressings).
- Excision of deeply burned devitalised tissue. Early 'total' burn excision within 48 hours of injury has been shown to have a significant positive effect in terms of recovery and morbidity.
- Wound closure with the patient's own skin (autograft). In large burns with limited donor site, this is done in a staged fashion over a number of weeks involving multiple operative procedures. In the intervening time, temporary wound closure with biological dressings or processed cadaveric skin (allograft) is frequently used. These provide a protective layer and, in the case of allograft, release local growth factors which prepare the wound for later autograft.
- Post-burn reconstruction. Often takes place following discharge to correct functional and cosmetic defects that reveal themselves as the child ages, often due to scar contraction. Children sustaining major burn injury may be under the care of the burns team for many years.

## Anaesthesia for Paediatric Burn Surgery

Burn centres in the United Kingdom are mandated to have a burns operating theatre available, preferably within the ICU. This minimises the infective risk associated with patient transfer and allows for better planning and coordination of surgical care. A large proportion of patients requiring burn surgery are children, often around one year of age, therefore it is vital the whole anaesthetic team are comfortable anaesthetising this age group. The majority of children are ASA 1–2 having a 'standard' anaesthetic for a single operation on a small area of burn – either sterile application of dressing or autograft (split skin graft). In the case of the latter, a painful donor site is created, often on the child's lateral thigh. These operations involve periods of intense stimulation, such as application of antiseptic solutions to raw areas or the taking of donor skin. In addition, surgical preparation often involves turning the patient, potentially dislodging a supraglottic airway. Securing the airway with a tracheal tube should be considered for these procedures. Short course, narrow spectrum, prophylactic dose antibiotics are administered. Pain is controlled using multimodal analgesics. Locoregional analgesic techniques can provide an invaluable way to treat wound and donor site pain. Young children will often need to return to theatre for dressing changes or staple removal, and hence psychological preparation is crucial.

Acute surgery for large burns can challenge even the most experienced of anaesthetists. These tend to be repeated, lengthy operations on children who may have limited sites for vascular access and monitoring and potentially difficult airways. Many of these children are already receiving intensive care and often have evidence of organ dysfunction, systemic sepsis and burn hypermetabolic syndrome. It is vital that there is preoperative coordination and a clear plan for the procedure amongst critical care, anaesthesia and surgical colleagues. Length of procedure, perioperative antimicrobial cover, estimation of possible blood loss, adequacy of vascular access and postoperative care needs should be discussed in the planning stage.

## Temperature Management and Feeding

Children with large burns are particularly prone to hypothermia during long operative procedures.

This is due to exposure and an increased surface area to weight ratio compared to adults. The ambient temperature of the operating room should be kept in the thermoneutral zone, which can be up to 32°C in infants. Active warming techniques, such as radiant heaters, may also be used in order to minimise heat loss and muscle catabolism from an already raised resting energy expenditure (REE) due to the burn hypermetabolic syndrome. It is common to enterally feed all patients with large burns intraoperatively, ideally through a post-pyloric feeding tube, in order to minimise calorie deficit. Ongoing dialogue between the anaesthetist and surgeon should take place. If the child becomes hypothermic, surgery should come to an end when it is safe to do so.

Blood loss during major burn surgery can be significant and is often hidden in pads and dressings. Infected wounds or delayed excision of deep wounds can result in up to three times the blood lost than if the excision is done early. An estimation of blood loss should be made preoperatively and blood and blood products be made available. Surgical techniques, including the use of tourniquets, diathermy, epinephrine containing infiltration and topical phenylephrine soaks, are commonly used intraoperatively. Avoidance of hypothermia and acidaemia is vital, and the administration of tranexamic acid is helpful. Blood and blood product administration should be guided by patient laboratory results where possible. Over-transfusion is associated with poor outcome in both adults and children. A haemoglobin concentration of 70 g $l^{-1}$ is adequate. A significant loss of blood can continue following surgery and should be carefully monitored and treated in the intensive care unit.

## Burn-Related Pharmacology

Burns can have a significant effect on the pharmacokinetic handling and pharmacodynamic action of many drugs. In the acute stages, burn oedema can lead to an increase in volume of distribution for water-soluble ionised drugs. Plasma proteins are acutely diluted by resuscitation crystalloid. Hepatic and renal clearance may also be a decreased due to hypovolaemia. In practical terms, these factors do not tend to change drug dosing at this stage. Later, however, various pathophysiological changes associated with large burns do have an impact:

- Altered gastrointestinal absorption (hyperchlorhydria, gastroparesis, increased gut permeability)
- Catabolism leading to hypoalbuminaemia and decreased acid/neutral drug binding
- Increased acute phase response (α-acid glycoprotein) leading to increased binding of basic drugs
- Reduced plasma-esterase concentration
- Increased hepatic and renal clearance of many drugs
- Hepatic phase 1 reactions impaired
- Hepatic phase 2 reactions induced
- Drug receptor population numbers change (often increase)
- Cellular secondary signalling altered and quantal release of acetylcholine at the neuromuscular junction increased

In practical terms, these changes manifest as a rapid clearance of non-depolarising muscle relaxants (NMDRs) and some antibiotics (e.g. piperacillin-tazobactam). Resistance frequently develops to the effects of opioids and NMDRs.

Extensive deep burns in particular can lead to a proliferation of extrajunctional nicotinic acetylcholine receptors. Administration of suxamethonium chloride can lead to acute life-threatening hyperkalaemia, and its use is relatively contraindicated 24 hours after a burn injury and for up to 18 months afterwards.

## Burn-Related Pain Management

> [Burn] pain is of a peculiar kind, resembling that from the continued application of fire to the part.
>
> Professor Jacob Bielow (1786–1879).

Burn pain management can be challenging and requires specialist knowledge when treating children. Conceptually, management should be viewed in terms of background pain, breakthrough pain and procedural pain. Pain scores should be frequently assessed in order to guide therapy according to a 'step-ladder' approach. Opioids are the mainstay of pain management as part of a multimodal approach. Non-standard opioids such as methadone and oxycodone have been used successfully for difficult to manage pain under specialist supervision. Pharmacological adjuncts are commonly used in non-opioid responsive pain. Common adjuncts currently used in our institution are clonidine, gabapentin and low-dose oral ketamine. As mentioned previously, NSAIDs are relatively contraindicated in patients with large burns in the acute stages. Non-pharmacological techniques are also important. Input from specialist children's nurses, play therapists and psychological therapy is often invaluable.

## Management of Painful Burn-Related Procedures

Children may undergo many painful procedures during the course of their inpatient stay ranging from physical therapy to extensive painful dressing changes and showers. Management options include short-acting analgesia, deep analgesia-sedation or general anaesthesia. Standards for monitoring and delivery of deep analgesia-sedation should be the same as for general anaesthesia. An example of a procedural pain management 'step ladder' from our institution is outlined in Table 40.1.

## Burn-Related Itch Management

Itching (pruritis) is very common after burn injury. It can be severe and debilitating. It can present during all phases of wound healing, the early inflammatory phase (zero to four days), the proliferative phase (4–20 days) and the late remodelling phase (21 days to 18 months). Most institutions have protocols in place for management of burn itch involving the use of pharmacological and non-pharmacological therapies. Commonly used medications are potent antihistamines, which tend to work better in the inflammatory, and early proliferative phases and gabapentin, which works well in the proliferative and early remodelling phases. Chronic itch going beyond the early remodelling phase tends to be poorly responsive to systemic pharmacotherapy; in these cases, psychological therapy can be effective, particularly in adults. Small case series and randomised controlled trials using novel topical therapies (colloidal oatmeal), laser therapy, transcutaneous electrical nerve stimulation (TENS) and intradermal botulinum toxin have shown some promise, particularly in adults, though their efficacy has not been reproduced in children.

**Table 40.1** An example procedural pain management 'step ladder'

| Management technique | Suitability of technique |
|---|---|
| Oral/intranasal opioids | Nurse-led on ward |
| Entonox | Nurse-led on ward |
| Oral midazolam and ketamine | Nurse-led protocol in sedation area of ward |
| 'Ketofol' (ketamine/propofol admixture) | Anaesthetist-led in the ICU/theatres |
| General anaesthesia | Anaesthetist-led in theatre |

## Critical Care Management of the Severely Burned Child

Intensive care for children with burns is a low-volume, high-intensity activity that requires careful coordination and close attention to detail. It should be delivered by a multidisciplinary team familiar with all aspects of burn care. A 'concertina of care' model works well, where facilities and staff can be expanded or contracted to meet the specific needs of the child.

Children who require tracheal intubation owing to airway oedema or respiratory insufficiency need adequate sedation and ventilation. Tracheal tubes should generally be uncut to allow for facial swelling, cuffed and fixed securely. This can be challenging in the presence of facial burns. Tracheal extubation can follow as oedema resolves. Elective tracheostomy is common in adults but less so in children due to an increased complication rate in comparison.

Children with suspected smoke inhalation injury should undergo diagnostic bronchoscopy and therapeutic bronchial lavage, if indicated, soon after admission. Frequent chest physiotherapy and 'inhalation injury' protocols consisting of nebulised drugs are commonly used. An alternating regimen of nebulised salbutamol, N-acetylcysteine and heparin used for five days has been shown to reduce complications following paediatric inhalation injury. Smoke inhalation injury, particularly if accompanied by a large cutaneous burn, may be complicated by acute respiratory distress syndrome necessitating prolonged respiratory support and lung-protective ventilation strategies.

Burn hypermetabolic syndrome is commonly seen in children with larger burns (>20% TBSA). The response appears to be driven by catecholamines, stress hormones and pro-inflammatory cytokines. The result is an elevated REE with augmented catabolism resulting in loss of lean body mass, bone density and the development of hepatic steatosis. Clinical manifestations are a hyperdynamic circulation, raised plateau temperature, hepatomegaly, weight loss, wound breakdown and infection. In addition to warming, physical therapy and feeding, propranolol and oxandrolone (a safe synthetic testosterone analogue) have been shown to maintain lean body mass, increase bone mineral content and prevent hepatomegaly in children with burns over 40%. Burn hypermetabolism can be evident up to three years following injury; the child's physical growth is often delayed as a result.

Sepsis is the main cause of organ failure and mortality in children with burns. Loss of physical barrier and injury-related immunosuppression leaves the child prone to systemic sepsis, often related to wound infection, vascular catheter sepsis and ventilator associated pneumonia. Gut dysfunction can also lead to bacterial translocation. Repeated exposure to antibiotics can eventually result in the emergence of multi-drug-resistant strains of bacteria, some being extremely difficult to treat. The diagnosis of sepsis is often challenging when the child has a hypermetabolic physiology and high plateau temperature. Careful evaluation of clinical, biochemical and haematological trends in addition to possible sources needs to be ongoing.

## The American Burn Association Have Produced Sepsis Criteria

At least three of the following should be present:

- Temperature >39°C or <36.5°C
- Progressive tachycardia (>2 standard deviation [SD] above age-specific norms)
- Progressive tachypnoea (>2 SD above age-specific norms)
- Thrombocytopenia (three days after initial resuscitation)
- Hyperglycaemia or insulin resistance
- Inability to tolerate enteral feeds >24 hours (abdominal distention, feed intolerance, diarrhoea)

These indications should appear alongside infection, demonstrated by one of the following:

- Culture positive infection
- Pathological tissue source identified
- Clinical response to antimicrobial therapy

## Staphylococcal Toxic Shock Syndrome

Special mention of burn-related TSS in children needs to be made. It is very common for children to have mild systemic illness following even a small burn injury. A small but significant proportion of young children will develop a fulminant TSS – a catastrophic systemic response. Some *Staphylococcus Aureus* isolates can produce a toxic shock syndrome toxin (TSST) which acts as a superantigen, causing a cytokine 'storm'. The degree of shock is unrelated to bacterial load and is associated with smaller burns presenting within a few days of injury. Children are particularly prone to this due to their immature immune systems. Diagnosis can be difficult. In addition to profound shock, children often present with the following:

- Pyrexia
- Diffuse macular rash
- Diarrhoea/vomiting (TSST is an enterotoxin)
- Lethargy/irritability
- Lymphopenia
- Hyponatraemia

In addition to resuscitation and supportive treatment, children should receive suitable anti-staphylococcal antibiotics (we use flucloxacillin, gentamicin and clindamycin). If this does not improve things rapidly, at the time of writing intravenous immunoglobulin (IVIG) is indicated for life-threatening staphylococcal TSS in the United Kingdom.

## Rehabilitation and Psychological Support

Holistic burn care is multidisciplinary. Physical rehabilitation happens from day one. The main goal of pain management is allowing this to happen. Psychological support is integral and is vital for the child, their family and occasionally the burn unit staff. Children with burns often have many procedures and can develop anxiety states and phobias. Anaesthetists need to be receptive and responsive to the individual needs of the child and develop strategies to prevent and deal with these issues.

## Safeguarding

Non-accidental injury (NAI) is thought to be involved with up to 10% of burns in children. Most involve unintentional neglect, but it is estimated that up to 1% may be intentional. Children with suspected NAI should be referred to the specialist burn service, irrespective of injury size. Delayed presentation or history inconsistent with the injury or degree of development should alert clinicians. Unusual or suspicious burn injury patterns and distribution should be recorded and discussed with the burn service involved.

## Outcome

Burns of any size can be fatal. Risk factors for morbidity and mortality in children are:

- Age less than two years
- Burn larger than 60%
- Smoke inhalation
- Delay of more than one hour before intravenous fluid replacement is started

There are very few survivors with a 90% burn, but children have better outcomes for massive burns than adults. Burns as small as 1% can be fatal if complications such as TSS occur. Most children with small partial thickness burns can be expected to recover within two weeks with minimal scarring. Larger burns will take three to six months; they need long-term burn wound management and often heal with lumpy unstable scars. Generally, parents should be advised that their child will need to stay in hospital for one or two days for each percentage of burn.

An experienced multidisciplinary burns team should manage all children with massive burns. Strong family support has a positive benefit on recovery, but children will inevitably be left with physical and psychological disabilities. Despite suffering severe injuries, it has been shown that children who survive massive burns can have a quality of life that is comparable to that of non-burned children.

### Key Points

- Burns are common in children, but large burn injuries are not.
- Formal fluid resuscitation is recommended in children with burns over 10%.
- Scald injuries are rarely airway threatening.
- Inhalational injuries are frequently airway threatening, and the risk increases over time, particularly when fluid resuscitation starts.
- Large burns are classic 'distracting' injuries – patients should undergo a full trauma evaluation.
- Hypotension and changes in conscious state are not features of an isolated burn injury. Beware of carbon monoxide or hydrogen cyanide poisoning from fires in enclosed spaces.
- Children with any safeguarding concerns should be referred to a specialist burn service.
- Sepsis is common and can be life threatening. It can present in patients with a small burn injury.
- Specialisation and improvements in burn care in recent decades have led to good treatment outcomes in burnt children.

## Further Reading


Desai MH, Mlcak R, Richardson J, Nichols R, Herndon DN. Reduction in mortality in pediatric patients with inhalation injury with aerosolized heparin/N-acetylcystine [correction of acetylcystine] therapy. *Journal of Burn Care Rehabilitation* 1998; 19:210–2.

Goutos I, Eldardiri M, Khan AA, Dziewulski P, Richardson PM. Comparative evaluation of antipruritic protocols in acute burns: the emerging value of gabapentin in the treatment of burns pruritus. *Journal of Burn Care and Research* 2010; 31:57–63. https://doi.org/10.1097/BCR.0b013e3181cb8ecf.

Jeschke MG, van Baar ME, Choudhry MA et al. Burn injury. *National Review Disease Primers* 2020; 6:11. https://doi.org/10.1038/s41572-020-0145-5.

Palmieri TL, Holmes JH 4th, Arnoldo B et al. Transfusion Requirement in Burn Care Evaluation (TRIBE): a multicenter randomized prospective trial of blood transfusion in major burn injury. *Annals of Surgery* 2017; 266:595–602. Available online: www.ncbi.nlm.nih.gov/pmc/articles/PMC5848498/. Accessed 13 April 2024.

Pardesi O, Fuzaylov G. Pain management in pediatric burn patients: review of recent literature and future directions. *Journal of Burn Care and Research* 2017; 38:335–47. https://doi.org/10.1097/BCR.0000000000000470.

Royal Collage of Paediatricians and Child Health. Child Protection Evidence. Systematic Review on Burns. 2017 July. Available online: https://childprotection.rcpch.ac.uk/child-protection-evidence/burns-systematic-review. Accessed 30 April 2024.

Chapter 41

# Principles of Paediatric Intensive Care*

Mae Johnson and James Diviney

## Introduction

Many hospitals with paediatric facilities will not have a paediatric intensive care unit (PICU) on site. Sick children presenting to these hospitals will need initial treatment and stabilisation in the emergency department (ED). Whilst in the ED, paediatric and ED staff will have already set in motion advanced life support measures, but often they will be looking for additional help.

The paediatric team will have experience in the intubation and ventilation of neonates but limited expertise in older children. The local anaesthetic team should be able to provide valuable support by understanding key elements of paediatric critical illness along with their skills in airway management. If intubated, the child will require transfer to a PICU unless potential extubation is imminent. This may be at another site, and transfer will generally involve a specialist paediatric intensive care retrieval team. For certain time-critical conditions, it may be necessary for the local anaesthetic team to undertake the transfer (see Chapter 42).

Anaesthetists are frequently involved in the management of children requiring intensive care, and this chapter will aim to cover some essential aspects of paediatric intensive care that will help the anaesthetist in these situations. There is also information on the management of the potential organ donor.

## How Much Paediatric Critical Care Is Out There?

Data from the Paediatric Intensive Care Audit Network (PICANet) indicates that there were approximately 60,000 PICU admissions in the United Kingdom in the three years from 2017 to 2019. Of these, approximately 18,300 patients were transferred to a PICU, nearly 1,500 of whom were transported by non-PICU teams. The current trend is for an increasing number and longer duration of admissions to PICU of children with life-limiting conditions, accounting for 58% of PICU admissions in 2018. PICU admissions are the tip of the iceberg; paediatric admissions overall continue to increase year on year, with around 5–10% of these requiring high-dependency care at their local hospital.

In the UK population of children requiring transfer to PICU in 2016 and 2018, the most common reason for admission was a respiratory condition (29% of transfers), with bronchiolitis representing a third of these cases. The next most common cause was cardiovascular conditions (27%). The children being transported are primarily young, with 50% $<1$ year and 75% $<5$ years old. A high proportion of the cohort were critically unwell, with an overall mortality of 6% and with 3% having experienced cardiorespiratory arrest prior to transfer.

## General Principles of Paediatric Intensive Care

### Why Infants Readily Develop Respiratory Inadequacy

Although children show significant tolerance to physiological challenges, they have anatomical and physiological attributes that pose disadvantages when compared to adults. They have small airways, and as the Hagen–Poiseuille equation (Flow = $\Delta P \pi r^{4}/8\eta l$) shows, any reduction in airway radius will have a marked effect on airflow and work of breathing. Smaller volumes of secretions are more likely to completely occlude small airways, with coughing being less effective in secretion clearance.

* Many thanks to Dr Ian Jenkins, who wrote the first edition of this book chapter, much of the content of which has been used in this revision.

**Table 41.1** Child Glasgow Coma Score

| | 1 | 2 | 3 | 4 | 5 | 6 |
|---|---|---|---|---|---|---|
| Eyes | No eye opening | Opens eyes to pain | Opens eyes to speech | Opens eyes spontaneously | | |
| Verbal | No verbal response | Inconsolable, agitated | Inconsistently consolable, moaning | Cries but consolable, inappropriate interactions | Smiles, follows objects and sounds, interacts | |
| Motor | No motor response | Extension to pain (decerebrate) | Flexion to pair (decorticate) | Withdraws from pain | Withdraws from touch | Infant moves spontaneously or purposefully |

*Note:* The lowest score possible is 3; anything below 8 is associated with poor outcomes and is the accepted level for mandatory intubation and ventilation.

Infants are much more dependent on diaphragmatic and abdominal muscles to breathe as their intercostal muscles are under-developed. Their muscles also fatigue more readily than in adults. Infants have horizontal and cartilaginous ribs, causing difficulty in increasing tidal volumes via rib movement. Overall, the chest wall is much more compliant, increasing the work of breathing. In conditions such as croup and bronchiolitis, attempts to significantly increase negative intrathoracic pressure result in mechanically inefficient subcostal or sternal recession. Lacking the ability to increase tidal volumes, infants must rely on an increased respiratory rate to increase ventilation.

## Clinical Indicators of Respiratory Inadequacy

- Tachypnoea
- Use of accessory muscles
- Subcostal and sternal recession
- Tachycardia
- Stridor – due to a smaller cricoid ring, which may become oedematous after tracheal intubation or in croup
- Deteriorating conscious level
- Rising $PaCO_2$
- Ultimately cyanosis

## Intubation

Apart from respiratory compromise, other indications for intubation include:

- Sepsis. This may be severe, necessitating large volumes of intravenous fluids, often >60 ml $kg^{-1}$. Pre-emptive support with intubation and ventilation is necessary to offset the development of respiratory compromise due to pulmonary oedema. This course of action, with aggressive fluid resuscitation, control of ventilation and administration of inotropes, is often inadequately managed. Early intubation for shock improves outcomes.
- Decreased conscious level. Conventionally, intubation is indicated with a Glasgow Coma Score of 8 or less (see Table 41.1) or AVPU score of 'Unresponsive'.
- Cardiovascular instability. Low cardiac output may be due to intrinsic congenital cardiac problems, myocarditis, cardiomyopathy or dysrhythmias.
- Smoke inhalation. Even when no respiratory effects are present initially, respiratory compromise can ensue quickly from airway swelling.

Intubation and ventilatory support also provide conditions for easier insertion of central venous and arterial catheters for monitoring and the central administration of inotropes where necessary.

## Drugs for Intubation in the Critically Ill Child

'Which drugs should be used?' is one of the most frequently asked questions when dealing with a seriously ill child. As in any other emergency situation, the potentially deleterious effects of anaesthetic induction agents on the circulation of a shocked patient still apply.

Agents that affect the systemic vascular resistance (SVR) the least and are less likely to exacerbate any obvious or occult hypovolaemia are the preferred option. Even when children appear normovolaemic, intrinsic cardiovascular compromise is present in sepsis, metabolic conditions, arrhythmias, cardiomyopathies and a number of cardiac lesions.

Particular care should be exercised in patients with a failing myocardium, as a fall in SVR results in decreased aortic root pressure and decreased coronary perfusion, resulting in myocardial ischaemia. Tachycardia and arrythmias must be avoided, as they can also cause decreased coronary perfusion.

In pulmonary hypertension, a fall in SVR results in decreased coronary blood flow to the hypertrophied right ventricle, resulting in rapid ischaemia due to its exquisite sensitivity to coronary hypoperfusion. Additionally, any increase in pulmonary vascular resistance (PVR) will reduce pulmonary blood flow, reduce left-ventricular preload and reduce cardiac output. An increase in the right-ventricular end diastolic pressure causes septal deviation, impairing left-ventricle function, which may also compromise cardiac output.

Those experienced with critically ill children, particularly children with cardiovascular compromise, find that agents such as ketamine combined with small doses of fentanyl along with a muscle relaxant cause less instability. Ketamine and pancuronium should be used with caution in tachydysrhythmias as they increase heart rate; a muscle relaxant such as rocuronium should be considered instead. Suggamadex should always be available for reversal of neuromuscular blockade, in case intubation is unexpectedly difficult. Ketamine has been shown to be safe in head injury. Propofol should be used with extreme caution in any child with cardiovascular compromise or suspected hypovolaemia, as the associated hypotension can lead to arrest on anaesthetic induction. Peripheral vasoactive infusions can reduce the risk of decompensation (see the section 'Fluids and Inotropes in Critically Ill Children'). Each hospital or local retrieval team should have guidance and checklists available.

## Respiratory Support in Children

There has been increasing use of high-flow nasal cannula (HFNC) oxygen therapy in the paediatric population over the last five years. Around 4 $cmH_2O$ of positive end expiratory pressure (PEEP) may be delivered, depending on the size of the cannulae compared to the diameter of the nostrils. The humidification of the inspired gases can help loosen secretions and aid in secretion clearance, reduce the metabolic work associated with gas conditioning and improve the conductance and pulmonary compliance. The washout of the nasopharyngeal dead space leads to improved alveolar ventilation. The evidence base to determine efficacy compared to other respiratory support modalities is still being established. HFNC is usually initiated at flow rates of 2 l $min^{-1}$ in children under 12 kg, plus 0.5 l $min^{-1}$ for each kilogram above 12 kg (to a maximum of 50 l $min^{-1}$). Appropriately sized nasal prongs need to be selected for both neonates and paediatric patients; these should not occlude more than 75% of the nares. Flow can be weaned once the $FiO_2$ is $<0.4$ by halving the flow rate initially and then removing HFNC support entirely if stability is maintained.

Continuous positive airway pressure (CPAP) provides respiratory support by maintaining airway patency, increasing the functional residual capacity and preventing alveolar collapse, thereby reducing the work of breathing. CPAP is frequently used in infants with less severe forms of croup, bronchiolitis and pneumonias and may obviate the need for intubation and ventilation. Interfaces and devices exist for all weights of children down to 500 g. Many devices allow escalation to bi-level positive airway pressure (biPAP). High respiratory rates and large leak relative to paediatric tidal volumes can make patient triggering difficult to maintain reliably. CPAP is initiated at pressures of 5–8 $cmH_2O$ and can be weaned once the $FiO_2$ is $<0.4$ by reducing the pressure to 4–6 $cmH_2O$ and then removing CPAP support entirely if stability is maintained.

In children under two years of age that require ventilation on the PICU, nasal tracheal intubation is better tolerated than oral, with decreased requirements for sedation. Additionally, nasal tubes are more stable, easier to fix and permit easier mouth care. Nasal tracheal intubation is associated with a lower rate of unplanned extubation in children under two years. It is a technically a more challenging procedure and associated with more complications, including bleeding and increased risk of sinusitis and ventilator-acquired pneumonia in the older patient groups.

Pressure-cycled ventilation is very commonly used in paediatric practice because leaks around traditionally used uncuffed tracheal tubes are rendered less significant, although changes in lung or thoracic compliance will alter alveolar ventilation. Volume-cycled ventilation is less vulnerable to compliance changes but is affected by the leaks around non-cuffed tubes. Current practice varies by centre but commonly includes provision of pressure support to spontaneous breaths in addition to the mandated minimal ventilation. Peripheral oxygen saturation and end-tidal $CO_2$ monitoring are essential, with specific paediatric devices available to minimise additional dead space.

The 'No Trace = Wrong Place' campaign from the Royal College of Anaesthetists emphasises that a capnography trace must be obtained after intubation and will be present, albeit attenuated, in cardiac arrest.

## Cuffed versus Uncuffed Tracheal Tubes in PICU

Cuffed tubes decrease leak by compensating for tube and larynx size mismatch. This permits greater use of volume-cycled ventilation modes as well as protecting against aspirated fluids. Improvements in endotracheal cuff design means that cuffed tubes are available down to size 3.0 mm and are now used in term infants. Available evidence suggests that tube size selection is much more important than whether a tube is cuffed or uncuffed in determining risk of subsequent laryngeal injury. Paediatric mucosal capillary occlusion pressures are lower than in adults, and thus cuff pressures should not usually exceed 20 $cmH_2O$, which may pose difficulties in high-pressure ventilation scenarios. Cuff pressures should be regularly monitored, especially in higher-risk situations such as when using inhaled nitric oxide, which will diffuse into the cuff and gradually increase cuff pressures.

In children with prolonged length of stay on the PICU, tracheostomies are less readily used owing to anatomical difficulties (short necks, short tracheal length) and their use being associated with longer-term problems such as local tracheomalacia or stenosis (even with more modern surgical techniques).

## High-Frequency Oscillatory Ventilation (HFOV)

The use of HFOV continues in children whilst its use in adult intensive care has declined. This decline followed evidence from the OSCAR and OSCILLATE studies, which showed HFOV use resulted in unchanged and worse mortality respectively. Its continued use in PICUs is supported mainly by evidence in neonates that HFOV reduces lung injury with no increase in mortality. Evidence in older children is less clear, but HFOV is used as a rescue therapy when conventional ventilation strategies are ineffective at the upper limit of support (e.g. peak pressures of $\geq$28 $cmH_2O$).

HFOV is recommended for paediatric patients with severe respiratory failure who are failing on conventional ventilation and as a second-line therapy for the management of a bronchopleural fistula. In the neonatal population, HFOV is indicated for patients with neonatal air leak syndrome, persistent pulmonary hypertension of the newborn (PPHN) and meconium aspiration syndrome (MAS).

HFOV is a mode of ventilation that delivers tiny tidal volumes (1–3 ml $kg^{-1}$) into the anatomical dead space at frequencies ranging from 7 Hz to 15 Hz. It is thought that the reduced tidal volumes avoid the shear stresses of pulmonary volutrauma whilst maximising alveolar recruitment and minimising atelectasis by maintaining a high mean airway pressure (MAP).

$CO_2$ elimination is dictated by the movement of gas in and out of the airway, driven by the action of a piston-powered diaphragm that oscillates at high frequency. This promotes gas exchange to the level of the alveoli through several mechanisms (convective streaming, radial mixing, pendelluft, asymmetric flow profiles and collateral ventilation) that differ significantly from those seen in conventional ventilation.

$CO_2$ elimination depends on the amplitude of the oscillation (how much the piston moves in each cycle, also referred to as $\Delta P$) and on the frequency set. Lower frequencies allow longer periods of time for gas exchange to occur, improving $CO_2$ clearance. If the waveform of piston movement is plotted (Figure 41.1), it is the area under the curve where gas exchange occurs. The desired elimination of $CO_2$ may be more readily achieved by reducing the frequency

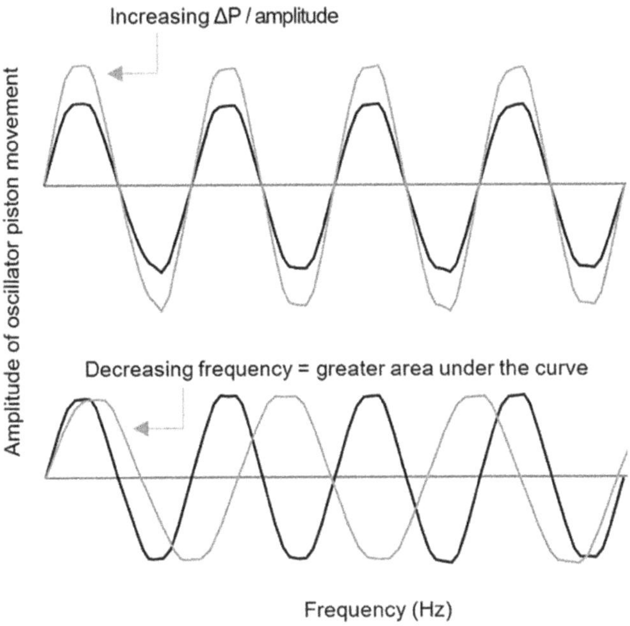


**Figure 41.1** Impact of amplitude and frequency changes on the oscillation waveform.

rather than increasing the amplitude of the piston movement.

Patient oxygenation depends on delivery of adequate oxygen to recruited alveoli, dictated by the MAP and composition of the gas flow ($FiO_2$). As the pulmonary condition improves, a constant MAP can cause over-inflation with pulmonary capillary compression and decreased gas exchange. Routine respiratory examination is limited on HFOV, and the paucity of variables measured by the ventilator means that regular chest radiographs are necessary to avoid over-inflation. The increased pulmonary vascular resistance from alveolar distension and increased intrathoracic pressure on HFOV can reduce cardiac preload and contribute to hypotension when HFOV is initiated. Care should be taken to ensure adequate filling before starting HFOV. Limitations of HFOV include the requirement for deep sedation and paralysis as well as the need to minimise ventilator disconnection, necessitating the use of smaller-lumen inline suction catheters.

Some portable ventilators can provide HFOV, but in practice it is very rare to transfer a patient on oscillatory ventilation, and conversion to conventional ventilation will be required for transfer for imaging or procedures.

A general approach to setting initial parameters is:

- MAP: 2–6 $cmH_2O$ above the MAP achieved using conventional ventilation.
- Frequency: set depending on age
  - Preterm infants: 15 Hz
  - Term infants: 12 Hz
  - Young children:10 Hz
  - Older child: 8 Hz
- Amplitude should be initially set at 50 $cmH_2O$ and adjusted until the characteristic body 'wobble' that is observed stops at the level of the patient's thigh.
- Percent of inspiratory time is set at 33% and rarely changed. This corresponds to an I: E ratio of 1:2.

Table 41.2 outlines the clinical impact of changing parameters.

## Extracorporeal Membrane Oxygenation (ECMO)

This comprises an extracorporeal circuit, draining blood from the venous system and returning it after gas exchange to either the arterial system (VA-ECMO, used in cardiac or cardiopulmonary failure) or the venous system (VV-ECMO, used in isolated respiratory failure). Apart from severe cardiac failure, e.g. cardiomyopathy or immediately after a cardiac surgical operation, the main indication for ECMO is severe respiratory failure. There are around 145 paediatric respiratory

**Table 41.2** Adjustment of HFOV parameters

| | | |
|---|---|---|
| **Under-oxygenation** | Increase MAP by 1–2 $cmH_2O$ (consider ECMO if >25) | Increase $FiO_2$ by 5% |
| **Over-oxygenation** | Decrease MAP by 1–2 $cmH_2O$ (consider conversion to conventional ventilation if <5) | Decrease $FiO_2$ by 5% |
| **Under-ventilation** | Increase amplitude by 2 $cmH_2O$ | Decrease frequency by 0.5 Hz |
| **Over-ventilation** | Decrease amplitude by 2 $cmH_2O$ | Increase frequency by 0.5 Hz |

ECMO runs and 80 cardiac ECMO runs in the United Kingdom annually.

ECMO can be considered in children over 2 kg in weight and 34 weeks of gestational age with reversible disease, for example, MAS, PPHN or congenital diaphragmatic hernia, and with no contraindication to systemic anticoagulation (such as intracranial haemorrhage), no lethal congenital abnormalities, no major immunodeficiency and no irreversible organ dysfunction including neurological injury.

Referral for ECMO should be made when one or more of the following are present:

- Severe hypoxia and/or hypercapnia with lack of response to conventional support measures (this may include high-frequency oscillation, inhaled nitric oxide, prone positioning and surfactant). Severe hypoxia in this context is usually defined as:
  - Oxygenation index (OI) >40,
    - ◇ Where OI = ($FiO_2 \times$ MAP ($cmH_2O$) $\times$ 100) / $PaO_2$ (mmHg)

or

  - P/F ratio <100
    - ◇ Ratio = $PaO_2$ (mmHg)/ $FiO_2$.
- Sustained elevated inflation pressures; for example:
  - >24 hours of MAP >20 on conventional ventilation
  - MAP >25 on HFOV
- Persistent air leak or interstitial air.

## Fluids and Inotropes in Critically Ill Children

Children, particularly infants, have greater insensible fluid losses and have greater maintenance requirements than adults. However, children are also more prone to developing inappropriate antidiuretic hormone (ADH) secretion, for example in respiratory conditions such as bronchiolitis. If given full IV fluid maintenance, as calculated from the Holliday–Segar formula (Table 41.3), they can develop severe hyponatraemia. In some circumstances, maintenance fluids are reduced to 80% of normal, and hypotonic fluids are not used. Balanced crystalloids are the fluid of choice for most clinical situations (see also Chapter 13).

**Table 41.3** Holliday–Segar maintenance fluid calculation

| Weight (kg) | Maintenance fluid requirement per day |
|---|---|
| 1–10 | 100 ml $kg^{-1}$ |
| 10–20 | 1,000 ml + 50 ml $kg^{-1}$ for each kg >10 |
| >20 | 1,500 ml + 20 ml $kg^{-1}$ for each kg >20 |

The cardiovascular system of infants differs from older children and adults:

- The heart is less compliant, with the result that cardiac output is less responsive to volume loading and is more dependent on heart rate.
- The Starling curve is flatter with an earlier downward inflection point at lower preloads.
- After term, myocyte β-receptor populations and response to catecholamines and phosphodiesterase inhibitors are normal.
- The infant heart is particularly sensitive to serum-ionised calcium levels; hypocalcaemia is not well tolerated.
- The liver is more distensible, with the result that fluid overload rapidly leads to hepatomegaly. A rise in blood pressure in response to external hepatic pressure can be used as a marker of hypovolaemia.

The most used inotropes in children are adrenaline and noradrenaline (0–1.0 mcg $kg^{-1}$ $min^{-1}$ for both), selected for central inotropy and peripheral vasoconstriction respectively. Hydrocortisone IV (1 mg $kg^{-1}$ every six hours to a maximum 100 mg, 2.5 mg $kg^{-1}$ every four hours in neonates) and vasopressin (0–0.002 u $kg^{-1}$ $min^{-1}$) are used in catecholamine resistant shock. In complex cases, cardiac output monitoring should be used to guide inotrope titration and choice. The inodilator properties of milrinone (0–0.75 mcg $kg^{-1}$ $min^{-1}$) are used in clinical situations with raised pulmonary vascular resistance, especially in children with congenital cardiac or lung disease.

There is increasing peripheral use of dilute inotrope infusions where central access is not available, with adrenaline used more frequently than noradrenaline. For both, an infusion made up with 0.3 mg $kg^{-1}$ (maximum 4 mg) in 50 ml can be used at as low a dose and for as short a time as possible. This is of particular use in settings where staff are not experienced in inserting central access in small children.

## Specific Respiratory Conditions

### Croup

Croup is one of the most frequent causes of respiratory distress in young children, with viral inflammation of the upper airway leading to a barking cough and stridor as the airway becomes obstructed. Obstructive symptoms can be temporarily relieved with nebulised adrenaline (400 mcg $kg^{-1}$ of 1:1,000, to max 5 mg) whilst allowing time for IV dexamethasone (0.15 mg $kg^{-1}$) to take effect. Biphasic stridor heralds severe obstruction and is one of the indications for intubation.

### Bronchiolitis

Bronchiolitis is a common viral respiratory condition associated with lower airway obstruction, air trapping and atelectasis affecting infants but seen up to two years of age. It is characterised by cough, tachypnoea, nasal flaring and subcostal recession. Usually there are widespread crepitations and a coarse wheeze. Patients are escalated through HFNC and then CPAP and infrequently require intubation. High-risk groups include those affected by prematurity, pre-existing respiratory conditions, neuromuscular conditions and immune deficiency. There is no evidence of benefit from any combination of inhaled or parenteral medication. Intubation and ventilation may be necessary for actual or impending respiratory fatigue, characterised by:

- $SpO_2$ <92% (despite $O_2$)
- Respiratory rate >70 bpm
- Signs of respiratory distress
- Apnoea
- Decreased level of consciousness

Pulmonary compliance is often very poor, so 'permissive' hypoventilation with modest hypercapnia, respiratory acidosis (pH $\geq$ 7.25) and $SpO_2$ 92–95% should be accepted. Current research is examining whether a conservative oxygen saturation target of 88–92% may be beneficial.

## Life-Threatening Asthma

Children usually present with respiratory distress, cough and wheeze. Life-threatening asthma is characterised by the following:

- Silent chest
- Cyanosis
- Hypotension
- $SpO_2$ <92% (despite high-flow $O_2$ therapy)
- Peak expiratory flow <33% best or predicted
- Poor respiratory effort
- Exhaustion or confusion
- Coma

Medical management of severe asthma includes:

- Nebulised bronchodilators:
  - Mixed ipratropium 250 mcg (125 mcg <2 years) every four to six hours and salbutamol nebulisers 2.5–5mg every 20–30 minutes.
- There is increasing use of nebulised magnesium sulphate in severe asthma:
  - 150 mg magnesium sulphate nebulised every 20 minutes for the first hour only (maximum of three doses) in patients two years or older.
- Steroids should be administered early, given an effect onset of three to four hours. In severe asthma, give hydrocortisone at 4 mg $kg^{-1}$ (max 100 mg).
- There is differing practice in the use of IV bronchodilators, with no clear superiority demonstrated for one approach:
  - Boluses of IV magnesium sulphate may be used at doses of 40–50 mg $kg^{-1}$, repeated

after one to two hours with monitoring of serum magnesium.
- IV salbutamol, loading dose 15 mcg $kg^{-1}$ given over 20 minutes (max 250 mcg), followed by infusion at 1 mcg $kg^{-1}$ $min^{-1}$ (max 20 mcg $min^{-1}$). Monitor for hypokalaemia and side effects such as tachycardia and lactic acidosis, which increase at higher doses.
- IV aminophylline, 5 mg $kg^{-1}$ loading dose (max 500 mg) over 20 minutes with electrocardiogram (ECG) monitoring, followed by infusion at 1 mg $kg^{-1}$ $h^{-1}$. Levels must be monitored, as there is a narrow therapeutic index.

Intubation and ventilation are indicated in the event of life-threatening asthma unresponsive to the aforementioned measures. Care needs to be taken during intubation, as there may be occult hypovolaemia secondary to decreased fluid intake. Fentanyl should be used in place of morphine, as it triggers less histamine release. Ketamine is useful in preserving blood pressure and for its bronchodilator action. A cuffed tube is essential, given the anticipated high ventilator inflation pressures. It should be remembered that the presence of the tracheal tube may be an ongoing stimulus for bronchospasm, and so the tube should be removed at the earliest opportunity, even if some wheeze persists.

For ventilation, adopt the following strategy:

- Pressure control mode with muscle relaxation
- Modest hypercapnia, accepting an arterial pH >7.2 (acceptable $PaCO_2$ 7–14 kPa)
- Tidal volume 5–7 ml $kg^{-1}$
- Inspiratory plateau pressures <35 $cmH_2O$
- Slow rate, 10–15 bpm (expiratory flow should reach zero before the next breath)
- Short inspiratory times to keep an adequate respiratory rate and avoid air trapping; I:E ratio of at least 1:2.
- Low PEEP (5 $cmH_2O$)

## Cardiovascular

Children may present to the ED or PICU in a low cardiac output state secondary to an undiagnosed cardiac disorder, an acute dysrhythmia or cardiomyopathy. The lack of out-of-hours paediatric echocardiography expertise in many centres can make management challenging.

In a baby who has been discharged entirely well from the maternity unit but re-presents to the hospital in a collapsed state in the first few days of life, congenital cardiac disease should be suspected. Most severe congenital cardiac lesions are identified on antenatal scanning, but occasionally these are missed. In some conditions, the patency of the ductus arteriosus compensates for the congenital abnormality immediately after birth by providing a shunt pathway. As the duct closes over the next few days, the change in haemodynamics can lead to a profound low-output state with severe metabolic acidosis and organ dysfunction. This can mimic severe sepsis.

Administering prostaglandins in this situation is essential. This may not re-open the duct fully but may allow time for transfer to a surgical centre for definitive diagnosis and management. During the infusion of prostaglandin, the newborn requires careful monitoring of heart rate, blood pressure, respiratory rate and core body temperature. In the event of a complication such as apnoea, profound bradycardia or severe hypotension, the infusion should be temporarily stopped and the complication dealt with; the infusion should be restarted at a lower dose. Recurrent or prolonged apnoea may require ventilatory support to allow the prostaglandin infusion to continue.

Total anomalous pulmonary venous drainage (TAPVD) is a rare congenital defect in which the pulmonary veins do not connect to the left atrium. Pulmonary venous blood instead drains into the right atrium via systemic veins and then to the left side via an atrial septal defect (ASD) and/or ventrical septal defect (VSD). It is frequently undiagnosed on antenatal scans. If pulmonary venous return is obstructed, infants will present within the first hours of life with tachypnoea, profound cyanosis, a plethoric chest X-ray and low cardiac output, and can be mis-diagnosed as sepsis, PPHN or MAS, especially if they have been compromised in utero and passed meconium during delivery. Obstructed TAPVD is a surgical emergency.

## PIMS-TS

Paediatric inflammatory multisystem syndrome temporally associated with SARS-CoV-2 (PIMS-TS) is a novel condition that was identified early in the SARS-CoV-2 pandemic. It has many similarities to Kawasaki disease, but also shares features of toxic shock syndrome, macrophage activation syndrome and haemophagocytic lymphohistiocytosis. The syndrome usually develops within four weeks of SARS-CoV-2 infection.

Common presenting features include fever, abdominal pain, vomiting, diarrhoea and shock, with shock necessitating PICU admission for vasoactive infusions in around two thirds of cases. Respiratory symptoms are not normally significant in these children. The mainstays of therapy are intravenous immunoglobulin and steroids, with some children requiring additional anti-inflammatory biologic therapies. The inflammation in PIMS-TS is prothrombotic, requiring prophylactic anti-coagulation in most cases.

Early echocardiography is mandatory, with the frequency of coronary artery abnormalities and left-ventricular impairment necessitating the close involvement of cardiology throughout the PICU admission. The shock is presumed to be secondary to a transient inflammatory vasoplegia, often requiring invasive blood pressure monitoring. Noradrenaline is used to counter the vasoplegia, with the addition of adrenaline if cardiac function is impaired.

## Gastrointestinal

Intussusception can present with lethargy and intermittent pain rather than the classical vomiting and redcurrant jelly stools, which are seen in only a third of cases. It can develop into a time-critical emergency where the viability of the intestine is at stake, with a marked systemic inflammatory response and circulatory failure.

Diarrhoeal conditions may go on to develop into haemolytic uraemic syndrome (HUS), particularly those associated with Shiga toxin-producing *Escherichia coli*, but also with *salmonella* and *campylobacter*. HUS is a condition caused by diffuse small vessel injury from thrombotic microangiopathy with a triad of haemolysis, thrombocytopenia and renal failure. Complications include seizures, coma, cardiac failure, pancreatitis and ischaemic colitis, where frank necrosis and perforation can occur. The treatment is to support the failing kidney with peritoneal dialysis or haemofiltration and, where possible, avoid platelet transfusion and systemic antibiotics, which may fuel the condition.

## Renal Failure and Support

The past few years have seen refinement in the equipment available for paediatric renal replacement therapy (RRT) in the PICU, and haemofiltration and haemodiafiltration have become relatively commonplace. Mortality is increased if the patients are hypotensive on initiation of RRT, particularly if receiving inotropic support or in secondary, rather than primary, renal failure.

RRT is also used as specific therapy in metabolic disease, particularly when there is marked hyperammonaemia, which is treatable by haemofiltration or haemodialysis. In certain cases, RTT may have to be used in neonates and is technically challenging.

Problems seen particularly in smaller patients include:

- Acute haemodynamic changes, exacerbated by the low circulating volume of neonates compared with circuit volumes. The smallest children may require initiation of peritoneal dialysis. There are current trials of devices designed for haemodialysis at weights <8 kg.
- Thrombocytopenia due to adsorption of platelets to the filter.
- A tendency to under-estimate insensible fluid losses.
- Hypothermia due to the patient's blood travelling through a circuit with a very high relative surface area.

## Neurology

### Seizures and Status Epilepticus

In a previously well child, the potential causes of seizures include infection, trauma, electrolyte derangement and tumours. Meningitis must be considered if the history is suggestive, but the most common cause of seizures in the six-month to six-year-old child is so-called febrile convulsions. These are classified as 'simple' if they are generalised tonic-clonic seizures lasting less than 15 minutes with recovery to baseline within one hour. Complex features include partial onset or focal features, duration >15 minutes, recurrence within 24 hours and incomplete recovery after one hour.

The trigger is cerebral irritation from inflammatory cytokines crossing the immature blood–brain barrier and the seizures are not secondary to fever itself. Control of temperature is not a primary treatment goal.

Should a presumed febrile convulsion last longer than five minutes, meeting the definition of status epilepticus, it is treated as for any other seizure. Children with complex febrile seizures are likely to be observed in hospital. CT imaging may be undertaken for focal seizures or persistent neurological deficit.

In status epilepticus, the usual cascade is:

- Two doses of benzodiazepines:
  - Midazolam 500 mcg $kg^{-1}$ buccally, or
  - Diazepam 500 mcg $kg^{-1}$ rectally, or
  - Lorazepam 100 mcg $kg^{-1}$ IV, then
- Phenytoin 20 mg $kg^{-1}$ IV over 20 minutes.
  - If already taking regular phenytoin, phenobarbital 20 mg $kg^{-1}$ IV.
- Paraldehyde 0.4 ml $kg^{-1}$ can be instilled rectally whilst preparing or infusing phenytoin.

Levetiracetam has been demonstrated to be as effective as phenytoin and is increasingly used in the management of status epilepticus. If these measures do not halt the seizure after 20 minutes, then intubation using IV thiopental should be undertaken. It may be necessary to continue a thiopental infusion at 1–8 mg $kg^{-1}$ $h^{-1}$ and proceed to continuous EEG recordings to detect ongoing seizure activity.

Neonatal seizures are managed with phenobarbital as the first line treatment.

## Traumatic Brain Injury (TBI)

Many patients with TBI will require time-critical transfer for imaging or to another centre for neurosurgery. This is likely to be undertaken by the local anaesthetic team.

Neuroprotection measures should be initiated as soon as possible:

- Keep the head in midline position with the bed 30° head up.
- Ventilation
  - Maintain oxygenation: $PaO_2$ >10–13 kPa.
  - Maintain $PaCO_2$ at 4.7 kPa (range: 4.5–5.0 kPa).
  - PEEP: 5 $cmH_2O$.
- Adequate sedation (fentanyl plus dexmedetomidine +/− vecuronium infusion initially)
- Normoglycemia: 3–12 mmol $l^{-1}$ .
- Haemoglobin: >70 g $l^{-1}$.
- Fluid restriction: 60%, maintain Na: 142–150 mmol $l^{-1}$.
- Maintain normothermia: 36–38°C.
  - 36.5°C if muscle relaxed and using a cooling blanket.
- Discuss with neurosurgery the initiation of prophylactic anti-epileptics.

Most centres that insert intracranial pressure (ICP) monitoring aim for an ICP of <20 mmHg with a minimal cerebral perfusion pressure (CPP) of at least 50 mmHg:

CPP = mean arterial blood pressure − ICP

For situations without ICP monitoring, empiric targets for MAP are used:

0–2 years >60 mmHg
2–6 years >70 mmHg
>6 years >80 mmHg

If there are difficulties maintaining ICP <20, then the initial approach is:

- Ensure sedation is adequate (avoiding the risk of hypotension with bolus sedation).
- Initiate the neuromuscular blockade.
- Administer bolus ± infusion of hypertonic saline.
- Consider CSF drainage via ventriculostomy.

If these interventions are insufficient, then surgical intervention for external ventricular drainage (EVD) or decompressive craniectomy may be required. Hyperventilation to $PaCO_2$ 3.7–4.5 kPa can be used as a temporising measure as can a barbiturate infusion or increasing hypertonic therapy (avoiding serum Na >160 mmol $l^{-1}$ or osmolality >360).

EVDs are inserted to decrease ICP by controlled release of cerebrospinal fluid and also for draining obstructive hydrocephalus in haemorrhagic brain injury. When transporting patients with EVDs the level of the drain must be controlled carefully. These are usually set 5–10 cm above a zero point (the midpoint between the lateral edge of the orbit and the tragus of the ear). Dropping the drain level may cause precipitous and excessive drainage. If the drain is lifted, then there may be some reflux back into the patient, leading to a rise in ICP and increasing danger of infection. Generally, it is safer to clamp these drains briefly for transfer but, once this is completed, to replicate their setting in PICU and maintain controlled drainage. Above all, it is important to remember to unclamp the drain and then ensure that free drainage has returned. If not, the drain may be blocked and will need attention.

# Metabolic Diseases

## Inborn Errors of Metabolism

These usually declare themselves in early childhood but may not manifest until young adulthood. Many conditions are insidious with 'failure to thrive', but there are a few that can present as medical emergencies, sometimes catastrophically. A trigger, such as infection, precipitates an acute collapse in a previously well child, with variable manifestations: lactic acidosis, hypoglycaemia and/or hyperammonaemia. The presentation is of a sick, drowsy, poorly perfused and sometimes encephalopathic child. Failure of energy regulation may cause single- or multi-organ impairment necessitating PICU admission. Where doubt exists, it is important to measure blood glucose, lactate and ammonia (which must go to the lab on ice).

Adequate carbohydrate administration will switch off protein and lipid metabolism, which may ameliorate the root cause of the crisis:

- A 10% glucose infusion must be started and run at a minimum of 5 ml $kg^{-1}$ $h^{-1}$ to give glucose delivery of 6–10 mg $kg^{-1}$ $min^{-1}$.
- All feeds must be stopped, as they may be substrates for toxic by-products that the child is failing to metabolise.

Once this is all accomplished, there will be time to set in motion more detailed metabolic investigations and to start ammonia scavenging medications and coenzymes. However, very high ammonia levels (>500 mcmol $l^{-1}$) will require haemofiltration as an emergency to clear this neurotoxic substance.

## Diabetic Ketoacidosis (DKA)

DKA in children differs significantly from in adults because of the increased risk of cerebral oedema. This disastrous complication is due to the rapidity with which deranged biochemistry is corrected, such as rapid changes in serum osmolality caused by the fluids used in rehydration, rapid control of hyperglycaemia or aggressive correction of the acidosis, particularly through use of bicarbonate, or any combination of these.

Consequently, paediatric management differs from adults and specifics vary between guidelines. Constant themes include:

- Cautious administration of fluids.
- Very gradual correction of glucose.
- No initial insulin bolus, with infusion rates kept to 0.05–0.1 units $kg^{-1}$ $h^{-1}$.
- Avoidance of bicarbonate.

Every patient should be given a 10 ml $kg^{-1}$ fluid bolus over one hour, with shocked patients given 20 ml $kg^{-1}$ over 15 minutes. Estimated fluid deficit (with the 10 ml $kg^{-1}$ bolus subtracted) should be corrected over the next 48 hours (body weight × % dehydration × 10). After an hour, a fixed-rate insulin infusion can be commenced. Thereafter, the glucose and potassium content of fluids is altered according to changes in serum values to achieve slow normalisation of acidosis and hyperglycaemia. The fluid calculations are complex and are frequently a source of errors. It is essential to refer to current guidelines for each patient.

If cerebral oedema is suspected, and there is a deteriorating Glasgow Coma Scale (GCS) rating, then mannitol 20% (2.5–5 ml $kg^{-1}$) or hypertonic saline 2.7% or 3% (2.5–5 ml $kg^{-1}$) should be given, fluids slowed to half maintenance and the deficit replaced over 72 hours. If this does not procure a lasting improvement, the child may need to be intubated.

Intubation in DKA can pose a significant risk from worsening acidosis secondary to an abrupt rise in $PaCO_2$. The decision to intubate should be discussed with the most experienced clinician available and is usually only undertaken in cases of ventilatory failure, airway compromise or decompensated shock. A CT scan should be performed to exclude cerebral venous thrombosis, a recognised complication of profound dehydration.

# Sepsis

In severe sepsis, where fluid volumes administered equal or exceed 60 ml $kg^{-1}$, it is advisable to consider intubation. Not only does this counteract the effects of the pulmonary oedema that often develops in these situations, but it also presents an opportunity to insert central venous and arterial catheters for more accurate haemodynamic monitoring and to facilitate the use of inotropes. It is a common mistake to underestimate the amount of fluid a child needs to maintain cardiac output in sepsis and not to intervene early enough with inotropes. See the section 'Fluids and Inotropes in Critically Ill Children'; for more detail, see the 'Further Reading' section.

## Non-accidental Injury and Child Protection ('Safeguarding')

Non-accidental injury may present as overt trauma but may 'masquerade' with seizures as 'failure to thrive' or as a 'collapse' in the emergency department. Anaesthetists and general intensivists must be alert to these possibilities, and all now have an obligation to have at least basic training in the recognition of abuse and in knowing what subsequent course of action to take. An ever-present index of suspicion is unfortunately necessary. See Chapter 5.

## Managing the Potential Organ Donor

When a child or young person has been subjected to a catastrophic brain injury with incipient brain death, it may not be in the child's (or the family's) best interests to move the child from a district general hospital (DGH) to a regional PICU. Good intensive care practice includes end-of-life care. All units have agreed triggers for referral to the specialist nurse for organ donation (SN-OD) team as part of end-of-life care, enabling assessment for organ and tissue donation in a timely manner. The triggers follow best practice as identified and supported in National Institute for Health and Care Excellence (NICE), United Kingdom Post-Intensive Care Syndrome (UKPICS) and National Health Service Blood and Transplant (NHSBT) guidance and strategies for organ donation. If donation is considered an option, the specialist team are then on hand to give all the information the family requires to make an informed choice and offer support through that process.

Donation of solid organs can occur following determination of death using either a neurological (donation after brainstem death, or DBD) or cardiopulmonary (donation after circulatory death, or DCD) determination. In the United Kingdom, for infants between 37 weeks corrected gestational age and two months of life, there is an agreed code of practice for the confirmation of neurological death (see 'Further Reading').

The majority of transplanted organs come from donors after neurological determination of death. Once neurological death is declared, a period of donor optimisation is carried out. This is important, as the potential organ donor is at high risk of instability due to the loss of CNS-dependent homeostasis. Haemodynamic instability and cardiac arrest after brain death accounts for the loss of up to 25% of potential donors; loss of hormonal and metabolic equipoise also contribute to physiological derangements.

The intensivist's role is to optimise potential organs for donation along with supporting the family. The goals for organ support are well established (see 'Further Reading'); Donor Optimisation Care Bundles include:

Respiratory:

- Lung protective strategies:
  - TV 8–10 ml $kg^{-1}$
  - PEEP 5–10 cm $H_20$
  - PIP <30 mmHg
  - $FiO_2$ <0.4, if able, keeping $PaO_2 \geq$ 10kPa
  - pH >7.25, $PaCO_2$ 5–6.5 kPa
- Fully inflated cuffed endotracheal tube.
- Measures to prevent ventilator-associated pneumonia (VAP).
  - Bed >20° head-up, lansoprazole, etc.

Cardiovascular:

- Normal blood pressure for age.
  - Use of inotropes or vasopressors as needed.
- CVP 4–10 mmHg.
- $SvO_2$ >70%.
- Cardiac output measurement where appropriate and possible.

Fluids and metabolic management:

- Urine output 1–2 ml $kg^{-1}$ $hr^{-1}$:
  - If >4 ml $kg^{-1}$ $hr^{-1}$, consider diabetes insipidus, and treat with DDAVP or vasopressin.
- Correct electrolyte abnormalities:
  - Maintain Na <150 mmol $l^{-1}$.
- Start insulin if necessary to keep blood sugar 4.0–12 mmol $l^{-1}$.
- Methylprednisolone and thyroid hormone replacement may be necessary.
- Continue NG feeding, if appropriate.

In recent years, there has been an increase in DCD organ donation. This involves the donation of solid organs, including heart and lungs, following active withdrawal of life-sustaining treatment and determination of death using standard cardiopulmonary criteria. The clinical team caring for the child must reach a consensus opinion that the withdrawal of life-sustaining treatment is indicated. It is important to note that imminent death should be expected at the time of treatment withdrawal. Patients who currently are expected to have a prolonged death or one way wean are not currently deemed potentials for organ donation. Potentially all patients that die can donate tissues, and this should be considered as part of normal end of life care.

## Key Points

- It is important that 'generalist' anaesthetists understand the principles of care of the critically ill child, as they are best placed to provide immediate care to a child presenting to the emergency department, working in conjunction with paediatricians.
- Ketamine maintains cardiovascular stability in the shocked child. Propofol should be used with caution in cardiovascular compromise.
- Cuffed tracheal tubes should be used in children over 28 days old, and the cuff pressure should be monitored.
- The need for fluid replacement and inotropic support is frequently underestimated in children with shock.
- Non-accidental injury should be considered in children presenting with trauma and in neonates with unexplained collapse.

## Further Reading


Academy of Medical Royal Colleges. A Code of Practice for the Diagnosis and Confirmation of Death. 2008. Available at: www.aomrc.org.uk/wp-content/uploads/2016/04/Code_Practice_Confirmation_Diagnosis_Death_1008.pdf. Accessed 25 April 2024.

Davis AL, Carcillo JA, Aneja RK et al. American College of Critical Care Medicine clinical practice parameters for hemodynamic support of pediatric and neonatal septic shock. *Critical Care Medicine* 2017 June; 45(6):1061–93.

Heddy N, British Society for Paediatric Endocrinology and Diabetes. Guideline for the Management of Children and Young People under the Age of 18 Years with Diabetic Ketoacidosis. 2021. Archives of Disease in Childhood – Education and Practice.

Healthcare Improvement Scotland. British Guideline on the Management of Asthma: A National Clinical Guideline. 2019.

Kotloff RM, Blosser S, Fulda GJ et al. Management of the potential organ donor in the ICU: Society of Critical Care Medicine/American College of Chest Physicians/Association of Organ Procurement Organizations consensus statement. *Critical Care Medicine* 2015; 43(6): 1291–325.

Murphy PJ, Marriage SC, Davis PJ. *Case Studies in Pediatric Critical Care*. Cambridge University Press. 2009.

Nichol DG, ed. *Rogers' Textbook of Pediatric Intensive Care*, 5th ed. Lippincott, Williams & Wilkins. 2016.

Pearson GA. Intensive care: because we can or because we should? *Archives of Disease in Childhood* 2018; 103(6):527–8.

PICANet, Universities of Leeds and Leicester. Paediatric Intensive Care Audit Network Annual Report 2020. 2021.

Royal College of Paediatrics and Child Health. The Diagnosis of Death by Neurological Criteria in Infants Less than Two Months Old. 2015.

Chapter 42

# Stabilisation and Transport of the Critically Ill Child

Daniel Lutman

## Introduction

Centralisation of specialist services, such as paediatric critical care, major trauma, cardiac surgery or neurosurgery, improves outcomes. For the critically ill child, accessing specialist critical care services may require transfer, either primarily by a 'front-line' ambulance (bypassing non-specialist centres) or secondarily by hospital teams after initial resuscitation and stabilisation in a non-specialist centre.

Children may be particularly vulnerable during transfer. Hospitals that admit children who may be critically ill or injured should be part of a clinical network involving paediatric critical care services and transport teams, with agreed guidelines for referral, immediate care and transport with appropriate audit and governance arrangements.

Transporting a critically ill child carries risks for the patient and requires the involvement of senior clinicians. For a critically ill child, the benefits of specialist services are usually greater than this risk, but each transport should be considered carefully.

This chapter describes general principles that specialist transport teams apply when undertaking the secondary transport of critically ill children and specific guidance for the transport of a child with a neurosurgical emergency, which may need to be undertaken by the referring hospital.

The need for transport of critically ill children is relatively predictable within a given geographical network or population. There are common diagnostic categories with predictable frequency and variation according to time of day and months of the year. Plans should therefore reflect the most commonly encountered scenarios. For example, airway emergencies are common in children, bronchiolitis is most common in the winter months and children are most involved in trauma out of school hours.

Support of respiratory and cardiovascular systems is similar for most of the commonly encountered diagnoses. Guidelines for the following commonly encountered emergencies should be available, ideally via the local paediatric critical care transport service website (for instance, from the Children's Acute Transport Service, CATS, www.cats.nhs.uk):

- Anaphylaxis
- Asthma
- Bronchiolitis
- Burns
- Coma
- Congenital heart disease
- Diabetic ketoacidosis
- Metabolic emergencies
- Neurosurgical emergencies
- Persistent pulmonary hypertension of the newborn
- Prospective planning
- Poisoning
- Sepsis
- Status epilepticus
- Trauma (now generally managed by primary or 'Front Line' responder networks)
- Upper airway obstruction

The secret to efficient stabilisation and transport of critically ill children is anticipation.

It is important to plan for transport in terms of resources, expertise and equipment before the need arises. This is important for both specialised transport services and for district hospitals who may be required to transport a child, for instance with a time-critical neurosurgical emergency.

## Referring a Child Needing Critical Care

Many regions of the United Kingdom now have a dedicated transport team for both children and neonates operating within a critical care network. Establishing the need for transport and the required time frame informs all other decisions.

There should be a close dialogue between the referring hospital and the transport team as soon as referral is considered. Specialist transport teams have dedicated consultant intensivists and are a valuable source of advice for the clinician involved in initial stabilisation of the child. Some referrals may resolve with advice from the intensive care team, avoiding the need for transport. Ideally, when a child is referred, the transport team will act as the liaison between the referring hospital and the specialist centre, leaving the referring doctor free to concentrate on the immediate clinical needs of the child.

The most senior clinician available at the referring hospital should assess the need for interventions once the decision to transport has been made. For instance, an arterial line and a central line may be indicated for a critically ill child, but is the time taken to insert them justified prior to the transport itself? If central venous access is technically difficult, how long should one persist and at what point should one abandon the attempt? Decisions about urgency of transfer also require an understanding of what will happen in the receiving hospital. Does the patient need emergency neurosurgery, or will they be transferred to the paediatric intensive care unit (PICU) for a period of ventilation and antibiotics?

Information for the transport team should be collated prior to referral.

In these complex situations, a checklist may be helpful to summarise information for referral (Table 42.1).

**Table 42.1** Referral checklist

| |
|---|
| Patient details |
| Referrer details |
| Reason for referral |
| Clinical details. Follow BAR format: |
| Situation |
| Background |
| Assessment |
| Recommendation |
| Allergies, medications, immunisations |
| Child protection issues |
| Trauma: details of injury, including timings |
| Status at referral: |
| Airway |
| Breathing |
| Circulation |
| Disability (AVPU: Alert, responds to Voice, responds to Pain, Unresponsive) |
| Everything else: blood results, blood gases, imaging, |
| microbiology results |
| Planned interventions |
| Summary of discussion |

## Acceptance and Agreement

It is vital that a critically ill child is taken to the correct receiving institution and that they are ready to receive the child. The child may be transported by a specialist transport team, or the local hospital team may be required to transfer the child themselves, depending on the availability of the transport team, the distances involved and the urgency of the clinical situation.

The transport team must know the name of the accepting consultant and the name of the receiving hospital. A member of the transporting team should contact the receiving unit immediately before departure. It is advisable to speak to someone who will be directly involved with the patient, for example the nurse in charge in the PICU. Describe the current condition of the child and any immediate needs of the patient, as well as how to get the patient from the ambulance entrance to the receiving ward.

## Generic Transport Rules

There are some accepted practice points that are common to most transporting teams and most scenarios:

- Before transport, interventions that improve patient outcome should be prioritised.
- Recognise the point at which the transport itself becomes the priority.
- Recognise there is a small risk to the health of the transporting team. The risk of an ambulance accident, for example, is small but present. Unnecessary risks (often involving adverse weather conditions or other external factors) should not be taken.

The point at which the transport becomes the priority sometimes occurs surprisingly quickly.

It is more easily recognised by someone who is 'hands off' in a leadership role. Unfortunately, in these situations the person with most clinical experience is frequently directly involved in clinical procedures. It is important that the team leader maintains a clear overview of the situation.

## Generic Goals: ABC

Physiological support may need to be instituted before a definitive diagnosis has been made.

If paediatric critical care transport is required, only perform investigations that change either clinical management decisions or the destination of the child.

### Airway

A clear airway needs to be maintained at all times.

It may be better to intubate a patient electively in the hospital environment rather than risk emergency intubation in the ambulance should the patient deteriorate en route.

Common indications for intubation include:

- Airway protection or to maintain a patent airway
- Respiratory failure
- Cardiovascular support
- Neuroprotection in severe head injury

It is important to maximise the chances of first attempt intubation success in this group of patients. Videolaryngoscope techniques offer some possible benefits to these patients when the clinician is familiar with them and should be considered.

The expected size and length of tracheal tube should be calculated for every transported patient, and one size larger and smaller should be carried for the transport.

It is not recommended to pre-cut the tracheal tube; instead, be aware and check the actual against the predicted length.

The aim should be to use a tracheal tube with a snug fit; if the tube has a large leak, it is almost always preferable to change it for one that fits more appropriately. Consider a cuffed tracheal tube, particularly in children with respiratory infection or sepsis, as lung compliance may deteriorate. The additional external diameter caused by the presence of a cuff can result in a smaller internal diameter tube being selected. Consider the risks of compromising gas flow and the risk of secretions blocking the tracheal tube on a transport in these circumstances, particularly if a very small-sized cuffed tube is selected.

Consider employing high-flow humidified nasal oxygen during emergency intubation (where an intravenous induction will be employed), as this may assist in maintaining patient oxygen saturation.

All children should have a gastric tube inserted after intubation, which should be left on free drainage.

If possible, put together an airway bag specifically for each patient transported. The airway bag should contain the following equipment:

- A functioning laryngoscope
- A replacement tracheal tube
- One larger tracheal tube, one smaller tracheal tube
- Magill's forceps
- Suction catheters
- Tape and scissors
- A face mask

The face mask is commonly forgotten if the patient is intubated prior to departure. Do not overload the airway bag, as this makes it difficult to use in an emergency.

## Failed Intubation

The Difficult Airway Society has produced helpful guidelines for these difficult situations (see https://das.uk.com/guidelines/paediatric-difficult-airway-guidelines).

In the context of critical illness, a 'cannot intubate and cannot ventilate' (CICV) situation could develop rapidly and may require consideration of rescue techniques with or without ENT expertise.

The priority is oxygenation; repeated attempts at laryngoscopy should be avoided. The main group at risk seems to be those under one year of age. It is important to consider transport early in any child in whom a difficult intubation is anticipated before their respiratory status becomes critical.

Although a supraglottic airway and breathing system has been used to transport patients successfully following failed intubation, this is not ideal, as sedation and paralysis are usually required to tolerate the airway and ventilation, which places the patient in a precarious position for the journey.

Hopefully the more widespread use and understanding of videolaryngoscopy and airway rescue techniques will make the management of these rare cases that require transport more straightforward.

## Breathing

Respiratory support can become a problem during a transport because the disease process may be evolving, and within that environment consumables such as oxygen and power are limited. The following precautions should be in place:

- A self-inflating bag should be available and in view at all times.
- An anaesthetic breathing system (bagging circuit) attached to an oxygen outlet should be ready at all phases of the transport.
- An adequate supply of oxygen should be calculated, and there should always be a backup supply; never carry all the oxygen in a single cylinder, for example.

If the patient is intubated, a mechanical ventilator is preferable to ventilation by hand. Hand ventilation uses a high fresh gas flow, and it may not be possible to deliver positive end expiratory pressure (PEEP) or control pressure as effectively as via a ventilator. Self-inflating bags are particularly difficult to use in this regard.

If a ventilator is used, the ventilator consumption of oxygen should be known and a calculation made to ensure that enough oxygen is available for the journey.

A calculation can be made using the following formula. It is safest to assume that the patient will require a $FiO_2$ of 1.0:

$$\begin{aligned}\text{Oxygen required (litres)} &= \text{ventilator consumption}\\ &\times \text{(litres per minute)}\\ &\times \text{journey length (minutes)}\\ &\times 2\end{aligned}$$

Most ventilators consume more gas than the minute volume delivered to the patient, and it is necessary to understand this excess to calculate the quantity of gas required for a journey.

Increasingly, ventilators use electrical power to operate and pressurise ambient air for patient ventilation. Battery life and access to en route power supplies are therefore additional considerations in most ventilated transports.

Understand, control and conserve gas and power supplies carefully during a transport. Plug in to wall supplies whenever possible. A common source of error is to fail to switch off a high-flow bagging circuit after unexpected use during the transport phase. Monitor actual oxygen consumption during a transport to make sure it approximately matches the amount calculated.

The transport ventilator and oxygen cylinders need to be secured so that they do not present a hazard to staff or the patient if the vehicle accelerates, brakes suddenly or is involved in an accident.

Use a bacterial/viral/humidifying filter in the circuit to retain heat and moisture if dead space allows. This is particularly important to prevent secretions obstructing a tracheostomy tube.

## CPAP/HFHO and HFOV

Oxygen consumption can be a distance- and time-limiting factor in transport involving continuous positive airway pressure (CPAP) and high-flow humidified oxygen (HFHO) because the gas consumption can be very high. An alternative strategy, such as invasive ventilation, can sometimes be required. Similarly, for a child requiring high-frequency oscillatory ventilation (HFOV), if conventional ventilation proves too risky, transport following initiation of extracorporeal membrane oxygenation (ECMO) prior to transport may be the best option for the patient.

## Oxygen Failure

Gas pressure alarms that are both auditory and visual are recommended for the transport environment. The self-inflating bag can provide emergency ventilation in the event of oxygen failure. The ambulance should then be diverted to the nearest emergency department.

## Ventilatory Problems during Transfer

At the point of transport, the physiology of a critically ill child is likely to be in evolution. This means that significant deterioration may occur during transport, and where possible this should be anticipated and planned for.

Consider the mnemonic 'DOPES' if ventilatory problems occur after intubation:

- Displaced?
- Obstructed?
- Pneumothorax?
- Equipment?
- Stomach?

Be ready to suction the airway at any stage in the transport (suctioning and a bolus of intravenous fluids are the two most frequent interventions during the transport phase).

## Ventilation Strategy

Ventilation strategy may differ between conditions; care should be taken to ventilate to normocapnia for the head injured child, but permissive hypercapnia (pH $\geq$ 7.25) is desirable in children with respiratory failure.

Children with acute severe asthma or bronchiolitis are at risk of dynamic hyperinflation and air-trapping, as expiration can be prolonged and require effort. When ventilated, this effort is eliminated, and these patients often require high inspiratory pressures and a long expiratory time to achieve expiration on the ventilator, which can limit available respiratory rate. Airway suctioning or respiratory physiotherapy can be very beneficial for these patients once sedation and bronchodilator therapy are optimal.

A child with chronic respiratory problems for whom target saturations are normally $\geq$ 88% is unlikely to benefit from attempts to ventilate to higher saturations.

It may be essential to target lower than normal saturations in some patients with congenital heart disease. In these rare cases, the greater risk to the patient is that of pulmonary over-circulation, at the expense of systemic circulation. Maintain a minimum of 75% saturations and seek expert opinion urgently.

## Circulation

Two secure intravenous lines are recommended for transport. A triple lumen central line counts as one site of vascular access.

Interosseous cannulation is a useful skill and should be considered until more definitive access can be obtained.

It is essential to monitor heart rate, rhythm and non-invasive blood pressure during any critical care transport, but they are crude surrogates for cardiac output, which is difficult to measure. Instead, a range of additional indicators are employed to evaluate the cardiovascular system. These include clinical history and anticipated clinical course, pulse volumes, capillary refill time, urine output, conscious level and response to therapeutic interventions such as the administration of a fluid bolus.

To achieve the necessary context, an understanding of age-appropriate heart rates and blood pressures is essential. This information is probably best incorporated as an aide memoire within the transport documentation.

Normal values should be targeted in most clinical situations. Exceptions include:

- Penetrating trauma where hypotensive resuscitation may be employed
- Head injury with raised intracranial pressure, when a higher blood pressure may be required to achieve adequate cerebral perfusion

## Monitoring Standards

The monitoring standards defined by the Association of Anaesthetists of Great Britain and Ireland are appropriate for all ventilated patients.

These include:

- Continuous ECG
- Blood pressure
- Pulse oximetry
- Capnography
- Temperature
- Ventilator alarms (minimum disconnect and high-pressure alarms)

Capnography is an essential component of respiratory monitoring and should be used for all transports. It is useful to monitor adequacy of ventilation, as it identifies correct tracheal tube placement (and displacement) and provides a useful indicator of cardiac output, particularly during cardiopulmonary resuscitation.

Non-invasive blood pressure monitors rapidly deplete the battery power of integrated monitors and become unreliable if there is a lot of movement. Blood pressure is most efficiently measured using intra-arterial monitoring, but time must not be wasted in failed attempts to insert an arterial line (this applies to any intervention). The time taken must not exceed the benefit of the line, and intermittent non-invasive blood pressure measurements may be the best option.

Central venous access is very useful for blood sampling as well as inotrope delivery, but again it is time consuming to insert, carries the risk of complications and it may not be possible to achieve. Recently, dilute inotropic solutions delivered through standard peripheral intravenous access have been employed successfully to achieve the desired physiological targets without risking either the time or complications of central access. This pragmatic approach has yet to be fully evaluated, but it has the advantage of simplicity, and initial experience in critically ill children is favourable.

## Documentation

An anaesthetic record is a good starting point for transport documentation. A contemporaneous record of the medical decisions and the physiological status should be made. A section summarising medical issues yet to be dealt with or any outstanding investigation results is essential. A copy of relevant documentation, scans and X-rays must be transferred either electronically or on paper to the receiving team and a copy returned to the referring hospital.

Ideally, transport documentation should be designed to facilitate decision-making processes by structuring assessment, providing information (drug calculations, tracheal tube size, normal physiological variables) and offering therapeutic goals.

Critical care transport can present many unusual situations, especially to ad hoc transport teams, and it is important to reduce the cognitive load wherever possible.

## The Transport Team

The skills of the transport team should match the requirements of the patient. A two-person team driven by an ambulance technician would be the most usual practice amongst specialist critical care transport teams in the United Kingdom for ventilated patients. Every hospital should develop a contingency plan for emergency paediatric transport, which should identify which personnel will form the transport team.

- Team leader. This should be someone with the ability to lead medical decisions, with the appropriate skills to undertake likely interventions. In practice, this is often a physician but may be an advanced clinical practitioner.
- Assistant. This should be someone able to assist the team leader in delivering the level of care required. In practice, this is often a children's nurse or operating department practitioner (ODP) but could be a paramedic with appropriate skills.
- Driver/technician. This should be someone capable of operating the transport ambulance equipment and driving the patient and team to the receiving facility in a safe, timely manner. In practice, the driver will often be an ambulance driver with training and experience in emergency response driving. The route to the receiving facility may be unfamiliar, or there may be a change en route, and the ambulance will need GPS and paper map backups.

The local ambulance service should not automatically be asked to supply a paramedic crew for the transport. The main role of the paramedic crew is for primary transport from home or roadside to a hospital facility, and a paramedic crew may be under-utilised in a physician-led secondary transport.

## Mode of Transport

### Road Transport

A 'frontline' NHS ambulance will have some of the equipment required for transport of a critically ill child. The essential requirements include oxygen, suction and a defibrillator suitable for the size of the child. Other equipment such as monitors, syringe pumps and airway/ventilation equipment may have to be sourced from the referring hospital for time-critical transfers; specialist children's transport ambulances will be fully equipped for the expected patient group.

Power sockets are usually available, and there are usually at least three seats. This will permit a parent or carer to accompany the patient if this is deemed clinically appropriate.

### Train Transport

For more stable patients, this may well prove to be a suitable mode of transport, especially given the environmental impact of other modes. At present in the United Kingdom, it has been used very rarely, but many services are hoping to develop this mode.

### Air Transport

The technical and logistical problems that accompany ad hoc secondary aeromedical transfer in the emergency setting are formidable. The main problem with aeromedical transport using fixed-wing aircraft or helicopter transfer is not the physiology of aviation, but coordination of multiple transfers, patient access and monitoring in unfamiliar, distracting, isolated, hazardous environments. Weather and landing site restrictions may reduce any potential time saved.

Road ambulances will be required to transport the patient to landing sites, and these will need to be coordinated with the aircraft. The local statutory ambulance service may be able to assist if an aeromedical transport is required.

Helicopter emergency medical service (HEMS) helicopters are limited in capacity, and it is likely that only one member of staff will be able to accompany the patient.

A search and rescue helicopter can be requested which has the capacity to transfer a medical team with the patient. In these circumstances, the transporting team should not expect any medical equipment, power or oxygen to be available. The dual pilots, navigator and winchman crew that accompany a search and rescue helicopter are an additional valuable resource for the transporting team, which may make this the best option for an ad hoc team.

## Aeromedical Transport: Altitude

It is important to liaise with the crew if altitude will cause clinical problems:

- All helicopters are unpressurised and often operate at or below 2,000 feet.
- Fixed-wing aircraft may be pressurised or unpressurised.
- A pressurised fixed-wing aircraft will not have a cabin pressure higher than 8,000 feet, even though the aircraft may fly at a higher altitude.

As a rule of thumb, at 8,000 feet (2,438 m) a healthy individual breathing air would experience a $PaO_2$ of 7 to 8.5 kPa ($SpO_2$ of 85–91%). A chartered air ambulance may be able to pressurise the cabin to sea level for the journey, but this will limit aircraft altitude and cause a fuel penalty.

Because a low ambient pressure causes expansion of trapped gases, the following issues should be considered:

- A pneumothorax will expand at altitude and should be drained pre-departure.
- Air transport is relatively contraindicated if the child has an open head injury or open eye injury.
- Air transport is relatively contraindicated for children with intestinal obstruction, as there is risk of perforation.
- Tracheal tube cuff pressures should be checked en route, and many recommend using water to fill the tracheal cuff, which will largely prevent expanded gas applying pressure to the tracheal mucosa.
- At altitude, minute volume from ventilators may increase, and end-tidal $CO_2$ monitoring must be used.
- Intravenous fluid bags containing gas may pressurise, increasing infusion rates unexpectedly.
- A vacuum mattress will soften at altitude as the gas within it expands.

## Parents and Carers

A parent or carer should accompany the patient. Unnecessary separation can add considerably to the distress of parents and carers at what is already a very difficult time. From the perspective of the transport team, parents are also an essential source of information, and it is helpful if they are present at the destination hospital when the transporting team arrives. It may be useful to re-examine the medical history with the parent or carer during the journey if circumstances permit.

The journey may also be a good opportunity to answer questions or provide explanations for parents or carers who may not have fully appreciated what has happened.

## Health, Safety and Insurance

The patient, parent or carer, equipment and staff must be adequately restrained when the vehicle is moving. Seat belts must be used. Some improvisation is usual in an emergency ad hoc transport, and inevitably there will be some risk to the team and patient from the transfer. Assessing risks and keeping them to an acceptable level is part of the overall process of transfer, and all members of the team need to participate. Oxygen cylinders are particularly dangerous, not just given the contents and pressure but also as heavy objects that need to be properly restrained when the vehicle is in motion.

Teams should consider a personal death or injury insurance such as that available to Association of Anaesthetists (AA), Intensive Care

Society (ICS) or Paediatric Intensive Care Society (PICS) members. All National Health Service (NHS) staff are eligible to benefit from the NHS Injury Benefits Scheme via the NHS Litigation Authority; however, this can be a legally complex and time-consuming process. As a result, the AA, ICS, PICS and allied organisations have arranged personal accident insurance for members undertaking patient transfers. Those likely to form part of a transport team should consider taking out this kind of insurance.

## Death of a Patient during Transport

If a child has suffered an irrecoverable head injury or major trauma, or brain stem death is inevitable, it is better to spare the family and the child the distress of a futile secondary transfer where no clinical benefit is likely.

If a child unfortunately succumbs during transport, it may be appropriate to continue to the planned destination to confirm death or divert/return to the nearest hospital accident and emergency department capable of managing the situation.

Emergency transfers will normally need to be referred to the coroner in the usual way.

## Time-Critical Neurosurgical Emergencies

The child requiring urgent neurosurgery, for instance because of extradural hematoma, blocked ventriculoperitoneal (VP) shunt or bleed into a previously undiagnosed cerebral tumour, should be transferred to a specialist neurosurgical centre as soon as possible. Transfer by the referring hospital team is usually the most clinically appropriate, but decisions should be made in joint consultation with the neurosurgeons and the specialist transport team. Transfer by an experienced anaesthetist is usually appropriate.

Useful pointers for urgent transfer include the following:

Following trauma:

- Rapid loss of consciousness
- Initial lucid interval followed by loss of consciousness
- Unequal pupils
- Cushing's triad – hypertension, bradycardia, abnormal respiration
- Focal neurological deficit, such as hemiparesis
- Obvious external injury, such as a depressed skull fracture

Non-traumatic:

- Suspected blocked VP shunt
- Rapid loss of consciousness in a previously well patient
- Unexpected cardiorespiratory arrest in a young infant (consider non-accidental injury)
- Focal neurological deficit, including focal seizures in an older child
- Antecedent severe headache and vomiting

Outcomes can be improved by reducing the time to surgery, but basic neuroprotection must be in place prior to transfer. Hypotension and hypoxaemia are associated with poor outcome and must be avoided at all times. Initial management of acute neurosurgical emergencies is in accordance with Advanced Paedeatric Life Support (APLS) guidelines:

- Set age-appropriate target values for mean arterial pressure (Table 42.2).
- Stabilise the airway (and cervical spine), breathing and circulation.
- Establish two points of IV access.
- Pass a urinary catheter and orogastric tube.

Indications for intubation:

- GCS $\leq$ 8 or rapid decrease in GCS
- Signs of raised intracranial pressure (ICP): unequal pupils, Cushing's triad
- Loss of airway reflexes
- Ventilator insufficiency
- Spontaneous hyperventilation ($PaCO_2 \leq$ 3.5 kPa)

Neuroprotection after intubation:

- Secure the tracheal tube and confirm bilateral air entry.
- Continue cervical spine immobilisation if indicated with sandbags and tape. Cervical collars are difficult to fit, especially to those under five years old, and an individual

**Table 42.2** Target values for mean arterial pressure in children with a neurosurgical emergency

| Age (years) | Target mean arterial pressure (mmHg) |
|---|---|
| <2 | >55 |
| 2–6 | >60 |
| >6 | >70 |

assessment will be required to assess benefit in the unconscious patient.

- Maintain oxygen saturation ≥94%, maintain normocapnia ($PaCO_2$ 4.7–5.3 kPa).
- Capnography is mandatory.
- Paralyse and sedate with morphine, midazolam and vecuronium infusions.
- Boluses of fentanyl 5 mcg $kg^{-1}$ may be useful to prevent responses to suction.
- Target adequate blood pressure to maintain cerebral perfusion pressure.
- Target mean arterial pressures according to the age of child are shown in Table 42.2.

Inotropes may be required:

- Dopamine 5–10 mcg $kg^{-1}$ $min^{1}$
- Noradrenaline 0.02–1 mcg $kg^{-1}$ $min^{-1}$
- Adrenaline 0.02–1 mcg $kg^{-1}$ $min^{-1}$

If there are concerns about raised ICP or rapid changes in clinical signs (e.g. pupillary changes or Cushing's triad), consider interventions to reduce ICP:

- Mannitol (0.25–0.5 g $kg^{-1}$ IV) and/or
- Hypertonic saline (2.8% saline, 3 ml $kg^{-1}$ IV) – target a serum sodium 145 mmol $l^{-1}$.
- Record pupil signs and vital signs every 15 minutes.
- Maintain central temperature 35–37°C. Avoid hyperthermia but do not target hypothermia.
- Identify and treat seizures with a loading dose of phenytoin 20 mg $kg^{-1}$.
- Fluid restrict to 50% maintenance.
- Use isotonic fluids only.
- Maintain normal blood sugar – for example, by adding dextrose to 0.9% saline:
    - For a child <2 years if blood glucose ≤4.4 mmol $l^{-1}$
    - For a child ≥2 years if blood glucose <3.9 mmol $l^{-1}$

Antibiotic prophylaxis is recommended for penetrating head injuries or when there is evidence of cerebrospinal fluid (CSF) leak. Consider associated injuries if there is hypotension and falling haemoglobin.

Ideally, associated injuries should be excluded or stabilised prior to transfer.

## Urgent CT Scan

A CT scan should be done within 30 minutes of suspicion of a mass lesion but does not take priority over neuroprotection and should only be carried out once neuroprotection goals are met.

If the CT scan indicates that urgent neurosurgery is required, transfer should take place immediately (target maximum <60 minutes from the end of the scan).

Indications for urgent CT scan in a child are:

- GCS <13 at any time since injury
- GCS equal to 13–14 at two hours after the injury
- Suspected open or basal skull fracture
- Post-traumatic seizure
- Focal neurological deficit
- >1 episode vomiting
- Amnesia >30 minutes of events before impact
- Dangerous mechanism of injury
- Coagulopathy

Although useful, insertion of a central line and arterial line should not delay transport.

In this situation, inotropes may need to be run via a peripheral cannula and the non-invasive blood pressure cuff used, such is the importance of timely surgery in this group of patients.

Table 42.3 provides a template checklist for non-specialist teams required to transport a child.

**Table 42.3** Checklist for non-specialist teams required to transport a child

| Checklist item to consider | Tick when completed/ considered |
| --- | --- |
| Receiving hospital staff spoken to by the responsible consultant. | |
| Ambulance service request (999 call or via duty controller). State ventilated neurosurgical emergency. Request ASAP response time. | |
| Estimated journey time from local ambulance service. | |
| *Airway equipment:*<br>Face mask<br>Ambu bag<br>Tape<br>Tubes<br>Laryngoscope<br>Scissors | |
| *Drugs:*<br>Fluid bolus<br>Mannitol | |

**Table 42.3** *(cont.)*

| Checklist item to consider | Tick when completed/ considered |
|---|---|
| Sedation<br>Paralysis<br>Inotropes | |
| Ventilator and oxygen calculation | |
| Infusion pumps | |
| Mobile phone with appropriate telephone numbers | |
| *Monitoring:*<br>ECG<br>$SpO_2$<br>Blood pressure (NIBP or arterial)<br>End-tidal $CO_2$ | |
| *Physiological targets:*<br>$SpO_2$ 96% or more<br>Blood pressure (NIBP or arterial) – age-appropriate target<br>End-tidal $CO_2$ required to achieve $PaCO_2$ 4.7–5.3 kPa | |
| Sedation | |
| Paralysis | |
| Torch | |
| Call receiving hospital immediately prior to leaving | |

## Penetrating Trauma

The majority of blunt trauma can be managed non-operatively and will respond to restoration of circulation attention to coagulation. A specialist transport team can then retrieve the patient after a full assessment has been made.

A child that presents to an adult trauma unit or other non-specialist hospital with penetrating trauma resulting in life-threatening haemodynamic instability requires special consideration.

The decision in this situation hinges on the surgical expertise at the non-specialist hospital at that moment, and damage limitation surgery may need to be attempted onsite if appropriate.

Immediate advice should be sought from the duty consultant at the nearest major trauma centre.

If damage limitation surgery cannot be attempted locally, the patient will need to be transported to the nearest major trauma centre or other specialist facility, and the best chance of survival probably lies with an immediate non-specialist team transfer or local HEMS provider.

The most senior clinician available should accompany the child on the transport. Aggressive fluid resuscitation in this situation may cause exsanguination and should be limited to achieve low-normal blood pressure.

Preplanning for this situation, usually as part of a trauma network, offers the best outcomes.

### Key Points

- The need for transport of a critically ill or injured child is predictable and should be planned within clinical networks.
- The retrieval team is an invaluable source of advice during initial stabilisation prior to transport.
- The airway should be secured early, prior to transport of critically ill children.
- Time-critical transfers may need to be undertaken by the referring hospital. Appropriate equipment and protocols should be prepared well in advance.
- Completion of a transport checklist reduces critical incidents during transport.

## Further Reading

Advanced Life Support Group (ALSG). *Advanced Paediatric Life Support: A Practical Approach to Emergencies*, 6th ed. Wiley-Blackwell. 2016.

Advanced Life Support Group (ALSG). *Neonatal, Adult and Paediatric Safe Transfer and Retrieval: A Practical Approach to Transfers*. Wiley-Blackwell. 2019.

Association of Anaesthetists of Great Britain and Ireland (AAGBI). Safety Guideline: Interhospital Transfer. February 2009. Available at: https://anaesthetists.org/Portals/0/PDFs/Guidelines%20PDFs/Guideline_interhospital_transfer_2009_final.pdf?ver=2018-07-11-163754-600&ver=2018-07-11-163754-600. Accessed 25 April 2024.

Children's Acute Transport Service (CATS). Available online: https://cats.nhs.uk/. Accessed 25 April 2024.

Martin T. *Aeromedical Transportation: A Clinical Guide.* MPG Books. 2006.

Paediatric Intensive Care Society. Quality Standards for the Care of Critically Ill or Injured Children, 6th ed. 2021. Available online: https://pccsociety.uk/wp-content/uploads/2021/10/PCCS-Standards-2021.pdf. Accessed 25 April 2024.

South Thames Retrieval Service (STRS). 24 Hour Emergency Referrals. Available online: www.evelinalondon.nhs.uk/our-services/hospital/south-thames-retrieval-service/overview.aspx. Accessed 25 April 2024.

# Index